Founda
for Nursi

Foundations

ESTHER LEVINE BRILL
R.N., M.S.N.

Assistant Professor, Nursing Department
Long Island University, Brooklyn Center

for Nursing

DAWN F. KILTS
R.N., M.A.

Assistant Professor, Nursing Department
Long Island University, Brooklyn Center

APPLETON-CENTURY-CROFTS
NEW YORK

Copyright © 1980 by Esther Levine Brill and Dawn F. Kilts
Illustrations copyright © 1980 by
APPLETON-CENTURY-CROFTS
A Publishing Division of Prentice-Hall, Inc.

All rights reserved. This book, or any parts thereof,
may not be used or reproduced in any manner without written
permission. For information, address
Appleton-Century-Crofts,
292 Madison Avenue, New York, N.Y. 10017.

80 81 82 83 84 / 10 9 8 7 6 5 4 3 2 1

Prentice-Hall International, Inc., London
Prentice-Hall of Australia, Pty. Ltd., Sydney
Prentice-Hall of India Private Limited, New Delhi
Prentice-Hall of Japan, Inc., Tokyo
Prentice-Hall of Southeast Asia (Pte.) Ltd., Singapore
Whitehall Books Ltd., Wellington, New Zealand

Library of Congress Catalog Card No. 80-7570

NOTICE: The authors and publisher of this book have made
every effort to ensure that drug dosages cited herein are accurate and in accord with standards accepted at the time of publication. The user is advised, however, to consult product information accompanying any drug they intend to administer to
ascertain that the recommended dosage or contraindications
for its use have not been changed.

Text design: Rodelinde Albrecht
Cover design: Susan Rich

PRINTED IN THE UNITED STATES OF AMERICA
08385-2687-x

To
our husbands, Edward and Doug;
our parents, Saul and Sophie Levine,
and Norman and Catherine Busfield;
and our students.

ABOUT THE AUTHORS

Esther Levine Brill, Assistant Professor of Nursing Long Island University, Brooklyn Center, received her Bachelor and Master of Science in Nursing degrees from Hunter College and is currently pursuing a Ph.D. in nursing at New York University. She has coordinated and taught fundamentals of nursing for the past several years. She is currently acting Assistant Chairperson for the Department of Nursing and Program Director for Continuing Education in Nursing. She has a wide background in clinical practice including medical-surgical nursing, cardiovascular nursing, and work on a research unit.

Dawn F. Kilts, Assistant Professor of Nursing at Long Island University, Brooklyn Center, received a Bachelor of Science degree from Adelphi University School of Nursing, a Master of Arts degree from New York University Division of Nursing and has completed her coursework for a Ph.D. in Nursing from New York University. She has taught fundamentals of nursing and coordinated Comprehensive Nursing-Crises and Repatterning throughout the Life Cycle. She is currently the interim Chairperson for the Department of Nursing. She has a varied background in clinical practice including oncology nursing, emergency room nursing, and nursing administration.

Both authors have presented a variety of workshops and seminars to professional interdisciplinary groups and lay groups. Both share a common interest in gerontological nursing and nursing research.

PREFACE

This text reflects our belief that:

A fundamentals of nursing book must provide a multifaceted approach to the increasingly complex practice of nursing; and a fundamentals textbook must provide the theoretical and scientific basis for nursing practice, as well as the concommitant psychomotor skills needed to make a positive difference in the health state of the individual.

In today's complex world, a nursing text cannot afford to address itself to a single group of individuals, but must consider the rich and varied groups of people who enter the variety of settings to be found within the health care system.

The simple explanation of the nursing process often found in textbooks does not allow the student to become proficient in the use of the nursing process through repeated exposure to diverse circumstances and situations, nor does it allow the student the opportunity to develop the creative and critical thinking skills necessary for effective problem solving.

The nurse works with unique individuals who actively participate, within the limits of their capabilities at a particular time and place, in planning and directing their own care. Using a human needs—life cycle approach is a logical method for the conceptualization and application of priority-

based interventions that are appropriate to the individual's health status and level of growth and development. One of the primary goals of nursing is to make a positive difference in the ability of the individual to meet his or her daily health needs through the process of change.

The physical, physiologic, and psychosocial components of the individual cannot be considered in isolation, but must be considered in relation to the whole. The person cannot be dealt with in isolation but must be considered in the context of his or her intimate social environment, be it a family or significant other group.

Summarization of previous learning must be readily available if this learning is to be integrated and synthesized with newly acquired skills and knowledge.

Based on these premises, this text incorporates the following elements:

The student is shown the theory base of each step of the nursing process, the practical applications, and the process of how to use each step. The use of each step is illustrated by the development and follow-through of the same situation in each chapter.

Each chapter which deals with individual health care needs is organized according to the nursing process format, so that there is a repeated exposure to the steps of the nursing process within a variety of settings and circumstances.

The term "individual" is used throughout the text to designate the person the nurse works "with" and cares "for." It is felt that terms such as client and "patient" label the person in the health care system and commit both the individual and the nurse to stereotypic roles and behaviors.

The term "family and/or significant others" is used as an entity to express the belief that individuals cannot be dealt with in isolation and that in today's complex, mobile society, all persons do not refer directly to the traditional family unit for support and intimacy.

The nurse deals with a variety of people with different ethnic and racial backgrounds. Thus, unique assessment factors relating to these groups are identified and incorporated into planning.

Related scientific principles are outlined at the beginning of each chapter to stress the scientific base of nursing care, to guide assessment and planning, and to reinforce previous learning.

We felt that by integrating theory, skills, previous learning, and other related material, this volume will not only serve as a comprehensive fundamentals text for the beginning nursing student, but will also serve as a valuable reference source throughout the student's course of study and professional practice.

ACKNOWLEDGMENTS

With thanks and appreciation to: Mark L. Levine for his advice and moral support; Sophie G. Levine for inspiring her children to write, and, among many other things, her typing and proofreading skills which were willingly given at all hours of the day and night; Saul Levine for inspiring a love for nursing; Ashna, Bernie, Stephen, Lisa and Michael Pincus for understanding their sister's and aunt's inattention during the writing of this book, and Edward H. Brill for his nourishment, nurturing and patience.

We would also like to thank Paul and Irene Snyder, Diane Marks, Frank MacNeil, Sadye and Harold Brill, Irving Sorgen, Donny and Vivien Resnicoff, Martha Chambers, and all those friends and colleagues who helped and supported us in ways too numerous to mention. Finally, we would like to thank Marcie Kipnees, Karen Emilson, Barbara Severs, John Morgan and the rest of the Appleton-Century-Crofts staff for their efforts and expertise; Irene Joos, University of Pittsburgh, for preparing the Teacher's Manual; Carl C. Graves Jr., University of Texas/Houston; Rosemarie Hogan, Cleveland State University; Margaret Hatfield, formerly at Jackson Community College; Anne E. Craig, Assistant Professor, University of Delaware/Newark; Virginia B. Byers, SUNY College of Technology/Utica; Susan Willis, Emory University; Renee N. Black, formerly at University of Massachusetts/Amherst; Rosalyn J. Watts, Assistant Professor of Nursing, University of Pennsylvania; Barbara Barton, Jackson Community College; Janice B. Lindberg, Assistant Professor, University of Michigan/Ann Arbor; and Vickie Lambert, University of California/San Francisco, all of whom kept us on the straight and narrow; and to the many authors, publishers, and firms for granting us permission to use material which has added to the depth of this book.

Esther Levine Brill
Dawn F. Kilts

CONTENTS

CHANGE AND THE NURSING PROCESS

UNIT II
THE NURSING PROCESS

Chapter 6
Introduction to the Nursing Process 107

Chapter 7
Assessment 121

HEALTH CARE NEEDS

INTERVENTION: THE NURSING PROCESS IN ACTION

Foundations for Nursing

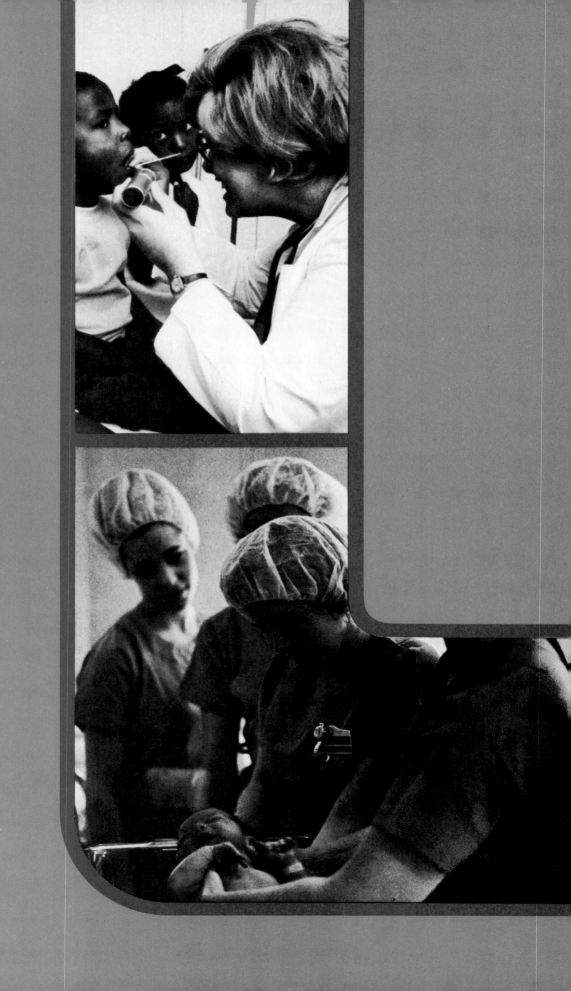

Change and the Nursing Process

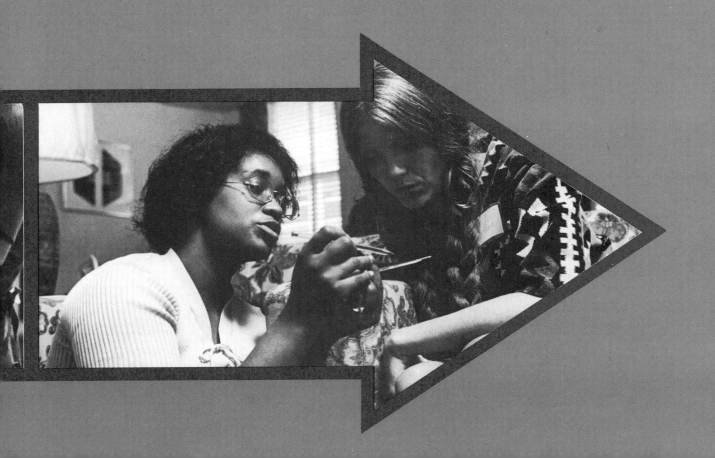

This part deals with the major concepts and methods utilized by the nurse to affect the health status of individuals within the context of their personal lives and the society of which they are members, to develop the nurse's expertise as a provider of health care, and to contribute to the advancement of the nursing profession.

Change is the first concept considered. Change is "to make a difference in the state or condition of a thing or to substitute another state or condition." Seen within this context change becomes a function of nursing.

One of the primary goals of nursing is to make a positive difference in the ability of the person to meet his or her daily health needs. To accomplish this the nurse must help in changing the person's pattern of functioning to one more compatible with environmental demands—both internal and external. This is done by creating an environment in which the person's needs, level of growth and development, and role in society are utilized in planning and implementing nursing care.

Since the individual's health status is in part a reflection of the health of a society, the parameters of nursing must also take into account and work toward making a difference in the general health goals and trends of subgroups, communities, and society as a whole.

In order for the student of nursing to meet the challenge inherent in bringing about change, he or she must build a foundation involving technical expertise, professional responsibilities, dynamics of health, patient advocacy, and interpersonal skills of leadership, teaching—learning, and communication.

In the latter section of Part I, nursing process is considered. Nursing process is seen as the method for systematically organizing the change process. It is viewed as a specialized form of problem solving. The skills of critical thinking and creativity are vital components of nursing process.

In learning to utilize the nursing process, the student may first be struck by its artificial, fragmentary nature. But one must deal with the parts first if one is to understand the whole. It is not until one has synthesized the parts that one can see the interdependent, cyclical nature of the whole.

Consideration of the nursing process begins with a holistic assessment of the individual within the context of his or her internal and external environments. A major focus of nursing process is the nursing diagnosis. Stress is placed on its difference from the medical diagnosis and its pivotal position in allowing the nurse to make a positive difference in the person's ability to meet daily health needs. The nursing diagnosis serves as the organizing principle around which data gathering can take place and planning decisions made. In turn, the goals and plan provide a base on which intervention can be instituted, evaluation of behavioral changes and nursing care methods made, and modification of care allowed for.

UNIT I

Change

1

Nothing endures but change.
—Diogenes Laertius

CHANGE—THE CONCEPT EXPLORED

Throughout his life man is constantly growing and developing. This process is a movement from one pattern of behavior to another and is known as change. Change is an everyday phenomenon occurring around us in biologic, chemical, social, and environmental ways. It is a subtle, continuous process pervading daily life and not just the dramatic, disruptive events with which it is most often associated. One is not the same person one was yesterday or even a few minutes ago. Some of a person's body cells have died, while others have replaced them; the new word learned yesterday is part of an individual's vocabulary today; the argument a person had with a roommate has upset what started out to be a good day; and even the atmosphere around a person has been chemically altered with every breath taken.

Change is a constant related to the interaction between people and their environment. An individual is continually reacting with internal and external stimuli to create a different state or condition of being. This interaction and the resultant change often occur without awareness or deliberation; what occurs is a covert change. In many instances, however, the recognition of the inevitable presence of covert change allows one to plan for and direct the change

and therefore take an active role in the change process. Once change is brought to the level of awareness, it can be termed overt.

CHANGE CONSIDERED

Whenever people are faced with overt change or become aware that change is occurring around them, they respond with diffuse feelings of apprehension, uneasiness, and tension—in short, anxiety. These feelings are related to individual perceptions of change as a threat to belief systems, values, and customary ways of doing things. In addition, they may feel a loss of autonomy, since change is often seen as an involuntary repatterning of behavior without regard for individual feelings, needs, or desires. These reactions to the idea of change result from viewing change as a single, revolutionary event rather than the continually occurring, dynamic process it actually is.

Reactions to change (Chart 1.1) stem from the

Chart 1.1
Reactions to Change

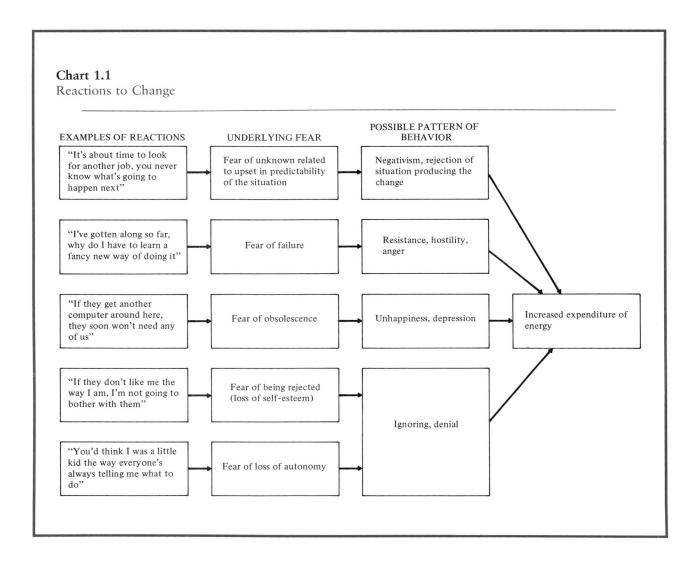

EXAMPLES OF REACTIONS	UNDERLYING FEAR	POSSIBLE PATTERN OF BEHAVIOR
"It's about time to look for another job, you never know what's going to happen next"	Fear of unknown related to upset in predictability of the situation	Negativism, rejection of situation producing the change
"I've gotten along so far, why do I have to learn a fancy new way of doing it"	Fear of failure	Resistance, hostility, anger
"If they get another computer around here, they soon won't need any of us"	Fear of obsolescence	Unhappiness, depression
"If they don't like me the way I am, I'm not going to bother with them"	Fear of being rejected (loss of self-esteem)	Ignoring, denial
"You'd think I was a little kid the way everyone's always telling me what to do"	Fear of loss of autonomy	

Increased expenditure of energy

basic human needs for self-esteem, safety, and security. Self-esteem needs are threatened when individuals feel that the change taking place is the result of their own inability to perform in an acceptable way. Self-esteem is related to a belief in one's self and one's abilities. Suppose an individual were chairperson of a school committee and the members decided to elect a new chairperson. The person would feel that the reason for the change in leadership was that he was inadequate and unable to meet the members' expectations. The reasons for the change could in reality be quite different. Whenever self-esteem is threatened, the person experiences feelings of rejection, worthlessness, and unhappiness with himself and the situation.

Threats to safety and security needs occur when the person's ability to predict what will happen next

in his environment is decreased. Predictability is the basis of one's ability to plan one's actions and to act accordingly, thereby feeling secure within one's own environment. Whenever situations occur that alter a person's ability to anticipate what will happen next, the person's response is one of dread, apprehension, and fear of loss of control. An example is the first day of class with a new teacher. Even though he or she gives a general outline of the course, students do not feel that they know what the teacher wants and really expects from them. The resulting feelings of anxiety and anticipation are linked to the need for predictability and, therefore, security. As the course progresses and the students become more familiar with the teacher's lecture methods, exam style, and personality, they feel more comfortable and in control.

Fear of the unknown and fear of a loss of autonomy may result when one's security is challenged. Fear of failure, obsolescence, rejection, and, again, fear of loss of autonomy may arise when self-esteem is attacked.

THE NURSE AND CHANGE

As change involves making a difference in the state or condition of being or as it involves substituting one state for another, so change becomes a function of the professional nurse. For the nurse, **change** can be defined as the planned and goal-oriented process of assisting the individual and groups in repatterning and modifying their internal and external environments. The change process enables the nurse to help the individual in changing his pattern of functioning to one more compatible with his environmental demands and therefore to make a positive difference in his ability to meet his daily health needs. (Illustration 1.1)

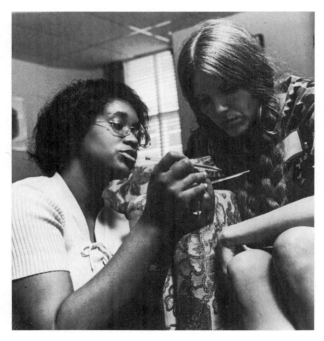

Illustration 1.1
A nurse teaches an individual to assist in meeting her own health needs in order to promote the individual's feelings of self-esteem, safety, and security. *(Photo © Watriss-Baldwin, from Woodfin Camp and Assoc.)*

A frequent situation encountered in which the nurse acts to change positively an individual's pattern of functioning is caring for the person with pain. The nurse may utilize such measures as modifying the external environment by dimming the lights and lowering the television volume, repatterning muscular sensations by massage and position change, modifying pain sources by medications, and repatterning or modifying the pain perception and interpretation through verbal interaction. Through these measures the nurse helps to positively change the individual's pattern of functioning within his internal and external environment so that he is better able to meet a health need—pain relief.

Any individual entering the health care system undergoes a change in his or her usual pattern of behavior. Hospitalization as an enforced change disrupts this pattern even further. Disruptions occur in such areas as autonomy, family roles, body function, and economic security. The nurse must recognize these inevitable changes, as well as those desired for positive repatterning of the individual's internal and external environments. This recognition enables the nurse to gather necessary information to plan and direct the change process in order to make a difference in the health status of the individual.

It is always easy enough to recognize change after it has occurred. The old adage "hindsight is better than foresight" is especially apt here. Change often takes place whether or not one intervenes, but for it to be most useful, change must be recognized as it is occurring, or the inevitability that it will occur must be recognized. Total recognition of change before it takes place is impossible. However, the nurse will want to identify as many factors contributing to change as possible so that the change can be planned and directed. Attention to clues that may indicate an individual is reacting to the change process assists the nurse in gathering information about the individual's level of awareness of the change and his response to it. Frequently conflict exists between the individual's perception of the change process and the nurse's perceptions of it. These differences may be accounted for in part by such things as variations in goals, belief systems, expectations, and culture. These differences are discussed in Chapter 3.

Nursing assessment related to bringing about effective change includes descriptions of:

■ What is the individual's perception of the change which is occurring?

- What is the nurse's perception of the change which is occurring?
- What related changes have already taken place?
- What related changes need to take place to make a positive difference in the health state of the individual?
- What needs are being interfered with?
- What is the individual's style of changing?
- How can the nurse use the ongoing change to plan for needed change?
- What are the stimuli for and against change?
- What plan is needed?

The nurse tries to build on the ongoing patterns of change within the individual so that resistance to change is decreased and movement toward positive health goals is facilitated. For example, in trying to set up a weight-reduction plan for the obese woman whose weight is affecting her physical health, the nurse will take into account such statements as "I can't seem to find any of today's clothes styles to fit me" or "My boyfriend doesn't find me as attractive as he used to when I was thin." These statements indicate that this woman's ongoing pattern of change is centered around her appearance. The nurse then structures the plan for weight reduction so that it includes the individual's goal of improved appearance as well as the ultimate goal of improved health. By identifying the woman's concern and incorporating it into her plan of care, the nurse decreases the individual's possible negative responses while increasing her participation and cooperation which are necessary for change. (Illustration 1.2)

Levels of Participation in Change

The nurse participates in change on many levels. The nurse may be the primary mover of change, a guide to change, or a sharer of change. The type of situation, the urgency of the situation, the level of knowledge and expertise of the nurse, the influence she has over other people, the availability of resources, and the setting all determine the role the nurse assumes.

As a primary mover of change, the nurse formulates the change, devises a plan to carry out the change, and intervenes to bring about the change. For example, when the individual he or she is caring for is unable to institute change for himself because he is critically ill, the nurse carries out changes for him.

The nurse helps guide change when he or she works with other people as a consultant to assist

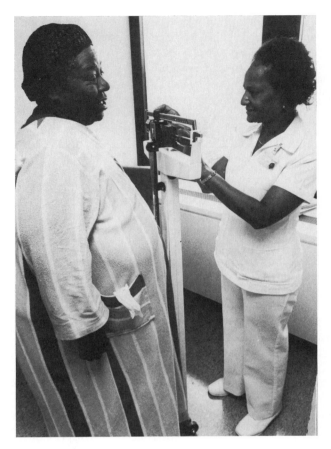

Illustration 1.2
Ongoing patterns of change are created through the cooperation of the nurse and individual. The nurse facilitates this change by incorporating the goal of improved health along with other personal goals of the individual. *(Photo © Leonard Speier, 1979)*

them in achieving the desired change. A community group, for instance, may devise a plan to institute a mobile health screening unit and ask the nurse to advise them about methods of facilitating their plan. (Illustration 1.3)

As a sharer of change, the nurse is a part of change which has been initiated by others but which influences the nurse. This type of change does not imply that the nurse is not a contributor to the change process, but that the nurse was not the major force behind it. An organizational change in the agency where the nurse works may be an example of this.

In all these situations, however, the nurse may assume any of the change roles. In the case of organizational change, the nurse may be the prime mover; while in the individual care situation, the nurse may

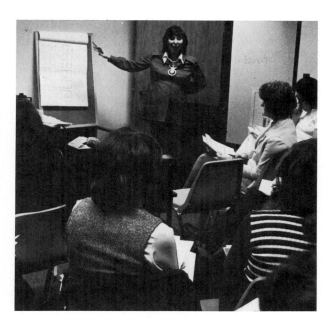

Illustration 1.3
As a guide to change, the nurse works with community groups to advise them about many health promotion topics such as family planning or any of a number of disease prevention programs. *(Photo © Lynn McLaren, 1975, from Rapho/Photo Researchers, Inc.)*

be the guide. Other factors influence the part she plays. The amount of time available for change contributes greatly to this. In some instances the nurse may have little or no time to collaborate with others about the change.

The nurse's level of knowledge and expertise affects the role he or she plays. The nurse may be the expert in some circumstances; while in others the nurse may not have the repertoire of professional responses to institute or guide change. Also, the degree of power or influence the nurse has over others greatly determines the role he or she plays in the change process. The nurse may have the expertise to carry out change but not the influence necessary to bring it about. For example, until the other members of the nursing team trust the nurse, they may not be willing to cooperate with the nurse in plans for change.

The type and degree of change and the level of participation of the nurse depend, in part, on the personnel, services, and equipment available. The available resources when used creatively increase the potential for change. The setting in which the change is to take place will influence the type of situation the

nurse encounters, the time and resources available to the nurse, the nurse's level of participation, and the degree of power he or she has. The types of settings may range from a nurse–individual interaction to a worldwide health interchange.

The degree of responsibility for initiating change that the nurse undertakes in the individual care situation is determined by the individual's state of well-being, his level of knowledge, his desire for change, and his recognition of the need for change to take place. The unconscious, severely ill or very young individual is more dependent upon the nurse to initiate change than is the individual whose ability to meet his own health care needs is less compromised.

Methods of Change

Change may be brought about in several ways. Change occurs passively through the passage of time. This type is unplanned, not goal directed, and unpredictable. Change takes place actively whenever learning occurs; when there is coercion; when there are modifications in the environment, when physiological, physical, or psychologic functioning alters; and when social interactions shift. Like passive change, active change may be unplanned, not goal-directed, and unpredictable. However, to be most effective, active change should be planned, goal-directed, and based on probable outcomes.

The nurse uses such tools as teaching; research; psychomotor, communication, leadership, and management skills; negotiation; and power to facilitate change. As the nurse's repertoire of professional responses increases, so does the nurse's ability to make a positive difference in the ability of individuals to meet their own daily health care needs.

Process of Change

In planning change, it should be recognized that no situation has a single cause. Thus as many contributing factors as possible must be identified before change is undertaken.

LEWIN'S MODEL

Lewin has identified six components of the planned change process.[1] The first is recognition of the area where change is desirable. The next element is the analysis of the situation to determine what forces exist to maintain the situation as it is (barriers) and what forces are working to change it (facilitators). When these forces are equal, Lewin says that "stable quasistationary equilibrium" exists and likens it to "a river which flows with a given velocity in a given direction during a certain time interval."[2]

The third component of planning change is the identification of methods by which change can occur. The first method is to increase the forces that facilitate change and the other is to reduce the barriers.

The fourth element in the process of planning change is the recognition of the influence of group mores or customs on change. The individual will be much more likely to change if his reference group encourages the change and is much less likely to change if the group resists. Closely tied is the fifth component, which is the identification of the methods that the reference group uses to bring about change.

The final component is the actual process of change. Unfreezing, movement and refreezing comprise long-term change. **Unfreezing** is the dissolution of the previously held patterns of behavior. **Movement** is the shift of behavior towards a new and more healthful pattern. **Refreezing** is the long-term solidification of the new pattern of behavior.

In unfreezing an imbalance between the facilitators and the barriers must be created. The facilitators must outweigh the barriers in order for the change to move in the direction desired. In other words, motivation for the change must be generated. Identification of what motivates individuals is the first step in the unfreezing phase. Individuals or groups have their own set of motivators which are determined by their perceived needs. Motivators include such things as praise, money, acknowledgment, comfort, or fear of bodily harm. Anything that threatens one's ability to meet a need or assists in meeting a need can act as a motivator.

The movement phase is the use of these motivating forces to enact the change. At this time the plan for change is put into effect and an attempt is made to reduce those forces which act against the change while increasing those which enhance the process.

Refreezing is the reinforcement of the new patterns of behavior to prevent a reversion to the previous patterns. Reinforcement of new patterns is achieved when the changes that have been made are in keeping with the individual's or group's needs, philosophy, and motivations and by continuing to reduce the barriers. Eventually, the goals will be met and the change will become the accepted pattern of behavior.

Establishing Goals

To ensure positive change, the nurse must establish goals which consider: (1) the desired direction of change, (2) the facilitators and barriers to change, (3) the time and resources available for the change, and (4) the setting in which the change will occur. These goals incorporate the person's or group's needs, level of growth and development, role in society, level of knowledge, motivation, and psychomotor and cognitive skills. (Chapter 9 discusses goal setting in detail.) From these goals a collaborative plan is devised which outlines the manner in which the change is to take place.

Facilitators of Change

▶ **Facilitators, or motivators, of change** are any factors which increase the probability that change will occur in the desired direction and that the change will be long term. Facilitators usually enhance the cohesiveness of a group and thus decrease its resistance to change. Facilitators provide support systems for the individual or group to reduce the anxiety brought about by change. They assist the individual or group in meeting their perceived needs. Chart 1.2 lists the major facilitators and briefly describes them.

Barriers to Change

Barriers to change are any factors which impede the attainment of a desired change. They increase one's resistance to change and decrease acceptance of projected goals. They are generally factors which threaten the individual's or group's ability to meet its basic needs for well-being, safety, and security. Barriers usually increase anxiety, stress, and feelings of loss of control. Chart 1.3 lists and describes the major barriers to change.

SUMMARY

The function of nursing thus becomes one of recognizing the continuous nature of change and planning and directing goal-oriented, positive change in the physical, psychosocial, and environmental spheres. Once the nature of change is recognized, nursing inter-

Chart 1.2
Descriptions of the Major Facilitators of Change

Assessment and planning help to identify the need for change, the forces for and against change, and the purposes of the change and assist in setting goals.

Collaboration is the active involvement of all participants affected by the change process in planning and implementing the change; for collaboration to occur, all members must be fully informed and knowledgeable throughout the entire change process.

Common goals are the mutually shared objectives for the outcome of change.

Similar health beliefs and attitudes are shared and there is a commitment to a philosophy of what is right or should be regarding health; this philosophy includes what the sick role is, what the health team role is, what is wellness, illness, appropriate reactions to stress, appropriate habits, and appropriate lifestyles; it is related to the individual's or group's culture, previous experience, level of knowledge, and level of growth and development.

Positive channels of communication provide for a common language, shared definitions, openness, trust, mutual respect, empathy, and flexibility.

Compromise is the ability to give and take to achieve mutually satisfying goals.

Resources include the manpower, equipment, finances, creativity, and and knowledge necessary to achieve the goals of change.

Preparation necessitates sufficient notification of all people involved in the change as to what is expected to occur, when and how.

Commitment is dedication to the achievement of a goal.

The use of previous patterns or methods is helpful because they are familiar and comfortable to the individual or group.

Teaching is a means by which new patterns of behavior may be learned.

A reward system provides a motivation for change; the reward is something the individual or group values highly.

Chart 1.3

Descriptions of the Major Barriers to Change

Threats to meeting needs that provide a sense of well-being, safety, and security.

Dissimilar health beliefs and values are philosophies which differ as to what is right or what should be regarding health; for example, what the sick role is, what the role of the health team is, what is wellness, illness, etc. The beliefs are related to the individual's or group's culture and previous experience.

Group mores are the customs or ways of doing things in the individual's reference group and offer security to an individual.

Conformity is adherence to the group mores.

Habits, long-term, repetitive patterns of behavior, are difficult to change.

Opposing goals, or objectives, at work in the change process which conflict with each other.

Unrealistic goals are unattainable within a given situation because of lack of time, resources, ability, or motivation.

Vested interests are special interests that individuals have in the existing system; they personally have more to gain by keeping things as they are.

Tunnel vision is focusing on a single facet of a situation rather than viewing the total picture.

Satisfaction with the present system is approval of the status quo.

Rigid organizational structure, with its highly structured, formalized approach, does not consider the input or needs of the individual within the system.

Secondary gains of illness may provide more benefits to the individual than the well role.

vention assists the individual, the nurse, and the profession to deal with the demands created by change. The nurse can initiate and take part in change within the nursing profession and in assisting the individual and groups to reach high-level wellness. The nurse uses a variety of change strategies to implement the nursing process in bringing about these changes. Knowledge is needed concerning the probable direction of changes in the profession and the individual's health, the nursing process, and expertise in using change strategies to bring about positive change and thus make a difference in the profession and the health care of individuals and groups.

NOTES

1. Kurt Lewin, "Quasi-stationary Social Equilibria and the Problem of Permanent Change," in *The Planning of Change,* Warren G. Bennis, Kenneth D. Benne, and Robert Chin, eds. Holt, Rinehart and Winston, 1962, p. 235.

2. *Ibid.*

SELECTED REFERENCES

Aschliman, D. D. "A Strategy for Planned Change." *Nurse Practitioner,* 1:121, January-February, 1976.

Aspres, Elsie. "The Process of Change." *Supervisor Nurse* 6:15, October, 1975.

Bennis, Warren G. *Changing Organizations.* New York, McGraw-Hill, 1966.

Bennis, Warren G., Benne, Kenneth D., and Chin, Robert, eds. *The Planning of Change.* 2nd ed. New York, Holt, Rinehart and Winston, 1968.

Bowman, Rosemary and Culpepper, Rebecca "Power: Rx for Change." *American Journal of Nursing,* 75:1053, June, 1974.

Brooton, Dorothy A., Hayman, Laura Lucia, and Naylor, Mary Duffin "Leadership for Change: A Guide for the Frustrated Nurse." *American Journal of Nursing,* 78: 1526, September, 1978.

Copp, Laurel Archer. "Inservice Education Copes with Resistance to Change." *Journal of Continuing Education in Nursing,* 6:19, March-April, 1975.

Dalton, Gene and Lawrence, Paul. *Organizational Change and Development.* Homewood, Ill., Richard Irwin, 1970.

Day, Harvey. "Change Can Be Planned and Effected." *Supervisor Nurse,* 5:47, March, 1974.

Deal, J. "The Timing of Change." *Supervisor Nurse,* 8:73, September, 1977.

Demereth, N. J. *System, Change, and Conflict.* New York, Free Press, 1967.

Garant, Carol. "The Process of Effecting Change in Nursing." *Nursing Forum* 17(2):152, 1972.

Gassett, H. "Participative Planned Change." *Supervisor Nurse,* 7:34, March, 1976.

Gordon, Marjory. "The Clinical Specialist as Change Agent." *Nursing Outlook,* 17:37, March, 1969.

Greenblatt, Milton et al. *Dynamics of Institutional Change.* Pittsburgh, University of Pittsburgh Press, 1971.

Guest, Robert. *Organizational Change.* Homewood, Ill., Dorsey Press, 1962.

Heineken, Jan and Nussbaumer, Beverly "Survival for Nurses Initiating Change." *Supervisor Nurse.* 7:52, October, 1976.

Kreuter, M. W. "An Interaction Model to Facilitate Health Awareness and Behavior Change." *Journal of School Health,* 46:543, November, 1976.

Lee, Irene. "Cope with Resistance to Change." *Nursing 73,* 3:6, March, 1973.

Levenstein, A. "Problem Solving Technics for Managing Change." *Hospital Topics,* 52:42, September-October, 1974.

Lewin, Kurt. "Quasi-stationary Social Equilibria and the Problem of Permanent Change," in *The Planning of Change,* Warren G. Bennis, Kenneth D. Benne, and Robert Chin, eds. New York, Holt, Rinehart and Winston, 1962.

Lippitt, Ronald. *The Dynamics of Planned Change.* New York, Harcourt, Brace, 1958.

Love, Lucille L. "The Process of Role Change," in *Behavioral Concepts and Nursing Intervention,* Carolyn E. Carlson, ed. Philadelphia, Lippincott, 1970.

Marriner, Ann. "Behavioral Aspects of Planned Change: Reorganization." *Supervisor Nurse,* 8:36, December, 1977.

Mauksch, I. G. "Paradox of Risk Takers." *AORN Journal,* 25:1289, June, 1977.

Morrow, J. T. *Developing Strategies to Effect Change.* National League for Nursing, Publication 52–1537, 1974, pp. 1–29.

Robinson, V. M. "How to Initiate Change in Practice." *AORN Journal,* 26:54, July, 1977.

Rodgers, J. A. "Theoretical Considerations Involved in the Process of Change." *Nursing Forum,* 12(2):160, 1973.

Stevens, Barbara. "Effecting Change." *Journal of Nursing Administration,* 5:23, February, 1975.

———. "Management of Continuity and Change in Nursing." *Journal of Nursing Administration,* 7(4):26, 1977.

Sullivan, M. E. "Processes of Change in an Expanded Role in Nursing in a Mental Health Setting." *Journal of Psychiatric Nursing,* 15:18, February, 1977.

Wiley, Loy. "The Safe Way to Introduce Change." *Nursing 76,* 6(12):65, 1976.

Zimmerman, Beverly M. "Changes of the Second Order." *Nursing Outlook,* 27:109, March, 1979.

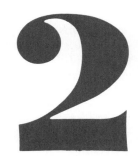

Between the amateur and the professional . . . there is a difference not only in degree but in kind.
— *Bernard De Voto,* Across the Wide Missouri

2 THE PROFESSION IN CHANGE

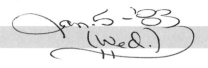

Modern technology, changes in social consciousness, and the reassessment of the quality and type of health care have placed new demands on the nurse and the nursing profession. There has been a shift of emphasis in health care today from acute, episodic, hospital-based care to preventive, community-based care. Concurrently, there has been an emergence of new and specialized units and services which require the development of new skills, new definitions of practice, and delineation of public and professional accountability.

HISTORICAL OVERVIEW

From a historical perspective the evolution of nursing has been one of movement from the dependent, hospital-trained nurse to the emergence of the independent, college-educated one. In the early Judeo-Christian era, women provided nursing services in the home as part of their ethical and humanitarian responsibilities. No formal education or training was expected, but rather the woman used her skills as a wife and mother to care for the ill on a person-to-person basis. Not until the Middle Ages (500–1500 A.D.) did nursing become an organized service. Most nurses were part of religious orders which were founded for ministering purposes. The nurses received training from the order itself, as well as from their practical experience in caring for the sick. Nurses at this time were better educated than other women since they came from the upper classes, where it was expected that women would devote time outside the home to care for the poor and the sick.

Nursing continued in the same fashion for many centuries until the time of the Protestant Reformation (early 1500s). With the onset of the Reformation, many religious orders were disbanded and women were expected to devote their time and energies to their own families and home. The nurses who did exist were criminals, debtors, and other social outcasts of the time. These women worked off jail sentences through nursing duties and had no training or preparation for the care of the sick. Historians refer to this period as the dark ages of nursing. This pattern of nursing care continued into the Industrial Revolution (1800s), until the time of Florence Nightingale. Ms. Nightingale was born into a prominent English family and had the benefits of an excellent education and a knowledge of the social conditions and reforms of the time. She believed that nursing should be a separate career and not part of religious responsibilities. In addition, Ms. Nightingale advocated the careful selection of educated, competent individuals as nurses, establishment of schools specifically for the education and training of nurses, and general reform of health and sanitary conditions. The "Nightingale Era" was the beginning of nursing as a profession. (Illustration 2.1)

Although Florence Nightingale set the stage for the evolution of professional nursing, the course has been neither smooth nor rapid. Nursing has traditionally followed a medical model approach in education, practice, and identification. This has meant that nursing school curricula were disease-oriented, based on treating signs and symptoms of pathologic states, with many courses designed, prepared, and taught by physicians. Emphasis was placed on the dependent role of the nurse in carrying out the physician's orders and following established routines and patterns of care. Nursing did not possess its own body of knowledge nor did it generate knowledge through nursing research. As late as 1959 a popular beginning nursing textbook read: "In many ways the nurse helps to build up the vast amount of data from which 'medical discoveries' are made, and this aspect of her work should offer incentive for better cooperation with members of the medical profession."[1]

This is not to imply that there were not any innovative, farsighted nurses who advocated the advance of nursing. Names such as Clara Barton, Lavinia L. Dock, Mary Breckinridge, Isabel Hampton Robb, Mary Mahoney, Annie Goodrich, Lillian Wald, Mary Adelaide Nutting, and Isabel Maitland Stewart are representative of those nurses who worked for increased education and standards for nursing. As early as 1912, Adelaide Nutting advocated the separation of nursing education from the hospital setting, but it was not until the 1960s that the number of nurses educated in institutions of higher learning outnumbered those prepared in hospital-based programs.

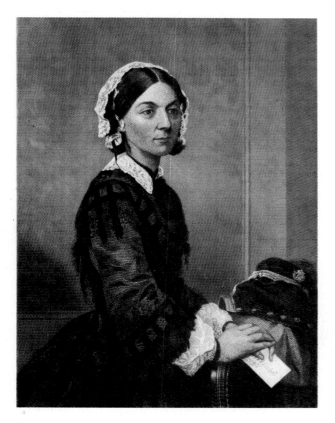

Illustration 2.1

Florence Nightingale (1820–1910). *(From Culver Pictures, Inc.)*

Reflection of Societal Change

The changes that have taken place in nursing and nursing education have paralleled and reflected changes in society and educational practices in general, technologic advances, increased focus on consumer rights, and trends toward specialization. A major societal change that has had a special impact on nursing has been the changing role of women in today's society. As more and more women entered the job market, the demand for equal pay, equal responsibilities, and equal job opportunities increased. Women began to reexamine their roles in relation to professional and personal responsibilities. Education was seen as a necessary requisite for developing skills and knowledge needed for advancement. Women in general no longer saw themselves as subservient and reliant on others for direction and leadership.

These societal trends have resulted in nursing's reassessment of itself as a profession. Examination of its aims and of its potential for meeting health care needs of individuals has led to a redefinition of nursing as a profession which has its own unique contribution to make to society.

Emergence of Wellness Promotion

In the past, nursing, following the medical model, has been disease oriented, either in terms of curing or preventing illness. This resulted in nurses working primarily in acute care settings or under the immediate direction of a physician. Today, however, the nurse is concerned not only with disease prevention and treatment, but also, more importantly, with wellness promotion. With this shift of emphasis, nurses now function not only in hospital settings, but also in independent practices, in the community, school, clinic, or any other setting where they can make a positive difference in the ability of individuals to meet their health care needs. Nursing can thus be defined as a process of assisting individuals in modifying and repatterning their internal and external environment in order to better meet their own health care needs and attain high-level wellness. This definition implies that the nurse no longer cares for, does for, or decides for the "patient," but rather that the nurse collaborates with the individual in mutually planning not only the type of care the individual receives, but also the way in which this care is carried out and by whom. This role requires that the nurse make decisions, communicate effectively, have a broad-based education, possess leadership abilities, make sound professional judgments, problem solve, and be accountable to the individual, his family and/or significant others, society, and the profession for the quality and quantity of health care given. (Illustration 2.2)

In addition, nursing leaders have begun to evolve conceptual bases for nursing practice which are separate and distinct from medical practices and which place nurses in a collaborative, rather than dependent, position within the health care system. While no single unified body of knowledge exists, nursing theorists have proposed many different but useful organizing conceptual models on which to base nursing practices. Among the leading nursing theorists are Virginia Henderson, Dorothy Johnson, Imogene King, Myra Estrin Levine, Dorothy Orem, Hildegarde Peplau, Martha E. Rogers, and Sister Callista Roy. Chart 2.1 briefly outlines their models.

Continuing Growth

Nursing's analysis and redefinition of itself is by no means complete or without controversy. Many unresolved questions still remain. However, as with any

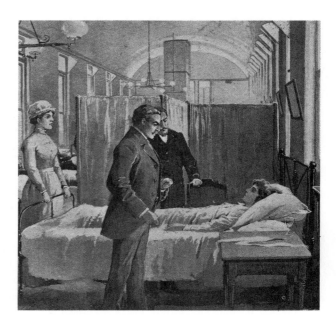

Illustration 2.2
In previous years, a nurse worked largely under the direction of the physician and the bulk of her duties was carried out in acute care facilities. *(From Culver Pictures, Inc.)*

change situation, these differences and uncertainties are to be expected and are, in fact, necessary for the continued growth and evolution of nursing as a profession. Some of the major issues which are still unresolved by the nursing profession are: Does nursing meet the criteria of a profession? What are the differences between the technical and professional nurse? What are the educational settings for the preparation of nurses? What new roles are nurses undertaking? What are the legal implications for a changing profession? What are the ethical implications for the changing profession?

NURSING AS A PROFESSION

Criteria for a profession

A **profession** has been defined by Etzioni as having certain characteristics.[2] First, it requires an extended educational and training period that is in addition to a basic liberal foundation. Second, it has a unique theoretical body of knowledge which results in well-

Chart 2.1
Major Conceptual Nursing Models

PROPONENT	DESCRIPTION OF MODEL
Henderson	Each person has the potential for wholeness and independence; nurse's role is to supplement those areas the individual is unable to do for self and encourage him or her to independence in meeting needs as rapidly as possible. Henderson identifies 14 basic activities of the individual with which the nurse assists when necessary. Empathy is a major component in identifying individual needs for assistance.
Johnson	Individual is integrated whole who must maintain behavioral stability. Any actual or potential threat to this stability is viewed as a nursing concern. The individual is composed of eight subsystems. Nursing process is considered the major tool for preventing behavioral instability or reestablishing stability.
King	Individual is a social being utilizing interpersonal relationships to maintain health. Individual's definition of health is based on his perceptions of interactions with others. Nurse facilitates individual's health through interaction process.
Levine	Man is an integrated whole constantly interacting with environment; concerned with conservation of energy, and structural, personal, and social integrity. Nurse helps individual to maintain wholeness through supporting and supplementing his adaptation in these areas.
Orem	Individual is concerned with self-care. Nurse's goal is to facilitate individual's ability to care for self.
Peplau	Man is an interpersonal being whose health can be facilitated through purposeful interpersonal interactions and reduction of tension and frustration
Rogers	Man is a unified whole in continuous mutual simultaneous interaction with his environment. Man is constantly increasing in complexity and expanding his interaction with the environment. There are five basic assumptions to model. Nurse helps facilitate man's interaction with environment.
Roy	Man is a biopsychosocial being who adapts to environment in four ways. Nursing helps individual to adapt successfully to changes.

defined skills, abilities, and norms. Next, a profession provides some type of service to individuals. Fourth, it is autonomous in its decision making and practice. Fifth, it has a code of ethics for practice which has been derived from within the profession itself. And finally, membership in a profession has a certain degree of status attached to it. Etzioni does not believe that nursing has fully attained these criteria, and thus does not qualify as a true profession but is instead a "semiprofession." Other definitions for a profession have been proposed which are similar in content to this one. An examination of the state of education for nursing, nursing theory, and practice; accountability in nursing, and ethical standards for practice provides a basis for evaluating the degree to which nursing meets the criteria for a profession.

Basic Education in Nursing

Looking at the first criterion, basic nursing education exists on three levels: the diploma program, the associate degree program, and the baccalaureate degree program. The diploma program varies in length from two to three years and may be affiliated with a college or university for the granting of nonnursing credits. This type of program is not part of a college or university, but may be hospital-based or an independent school of nursing. On graduation from the diploma program, the graduate is awarded a diploma in nursing.

The associate degree program is usually a two-year course of study which is part of an institution of higher learning. The setting may be a community, junior, or senior college or university. Baccalaureate degree programs are four to five years in length and are found in senior colleges or universities. Charts 2.2, 2.3 and 2.4 compare and contrast the characteristics of these three programs.

A relatively new alternative type of nursing education is the external degree program. While it is conducted under the auspices of institutions of higher learning, students may obtain credit through independent study and life experiences rather than through classroom attendance. These programs presently grant associate or baccalaureate degrees.

Issues of Practice

TECHNICAL AND PROFESSIONAL NURSING

In 1965 the American Nurses' Association presented a position paper which distinguished two types of nursing practice: professional and technical. According to the paper, the professional nurse is a graduate of a baccalaureate program of nursing, while the technical nurse is educated in an associate degree program. The controversy still continues as to the differentiation between professional and technical nursing; and as yet no definitive differentiation has been agreed on. An example of one proposal which has created much debate and dialogue among the nursing leadership is a bill from the New York State Nurses Association commonly called the 1985 Resolution, which would provide for two separate licensure exams, with baccalaureate nursing being the entry point for professional nursing. Under this proposal, diploma programs in nursing would cease to exist in New York State, while existing diploma program and associate degree graduates would continue to be licensed as professional nurses.

CAREER LADDER APPROACH

Another educational issue that has resulted from the changing definitions and concepts of nursing is the career ladder approach to nursing education. The

career ladder concept evolved out of the desire of many associate degree and diploma program graduates to use their educational and experiential backgrounds as a foundation for acquiring a baccalaureate degree in nursing. Within the career ladder approach, these graduates can gain credit for previous education and experience toward the attainment of an advanced degree.

CONTINUING EDUCATION

Continuing education is another issue of practice. Continuing education in nursing has been developed in order to expand and update nursing skills and knowledge. While few persons will argue against the need for ongoing education, the question has arisen as to whether it should be mandatory for relicensure or voluntary. Some states have currently enacted laws which make a certain number of continuing education credits necessary for renewal of licenses, and other states are considering this. Another aspect of the continuing education issue is what kind of educational program will be considered valid.

Nursing Theory, Practice, and Roles

As previously discussed, many nursing conceptual models for nursing practice have been proposed. While no single model has been accepted as a unifying framework, these models are providing the basis for nursing research. Nursing research will further define and refine the unique skills and abilities of nurses and evolve a separate and distinct theory of nursing. These nursing theories will help to identify more clearly what constitutes professional nursing practice, the skills that are necessary, and the roles which are required of the nurse to carry out these practices. As an outgrowth of the attempt to define practice skills and abilities, new roles have evolved for the nurse. In part, these new roles have been in response to technologic advances, consumer demands, and the redefinition of nursing as separate from the medical model.

Some of the newer roles that have developed are the primary care nurse, the independent practitioner, and the clinical specialist. While some persons may argue that these roles are not new, but merely redefinitions of old ones, increased attention has been focused on them.

Chart 2.2

Characteristics of Baccalaureate Education in Nursing*

The baccalaureate program in nursing, which is offered by a senior college or university, provides students with an opportunity to acquire: (1) knowledge of the theory† and practice of nursing; (2) competency in selecting, synthesizing, and applying relevant information from various disciplines; (3) ability to assess client needs and provide nursing interventions; (4) ability to provide care for groups of clients; (5) ability to work with and through others; (6) ability to evaluate current practices and try new approaches; (7) competency in collaborating with members of other health disciplines and with consumers; (8) an understanding of the research process and its contribution to nursing practice; (9) knowledge of the broad function the nursing profession is expected to perform in society; and (10) a foundation for graduate study in nursing.

Nurses are prepared as generalists at the baccalaureate level to provide within the health care system ‡ a comprehensive service of assessing, promoting, and maintaining the health of individuals and groups. These nurses are prepared to: (1) be accountable for their own nursing practice; (2) accept responsibility for the provision of nursing care through others; (3) accept the advocacy role in relation to clients; and (4) develop methods of working collaboratively with other health professionals. They will practice in a variety of health care settings—hospital, home, and community— and emphasize comprehensive health care, including prevention, health promotion, and rehabilitation services; health counseling and education; and care in acute and long-term illness.

Baccalaureate nursing programs are conceptually organized to be consistent with the stated philosophy and objectives of the parent institution and the unit in nursing. These programs provide the general and professional education essential for understanding and respecting people, various cultures, and environments; for acquiring and utilizing nursing theory upon which nursing practice is based; and for promoting self-understanding, personal fulfillment, and motivation for continued learning. The structure of the baccalaureate degree program in nursing follows the same pattern as that of baccalaureate education in general. It is characterized by a liberal education at the lower division level, on which is built the upper division major. In baccalaureate nursing education, the lower division consists of foundational courses drawn primarily from the scientific and humanistic disciplines inherent in liberal learning. The major in nursing is built upon this lower division general education base and is concentrated at the upper division level. Upper division studies include courses that complement the nursing component or increase the depth of general education.

Consistent with the foregoing characteristics and directly related to the *Criteria for the Appraisal of Baccalaureate and Higher Degree Programs*

---

*This statement by the Council of Baccalaureate and Higher Degree Programs is a revision of a 1974 statement and was approved at the Council's November 1978 meeting. It is reproduced from "Characteristics of Baccalaureate Education in Nursing," © 1978 by the National League for Nursing.
†Throughout this statement, theory is used in the universal sense as it applies to all disciplines.
‡The health care system includes social, cultural, economic, and political components. It can be conceptualized from an individual perspective of nurse and client/family to the broad, national health care scene. For the most part, the graduates of baccalaureate programs in nursing work within the local health care system although fully aware of the regional and national health care scenes. The master's graduates in nursing are proficient in working within the local health care system and have learned to extend their influence and effectiveness to and through the regional and national levels.
From: Characteristics of Baccalaureate Education in Nursing," © 1978 by the National League for Nursing. In Nursing Outlook, 27:51, January, 1979.

Chart 2.2

Characteristics of Baccalaureate Education in Nursing* (Cont.)

---

in Nursing, the graduate of the baccalaureate program in nursing is able to:

- Utilize nursing theory in making decisions on nursing practice.
- Use nursing practice as a means of gathering data fro refining and extending that practice.
- Synthesize theoretical and empirical knowledge from the physical and behavioral sciences and humanities with nursing theory and practice.
- Assess health status and health potential; plan, implement, and evaluate nursing care of individuals, families, and communities.
- Improve service to the client by continually evaluating the effectiveness of nursing intervention and revising it accordingly.
- Accept individual responsibility and accountability for the choice of nursing intervention and its outcome.
- Evaluate research for the applicability of its findings to nursing actions.
- Utilize leadership skills through involvement with others in meeting health needs and nursing goals.
- Collaborate with colleagues and citizens on the interdisciplinary health team to promote the health and welfare of people.
- Participate in identifying and effecting needed change to improve delivery within specific health care systems.
- Participate in identifying community and societal health needs and in designing nursing roles to meet these needs.

These characteristics were developed by the professional nurse membership of the Council of Baccalaureate and Higher Degree Programs and are an expression of professional accountability to the consumer, both student and client.

PRIMARY CARE NURSE

A **primary care nurse** coordinates nursing care for the individual from the time of admission until discharge. The primary care nurse actually provides the care for the individual or directly supervises it during his or her working hours and plans, and is responsible for, the care given at other times. Primary care is an attempt to give holistic nursing to the individual within the context of his or her family and/or significant others system. The primary care nurse assesses, plans, and intervenes for all of the health care needs of the individual. And he or she collaborates with other health care professionals to maintain a continuity for meeting these needs.

INDEPENDENT PRACTITIONER

The **independent practitioner** is a nurse who functions in settings other than traditional, organized health care systems. This nurse usually has educational preparation beyond the basic education for nursing and may specialize in such areas as the nursing care of the child or the elderly person. Such a nurse may set up a private practice or work in a joint practice with other nurses or health care professionals. The independent practitioner usually collaborates with a physician for purposes of medical referrals and treatment. The specific activities of independent practitioners are determined by the nurse practice act of the state within which they practice.

CLINICAL SPECIALIST

The **clinical specialist** is a nurse who is an expert in a particular area of nursing practice such as the care of the critically ill adult, community health care, or rehabilitation, and usually holds a Master's Degree. As with the independent practitioner, the nurse has specialized educational preparation. The clinical specialist provides direct nursing care, serves as a role model for other nurses, and coordinates the care of individuals within the nurse's specialized category. The specialist is often responsible for staff development and educational programs within his or her area of expertise. The clinical specialist may practice within the hospital, long-term care facility, community, school, or work place, or within any other area in which the nurse's skills and expertise are needed. (Illustration 2.3)

Chart 2.3

Associate Degree Education in Nursing |N/A|

CHARACTERISTICS OF ASSOCIATE DEGREE EDUCATION IN NURSING

Associate degree education in nursing is a well-established part of the system of higher education in the United States. Three-fourths of the programs are located in community or junior colleges and one-fourth are in senior colleges or universities. Associate degree nursing education provides both liberal and technical education for an individual who will contribute to the provision of nursing services needed by society.

An associate degree program in nursing is flexible and progressive, meets the changing needs of society, and is based on sound educational methods and a humanistic approach.

CHARACTERISTICS OF ASSOCIATE DEGREE PROGRAMS IN NURSING

1. The unit in nursing is an integral part of the parent institution and is structured, controlled, and financed as is any other unit of the institution.
2. Faculty members in the unit in nursing have the same privileges and responsibilities as other faculty of the institution. They are responsible for development, implementation, and evaluation of the program of learning.
3. The program of learning is usually organized for completion within a two-year period. It is based on a clearly stated rationale and a conceptual framework which are derived from its philosophy and objectives. The program of learning meets the requirements of the parent institution for granting an associate degree and of the state licensing agency for eligibility to write the State Board Test Pool Examination.

4. Students meet the requirements of the institution and its nursing program for admission, continuation of study, and graduation. They share in the responsibilities and the privileges of the total student body.

CHARACTERISTICS OF GRADUATES OF ASSOCIATE DEGREE PROGRAMS IN NURSING

The graduates of associate degree programs, given the opportunity to develop their potential, are prepared to:

1. participate with the other members of the health team in rendering care to individuals.
2. use principles from an ever-expanding body of knowledge.
3. assess the individual's nursing needs.
4. plan day-to-day care of individuals.
5. select appropriate nursing measures with knowledge and precision.
6. implement measures to alleviate distress.
7. perform nursing and other therapeutic measures with a high degree of skill.
8. evaluate the individual's reaction to therapy.
9. supervise other workers in the technical aspects.

Because career goals may change or often a student is unable to attain his ultimate goal without interruption, associate degree programs accept applicants with varying educational backgrounds and experiences by giving recognition to proficiencies already acquired. Also, if an associate degree graduate wishes to pursue his education further, he is provided an opportunity to validate his education and experience.

From: *Council of Associate Degree Programs, National League for Nursing, Publication No. 23-1500, 1973. In* Nursing Outlook, 26:457, July, 1978. Copyright © *National League for Nursing, 1973.*

LEGAL CHANGES

As roles change and are redefined, the laws which regulate nursing practice have also changed and continue to change. Each state in the United States has a nurse practice act which defines nursing, categorizes its various levels, and states the activities in which the nurse may legally engage. More and more, nurse practice acts are being expanded to include new modes of practice or to clarify previous practice pat-

Chart 2.4
Role and Competencies of Graduates of Diploma Programs in Nursing*

The graduate of the diploma program in nursing is eligible to seek licensure as a registered nurse and to function as a beginning practitioner in acute, intermediate, long-term, and ambulatory health care facilities. In order to fulfill such roles, graduates should demonstrate the following competencies.*

ASSESSMENT

- Establishes a data base through a nursing history including a psychosocial and physical assessment.
- Utilizes knowledge of the etiology, pathophysiology, usual course, and prognosis for the prevalent illnesses and health problems.
- Establishes priorities when providing nursing care for one or more patients.
- Recognizes the significance of non-verbal communication.

PLANNING

- Formulates a written plan of nursing care based on the assessment of patient needs.
- Includes in the nursing care plan the effects of the family or significant others, life experiences, and social-cultural background.
- Involves the patient, family, and significant others in the development of the nursing plan of care.
- Incorporates the learning needs of the patient and family into an individualized plan of care.
- Applies principles of organization and management in utilizing the knowledge and skills of other nursing personnel.

IMPLEMENTATION

- Meets the health needs of individuals and families.
- Utilizes concepts, scientific facts and principles when providing nursing care.
- Performs technical nursing procedures.
- Initiates appropriate intervention when environmental and safety hazards exist.
- Initiates preventive, habilitative, and rehabilitative nursing measures according to the needs demonstrated by patients and families.
- Performs independent nursing measure and/or seeks assistance from other members of the health team in response to the changing needs of patients.
- Collaborates with physicians and members of other disciplines to provide health care.
- Documents nursing interventions and patient responses.
- Utilizes effective verbal and written communication.
- Communicates pertinent information related to the patient through established channels.
- Assists the physician in implementing the medical plan of care.
- Applies knowledge of individual and group behavior in establishing interpersonal relationships.
- Teaches individuals and groups to achieve and maintain an optimum level of wellness.
- Utilizes the services of community agencies for continuity of patient care.
- Protects the rights of patients and families.

EVALUATION

- Evaluates the effectiveness of nursing care and takes appropriate action.
- Initiates and cooperates in efforts to improve nursing practice.

PROFESSIONALISM

- Recognizes the legal limits of nursing practice.
- Demonstrates ethical behavior in the performance of nursing.
- Practices nursing in a nondiscriminatory and nonjudgmental manner.
- Respects the rights of others to have their own value systems.
- Accepts responsibility and accountability for professional practice.
- Pursues independent study and continuing education.
- Demonstrates flexibility in functioning in a changing society.
- Adjusts with minimal difficulty to the role of employee.

This revised statement by the Council of Diploma Programs in Nursing, National League for Nursing, was approved at the Council's April 1978 meeting.

---

*Competency, as used in this document, is the ability to apply in practice situations the essential principles and techniques of nursing and to apply those concepts, skills, and attitudes required of all nurses to fulfill their role, regardless of specific position or responsibility. *Reproduced from "Role and Competencies of Graduates of Diploma Programs in Nursing."* © 1978 by the National League for Nursing.

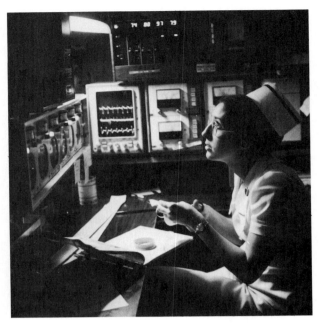

Illustration 2.3
A clinical specialist working here in an intensive care unit has received specialized education in order to execute her expanded nursing role. *(Photo © Sherry Suris)*

terns. Chart 2.5 outlines some of the trends in revision of nurse practice acts. Chart 2.6 gives an example of one state's nurse practice act. Each nurse needs to be fully familiar with his or her own state's practice acts and the ramifications and implications for practice.

CONCURRENT EDUCATION CHANGE

Education for nursing has evolved concurrently with nursing practice. In addition to the basic education programs previously mentioned, a wide scope of certification programs, master's degree programs, and doctoral programs have emerged. Certification programs are usually aimed at providing knowledge and skills for specialty areas. Certification is now given in such areas as midwifery, gerontologic nursing, care of the premature infant, and school nurse teaching. Master's degree programs are available in all the specialty areas, as well as in generalized nursing practice and nursing administration and education. Doctoral education can be pursued in the areas of nursing research, theory development, education, practice, and administration.

Personal obj. 4

Accountability in Nursing

In providing for the health care needs of individuals and groups, nurses are accountable to the individual, themselves, the profession, and society for their actions and the actions of those they supervise. **Accountability** for the nurse is being responsible for maintaining safe, competent skills; protecting the individuals being cared for from harm and promoting their well-being; understanding the implications of care that is provided; improving professional standards of practice; and advocating societal well-being. The nurse is accountable by continually expanding and updating his or her knowledge base and skills, being aware of professional and health care trends, participating in peer review, using mangement and leadership skills with those under his or her supervision, actively participating in professional organizations, and using advocacy skills.

CREDENTIALING

The professional process for determining and maintaining competency in the practice of professional nursing is **credentialing.** The credentialing process is one way in which the profession is accountable for the types and level of education provided, the minimum standards for beginning practice, and the proficiencies and competencies necessary for advanced practice. The credentialing process includes licensure, registration, certification, and accreditation.

Obj. 7 r. 2

Licensure

Professional **licensure** is a governmental and legal process to establish minimal criteria for practice within a profession and to protect the public from unsafe practitioners. Licensing is a mandatory procedure for the practice of nursing. However, it is not under the direct control of the nursing profession. In order to carry out this licensing process, each state has a state board of nursing which serves to regulate and coordinate the enactment of the state's nurse practice act. These boards of nursing may be composed of physicians, lay persons, and nurses. However, in some states it is not necessary for there to be a nurse as a member of the board of nursing. According to Stahl, there are eight responsibilities of these boards of nursing:

Chart 2.5

Trends in Revising Nurse Practice Acts: A State-by-State Review

State	Traditional Statute	Traditional/Broad Interpretation	Traditional/Broad Interpretation (currently revising)	Authorization Statute	Administrative Statute
Alabama					X
Alaska					X
Arizona					X
Arkansas	X				
California				X	
Colorado			did not respond to information request		
Connecticut				X	
Delaware			X		
Florida					X
Georgia			X		
Hawaii	X				
Idaho					X
Illinois	X				
Indiana					X
Iowa					X
Kansas					X
Kentucky					X
Louisiana					X
Maine					X
Maryland					X
Massachusetts					X
Michigan	X				
Minnesota				X	
Mississippi					X
Missouri	X				
Montana		X			
Nebraska					X
Nevada					X
New Hampshire					X
New Jersey				X	

(continued)

1 Establish minimal standards for schools of nursing.

2 Survey programs in nursing to determine whether the minimal standards are being met.

3 Place programs meeting the standards on the state's approved or accredited list.

4 Select, administer, and determine the passing score on the licensing examination.

5 Grant licenses by examination and by interstate endorsement.

6 Renew licenses.

7 Prosecute violators of the law.

8 Revoke or suspend license for cause.[3]

Registration

Registration, in contrast to licensure, is a voluntary process for demonstrating basic competencies in areas of professional practice. The process for registration is determined by the profession itself. At present this process is not generally used by the nursing

Chart 2.5
Trends in Revising Nurse Practice Acts: A State-by-State Review (Cont.)

State	Traditional Statute	Traditional/Broad Interpretation	Traditional/Broad Interpretation (currently revising)	Authorization Statute	Administrative Statute
New Mexico		X			
New York				X	
North Carolina					X
North Dakota					X
Ohio	X				
Oklahoma				X	
Oregon					X
Pennsylvania					X
Rhode Island		X			
South Carolina					X
South Dakota					X
Tennessee	X				
Texas	X				
Utah					X
Vermont					X
Virginia					X
Washington					X
West Virginia			X		
Wisconsin	X				
Wyoming					X

EXPLANATION OF TERMS:
Traditional — original nurse practice act remains in effect
Traditional/Broad Interpretation — statute modification through addition of clauses to original act
Authorization — refined nursing through use of language authorizing nurses to perform additional acts beyond the standardized definition
Administrative — redefined nursing by allowing nurses to perform such additional tasks as may be authorized by appropriate regulatory state agencies.
From Darlene Trandel-Korenchuk and Keith Trandel-Korenchuk: "How State Laws Recognize Advanced Nursing Practice." Nursing Outlook, 26:(11)716, November, 1978. Copyright 1978, American Journal of Nursing Company. Reproduced with permission.

profession. Recently, however, the Committee for the Study of Credentialing in Nursing of the American Nurses' Association advocated a process of national registration for nurses.

Certification

The professional process for determining and evaluating the minimum standards for specialty-area nursing practice is **certification**. An example of this type of credentialing is the American Nurses' Association Certification Program in such areas as gerontology and maternal–child health.

Accreditation

The credentialing of professional educational programs by a recognized professional organization is **accreditation**. In nursing the accrediting body for basic education programs is the National League for Nursing. Educational programs in specialty practice areas are accredited by the appropriate specialty or-

Chart 2.6
Excerpts from the New York State Nurse Practice Act

LEGAL DEFINITION OF NURSING
PRACTICE EFFECTIVE MARCH 15, 1972

The following amendments to Article 139 of the Education Law in relation to the practice of nursing, sponsored by the New York State Nurses Association, were enacted into law on March 15, 1972:

Section 6901:

Definitions. As used in Section 6902:

1. "Diagnosing" in the context of nursing practice means that identification of and discrimination between physical and psychosocial signs and symptoms essential to effective execution and management of the nursing regimen. Such diagnostic privilege is distinct from a medical diagnosis.

2. "Treating" means selection and performance of those therapeutic measures essential to the effective execution and management of the nursing regimen, and execution of any prescribed medical regimen.

3. "Human Responses" means those signs, symptoms and processes which denote the individuals interaction with an actual or potential health problem.

Section 6902:

Definition of the practice of nursing.

1. The practice of the profession of nursing as a registered profession nurse is defined as diagnosing and treating human responses to acute or potential health proglems through such services as casefinding, health teaching, health counseling, and provision of care supportive or restorative of life and well-being, and executing medical regimens prescribed by a licensed or otherwise legally authorized physician or dentist. A nursing regimen shall be consistent with and shall not vary any existing medical regimen.

2. The practice of nursing as a licensed practical nurse is defined as performing tasks and responsibilities within the framework of casefinding, health teaching, health counseling, and provision of supportive and restorative care under the direction of a registered professional nurse or licensed or otherwise legally authorized physician or dentist.

Section 6906:

2. Nothing in this article shall be construed to confer the authority to practice medicine or dentistry.

---

ganization. Like registration, accreditation is a voluntary process. The educational program requests the accrediting body to examine its program and determine its eligibility for accreditation.

ACCOUNTABILITY UNDER THE LAW

The nurse is not only morally and legally accountable in terms of licensure, but also through the legal codes, statutes, and laws of society. The legal system protects the rights and determines the responsibilities of all individuals in civil and criminal matters. **Civil law** deals with the protection of individual rights and property, while **criminal law** applies to the welfare of society as a whole. The nurse needs to be aware of these laws and the implications that they have for practice, as the nurse is held legally liable for all the activities carried out in a professional capacity.

Specific areas in which legal situations may arise include the nurse's own care, the care given by others, informed consent, confidentiality, and emergency care situations. Any acts of the nurse that harm, injure, or distress the individual may result in legal action. The nurse is responsible for providing safe, competent care that is carried out in a manner consistent with his or her educational preparation, professional standards, and the appropriate nurse practice laws.

Acts of Commission and Omission

Negligence and malpractice can occur through acts of both omission and commission. Activities of care the nurse performs which result in damage to the individual or the individual's property are referred to as **acts of commission,** while activities the nurse fails to perform are **acts of omission.** For example, if the nurse gives the wrong medication that is an act of commission. Failure to give a prescribed medication, on the other hand, is an act of omission. The nurse is also liable for activities that he or she performs and knows to be wrong or unsafe whether it is under the order of someone else or not. The nurse is also liable for the activities of those under his or her supervision if the nurse knows that those persons are incapable of carrying out the activities or are prevented by law from doing so.

The nurse, in witnessing consents for treatment, may be held liable if he or she does not know what the individual has been told about the procedure, its implications, ramifications, and risks. If the nurse is aware of the individual's lack of knowledge when that person signs the consent and proceeds to witness the document, the nurse can also be held liable. Thus the nurse needs to give serious consideration to participation in the often "routine" witnessing of consents.

Any information the nurse obtains from or about the individual is confidential, and disclosing this information to anyone not involved in the actual care of the individual may result in the nurse's being held liable for invasion of privacy. In addition, any untrue or inaccurate information given about the individual may be considered defamation through libel or slander. The nurse should not promise to keep information "secret" when the nurse knows that it will be necessary to share this information with members of the health team. The nurse, however, must inform the individual that any information the nurse receives will not be shared with persons not directly involved in the individual's care without that individual's consent.

Many states have laws which protect various health care professionals from liability in providing emergency care outside the health care system. These laws are commonly called "good Samaritan laws" and vary greatly in their content. The nurse should be aware of the pertinent good Samaritan law, whom it covers, and the possible implications for practice.

In addition to being held liable, the nurse can be called on as a witness to validate the care given by others. This is often necessary to determine whether the individual in question acted in a manner consistent with the acts of others with similar preparation and experience. The nurse may also be asked to tes-

tify as to the sequence of events in a care situation. Written records may be introduced to clarify and verify what happened in the care situation in question. Thus records should be clear, concise, accurate, and objective. Chart 2.7 defines common legal terminology.

Ethical Standards for Practice

The nurse is not only legally responsible for his or her actions, but is also morally and ethically responsible for the quality and competency of care. (Illustration 2.4)

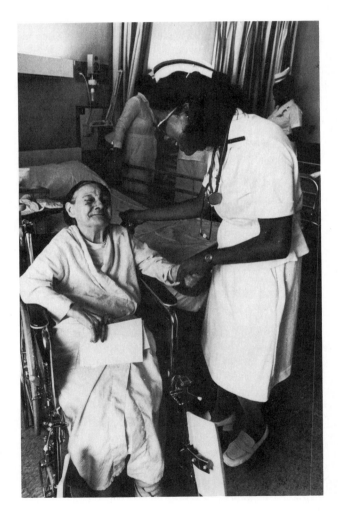

Illustration 2.4
In providing for the health needs of individuals, the nurse is morally and legally accountable to see that safe, competent care is given. *(Photo © Leonard Speier, 1979)*

Chart 2.7

Common Legal Terminology

Assault	Threat of bodily injury	**Fraud**	Intentional misrepresentation
Battery	Commission of bodily injury	**Invasion of privacy**	The encroachment on aspects of an individual's life that person considers personal and which leads to embarrassment or distress
Breach of contract	Failure to carry out the terms of a contract		
Caveat	Warning		
Common law	Laws based on judiciary decisions, traditions, precedents	**Liability**	Responsibility or obligation
Consent	Voluntary permission by one person to another	**Libel**	Defamation through written means
Contract	A written or oral agreement between or among individuals	**Malpractice**	Criminal, civil, or ethical violations of professional responsibilities without due care
Crime	Violation of law enacted in society's behalf	**Negligence**	Failure to take due care
Defamation	Injuring reputation of another through false or malicious statements	**Respondeat superior**	Employer's responsibility for an employee's actions as defined by the work contract
Due care	The expected action under a given set of circumstances	**Slander**	Oral defamation
False imprisonment	Restraining or withholding someone for no legal reason against his or her will and without consent	**Tort**	Legal or civil wrong by one person against another or another's property

PERSONAL CODE

All individuals have their own moral standards and philosophy of life which determine personal values and attitudes. These beliefs influence the manner in which one individual interacts with another and the sense of responsibility one has about professional obligations. When these beliefs conflict with those of the individual in the nurse's care, they can interfere with the quality and quantity of care given. Each nurse needs to explore his or her own value system and determine the impact of these values on the care given.

Each nurse, regardless of personal beliefs, is responsible for upholding the professional standards of conduct and ethics. The nursing profession is continually reviewing and modifying its ethical code in keeping with societal demands and changing times. Chart 2.8 gives the most current code of ethics developed by the American Nurses Association.

PROFESSIONAL ORGANIZATIONS

Standards for nursing practice and education are also maintained through professional organizations.

Chart 2.8
The Code for Nurses

PREAMBLE

The *Code for Nurses* is based on belief about the nature of individuals, nursing, health, and society. Recipients and providers of nursing services are viewed as individuals and groups who possess basic rights and responsibilities, and whose values and circumstances command respect at all times. Nursing encompasses the promotion and restoration of health, the prevention of illness, and the alleviation of suffering. The statements of the *Code* and their interpretation provide guidance for conduct and relationships in carrying out nursing responsibilities consistent with the ethical obligations of the profession and quality in nursing care.

1 The nurse provides services with respect for human dignity and the uniqueness of the client unrestricted by considerations of social or economic status, personal attributes, or the nature of health problems.

2 The nurse safeguards the client's right to privacy by judiciously protecting information of a confidential nature.

3 The nurse acts to safeguard the client and the public when health care and safety are affected by the incompetent, unethical, or illegal practice of any person.

4 The nurse assumes responsibility and accountability for individual nursing judgments and actions.

5 The nurse maintains competence in nursing.

6 The nurse exercises informed judgment and uses individual competence and qualifications as criteria in seeking consultation, accepting responsibilities, and delegating nursing activities to others.

7 The nurse participates in activities that contribute to the ongoing development of the profession's body of knowledge.

8 The nurse participates in the profession's efforts to implement and improve standards of nursing.

9 The nurse participates in the profession's efforts to establish and maintain conditions of employment conducive to high quality nursing care.

10 The nurse participates in the profession's effort to protect the public from misinformation and misrepresentation and to maintain the integrity of nursing.

11 The nurse collaborates with members of the health professions and other citizens in promoting community and national efforts to meet the health needs of the public.

From: Code for Nurses with Interpretive Statements. *Kansas City, Missouri, American Nurses' Association, 1976. Used with permission.*

The International Council of Nurses (ICN), the American Nurses' Association (ANA), the National League for Nursing (NLN), and the National Student Nurses' Association (NSNA) are the major professional organizations which help to scrutinize and improve nursing practice and education. These organizations also help to protect and educate the public. The ICN is an organization made up of nurses from 79 different countries developed to look at nursing and health standards throughout the world.

The ANA sets the standards of nursing practices within the United States and engages in advocacy for nurses. Membership is open to all registered nurses in the United States. The official publication of the ANA is the *American Journal of Nursing*. Through its various programs the ANA lobbies for legislation benefiting nurses and the health care of society, develops certification standards, serves as the representative for many nurses in labor relations, funds research, and advances nursing practice.

The NLN is the official accrediting body for all educational programs and community health nursing services in the United States. In addition it works to improve the standards of nursing practice, education, and health care; and it provides achievement examinations in various areas of nursing education. Membership in the NLN is open to all interested individuals, particularly those within the health care area.

The NSNA is the national organization for students of nursing. It helps advocate for the rights of students of nursing, works to improve professional care standards, and provides avenues for the contribution of students to the profession at large. Its membership is open to all student nurses in recognized schools of nursing. *Imprint* is the NSNA's official publication.

A variety of other professional organizations exist. Some are political action groups, while others represent various specialty groups and special interest groups. All of these professionals serve to inform their membership of issues related to the group and the health care of the nation. In addition, professional societies exist which recognize excellence in nursing practice and education, such as the Academy of Nursing, National Nursing Honorary, and Sigma Theta Tau. (Illustration 2.5)

A PERSONAL EXAMINATION

The many issues that continue to arise as a result of the flux in nursing have created the need for the nurse to engage in a self-examination, as looking at the profession from four perspectives: (1) what the public thinks the nurse does; (2) what the nurse is hired to do by way of contract or job description; (3) what the nurse actually does that is a nonnursing function; and (4) what the law states the nurse is allowed to do. There is much confusion and conflict among these views which add to the challenge of the changing nursing profession today. Awareness of these perspectives and the impact on and implications for the profession is necessary for the nurse to anticpate and facilitate the change process.

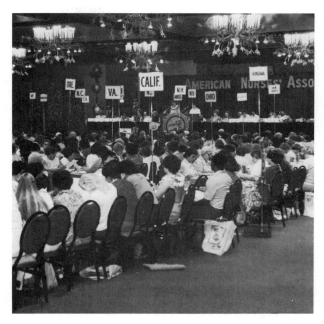

Illustration 2.5
A number of nursing organizations whose memberships represent nurses from all over the U.S., as well as some with international representation, work to establish professional standards of education, practice, and ethics. *(Photo courtesy of American Nurses' Association)*

NOTES

1. Alice L. Price. *The Art, Science and Spirit of Nursing.* Philadelphia, Saunders, 1959, p. 19.
2. Amitai Etzioni. *The Semi Professions and Their Organizations,* New York, The Free Press, pp. v–xvii.
3. Adele G. Stahl. "State Boards of Nursing: Legal Aspects." *Nursing Clinics of North America,* 9:508, September, 1974.

SELECTED REFERENCES

Bandman, Bertram. "Do Nurses Have Rights?" *American Journal of Nursing,* 78:84, January, 1978.
"BSN Students Taking Early State Boards in California Find Reciprocity Difficult." *American Journal of Nursing,* 7:351, March, 1977.

Bullough, Bonnie. *The Law and the Expanding Nursing Role.* New York, Appleton, 1975.

Bullough, Bonnie and Bullough, Vern, eds. *Expanding Horizons for Nurses.* New York, Springer, 1977.

Bush, Patricia J. "The Male Nurse: a Challenge to Traditional Role Identities." *Nursing Forum,* 15:390, 1976.

Churchill, Larry. "Ethical Issues of a Profession in Transition." *American Journal of Nursing,* 77:873, May, 1977.

Ciske, Karen L. "Accountability—The Essence of Primary Nursing." *American Journal of Nursing,* 79:890, May, 1979.

Cleland, Virginia. "Sex Discrimination: Nursing's Most Pervasive Problem." *American Journal of Nursing,* 75:1542, August, 1971.

———. "To End Sex Discrimination." *Nursing Clinics of North America,* 9:563, September, 1974.

Colleta, Suzanne Smith. "Values Clarification in Nursing." *American Journal of Nursing,* 78:2057, December, 1978.

Creighton, Helen. *Law Every Nurse Should Know,* 3rd ed. Philadelphia, Saunders, 1975.

———. "The Malpractice Problem." *Nursing Clinics of North America,* 9:425, September, 1974.

Curtin, Leah L. "Nursing Ethics: Theories and Pragmatics." *Nursing Forum,* 17(1):4, 1978.

Donaldson, Sue K. and Crawley, Dorothy M. "The Discipline of Nursing." *Nursing Outlook,* 26:113, February, 1978.

Driscoll, Veronica. "Liberating Nursing Practice." *Nursing Outlook.* 20:24, January, 1972.

Elms, Rosyln R. and Moorehead, Jean M. "Will the 'Real' Nurse Please Stand Up: The Stereotype vs. Reality." *Nursing Forum,* 16(2):112, 1977.

Fagin, Claire. "Nurses' Rights." *American Journal of Nursing,* 75:82, January, 1975.

"Final Report of the Task Force on Organizational Implications of the 1985 Proposal." *Journal of the New York State Nurses Association,* 9:6, 1978.

Fried, Charles. "An Analysis of 'Equality' and 'Rights' in Medical Care." *Hospital Progress,* 16:44, February 1976.

Gamer, Mary. "The Ideology of Professionalism." *Nursing Outlook,* 27:108, February, 1979.

Gray, Judith E. Gray, Murray, Barbara L., Roy, Judith F. and Sawyer, Janet R. "Do Graduates of Technical and Professional Nursing Programs Differ in Practice?" *Nursing Research,* 26:365, September/October, 1977.

Guy, Joan S. and Peterson, Paul. "Should Institutional Licensure Replace Individual Licensure?" *American Journal of Nursing,* 74:444, March, 1974.

Hassenplug, Lulu. "Nursing Can Move From Here to There." *Nursing Outlook,* 25:432, July, 1977.

Heide, Wilma. "Nursing and Women's Liberation—A Parallel." *American Journal of Nursing,* 73:824, May, 1973.

Hemelt, Mary and Mackert, Mary. *Dynamics of Law in Nursing and Health Care.* Reston, Va., Reston Publishing, 1978.

Henderson, Virginia. *The Nature of Nursing.* New York, MacMillan, 1966.

Hillsmith, Katherine E. "From RN to BSN: Student Perceptions." *Nursing Outlook,* 26:98, February, 1978.

Hinsvack, Inez. "Implications for Action in the Expanded Nurse Role." *Nursing Clinics of North America,* 9:411, September, 1974.

Hogstel, Mildred O. "Associate and Baccalaureate Degree Graduates: Do They Function Differently?" *American Journal of Nursing,* 77:1598, October, 1977.

Hott, Jacqueline Rose. "Nursing and Politics: The Struggles Inside Nursing's Body Politic." *Nursing Forum,* 15(4):325, 1976.

Hughes, Elizabeth and Proulx, Joseph. "Learning About Politics." *American Journal of Nursing,* 79:494, March, 1974.

Ingles, Thelma and Montag, Mildred. "Debate: Ladder Concept in Nursing Education—Pro and Con." *Nursing Outlook,* 19:726, November, 1971.

Jacox, Ada. "Address to the Next Generation." *Nursing Outlook,* 26:38, January, 1978.

Kalish, Beatrice. "The Promise of Power." *Nursing Outlook,* 26:42, January, 1978.

Kalish, Beatrice and Kalish, Philip. "Slave, Servants or Saints? (An Analysis of the System of Nurse Training in the United States 1873–1948)." *Nursing Forum,* 14(3):222.

Kelly, Lucie Young. "Institutional Licensure. *Nursing Outlook,* 21:566, September, 1973.

———. "Credentialling of Health Care Personnel." *Nursing Outlook,* 25:562, September, 1977.

King, Imogene. *Toward a Theory for Nursing.* New York, Wiley, 1971.

Kinlein, M. Lucille. *Independent Nursing Practise With Clients.* Philadelphia, Lippincott, 1977.

———. "Self Care Concept." *American Journal of Nursing,* 77:598, April, 1977.

Kohnke, Mary. "The Nurse's Responsibility to the Consumer." *American Journal of Nursing,* 78:440, March, 1978.

Kritek, Phyllis and Glass, Laurie. "Nursing: A Feminist Perspective." *Nursing Outlook,* 26:182, March 1978.

Lawrence, John C. "Confronting Nursing's Political Apathy." *Nursing Forum,* 15(4):363, 1976.

Lysaught, Jerome, *Action in Nursing.* New York, McGraw-Hill, 1974.

Mancini, Marguerite. "The Legal Side: Laws, Regulation and Policy." *American Journal of Nursing,* 78:681, April, 1978.

Mass, Meridean, Specht, Janet, and Jacox, Ada. "Nurse Autonomy: Reality, Not Rhetoric." *American Journal of Nursing,* 75:2201, December, 1975.

McClure, Margaret. "The Long Road to Accountability." *Nursing Outlook,* 26:47, January, 1978.

McGriff, Erline and Simms, Laura. "New York Nurses Debate the NYSNA 1985 Proposal." *American Journal of Nursing,* 76:930, June, 1976.

Michelmore, Ellen. "Distinguishing Between AD and BS Education." *Nursing Outlook,* 25:506, August, 1977.

Mullane, Mary. "Nursing Care and the Political Arena. *Nursing Outlook,* 22:699, November, 1975.

Murphy, Catherine P. "The Moral Situation in Nursing," in *Bioethics and Human Rights,* Elsie L. Bandman and Bertram Bandman, eds. Boston, Little, Brown, 1978, pp. 313–320.

National League for Nursing. "Report of the Task Force to Study the Implications of the Recommendations Presented in *An Abstract for Action." Nursing Outlook,* 21:111, February, 1973.

Notter, Lucille E. and Spalding, Eugenia K. *Professional Nursing: Foundations, Perspectives and Relationships,* 9th ed. Philadelphia, Lippincott, 1976.

Orem, Dorothea. *Nursing: Concepts of Practice.* New York, McGraw-Hill, 1971.

Padilla, Geraldine, ed. "The Clinical Nurse Specialist and Improvement of Nursing Practice." *Nursing Digest,* 6(4), Winter, 1979.

Powell, Diane J. "Nursing and Politics: The Struggles Outside Nursing's Body Politic." *Nursing Forum,* 15:341, 1976.

Rahoja, Krishna. "Nursing in Transition," *Nursing Forum,* 15(4):413, 1976.

"Reference Sources for Nursing." *Nursing Outlook,* 26:325, May, 1978.

Riehl, Joan P. and Roy, Sister Callista. *Conceptual Models for Nursing Practice.* New York, Appleton, 1974.

Rines, Alice R. "Associate Degree Education: History, Development and Rationale." *Nursing Outlook,* 25:496, August, 1977.

Rogers, Martha. *An Introduction to the Theoretical Basis Of Nursing.* Philadelphia, F. A. Davis, 1970.

———. "Nursing: To Be or Not To Be?" *Nursing Outlook,* 20:42, January, 1972.

Rotkovitch, Rachel. "The AD Nurse: A Nursing Service Perspective." *Nursing Outlook,* 24:234, April, 1976.

Roy, Sister Callista. *Introduction to Nursing: An Adaptation Model.* Englewood Cliffs, N.J., Prentice-Hall, 1976.

Roy, Sister Callista and Obloy, Sister Marcia. "The Practitioner Movement—Toward A Science of Nursing." *American Journal of Nursing,* 78:1698, October, 1978.

Rozovsky, Lorne E. "Answers to the Fifteen Legal Questions Nurses Usually Ask." *Nursing 78,* 8:73, July, 1978.

Scholtfeldt, Rosella. "On the Professional Status of Nursing." *Nursing Forum,* 13(1):16, 1974.

Sheahan, Sister Dorothy. "Degree Yes—Education, No." *Nursing Outlook,* 22:22, January, 1974.

Simms, Elsie. "Preparation for Independent Practice." *Nursing Outlook,* 25:114, February, 1977.

Sorenson, Gladys. "Sounding Board: In Support of the Generic Baccalaureate Degree Program in Nursing." *Nursing Outlook,* 24:384, June, 1976.

Stahl, Adele B. "State Boards of Nursing: Legal Aspects." *Nursing Clinics of North America,* 9:505, September, 1974.

Stanton, Marjorie. "Political Action and Nursing." *Nursing Clinics of North America,* 9:579, September, 1974.

Styles, Margretta M. "Dialogue Across the Decades." *Nursing Outlook,* 26:28, January, 1978.

Styles, Margretta and Gottdank, Mildred. "Nursing's Vulnerability." *American Journal of Nursing,* 76:1978, December, 1976.

"The Study of Credentialling in Nursing: A New Approach." *Nursing Outlook,* 27:263, April, 1978.

Trandel-Korenchuk, Darlene and Keith. "How State Laws Recognize Advanced Nursing Practice." *Nursing Outlook,* 26:713, November, 1978.

Uustal, Diane B. "Values Clarification in Nursing: Application to Practice." *American Journal of Nursing,* 78: 2058, December, 1978.

Wheelock, Alan. "The Tarnished Image." *Nursing Outlook,* 24:509, August, 1976.

Winstead-Fry, Patricia. "The Need to Differentiate a Nursing Self." *American Journal of Nursing,* 77:1452, September, 1977.

Wooley, Alma S. "From RN to BSN: Faculty Perceptions." *Nursing Outlook,* 26:103, February, 1978.

Young, Kenneth E. "Issues in Accreditation." *Nursing Outlook,* 24:622, October, 1976.

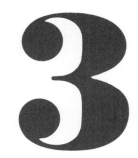

3

Health is when you have the same disease as everyone else.
−Quentin Crisp, The Naked Civil Servant

DYNAMICS OF HEALTH

HEALTH

Definitions

▶ **Health** is a dynamic process which continually changes as the interactions between individuals and their internal and external environments change. Health in itself is not innately negative or positive, but a reflection of the individual's physical, physiological, or psychosocial state at any given time.
▶ The individual's **physical state** refers to the structure
▶ and form of body tissues, while **physiologic state** refers to the function of body tissues and the biochemical interactions which occur within the body. The
▶ **psychosocial state** includes the interactions between the individuals and their environment, mood, emotional makeup, personality, and cognitive and interaction styles. Health may be viewed as being on a relative continuum, with wellness and illness as the polar end points. At any point on this continuum the individual has positive attributes of wellness simultaneously with negative attributes of illness.

The individual's state of health is not static, but constantly changing as he or she moves along the continuum. The proportional balance of positive (well) and negative (ill) attributes at any point in time determines the individual's relative state of health. The most positive state of health or the highest level
▶ of **wellness** is the maximum level of functioning of a person at that time and place. This occurs when the physical, physiologic, and psychosocial needs of people are met in a manner and degree which are
▶ satisfactory to them. Severe **illness,** on the other hand, is the inability of the individuals to meet their needs in a way which allows them to function. Between these two points are various stages of wellness and illness. Wellness states are those in which the well aspects outweigh the ill aspects, while illness states are those in which ill aspects outweigh the well ones. Based on these definitions, the nurse's role is one of identifying the positive and negative aspects of health, building on those positive attributes, reducing the negative ones, and helping to create an environment that enables the individuals to reach their highest level of wellness.

Throughout history, health has been defined according to the prevailing levels of knowledge, philosophical theories or views, and cultural and religious beliefs. However, most definitions were in terms of disease and its causes, both natural and supernatural, with little, if any, emphasis on the well state. The World Health Organization (WHO) proposed one of the first wellness-oriented definitions in 1946. This definition views health as "a state of complete physical, mental, and social well being, not merely the absence of disease or infirmity."[1] While this definition moves away from early concepts of health as simply the lack of disease, it fails to encompass the dynamic and ever-changing nature of health.

THE DUNN MODEL

In contrast, Dunn emphasizes high-level wellness rather than health. He views health as simply the absence of disease, while high-level wellness is "an integrated method of functioning which is oriented toward maximizing the potential of which the individual is capable, within the environment where he or she is functioning."[2] Dunn's approach to high-level wellness recognizes individuals as holistic beings in interaction with their internal and external environments. This conceptualization is consistent with the definition of wellness previously mentioned.

Five premises are basic to Dunn's model. These are totality, uniqueness, energy, inner and outer worlds, and self-integration and energy use. Totality is the integration of the physical, physiologic, and psychosocial components into a unified whole. This implies that one component of the individual must be viewed in the context of the other components. Separation of these fails to recognize the total interdependency of one with the others, since a change in any aspect of the individual creates a change in all other aspects.

The way in which these components are integrated in each individual determines his or her uniqueness. Each individual's genetic background, biochemical makeup, structure, function, and experience coalesce to form an individual who is different from any other individual. Although all individuals have similar basic needs, the way each focuses on these needs and strives to fulfill them varies, thus reflecting a uniqueness.

Individuals require a constant source of energy for survival. This energy is found in the physical realm in such things as food and oxygen, physiologically from the complex biochemical reactions in the body, and psychosocially in terms of verbal and nonverbal communications and in interactions with the external environment. Energy can be either beneficial or destructive to the individual. The same source of energy can be beneficial to the individual at one time

and destructive at another, depending on the concentration, length of exposure, condition of the individual, and the interactions between the physical, physiologic, and psychologic components of the individual at that given time. For example, the thin, malnourished individual who consumes a well-balanced 3000-calorie daily diet will benefit from this intake and use this energy to rebuild and maintain tissue, while the obese individual receiving the same diet will store some of the energy, thus further increasing the obese state.

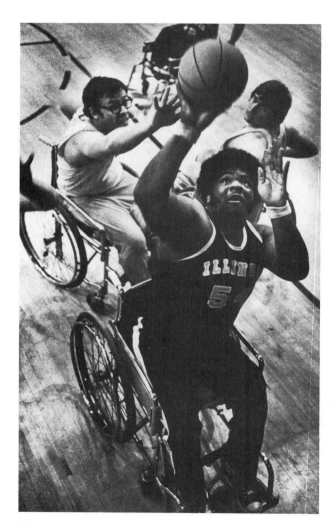

Illustration 3.1
Often, to maintain high level wellness, persons must change how they integrate the physical, physiological, and psychological components of their every day functioning. *(Photo © Jose A. Fernandez, 1979, from Woodfin Camp and Assoc.)*

The interactions of individuals with the external environment are a reflection of their present and previous experiences with the external and internal environments, their inner and outer worlds, and the perceptions of these arising from such experiences form patterns of behavior. Throughout the individual's life these behavioral patterns are modified as more and different interactions occur. However, previous patterns of interactions are stored and may be evoked by a stimulus similar to the original situation which formed the pattern. For example, the person who as a child was afraid of the dark may react to an electrical failure in a manner similar to that when he or she was young, despite newer patterns learned to respond to crises.

In order for the individual to use energy in maintaining high-level wellness, the person's physical, physiologic, and psychosocial components must be integrated. When one of these components changes, the individual must learn new patterns of integration to restore or maintain high-level wellness. It is often necessary to unlearn longstanding behavioral patterns and replace them with new ones in order to accomplish this. The person who cannot reintegrate components will not be able to use energy efficiently and effectively and may, as a result, become ill or die. (Illustration 3.1)

Dunn's five premises can be utilized to form the basis for nursing assessment, planning, and intervention since they provide a framework from which other concepts related to the individual's health can be viewed. These concepts include the individual's personal definition of health, agent—host—environment interactions, basic human needs, the interactions of living system, and stress adaptation.

DYNAMIC CONCEPTS RELATED TO HEALTH

Interactions of Living Systems

When considering the holistic responses of the individual, the nurse looks at the individual, not only as an integrated system, but also as a part of other systems such as the family and society as a whole. An ▶ **open system** is any grouping of living organisms which are in constant interaction with each other to form a unified whole.

THE SIX CHARACTERISTICS OF A SYSTEM

All systems demonstrate six basic characteristics. The first is that the sum of a system is greater than and different from its parts. This means that the different parts interacting together to form a whole have characteristics and properties that are unique from any component taken by itself. A family, for instance, while composed of individual members, each with his or her own individual characteristics, has unit traits that are different from and wider in scope than those of each member taken separately.

A second characteristic of a system is that a change in any one part of the system affects the system as a whole. This can be illustrated by looking at the individual system. Whenever a change occurs in either the physical, physiologic,' or psychosocial component of the individual, a change will automatically occur in the other two components. Thus the nurse assesses how changes in one component influence the other components.

Although a change in one part of the system is frequently more evident than changes in the entire system, the system does respond as a whole, no matter how subtly other changes occur. This holistic change in the total system is the third characteristic of systems. When any part of a system is removed, the system can no longer exist in its original form, but must reintegrate and reorganize to create a new system with its own unique characteristics. For example, if a family member leaves the family through death, divorce, or any other means, the previous family unit will cease to exist and a new family system must evolve or the system will disintegrate.

A system cannot remain static, but is continually changing as it constantly interacts with the environment to exchange energy. This energy flow is necessary if the system is to remain viable. Any interference with the flow of energy, either to or from the system, will bring about a change or adaptation in the system.

As a result of the unique energy interchange of each system, another characteristic of a system, equifinality, occurs. Equifinality is the attainment of similar, generalizable characteristics among systems through different means and patterns of organization. Thus two different systems within a category can, through differing uses of energy, reach the same degree of organization and integration. For example, a premature infant may reach the same level of growth and development as a full-term infant even though it may take a longer time, require different uses and types of energy, and begin at a different gestational age.

The final characteristic of systems is that they organize into multilevel hierarchies. This implies that each system is subsumed under a larger and more complex system. Thus each system can be viewed in two ways—as a unique, holistic system made up of interacting subsystems and as a subsystem which integrates with other subsystems to form a larger whole. For example, the individual person functions as a unique system but is also a component of the larger, more complex system of family and/or significant others which, in turn, interacts with other family and/or significant other systems to form a still larger, multicomplex system of a community.

NURSING ASSESSMENT

The nurse identifies the systems which are significant to the individual in order to intervene most effectively. This is necessary because if the individual is to reach his or her highest level of wellness, that individual will need to function maximally within each system of which he or she is part. The nurse assesses the individual as a separate and unique system, as part of a family or significant others system, as part of a cultural system, as part of a social system, as part of the health care system, and as part of any other system which directly influences or has relevance to the individual's health state.

When assessing the individual as a system, the nurse looks at how a change in either a physical, physiologic, or psychosocial subsystem changes and influences the whole system, other subsystems, energy use, and integration of the whole system. The nurse also looks at how these changes affect the manner in which the individual interacts with other systems to which he or she belongs. The primary system to which individuals belong is the family or significant others system. This system can consist of a group of persons related by blood or marriage, or persons who are bound to one another by intimate, meaningful re-
▶ lationships. This latter type of relationship is a **significant others system** and can act in place of or in addition to a family system. When the significant others system acts in place of the family system, it may be either because there is no family system or because the family system does not provide the support or meaning needed by the individual. Significant others may be nontraditional in the sense that they do

not have to reside with the individual, may not be of the opposite sex or have any legal relationships, or even be human beings. Pets frequently serve as significant others. Significant others must be seriously considered as having a great influence on the individual by the health professional if the individual's needs are to be met.

Stress-Adaptation

Changes which occur in the individual system's internal or external environment create stress and can ac-
▶ tivate the stress mechanism. **Stress** is the tension which results when changes occur in any component of the individual and to which he or she responds holistically. Any force, agent, or threat to the individual's ability to meet his or her needs satisfactorily,
▶ which results in stress, is a **stressor.** Stressors can be physical (e.g., burns), physiologic (e.g., increased blood glucose level), or psychosocial (e.g., a new job). Stress is continuously present in the living system and is, in fact, necessary for survival. In itself stress is neither negative nor positive. Stress states result from both pleasant and unpleasant experiences or changes. The same processes are activated in either situation.

It is only when the body cannot compensate for the stress that illness occurs. The process of compen-
▶ sation is **adaptation.** Adaptation can support wellness and thus be positive, or it can decrease the individual's ability to function and be negative. When the individual is adapting to the stress state, that person brings into play coping behaviors which attempt physically, physiologically, and psychosocially to deal with the stress. (Illustration 3.2)

GENERAL ADAPTATION SYNDROME

Selye has identified the physical and physiologic coping behaviors to the stress state as the General Adaptation Syndrome (GAS).[3] The syndrome has three stages.

Alarm Phase
▶ The first stage of GAS is the **alarm phase.** The body responds to a stressor by activating the sympathetic nervous system. This is commonly called the "fight-or-flight" stage. Figure 3.1 describes the responses which occur during this stage. This phase prepares the individual to adapt to the stressor.

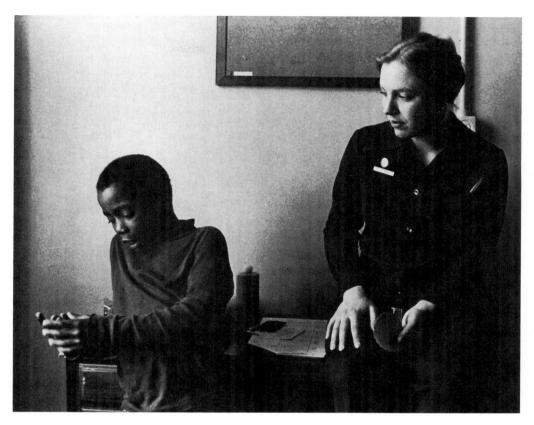

Illustration 3.2

The nurse has many opportunities to guide an individual's efforts to compensate for stress. The nurse assists a person in such a way that the adaptation that occurs will support wellness, not illness. *(Photo © L. Fleeson, from Stock, Boston)*

Resistance Phase

Holistic body responses to cope with the stressors and limit their effects occur during the **resistance phase.** At this point the body actually compensates or adapts. Changes in the internal and external environment take place to support the adaptive process and help the individual attain and maintain his or her highest level of wellness. As the body successfully adapts, processes will return to previous levels. However, each time individuals undergo adaptation, they acquire new behaviors which will better prepare them to deal with succeeding situations.

Phase of Exhaustion

If the individual's adaptive resources are depleted, overwhelmed, or insufficient to deal with the stressors, the **phase of exhaustion** will occur and illness may result. Unless the individual is able to replenish adaptive energy at this point, through either internal processes or external supports and interventions, death will occur.

PSYCHOSOCIAL ADAPTATION

In addition to the physical and physiologic aspects of the stress mechanism, behaviors which are predominantly psychosocial are also activated. Throughout life the individual develops characteristic modes of psychosocially dealing with the stress states. Each time the individual successfully adapts, the behaviors used are reinforced and further integrated into the adaptive style. Some of the most commonly used psychosocial coping behaviors are outlined in Chart 3.1. At times when these behaviors are insufficient or inappropriate to adequately assist the individual to deal with stress, crisis can occur. (Chapter 25 describes crisis.)

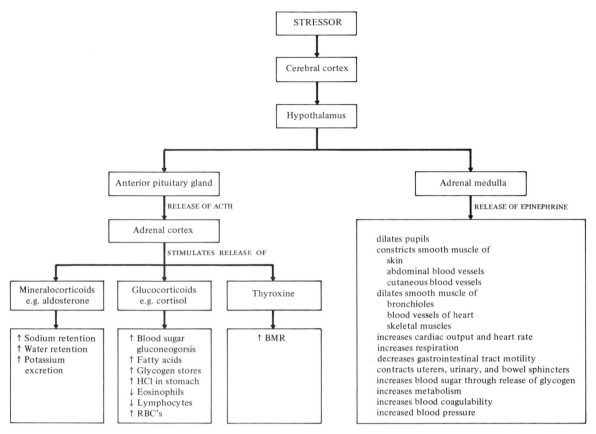

Figure 3.1
Alarm phase of general adaptation syndrome.

FEEDBACK

The principle of feedback is essential to the stress-adaptation process. **Feedback** is a cyclic process whereby a stimulus results in a response or series of responses which modify the recipient's reaction to the initial stimulus. For example, a heating system has a thermostat which is set for 72 F. When the environmental temperature drops below 72 F, the mechanism in the thermostat triggers the furnace to produce heat. When the environmental temperature again reaches 72 F, the thermostat mechanism turns off and the furnace stops producing heat. This cycle is repeated each time the environmental temperature goes below 72 F.

In stress-adaptation, the stressor serves as a stimulus to which the individual responds by adapting physically, physiologically, and/or psychosocially. Once adaptation has taken place the individual is prepared to respond to the same stressor, if it is still present, or to other stressors in a continuous feedback cycle. In the individual this feedback process can be seen in the body's response to decreased water and raised sodium levels in the blood. When this occurs, the posterior pituitary is stimulated to produce antidiuretic hormone so that water will be reabsorbed by the renal tubules, thus decreasing the sodium concentration of the blood. When the sodium concentration reaches the body's expected levels, the posterior pituitary shuts off its production of antidiuretic hormone until such time when sodium levels again rise.

ANXIETY

When there is an actual or perceived threat to the individual's ability to meet any need, anxiety occurs. **Anxiety** is a diffuse feeling of dread and apprehension. It cannot be focused on any specific event, but can be associated with a generalized situation or sequence of events. Anxiety activates the stress mechanism and thus can produce any of the adaptive

Chart 3.1
Psychosocial Coping Behaviors

BEHAVIOR	DESCRIPTION	BEHAVIOR	DESCRIPTION
Aggression	Physical or psychologic release of energy directed at a specific target (person or object); forceful and hostile	Intellectualizing	An attempt to explain behavior and actions in terms of intellectual or cognitive rationales
Anger	Feelings of animosity and malevolence toward people and objects	Magical thinking	Assigning of unrealistic or fantasized power or ability to person or object
Compensation	The attempt to defend the ego by offsetting actual or perceived deficiencies with other behaviors	Projection	Attributing of negative feelings about self to others
Denial	Lack of conscious recognition of facts or situation	Rationalization	Conscious attempt to explain behavior through causes other than actual ones
Depression	Sense of sadness, dejection, self-doubt	Somatization	Expression of negative feeling of self through physical or physiologic symptoms
Displacement	The transference of feelings toward persons or objects to a different person or object	Sublimation	Displacement of unacceptable or unattainable drives into more acceptable or attainable behaviors
Hostility	Same as anger, accompanied by a desire to do harm or damage to target of feeling	Withdrawal	The removal of one's self, either physically or psychosocially, from active interaction with external environment
Identification	The investing of desirable characteristics of others to self		

behaviors. A certain amount of anxiety is necessary to motivate the individual to seek need fulfillment. However, when it becomes excessive, it overwhelms the individual and results in disorganized thinking and behavior. Reality-oriented perception of events and situations decreases as anxiety increases. Cognitive abilities are altered, and the individual experiences a decrease in attention span, judgment, problem-solving ability, and decision-making skills.

Severe anxiety results in panic and loss of functional abilities.

NURSING INTERVENTION

The individual's response to stress is determined by the type, degree, and duration of stressor, the number of concurrent stressors, familiarity with and exposure to the stressor, previous success in dealing with the stressor, perception of the stressor, and the relevance of the stressor to the individual. By identifying possible stressors to the individual and circumstances under which they are likely to occur, the nurse can assist the individual to eliminate some stressors, develop new behaviors to cope with them, provide supports and interventions to supplement adaptation, and help the individual to anticipate potential experiences with stressors. In this way the individual will be able to adapt more positively and attain and maintain higher levels of wellness. (See Chap. 12 for a further description of anxiety)

Agent–Host–Environment Interactions

When systematically looking at concepts related to the interactions of living systems and the resulting nursing interventions, it is useful to analyze the agent–host–environment interactions. These interactions are dynamic in nature and help to determine the individual's place on the wellness–illness continuum. An **agent** is any biologic, chemical, physical, mechanical, or psychosocial mechanism which has the potential for creating illness. The **host** refers to the individual who is susceptible to the forces of an agent. The **environment** is the internal or external milieu of the host, which can either facilitate or hinder the individual's level of wellness.

Living organisms such as bacteria, viruses, or amoebas are examples of biologic agents. Chemical agents include nutrients, drugs, noxious gases, toxins, or other compounds. Heat, atmospheric alterations, radiation, and sound are types of physical agents. Mechanical agents are forces such as friction or increased pressure which produce alterations in body tissues. Psychosocial agents are those nonphysical forces resulting from interpersonal and social interactions.

During well states the dynamic interaction between the agent, host, and environment is such that the host is able to resist any threat from the agent, and the environment supports the host's defenses while reducing the illness-producing potential of the agent. Many combinations of circumstances can produce a change in the health state of the individual. Figure 3.2 illustrates how alterations in any of these factors can change the individual's health state. These changes are not as simplistic as they appear, since many characteristics of each factor are interacting simultaneously. Thus assessment of factors related to the individual's health state is a complex, multifa-

ceted one which cannot be achieved by simply analyzing each factor separately. This dynamic process is a direct reflection of the holistic nature of human beings and their social relationships.

Basic Human Needs

Every individual has essential requirements to maintain life, promote physical and physiologic growth and psychosocial development, and achieve and maintain wellness. These requirements are the individual's **basic human needs.** Many different categorizations of these needs exist. Two of the most widely used are Maslow's hierarchy of needs and Dunn's basic needs of man. While similar in overall content, Maslow's hierarchy is a vertical building-block schema, while Dunn's needs are a horizontal model of interdependent requirements. Figure 3.3 shows Maslow's hierarchy of needs.

MASLOW'S HIERARCHY OF NEEDS

The first level of Maslow's needs are those requirements necessary for physiologic survival. Oxygen, food, elimination, temperature control, sex, movement, rest, and comfort are the physiologic needs included at this level. According to Maslow, these needs supersede all others and must be met before other needs emerge. This concept is true for all levels of the hierarchy—lower level needs must be satisfied before the individual can invest energy in the next level. (Illustration 3.3)

Safety and security needs, the second level, refer to both the physical and psychologic well-being of the individual without threat to existence. Predictability of outcomes, continuity, and stability are aspects of these needs. Love and belonging needs comprise the third level. Affiliation, affection, closeness to others, intimacy, support, and reassurance are all components of this third level. Self-esteem needs emerge next. These involve the need to feel a sense of self-worth and one's significance and meaning in the world. The concepts of dignity, privacy, and self-reliance are integral parts of self-esteem.

The final level is that of self-actualization needs. These needs concern the individuals' recognition and realization of their own potential, functioning at their highest possible level, and realization of their innate capabilities. Maslow's hierarchy of needs is further discussed in Chapter 5. When assessing the individual using Maslow's framework, the nurse begins at the

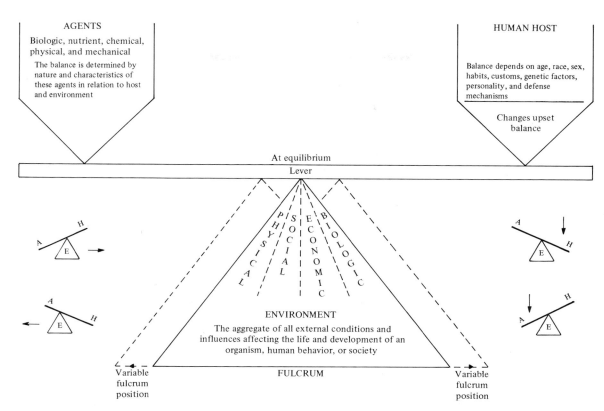

Figure 3.2
Schema of agent–host–environment interaction. *(From: Hugh Rodman Leavell and E. Gurney Clark,* Preventive Medicine for the Doctor and His Community, *3rd ed. (New York, McGraw-Hill, 1958)*

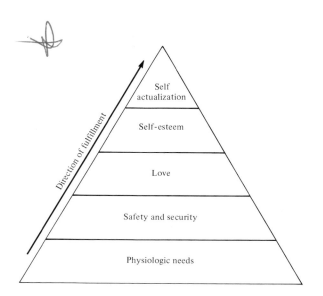

Figure 3.3
Maslow's hierarchy of needs. *(From: Abraham H. Maslow,* Motivation and Personality, *2nd ed. New York, Harper and Row)*

lowest level of priorities and plans to meet first any unsatisfied physiologic needs before moving on to the next higher level.

DUNN'S BASIC NEEDS OF MAN

Dunn's horizontal model of needs represents the basic characteristics of the individual. When all of these needs are satisfactorily met, the individual is in a state of high-level wellness. When need satisfaction decreases, so does the individual's state of health. Dunn's basic needs are survival, communication, fellowship, growth, imagination, love, balance, environment, communion with the universal, way of life, dignity, and freedom and space. Chart 3.2 describes these needs. At any given time some of these needs may be of greater importance to the individual than others; however, their fulfillment motivates the individual toward a maximum level of functioning and of high-level wellness.

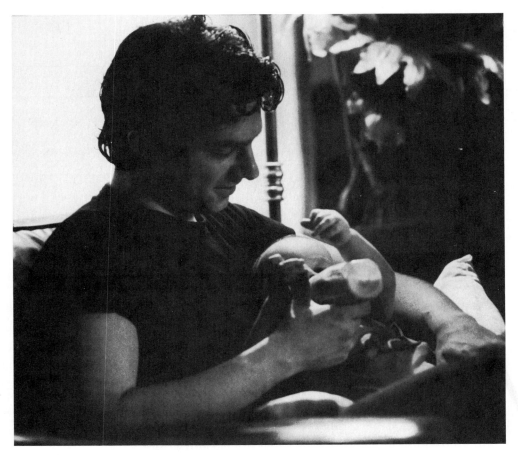

Illustration 3.3
Among the basic human needs of all individuals are the requirements for food, security, and love. *(Photo © Joel Gordon, 1979)*

When utilizing Dunn's model as the basis for nursing care, the nurse, recognizing the concurrent nature of these needs, determines which ones are being met to the individual's satisfaction and identifies what supports are necessary to facilitate the individual's reaching his or her highest level of wellness.

BASIC HEALTH CARE NEEDS

No matter what model of basic human needs is used, those which relate to the individual's state of health fall within the nurse's domain and are considered **basic health care needs.** Behaviors the individual demonstrates—whether physical, physiologic, psychosocial, or cognitive—are the only observable way the nurse can identify and analyze health care needs.

Health Behaviors
Health behaviors represent the negative and positive aspects of the individual's health state and can, in themselves, be either positive or negative. **Health behaviors** include both the overt, consciously learned activities which the individual carries out and the automatic, involuntary, internal mechanisms of the individual. An example of the overt, learned behavior is the individual's eating habits, while an example of an involuntary, internal behavior is a change in blood pressure. The nurse assists the individual in supporting positive health behaviors which promote high-level wellness and helps the individual to change those negative behaviors which hinder wellness.

Chart 3.2
Dunn's Basic Needs of Man

NEED	DESCRIPTION	NEED	DESCRIPTION
Survival	Basic physical and physiologic energy requirements; reduction of harmful energy sources	Balance	Use of energy to maintain direction, action, and purpose without exhausting available energy supplies
Communication	Need for communication on all levels, from cellular upward; involves input, output, and integration of energy between systems	Environment	The energy field in which the individual functions must be motivating without overdepleting or conserving energy
Fellowship	A sense of intimacy and belonging between individuals through empathy	Communion with the universal	Sense of place and historicity within the universe; a sense of oneness with the rest of humanity
Growth	Use of energy to develop and expand physically, physiologically, and psychosocially in order to meet one's highest potential	Philosophy of living	The personally derived set of rules by which the individual governs his or her life; must be consistent with the overall social order
Imagination	Release of energy to use one's creativity in expressing the inner self	Dignity	A feeling of personal worth; reflection of integration of components of self into unique being
Love	Sense of altruism without concern for selfish ends	Freedom and space	The ability to interact with environment and others in own unique pattern with place for one's own energy field

From Halbert H. Dunn, High Level Wellness. *Arlington, Va., Beatty, 1973, and H. H. Dunn, "What High Level Wellness Means."* Canadian Journal of Public Health *50:447-57, November, 1959.*

Personal Definitions of Health: Influencing Factors

The definitions of health, wellness, and illness of people ultimately determine the way they utilize the health care system, the health practices they engage in, their reactions to changes in physical, physiologic, and psychosocial status, and their expectations of the outcomes of health care. Frequently the individual's view of health, wellness, and illness is not consistent with those held by health professionals. Since each individual is unique, perceptions, experiences, values, and attitudes differ from person to person and combine in varying ways to form an individual's definitions of health, wellness, and illness. These definitions are influenced by a person's level of growth and development, cognitive abilities, culture, family and social interactions, previous wellness—illness experience, level of knowledge, functional expectations, and perceptions of self.

LEVEL OF GROWTH AND DEVELOPMENT

The individual's ability to conceptualize and abstract his or her state of health and the ability to respond to and deal with changes in state of health are directly related to the individual's level of growth and development. The individual's **level of growth and development** describes his or her physical, physiologic, and psychosocial behaviors at a point in time on the life process continuum. Growth refers to the physical and physiologic aspects of the person's behavior, while development encompasses the psychosocial and cognitive behaviors. Knowledge of growth and development enables the nurse to assess the appropriateness of the individual's behavior at any given stage of growth and development and to predict expected behaviors. Thus the nurse can plan interventions which are congruent with the individual's level and provide opportunities for the individual to meet developmental tasks. (Illustration 3.4)

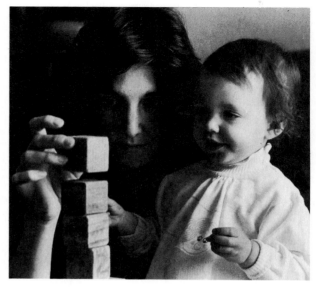

Illustration 3.4

An individual's level of growth and development is a valuable index, at any age, for determining the appropriateness of his health behaviors. Here, a toddler pursues her lessons in self-reliance by developing psychomotor skills. *(Photo by Jean-Claude LeJeune, from Stock, Boston)*

Chart 3.3

Havighurst's Developmental Tasks*

STAGE	TASK	STAGE	TASK
Infancy and early childhood (0–6 years)	Learning to walk Learning to take solid foods Learning to talk Learning to control elimination of body wastes Learning sex differences and sexual modesty Achieving physiologic stability Forming simple concepts of social and physical reality	Infancy and early childhood (0–6 years) (cont.)	Learning to relate oneself emotionally to parents, siblings, and other people Learning to distinguish right and wrong and developing a conscience
		Middle childhood (6–12 years)	Learning physical skills necessary for ordinary games Building wholesome attitudes toward oneself as a growing organism

---

*Throughout the life process Havighurst considers the biologic, psychologic and cultural basis, and educational implications of each task.
From: Robert J. Havighurst, Developmental Tasks and Education, *2nd ed. New York, Longmans, Green, 1952; and R. J. Havighurst,* Human Development and Education. *New York, Longmans, Green, 1953.*

(continued)

Chart 3.3 (Con't.)
Havighurst's Developmental Tasks*

STAGE	TASK	STAGE	TASK
Middle childhood (6–12 years) (cont.)	Learning to get along with agemates Learning an appropriate masculine or feminine social role Developing fundamental skills in reading, writing, and calculating Developing concepts necessary for everyday living Developing conscience, morality, and a scale of values Developing attitudes toward social groups and institutions Achieving personal independence	Early adult (18–30 years)	Selecting a mate Learning to live with a marriage partner Starting a family Rearing a family Managing a home Getting started in an occupation Taking on civic responsibility Finding a congenial social group
Adolescence (12–18 years)	Achieving new and more mature relationships with agemates of both sexes Achieving a masculine or feminine social role Accepting one's physique and using the body effectively Achieving emotional independence of parents and other adults Achieving assurance of economic independence Selecting and preparing for an occupation Preparing for marriage and family life Developing intellectual skills and concepts necessary for civic competence Preparing and achieving socially responsible behavior Acquiring a set of values and an ethical system as a guide to behavior	Middle age (30–55 years)	Achieving adult civic and social responsibility Establishing and maintaining an economic standard of living Assisting teenage children to become responsible and happy adults Developing adult leisure time activities Relating oneself to one's spouse as a person Accepting and adjusting to the physiologic changes of middle age Adjusting to aging parents
		Later maturity (55–)	Adjusting to decreasing physical strength and health Adjustment to retirement and reduced income Adjusting to death of spouse Establishing an explicit affiliation with one's age group Meeting social and civic obligations Establishing satisfactory living arrangements

Chart 3.4
Erikson's Eight Stages of Human Development

STAGE	TASK	DESCRIPTION OF SUCCESSFUL COMPLETION
Infancy	Trust vs. mistrust	Through interactions with significant others and the environment, infant develops a sense of security in self, others, and the environment
Toddler	Autonomy vs. shame and doubt	Learns sense of self-reliance and independence through exploration of environment and mastery of basic skills
Preschool	Initiative vs. guilt	Further exploration of environment and increased scope of interaction leads child to feelings of enterprise and energy
School age	Industry vs. inferiority	Through school, interactions with peers and significant others, feelings of ability, adequacy, and self-sufficiency develop
Adolescence	Identity vs. identity diffusion	Physical, physiologic, and psychosocial changes along with the assumption and testing of adult role results in crystallization of self-concept
Young Adulthood	Intimacy vs. isolation	Establishment of long-term close ties with a significant other, resulting in a sense of belonging and love, furthering feelings of self-worth.
Adulthood	Generativity vs. self-absorption	Through participation in family and society, individual feels sense of creativity and immortality and of having contributed to well-being of succeeding generations.
Late adulthood	Integrity vs. despair	Acceptance of one's place in the world and role unit leads individual to continued feelings of self-respect and self-esteem.

Many theorists have developed conceptualizations of the process of growth and development. Three of the major theorists are Havighurst, Erikson, and Piaget, whose expected stages are outlined in Charts 3.3, 3.4, and 3.5, respectively. (Illustration 3.5)

Havighurst emphasizes the physical development and changes in the individual and the concurrent social forces or events. Erikson focuses on the psychosocial tasks that the individual needs to complete in order to successfully achieve and retain his or her identity. In contrast, Piaget centers on cognitive development and the related sensorimotor aspects of the life process. All of these are generalized or averaged expectations and individuals may actually vary considerably from these norms.

COGNITIVE ABILITIES

In order to determine nursing strategies which will be the most effective for the individual, the nurse needs an understanding of the person's cognitive abilities. The individual's cognitive abilities affect that person's definitions of health, wellness, and illness, the scope of these definitions, the degree of concreteness or abstraction of these definitions, and the implications of these definitions on behavior. **Cognitive abilities** are those higher associative and interpretive capabilities which allow the individual to learn new behaviors and modify old ones, to reason, conceptualize, and utilize and generate knowledge. These abilities are reflected in the individual's ability to un-

Chart 3.5
Piaget's Stages of Cognitive Development

STAGE	DESCRIPTION
Stage I Sensorimotor (0–2 years)	Divided into six stages, infant moves from a sense of diffusion with external world to identity as a separate person; learns basic psychomotor coordination and skills; begins to conceptualize time, space, and cause and effect
Stage II Preoperational thought (2–7 years)	Divided into two phases: preconceptual (2–4 years) and intuitive thought (4–7 years); develops basic language skills; increases in complexity of thought and action; does not conceptualize wholeness in relationship to parts of whole either in the abstract or the concrete; avid information and experience gatherer
Stage III Concrete operator (7–11 years)	Acquires understanding of relationship of parts to whole; can problem solve concrete situations; begins to understand dynamics of weight, volume, and size Develops awareness of conservation, i.e., shape may change but volume or weight remain constant Begins to understand that there are many routes to the same end (associatively)
Stage IV Formal operations (12–15 years)	Develops ability to use abstract reasoning; integrates all aspects of problem solving and conceptualization; can see things in perspective of past, present, and future

derstand the meaning of events and situations, recognize relationships between concepts and ideas, retain information, solve problems, and make decisions.

CULTURAL INFLUENCES

The individual's exposure to situations, events, ideas, attitudes, and values are, in part, a function of the individual's culture, family, and social interactions. The individual's definitions of health, wellness, and illness are rooted in these experiences. Each culture derives its own health definitions and expectations, which are most often, but not always, transmitted through the family. **Culture** is the sum total of traditions, experiences, practices, beliefs, and values developed by a group of persons and passed on from generation to generation. Such things as art, religion,

folklore rituals, and patterns of eating, dress, and language are all components of culture.

The individual is exposed to these modes of behavior for as long as he or she is under the influence of the culture. As social interactions increase, the individual may hold onto these beliefs or modify or reject them. The more important and relevant the cultural, family, and social interactions are to the individual, the more strongly that individual will hold onto the traditions and mores of these groups. If these groups are highly significant to the individual, the individual will strongly resist opposing views from less significant sources. For example, when the individual holds a culturally and socially based definition of health that is inconsistent with that of the health care professional, the individual will be less likely to follow health care practices proposed. However, if the health care professional can, in some way, put the in-

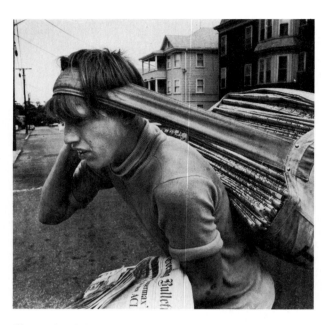

Illustration 3.5
In the American culture, adolescence is a period when young people begin to achieve, among other developmental tasks, emotional independence from adults and assurance of economic independence. *(Photo by Anestis Diakopoulos, from Stock, Boston)*

formation in the context of the individual's cultural and social frame of reference, the likelihood of its acceptance is increased.

HEALTH EXPERIENCES

The individual's previous wellness and illness experiences also contribute to the formulation of definitions of health, wellness, and illness. The implications of certain kinds of pain or dysfunctions, the relevancy of the illness or wellness to life-style, the reactions of family and/or significant others and society to these previous health states, and observations of well and ill states in significant others are among those influences which affect these definitions. In addition, the individual's level of knowledge resulting from these experiences, as well as from other interactions, will also help determine individual definitions. The individual with a limited level of knowledge is more likely to define health, illness, and wellness in terms of the observable, the concrete, cultural and social expectations and personal experience than is the individual with a greater scope of knowledge and information at his disposal.

PERCEPTIONS OF SELF

The individual's perceptions of self at any given time will influence personal definitions of the health state. These perceptions include the individual's feelings and interpretations about such aspects of self as abilities, function, worth, needs, roles, control over events, power, and body image. Any circumstance which alters the individual's perception of self will create some degree of anxiety within and therefore lead to a reaffirmation or redefinition of the individual's level of wellness. For example, if a woman views herself as strong, independent, and self-reliant, any condition which decreases her ability to perform in a manner consistent with these perceptions may be considered illness. On the other hand, the individual whose view of self is opposite from this may, under the same circumstances, consider himself well.

VIEW OF FUNCTIONAL ABILITIES

One outgrowth of all the previously mentioned factors is the individual's expectations of his or her functional abilities in relation to his or her definitions of health, wellness, and illness. Some individuals feel that their physical, physiologic, and psychosocial functioning must be at the highest possible level in order to define themselves as well. Others, however, describe themselves as well if they can even minimally carry out their activities of daily living. Still other persons define themselves as well if their health state has slightly improved or even remained the same in the face of a serious pathophysiologic, physical, or psychosocial interference.

RESULTING HEALTH BELIEFS AND PRACTICES

All these factors interact to form health state definitions and to influence health beliefs and practices. **Health beliefs** are convictions the individual holds related to health which are not necessarily based on fact or reality. A **health practice** is an activity the individual carries out as a result of personal health beliefs and definitions. While these beliefs or practices may, in fact, either support wellness or negatively affect health, the individual considers them vital to the maintenance of wellness. They may lead the individual to resist entry into the health care delivery system or reject the treatments initiated by

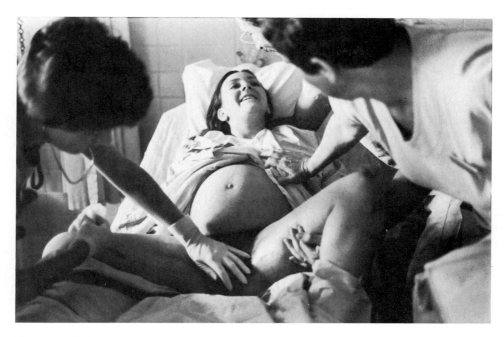

Illustration 3.6
Expressions of pain vary among individuals, depending upon a person's definition of health, the cultural expectations, and one's previous experience. This mother's feelings of self-worth and happiness at giving birth have also influenced her perception of pain. *(Photo © Suzanne Arms/Jeroboam, 1978)*

health care professionals unless these beliefs and practices are taken into consideration in the care that is provided. For example, if the individual believes that the hospital is the place where one goes to die, that individual may refuse to be admitted to the hospital even in life-threatening situations. In any assessment of the individual, his or her definitions of the health state, factors contributing to it, health beliefs, and the resulting practices must be identified and integrated into a plan for care if health care interventions are to be successful and meaningful to the individual. Any attempt to change negative health practices must also be carried out within the context of the individual's definitions, practices, and beliefs concerning the health state. Failure to do so often results in the individual's dissatisfaction with and rejection of health care. (Illustration 3.6)

THE SICK ROLE

If, based on the individual's personal definitions of health, physical, physiologic, and/or psychosocial signs and symptoms demonstrate to the individual

that he or she is ill, the individual can assume what is known as the sick role. The **sick role** can be defined as the utilization of patterns of behaviors which the individual sees as being consistent with "being sick." In our society it is commonly accepted that people who are ill will have an increased degree of dependence on others, be released from responsibilities and roles, have a desire to get well, seek established types of health care, and be self-centered and egocentric. However, many people may not personally define the sick role in these terms and will thus be in conflict with the family and/or significant others, society, and even the health care system itself. However the individual defines himself within the sick role, the nurse needs to assess whether the individual's definitions are consistent with those of others around the individual, what anxieties are created by possible conflicts among definitions, and how the individual can best be helped to support coping behaviors and maximize his level of wellness.

The contract the nurse establishes with the individual will, in part, be determined by the person's sick role behaviors and beliefs. A **contract** is a collaborative agreement between the nurse and the individual which defines what the nature of the interaction will be, who will assume what activities of care, what methods will be utilized to carry out care, and what mode of negotiation will be used for future changes in plans of care. A contract at any given time will be determined by the individual's state of health, setting, time available, definitions of health and sick role (of both the nurse and the individual), and the expectations of the outcomes of health care. (Illustration 3.7)

These contracts are established at the individual's entry into the health care system and are continually reassessed and revised as necessary while the individual remains within the health care system. Contracts can be either formal or informal. The care plan becomes the written form of this agreement.

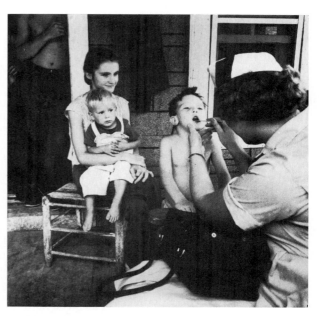

Illustration 3.7
Contracts that the nurse "negotiates" with individuals may be informal, as well as formal, depending upon such factors as the setting and the individual's health state. Here, a nurse functions to promote wellness among family members in an informal rural setting. *(Photo by Ken Heyman)*

WELLNESS PROMOTION

The nurse has a unique role in helping individuals attain and maintain a level of wellness compatible with their health status at that point in time, regardless of their position on the wellness–illness continuum. Through this process, nurses utilize their knowledge of nursing process, growth and development, dynamic concepts related to health, and change strategies to promote wellness.

Levels of Prevention

A useful framework for wellness promotion is the levels of prevention as identified by Leavell and Clark.[4] Although these levels of prevention are disease-oriented, they provide guidelines for the nurse to follow in making effective, positive changes in the health status of the individual. The levels of
► prevention are **primary prevention,** which includes general wellness promotion and specific protection
► against disease; **secondary prevention,** which includes early diagnosis and prompt treatment of illness and disability limitation through prevention of
► illness sequelae; and **tertiary prevention,** which encompasses rehabilitation.

PRIMARY PREVENTION

Because the nurse sees wellness promotion in a positive light, the nurse expands the levels of prevention to provide his or her own unique role. The nurse uses wellness promotion skills in a variety of settings, including the community, home, school, industrial situations, clinic, private office, and hospital. These skills may be applied in global ways by the nurse acting to change wellness-related laws, in a more specific manner by promoting wellness with groups of people, or very specifically in one-to-one interactions with individuals.

In primary prevention such activities as nutrition education, establishing well-baby clinics, sex education, and prenatal classes are evidence of the nurse's concern for wellness promotion. These activities serve to help individuals and groups maintain high-level wellness by acquiring positive health behaviors and providing environmental conditions which support wellness. By identifying populations potentially at risk and intervening before health is negatively affected, the nurse further promotes wellness.

SECONDARY PREVENTION

Insightful recognition of illness sequelae; independent nursing measures such as body alignment, skin care, and fluid maintenance; and recognition of mainfestations of coping mechanisms in the person and his family are indications that the nurse is acting in the role of wellness promoter at the secondary level of prevention. In addition, collaboration with other health care professionals to assist the individual during the acute phase of illness is part of secondary prevention.

TERTIARY PREVENTION

At the tertiary level of prevention, the nurse promotes wellness by assessing abilities and disabilities to prevent further debilitation and promote function. The nurse can then assist the individual and his family and/or significant others to set short- and long-term wellness goals. Through nursing interventions such as teaching the person and family and/or significant others, helping them through stages of death and dying, and acting as liaison for the myriad agencies and services they can utilize, the nurse can further promote high-level wellness on the tertiary level.

HEALTH CARE DELIVERY PATTERNS

The health care delivery system is a multifaceted, interdependent network which provides health-related supports and services. Many different health profes-

sionals and paraprofessionals work together in an attempt to meet the health care needs of individuals and groups. These services may be organized around federal, state, or community health care needs and include wellness promotion, treatment of illness, restoration of wellness, and research. The health care system is supported by federal, state, and local taxes, private contributions, and receipt of payment for services rendered. Agencies which are supported and controlled by public funds are known as **public** or **official;** those which are nonprofit, community-funded, and -controlled agencies are known as **voluntary.** And those agencies which are owned by individuals and run for profit are known as **proprietary,** or **private.**

The emphasis on delivery of health care has begun to shift from acute, episodic treatment of pathologies within the hospital to lifelong distributive wellness promotion. This shift has occurred in response to the recognition of the relationships between health promotion and the prevention of disease and its sequelae and the realization that prolonged hospital stays are often unnecessary when support systems exist in the community. Hospitalization is not only expensive; it disrupts the individual's patterns of economic, cultural, social and psychologic life. (Illustration 3.8)

Distributive care can result in decreased personal and societal economic expenditures, better utilization of services and personnel, provision of health care options for the individual, and an increased level of

Illustration 3.8
Wellness promotion includes providing specific protection against disease. In clinics, primary prevention programs are established to inoculate certain populations against outbreaks of a disease. *(Photo by Arthur Grace, from Stock, Boston)*

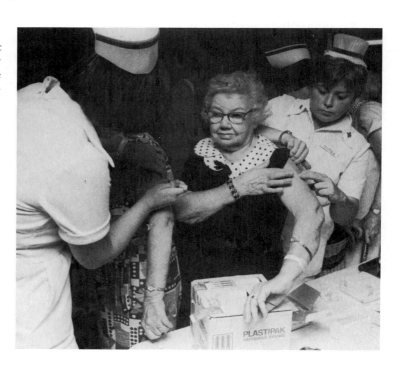

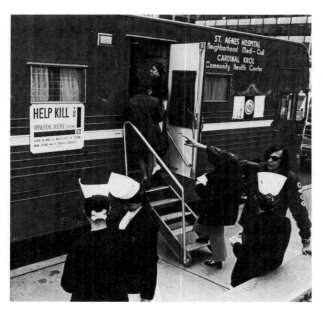

Illustration 3.9
Many programs that promote wellness include all levels of prevention. For example, in dealing with venereal disease it is necessary to provide primary prevention through education and secondary prevention by means of early diagnosis and prompt treatment. *(Photo by Daniel S. Brody, from Stock, Boston)*

wellness for society in general. Viewing health care in terms of the community provides the opportunity to determine individual and group needs based on the characteristics of the population and environment. In this way appropriate, necessary services can be provided and utilized to their fullest and fragmentation of services avoided while continuity of care is maintained. (Illustration 3.9)

Entry into the System

A multiplicity of factors influences an individual's entry into the health care system. Among the most significant factors are the availability of resources and agencies, the individual's knowledge about the existence and use of these resources, the individual's perception of wellness and illness, the individual's health beliefs and practices and expectations of the health care system, and the individual's actual state of health. The availability of resources to the individual depends on federal and private funding, community needs, population distribution, geographic location, political structure of the community, and the

socioeconomic status of the individual. These factors determine the number and nature of health care facilities in a given area and the individual's access to them. By being aware of the forces which influence the availability of health care resources, the nurse can play a part in determining the availability and distribution of services. The nurse can help improve available health care through such activities as opening a private practice, lobbying for political change, serving on health care-related task forces, and working with community groups to maximize efforts. (Illustration 3.10)

The individual's knowledge of these resources can come from family, friends, health professionals, work associates, or the mass media. Frequently, facilities exist within the individual's environment and the individual is unaware of them, uses them inappropriately, or has misconceptions about their purposes. The nurse needs to be aware of what the available resources are, what services they provide and to whom, and the ways an individual can best make use of these services. In this way the nurse can not only provide primary care but also act in a referral and resource capacity.

Our individual perceptions of our health care needs, our health beliefs and practices, and our expectations of the outcomes of health care play a great role in the way we use available resources. For example, one person with a cold might visit a health professional and another utilize home or patent remedies, depending on personal beliefs about the appropriate treatment for this condition and whether or not the person believes the health care system has anything to offer. Factors such as economics, available time, significance of the symptoms to the individual, previous experiences with similar symptoms, and family and/or significant others' validation or rejection of the symptoms as significant will also influence the individual's course of action. The nurse, through health teaching and role model behaviors, can assist the individual in taking the appropriate courses of action.

In addition, the actual state of the individual's health determines the resources available to that individual and the benefits to be derived from their use. A critically ill person will need different types of services than the individual who is seeking wellness maintenance information. If the individual is not aware of these differences, time, money, and energy may be wasted, and the individual may become disillusioned and frustrated with the health care system and compromise his or her health state. For example,

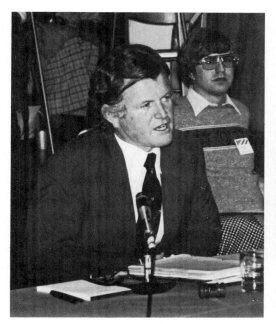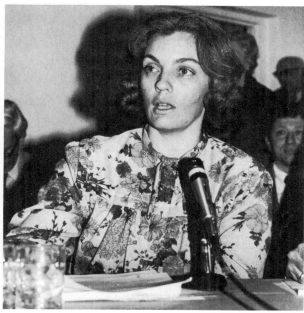

Illustration 3.10
One way that nurses can improve the quality of health care is to influence the political structure within which legislation is developed that affects the health care system. *(Photos by Christine Quinn, courtesy of American Nurses' Association)*

the individual who needs an annual physical for work may go to the local hospital's emergency room. There the individual may experience a lengthy registration period and later get billed for use of the emergency room even though he or she never received a physical because it was not within the scope of services of the emergency room.

Resources at the Levels of Prevention

At each level of wellness promotion, the individual may utilize resources and agencies which focus on that level. Clinics, private nurse practitioners and physicians, health maintenance organizations (HMOs), health stations, screening centers, day-care centers, and information distribution services are examples of primary level services. The general and specialty hospital is the major setting for care during the secondary level of prevention. However, depending on the severity of the illness and the services the individual requires, the individual may remain in the home environment and be treated at a clinic or private physician's office or be seen by a community health nurse.

Rehabilitation centers, halfway houses, nursing homes, extended care facilities, and specialty interest groups such as Cancer Care or the United Cerebral Palsy Association provide services and supports at the tertiary level of prevention. Many of these services may be provided in either the home or institutional settings. The individual's use of and satisfaction with any of the levels of health care delivery system depends on the degree to which these services meet perceived and actual needs, the congruity between expected and actual outcomes, and whether the individual is treated as worthy of dignity and respect.

Enforced Changes

Any time the individual enters the health care delivery system, varying degrees of enforced changes occur in the individual's life-style, roles, patterns of daily living, family and/or significant others' interactions, and levels of independence. These changes act as stressors to the individual in addition to those stressors which necessitated admission to the facility in the first place. The individual's specific reaction to hospitalization will be determined by such factors as the individual's level of growth and development, his role perception, the roles of the people around him, and the individual's state of health and usual coping behaviors. Anxiety is the most frequently seen reaction to hospitalization. The family and/or significant others may also undergo similar changes and react in similar ways.

The nurse's interventions will depend on the specific reactions of the individual and those of the family and/or significant others; however, certain basic interventions will help relieve their anxieties. Familiarizing the individual and the family and/or significant others with the surroundings, basic routines, personnel, and equipment in the immediate environment is one way anxiety may be lessened. The nurse also explains all procedures, the individual's role in the procedures, and the expected sequence of events, to allay anxiety about the unknown and to increase the individual's cooperation, participation, and feeling of control. Answering all questions honestly, collaborating with the individual on all care goals and plans, and respecting the individual's confidentiality and privacy help the individual to have confidence in and security about the care that will be provided.

The Complex Concept of Health

The concept of health is a complex one which depends on many individual and environmental variables. Each individual has a personal definition of health and reacts to changes in health state in a unique and holistic manner. In order to create change and promote wellness, the nurse must recognize individual differences and provide for ways in which individuals can satisfactorily meet their basic needs within the context of their culture, interaction patterns with the family and/or significant others, level of growth and development, and cognitive abilities. In this way, each individual can reach a maximum level of wellness at any given point on the health continuum.

NOTES

1. Preamble, Constitution of the World Health Organization.
2. Halbert L. Dunn, "What High Level Wellness Means." *Canadian Journal of Public Health,* 50:447, November, 1959.

3. Hans Selye, *The Stress of Life.* New York, McGraw-Hill, 1956.
4. Hugh Rodman Leavell and E. Gurney Clark, *Preventative Medicine for the Doctor in His Community,* 3rd ed. New York, McGraw-Hill, 1958, p. 204.

SELECTED REFERENCES

Anonymous. "A Consumer Speaks Out About Hospital Care." *American Journal of Nursing,* 76:1443, September, 1976.

Battistella, Roger M. "The Right to Adequate Health Care." *Nursing Digest,* 4:52, January-February, 1976.

Bell, Robert. "The Impact of Illness on Family Roles," in *A Sociological Framework for Patient Care,* Jeanne Folta and Edith S. Deck, eds. New York, Wiley, 1966.

Bellack, Janis P. "Helping a Child Cope with the Stress of Injury." *American Journal of Nursing,* 74:1491, August, 1974.

Benson, Evelyn R. "The Consumers Right to Health Care: How Does the Nursing Profession Respond?" *Nursing Forum,* 16(2):138, 1977.

Bernal, Henrietta. "Levels of Practice in a Community Health Agency." *Nursing Outlook,* 26:364, June, 1978.

Bernhard, Robert. "The Dehumanized Hospital Hurts You and Your Patients." *Nursing Digest,* 1:39, Spring, 1977.

Bertalanffy, Ludwig von. *General Systems Theory. Foundations, Development and Applications.* New York, Braziller, 1968.

Brell, Christena and Dracup, Kathleen. "Helping the Spouses of Critically Ill Patients." *American Journal of Nursing,* 78:50, January, 1978.

Bullough, Bonnie and Bullough, Vern. *Poverty, Ethnic Identity and Health Care.* New York, Appleton, 1972.

Chaney, Patricia, ed. "Ordeal." *Nursing 75, 5*:27, June, 1975.

Colt, Avery, Anderson, Norma, Scott, H. Denman and Zimmerman, Harvey. "Home Health Care Is Good Economics." *Nursing Outlook, 25*:632, October, 1977.

Dunn, Halbert. "High Level Wellness." *American Journal of Public Health,* 49:786, June, 1959.

———. *High Level Wellness.* Arlington, Va., Beatty, 1973.

Erikson, Erik H. *Identity, Youth and Crisis.* New York, Norton, 1968.

———. *Childhood and Society.* New York, Norton, 1963.

French, Jean G. "This I Believe About Community in the Future." *Nursing Outlook,* 19:173, March, 1971.

Glittenberg, Joan. "Adapting Health Care to a Cultural Setting." *American Journal of Nursing,* 74:2118, December, 1974.

Hall, Joanne and Weavor, Barbara, eds. *Distributive Nursing Practice.* Philadelphia, Lippincott, 1977.

Havighurst, Robert. *Developmental Tasks and Education,* 2nd ed. New York, Longmans, Green, 1952.

————. *Human Development and Education.* New York, Longmans, Green, 1953.

Hein, Eleanor and Leavitt, Maribelle. "Providing Emotional Support to Patients." *Nursing 77,* 7:38, May, 1977.

Hover, Julie and Juelsgard, Nancy. "The Sick Role Reconceptualized." *Nursing Forum.* 17(4):406, 1978.

Isaacs, Marion. "Toward a National Health Policy: A Realist's View." *American Journal of Nursing,* 78:848, May, 1978.

Jacox, Ada and Norris, Catherine, eds. *Organizing for Independent Practice.* New York, Appleton, 1977.

Langford, Teddy. "Establishing a Nursing Contract." *Nursing Outlook,* 26:386, June, 1978.

Larsen, Virginia L. "What Hospitalization Means to Patients." *American Journal of Nursing,* 61:44, May, 1961.

Leavell, Hugh Rodman and Clark, E. Gurney. *Preventive Medicine for the Doctor in His Community,* 3rd ed. New York, McGraw-Hill, 1958.

Long, Edna. "How to Survive Hospitalization." *American Journal of Nursing,* 74:486, March, 1974.

Love, Lucille L. "The Process of Role Change," in *Behavioral Concepts and Nursing Intervention,* Carolyn E. Carlson, ed. Philadelphia, Lippincott, 1970.

Maslow, A. H., *Motivation and Personality,* 2nd ed. New York, Harper & Row, 1970.

Mauksch, Ingeborg G. "On National Health Insurance." *American Journal of Nursing,* 78:1323, August, 1978.

McCarthy, Elaine. "Comprehensive Home Care for Earlier Hospital Discharge." *Nursing Outlook,* 24:625, October, 1976.

McClure, Walter. "National Health Insurance and H.M.O.'s." *Nursing Outlook,* 21:44, January, 1973.

Mills, John S. "Primary Care: Definition of and Access To." *Nursing Outlook,* 25:443, July, 1977.

Murray, Ruth and Zentner, Judith. *Nursing Assessment and Health Promotion Through the Life Span,* 2nd ed. Englewood Cliffs, N.J., Prentice-Hall, 1979.

————. *Nursing Concepts for Health Promotion.* 2nd ed. Englewood Cliffs, N.J., Prentice-Hall, 1979.

Navarro, Vicente. "From Public Health to Health of the Public." *American Journal of Public Health,* 64:591, June, 1974.

Oelbaum, Cynthia H. "Hallmarks of Adult Wellness." *American Journal of Nursing.* 74:1623, September, 1974.

Parsons, Talcott. "On Becoming a Patient," in *A Sociological Framework for Patient Care,* Jeanne Folta and Edith S. Deck, eds. New York, Wiley 1966.

Piaget, Jean. *The Growth of Logical Thinking from Childhood to Adolescence.* New York, Basic, 1961.

Porter, Anne L., Moschel, Patricia, Luderman, Barbara and Pope, Marge. "Patient Needs on Admission." *American Journal of Nursing,* 77:112, January, 1977.

Selye, Hans. *The Stress of Life.* New York, McGraw-Hill, 1956.

Schenk, Katherine. "Teaching Distributive Nursing." *Nursing Outlook,* 24:574, September, 1976.

Spector, Rachel E. *Cultural Diversity in Health and Illness.* New York, Appleton, 1979.

Standeven, Muriel. "Social Sensitivity in Health Care." *Nursing Outlook,* 25:640, October, 1977.

Stephenson, Carol A. "Stress in Critically Ill Patients." *American Journal of Nursing,* 77:1806, November, 1977.

Sutterly, Doris Cook and Donnelly, Gloria. *Perspectives in Human Development: Nursing Throughout the Life Cycle.* Philadelphia, Lippincott, 1973.

Topia, Jane A. "The Nursing Process in Family Health." *Nursing Outlook,* 19:267, April, 1971.

Turnbull, Sister Joyce. "Shifting the Focus to Health." *American Journal of Nursing,* 76:1985, December, 1976.

Vincent, Pauline. "The Sick Role in Patient Care." *American Journal of Nursing,* 75:1172, July, 1975.

Valke, Maryann K. "When a Patient Needs to Unburden His Feelings." *American Journal of Nursing,* 77:1164, July, 1977.

Williams, Carolyn A. "Community Health Nursing— What Is It?" *Nursing Outlook,* 25:250, April, 1977.

*He is eyes for the blind, strength for the weak,
and a shield for the defenseless.*

—*Robert Green Ingersoll,* Liberty

ADVOCACY IN CHANGE

THE NURSE, THE ADVOCATE

In effecting change and promoting wellness, the nurse works as an advocate. An **advocate** is defined as one who works with or on behalf of a person or system to bring about a positive difference in the system's state or the individual's condition of health. It is the construct of advocacy which gives direction to the nurse's goals and promotes the organized direction of planning in order to bring about positive change. Advocacy is not a happenstance occurrence, but rather results from a conscious, organized, and thorough plan to assess the needs of the individual or system and a commitment to change.

The nurse acts as an advocate whenever attempting to bring about a change, whether in giving direct care to an individual on a one-to-one basis or working as a representative of the individual to others in the health care system and to the family and/or significant others. Advocacy also includes the nurse's accountability for his or her own actions and the actions of those the nurse supervises, as well as acting as a spokesperson for the individual and the nursing profession in providing health care. In the one-to-one direct care situation, the nurse assists the individual in exploring options for health care and supports those informed choices that the individual ultimately makes.

Providing Options

Options are those alternatives or choices that the individual has within a given situation. Every situation can be dealt with in a variety of ways using a variety of techniques. Frequently the individual is unaware of the multiplicity of choices that are available. For example, the individual who wants to lose weight may feel that the only way to do this is by drastically cutting the intake of all foods. However, other methods such as changing food patterns, increasing exercise, hypnosis, and biofeedback, all may contribute to weight reduction.

Presenting options alone is not sufficient for the nurse in acting as an advocate. Choices that are not explored in terms of their negative and positive components and probable outcomes or those which are representative of the nurse's own biases do not provide for an informed choice. An informed choice means that a complete picture has been presented to the individual. A simple statement of "You can do this, that, or something else" is not providing for an informed choice. In addition, the individual has the option of not considering any option which is presented.

The Individual's Freedom to Act

Inherent in the concept of option giving is the belief that once the individual has been presented with sufficient information to make informed choices, the individual has the right to follow through on the option which he or she chooses. Advocacy, therefore, continues when the nurse supports whatever choice the individual has made. This does not imply that the nurse cannot disagree or attempt to speak on behalf of the nurse's preferred options. However, it does mean that the nurse assists the individual in carrying through with choices made. For example, the individual who, after careful presentation and consideration of all available alternatives and information, has chosen one option over the others is helped to carry out this choice and is referred to appropriate resources, whether the nurse agrees with the choice or not.

Representing the Individual

Many times, as a result of the option process, the nurse then acts in the advocate role to represent the individual to his or her family and/or significant others and to other members of the health care system. Frequently the family and/or significant others may have perceptions and needs different from the individual's. Thus they may not be able to understand and accept automatically the individual's point of view or choices. Because of the individual's state of health, energy levels, or interaction patterns, the individual may not be able to act fully in his or her own behalf and thus designates the nurse to do so. Many times the family and/or significant others will also need assistance in carrying out these choices.

Since the health care system contains so many components, the nurse often acts as an advocate for the individual to help him or her carry out choices in the most efficient and effective manner. This process may involve such actions as referring the individual to the appropriate resources, manipulating schedules, and acting as a spokesperson. For example, the individual who is scheduled for a series of diagnostic tests, one right after another, may not have the endurance to undergo all these tests. The nurse

can talk with various persons involved in the testing processes to reschedule the tests with periods of rest in between.

THE ETHICS OF ADVOCACY

Advocacy is not the usurping of an individual's rights, but the supplementing of the person's ability to meet personal goals. The individual's needs in a particular situation, level of growth and development, functional abilities and level of awareness help determine the degree of advocacy required. Integral to advocacy is the ability of the person to designate the nurse as advocate. The individual who is unconscious or unable to make decisions because of immaturity, level of awareness, or functional disability cannot in reality designate an advocate. In this case, the nurse still works on behalf of the individual; however, the nurse determines what actions to take according to his or her own perceptions of the individual's needs and the desires of the family and/or significant others.

The Law

Laws vary from state to state as to the types of options the nurse can give and the form that advocacy will take. Many of these laws are in a state of flux and are not clearly spelled out. Therefore, the nurse, must be familiar with the law of his or her own state and the policies of the setting where the nurse is working.

Collaboration

The nurse who acts as the appointed advocate of an individual does so through collaboration with others rather than through confrontation. Advocate and adversary are not synonymous terms or components of each other. When acting as advocate for the individual, the nurse informs others in the health care system of the action; confers with others to find means of carrying out the individual's informed choices; seeks information and clarification; and respects others' opinions, viewpoints, and expertise in the option process.

To act as an advocate for the individual the nurse needs to realize that others may be simultaneously advocating for the individual and thus plans, goals, and interventions need to be coordinated. There may be differences of opinions and times when positions must be negotiated, and the situation may be such that the time and circumstances are not appropriate for a change to occur. Principles of change need to be considered and incorporated into the process of advocacy. In order to be an effective advocate, the nurse will need to use judgment, creativity, problem-solving skills, and all the change strategies (Chap. 5) at his or her disposal.

CONSUMERISM AND ADVOCACY

As the trend toward consumerism increases in the United States, the public is making more demands on the nurse to act as an advocate. **Consumerism** is the

process which individuals use to increase the control they have over decisions in their lives and to choose the products and services which they utilize. Increasingly, the general public is becoming better informed about health care, the availability of options, and the services which should be provided by individuals within the health care system. As a result, individuals are questioning the quality, quantity, and type of care they are receiving within the health care system and are demanding their rights in decisions regarding health care. (Illustration 4.1)

One outgrowth of health care consumerism is the formulation of so-called patients' bills of rights. They are written statements of the guaranteed rights of an individual within a given health care setting. For the nurse, these bills of rights can often serve as a guideline on which to build a foundation for advocacy. Charts 4.1 to 4.3 are examples of various bills of rights. Generally these bills protect the individual's confidentiality, privacy, access to health care

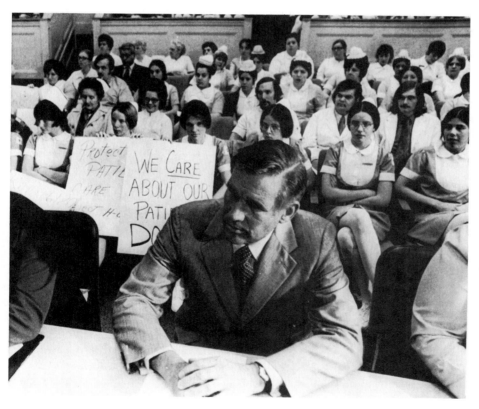

Illustration 4.1
Being aware of the impact of the political environment on the health care system will assist the nurse as an advocate for the individual and the nursing profession. *(Photo from United Press International)*

Chart 4.1
American Hospital Association Patient's Bill of Rights

1. The patient has the right to considerate and respectful care.

2. The patient has the right to obtain from his physician complete current information concerning his diagnosis, treatment, and prognosis in terms the patient can be reasonably expected to understand.

3. The patient has the right to receive from his physician information necessary to give informed consent prior to the start of any procedure and/or treatment. . . . Where medically significant alternatives for care or treatment exist, or when the patient requests information concerning medical alternatives, the patient has the right to such information [and] to know the name of the person responsible for the procedures and/or treatment.

4. The patient has the right to refuse treatment to the extent permitted by law, and to be informed of the medical consequences of his action.

5. The patient has the right to every consideration of his privacy concerning his own medical care program.

6. The patient has the right to expect that all communications and records pertaining to his care should be treated as confidential.

7. The patient has the right to expect that within its capacity a hospital must make reasonable response to the request of a patient for services.

8. The patient has the right to obtain information as to any relationship of his hospital to other health care and educational institutions insofar as his care is concerned . . . [and] any professional relationships among individuals, by name, who are treating him.

9. The patient has the right to be advised if the hospital proposes to engage in or perform human experimentation affecting his care or treatment . . . [and] has the right to refuse to participate. . . .

10. The patient has the right to expect reasonable continuity of care.

11. The patient has the right to examine and receive an explanation of his bill regardless of source of payment.

12. The patient has the right to know what hospital rules and regulations apply to his conduct as a patient.

Reprinted with permission of the American Hospital Association, copyright, 1975.

records and information, and the right to informed consent. Nurses need to make individuals aware of these bills, their implications, and how to obtain their rights.

The Nurse's Accountability

The nurse as an advocate is accountable to the individual, the public, and the profession for his or her own actions and the actions of those the nurse supervises. Accountability is part of advocacy, since the nurse, in representing the individual, must insure that the individual receives qualified, competent care. This is done through self-evaluation and peer review. (Chapter 2 discusses accountability.)

In addition, the nurse works on behalf of the individual to improve health care by recognizing the changes that are necessary in the health care system and the profession and by taking an active part in promoting those changes. An awareness of the political environment and its impact on health care is a necessary component of advocacy. Speaking to issues that affect nurses, nursing, and health is a way that awareness can be utilized to improve health care delivery at all levels.

The nurse is frequently in a position to work as a resource person for consumer groups who are at-

Chart 4.2

United Nations Declaration of
the Rights of the Child

The right to affection, love, and understanding.

The right to adequate nutrition and medical care.

The right to free education.

The right to full opportunity for play and recreation.

The right to a name and nationality.

The right to special care, if handicapped.

The right to be among the first to receive relief in times of disaster.

The right to learn to be a useful member of society and to develop individual abilities.

The right to be brought up in a spirit of peace and universal brotherhood.

The right to enjoy these rights, regardless of race, color, sex, religion, or national or social origin.

United Nations, 1979.

Chart 4.3

The Rights of Senior Citizens

1. The right to be useful.

2. The right to obtain employment, based on merit.

3. The right to freedom from want in old age.

4. The right to a fair share of the community's recreational, educational, and medical resources.

5. The right to obtain decent housing suited to needs of later years.

6. The right to the moral and financial support of one's family so far as is consistent with the best interests of the family.

7. The right to live independently, as one chooses.

8. The right to live with dignity.

9. The right of access to all knowledge available on how to improve the later years of life.

The Nation and Its Older People, Report of the White House Conference on Aging, January 1961, United States Department of Health, Education and Welfare.

tempting to make changes directly related to health care and health care services. By providing information on change strategies and areas of concern being considered by other health groups, the government, and the nursing profession, the nurse can assist consumer groups to meet their health care goals. In the community, the nurse can often point out ways that health is being compromised or promoted, and in this way assist people to utilize available facilities or help them to form action groups to attain needed services.

Within the community the nurse can promote the image of the nurse as an informed professional who is pivotal in providing quality health care. By acting as a role model and dispelling the myths and misconceptions the public holds as a result of misinformation transmitted by the mass media and past experiences within the health care system, the nurse advocates not only for the public but also for the profession. Many times the nurse is asked to speak before community groups, serve on committees, or participate in setting up community projects. By engaging in these activities, the nurse can further promote the image of the profession and ultimately improve health care. The more the nurse is seen as a valuable resource person and as a provider of quality health care and with his or her own area of expertise, the more the nurse can be recognized as an advocate for health rights.

Within the profession the nurse represents not only himself or herself but also the individual. Therefore the nurse supports movements within the profession to increase quality assurance, promote professional activities, and develop an independent theory of nursing. By joining professional organizations the nurse has a voice in the policies and standards which are set forth for the profession and which relate to improvement of health care delivery.

The Construct of Advocacy

The construct of nursing advocacy is one which is in the process of definition and refinement, and the specific role of the nurse as an advocate is still developing. However, any advocacy role the nurse takes on will require a broad and deep knowledge base, creativity, and judgment. Consideration of the needs of the individual, profession, and society guides the nurse in the role of advocate. Advocacy requires the consent of the individual and the nurse's taking both personal and professional risks.

SELECTED REFERENCES

Abrams, Natalie. "A Contrary View of the Nurse as Patient Advocate." *Nursing Forum,* 17(3):258, 1978.

Bandman, Elsie L. "The Rights of Nurses and Patients: A Case for Advocacy," in *Bioethics and Human Rights,* Elsie L. Bandman and Bertram Bandman, eds. Boston, Little, Brown, 1978, pp. 332–338.

———— and Bandman, Bertram. "There Is Nothing Automatic About Rights." *American Journal of Nursing* 77:867, May, 1977.

Besch, Linda Briggs. "Informed Consent: A Patient's Right." *Nursing Outlook,* 27:32, January, 1979.

Dodge, Joan S. "What Patients Should Be Told: Patients' and Nurses' Beliefs." *American Journal of Nursing,* 72:1852, October, 1972.

Donahue, M. Patricia. "The Nurse—A Patient Advocate?" *Nursing Forum* 17(2):143, 1978.

Fay, Patricia. "In Support of Patient Advocacy as a Nursing Role." *Nursing Outlook,* 26:252, April, 1978.

Kalish, Beatrice J. "Of Half Gods and Mortals: Aesculapian Authority." *Nursing Outlook,* 23:22, January, 1976.

Kelly, Lucie Young. "The Patient's Right to Know." *Nursing Outlook,* 24:26, January, 1976.

Kosik, Sandra Henry. "Patient Advocacy or Fighting the System." *American Journal of Nursing,* 72:694, April, 1972.

Langford, Teddy. "Establishing a Nursing Contract." *Nursing Outlook,* 26:836, June, 1978.

Lewis, Edith P. "The Right to Inform" (Editorial). *Nursing Outlook,* 25:561, September, 1977.

Quinn, Nancy and Somers, Anne R. "The Patients' Bill of Rights: A Significant Aspect of the Consumer Revolution." *Nursing Outlook,* 22:240, April, 1974.

Ryden, Muriel. "An Approach to Ethical Decision Making." *Nursing Outlook,* 26:705, November, 1978.

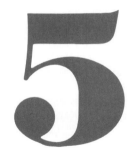

Man is a tool-using animal . . . without tools he is nothing, with tools he is all.
—Thomas Carlyle

CHANGE STRATEGIES

To meet the challenge inherent in bringing about change and promoting advocacy, the nurse builds a foundation which includes interpersonal skills of communication, leadership, use of power, management, group process, and teaching–learning; psychomotor skills; and research. The nurse must become proficient in utilizing these tools and be able to identify their appropriate use in a variety of settings. These skills are the tools which provide the nurse with the means to put the concepts of change and advocacy into action. These learned behaviors are the bridge between theory and practice.

COMMUNICATION

▶ **Communication** is defined as the dynamic, multisensory interchange between two or more persons. The interchange is a continuous phenomenon where it is impossible not to communicate. All behavior is a form of communication, and therefore, it is imperative for the nurse to be able to identify and utilize the communication process.

All the senses—auditory, visual, tactile, olfactory, and taste—take part in communication. When a person speaks, the receiver not only hears the words, the intonation, language usage and structure, accents, and emotional content, but also sees the speaker's facial expression, posture, gestures, appearance, and the distance he places between himself and the receiver, and feels the vibrations set off by the sound waves he produces when speaking. In addition, if the speaker touches the receiver, the receiver feels thermal sensations, the degree of moisture on the skin, the sensations evoked, and the character, appropriateness, and intimacy of the touch. The sense of smell also comes into play as the receiver smells the odors given off by the speaker. Although the sense of taste is not commonly used in formal social interactions, it is utilized in intimate interactions such as kissing and sexual foreplay.

These interactions of the senses occur almost simultaneously and usually unconsciously. They may either support or contradict each other, making communication a multisensory, dynamic experience. For example, when a person says, "What are you doing?" the receiver may interpret this as a polite inquiry, an accusation, an invasion of privacy, or a rhetorical question, depending on the context in which it is spoken, the tone of voice used, the gestures or facial expressions used, and the type of touch involved. Thus the communication process involves not only verbal (spoken or written) messages, but also nonverbal (sight, touch, smell, and taste) cues.

The manner in which communication is interpreted by the individual is determined by the individual's level of growth and development, previous experience, culture, attitudes, cognitive level, own interaction style, intact sensory organs, and level of anxiety. Chapter 12 details these influences and how they may be assessed by the nurse.

Functions of Communication

Communication is used for gathering and transmitting knowledge and information, expressing emotions, social intercourse, transferring culture, influencing behavior, entertainment, and self-expression. In other words, communication is the mode of transmission of all human social interactions.

The individual utilizes the communication process for self-validation. As he expresses thoughts, ideas, values, and emotions, he receives feedback from the people in his environment. This feedback provides either negative or positive reinforcement for his behavior. This does not mean that the individual will automatically modify his behavior based on this feedback, but his self-concept and future interactions are influenced. The impact of communication feedback depends, in part, on how the individual views the message and the sender, his basic personality, his reliance on personal validation, and the context in which the interaction took place.

Process of Communication

Communication between people basically occurs when one person has information he wants to trans-

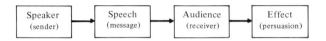

Figure 5.1
Aristotle's communication model

mit to others. He sends the message either verbally or nonverbally to another person (or persons) who receives it by one or more of the recipient's sense organs. The communication stimulus is then sent to the brain, where it is perceived (decoded and interpreted). The perception process results in some type of response from the receiver. This response may be a behavior or a filing away of the information for use at another time.

Various theories have evolved to explain the process of communication. Figures 5.1 through 5.8 illustrate some of the major communication models.

THE COMPONENTS

In viewing the process of communication, the nurse needs to look at the components of communication—the vocabulary, syntax, content, context, and the mode of transmission. The **vocabulary** is the symbolic representation of ideas, thoughts, and feelings. Vocabulary includes words, letters, and numbers. Each language, discipline, and culture has its own vocabulary which is meaningful to the people using it.

The **syntax** of communication is the way the vocabulary is structured into meaningful messages. The **content** of communication is a combination of the vocabulary and syntax. It is the message which the sender is transmitting to the receiver.

The environment, atmosphere, intent, and state of the receiver determines the context of the communication. The **context** is the approach of the communication. The method the individual uses to

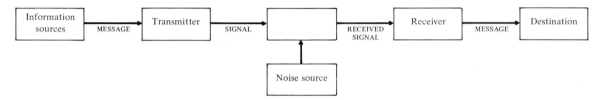

Figure 5.2
Shannon and Weaver communication model. *(From Claude E. Shannon and Warren Weaver. The Mathematical Theory of Communication. Urbana, Ill., University of Illinois Press, 1949)*

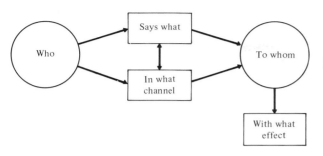

Figure 5.3
Lasswell's communication model. *(Based on data from "The Structure and Function of Communication in Society" by Harold D. Lasswell, in* The Communication of Ideas, *ed. Lyman Bryson. Copyright 1948 by Institute for Religious and Social Studies. Reprinted by permission of Harper and Row, Publishers, Inc.)*

► send the communication is the **mode of transmission.** Modes range from the spoken word to the mass media to literature.

A disturbance in any one of these components will cause a distortion in communication. The disturbance may emanate from either the sender or the receiver. For example, the nurse may use professional language (jargon) when attempting to transmit information to an individual. In that case, the nurse uses the correct vocabulary and syntax for professional to professional communication but has not considered the context, and the layman is unable to understand the meaning of the message. Therefore, when the nurse tells an individual, "You will be kept N.P.O. after midnight," that individual probably will not know that he can't have any food, fluid, or medication orally after the hour of midnight.

Communication for Change

Although communication is always occurring, **therapeutic communication** within the health care setting is a conscious, goal-oriented, and planned process. The nurse is aware of the effects of his or her behavior on others and vice versa, the desired outcomes, and the purpose of the communication. With these factors in mind, the nurse formulates goals or objectives which focus the communication process and then proceeds to plan for the most effective and efficient way of meeting those goals.

Therapeutic communication is not merely random conversation, a way to pass time, or busywork. It is, however, a way to facilitate change by allowing for expression of feelings, transference of information, teaching and learning, and clarification of attitudes and values. Through therapeutic communication the nurse helps the individual to make a positive difference in his ability to meet his daily health needs. This does not imply that social conversation does not have a place in therapeutic communication, but rather that conversation is a means to therapeutic communication and not the goal.

Facilitators of Communication

► **Facilitators of communication** are those factors which enhance the effectiveness of the process. Common attitudes, values, and beliefs; similar culture; therapeutic techniques; an environment in which the individual feels free to express himself; words which have the same connotation and denotation to both the sender and the receiver; trust, open-

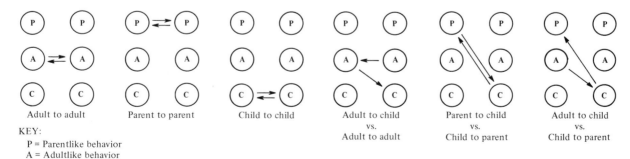

KEY:
P = Parentlike behavior
A = Adultlike behavior
C = Childlike behavior

Figure 5.4
Examples of transactional analysis interactions. *(Based on Thomas A. Harris.* I'm O.K., You're O.K. *New York, Harper and Row, Publishers, Inc., 1969)*

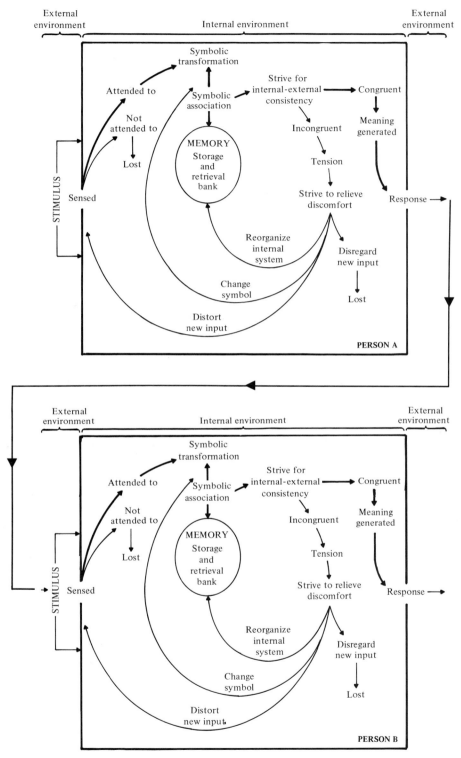

Figure 5.5

Interpersonal communications model. The response of Person A is the stimulus for Person B.
(Reprinted with permission from Margaret L. Pluckman, Human Communication: The Matrix of Nursing. *New York, McGraw-Hill, 1978)*

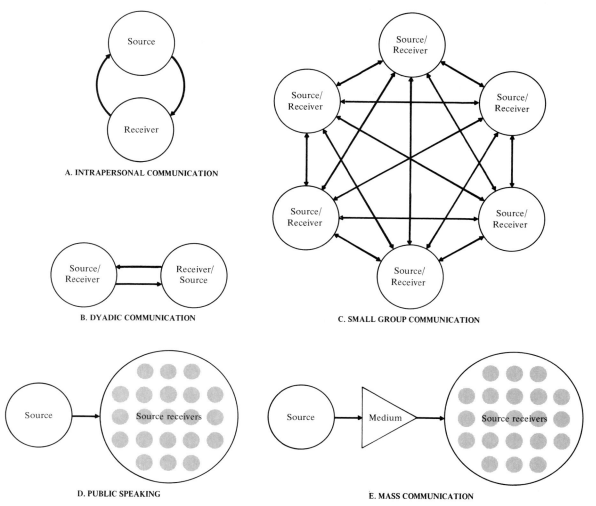

A. INTRAPERSONAL COMMUNICATION

B. DYADIC COMMUNICATION

C. SMALL GROUP COMMUNICATION

D. PUBLIC SPEAKING

E. MASS COMMUNICATION

Figure 5.6

Five forms of communication. (*From* The Interpersonal Communication Book *by Joseph A. DeVito. Copyright © 1976 by Joseph A. DeVito. Reprinted by permission of Harper and Row, Publishers, Inc.)*

ness, and flexibility; mutual respect; acceptance; self-awareness; and objectivity, a nonjudgmental attitude, and an awareness of the effect of one's behavior on others are some of the facilitators to effective communication.

Some interaction techniques which are useful in promoting communication are outlined in Chart 5.1. These techniques can form the framework from which the nurse develops an effective style of interaction. They do not, in and of themselves, ensure communication that is effective and therapeutic, but serve as guidelines. Often it is the context and the mode in which the communication takes place that determine the resulting interaction, rather than the actual vocabulary and syntax used. Since these techniques are

labeled therapeutic, they are often overused and restrict the communication process.

Barriers to Communication

▶ **Barriers to communication** are those factors which hinder the process. Communication can be hindered by dissimilar attitudes, values, beliefs, cultures, and expectations; nontherapeutic techniques; a restrictive, judgmental atmosphere; words which do not have the same connotation and denotation to the sender and receiver; distrust, close-mindedness, rigidity and biases; lack of mutual respect and rejection; language differences; lack of self-awareness; subjectivity; lack of awareness of the effect of one's be-

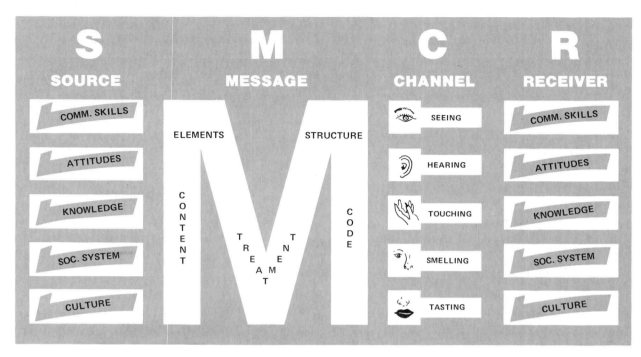

Figure 5.7

A model of the ingredients in communication. *(From* The Process of Communication: An Introduction to Theory and Practice *by David Berlo. Copyright © 1960 by Holt, Rinehart and Winston, Inc. Reprinted by permission of Holt, Rinehart and Winston)*

havior on another and vice versa; and inattention. These barriers, as well as the facilitators and the related nursing assessment, are discussed in Chapter 12. These barriers can influence the interaction process to such an extent that effective communication can be blocked.

Just as there are useful interaction techniques to promote therapeutic communication, there are nontherapeutic techniques. Some of them are listed in Chart 5.2. These techniques are commonly used in everyday situations; however, their use in therapeutic communication may result in unexpected and undesired reactions such as stopping the interaction. Like therapeutic techniques, it is often not the fact that these approaches are used, but rather the manner in which they are used which determines the nature of the interaction. When used in the regular context and mode, they may be appropriate.

Skill Development

Communication is an all-pervasive concept which can be utilized therapeutically by the nurse to effectuate positive change. Effective communication is an

acquired skill which is continuously being refined and reexamined through use in a wide variety of situations. As the nurse increases her experience in therapeutic communication, she develops her own interaction style which effectively balances a wide variety of techniques in a manner in which both the nurse and the individual whom the nurse is working with are comfortable.

TEACHING–LEARNING

Teaching–Learning Process

One of the major change strategies the nurse utilizes
► is the **teaching–learning process.** It is a planned interaction which produces a relatively permanent change in behavior not brought about by maturation
► or any chance circumstances. **Learning** is the resul-
► tant behavioral change, while **teaching** is that part of the process which facilitates the change. Thus the teaching–learning process is a basic method the nurse

utilizes to assist individuals in acquiring behaviors necessary to make a positive difference in their ability to meet their health care needs. Nurses also increase their own professional knowledge and skills through use of the teaching–learning process.

This process is a dynamic interaction between the teacher and the learner to which each of the participants brings beliefs, values, and communication and learning styles. The exchange that results is a reciprocal interaction in which the teacher communicates with the learner and the learner communicates with the teacher. Information, emotions, and perceptions are among those things transmitted back and forth. Thus the teaching–learning process is not simply the teacher imparting information to the learner and the learner receiving that information.

Figure 5.8
Johari Window

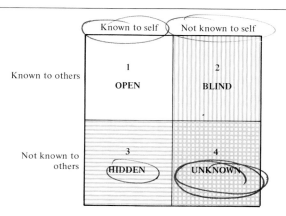

INTERPRETATION OF JOHARI WINDOW

1. A change in any one quadrant will affect all other quadrants.

2. It takes energy to hide, deny, or be blind to behavior which is involved in interaction.

3. Threat tends to decrease awareness; mutual trust tends to increase awareness.

4. Forced awareness (exposure) is undesirable and usually ineffective.

5. Interpersonal learning means a change has taken place so that Q1 is larger and one or more of the other quadrants has grown smaller.

6. Working with others is facilitated by a large enough area of free activity. An increased Q1 means more of the resources and skills in the membership can be applied to a task.

7. The smaller the first quadrant, the poorer the communication.

8. There is universal curiosity about the unknown area, but this is held in check by custom, social training, and diverse fears.

9. Sensitivity means appreciating the covert aspects of behavior, in quadrants 2, 3, and 4, and respecting the desire of others to keep them so.

10. Learning about group processes as they are being experienced helps to increase awareness (enlarge Q1) for the group as a whole as well as for individual members.

11. The value system of a group and its membership may be noted in the way unknowns in the life of the group are confronted.

12. A centipede may be perfectly happy without awareness, but after all, he restricts himself to crawling under rocks.

From Group Processes: An Introduction to Group Dynamics *by Joseph Luft, by permission of Mayfield Publishing Company (formerly National Press Books). Copyright © 1963, 1970 Joseph Luft. See also* Of Human Interaction.

Chart 5.1
Therapeutic Communication Techniques

TECHNIQUE LABEL AND DESCRIPTION   EXAMPLES

Using Silence

Refraining from verbal comments while conveying an attitude of care and interest toward the patient; being alert to the feeling tone communicated by the patient through posture, gesture, facial expression, voice tone, and inflections.

Sitting or walking with a patient who is unable or unwilling to communicate with words. Resisting the temptation to make immediate responses or to ask questions when a prolonged verbal pause occurs during an interaction.

Offering Self

The nurse offers his or her presence, interest, and desire to understand without making any demands on the patient. The patient is not made to feel he must "give" in order to receive attention. No "condition" is attached to the offer.

"I'll stay with you while you wait for your treatment."
"I'll help you make your bed."
"We can sit here quietly; there's no need to talk unless you want to."

Giving Broad Openings and/or
Offering General Leads

Providing the opportunity for the patient to take the initiative in introducing a topic and determining the direction of conversation. Giving encouragement for the patient's continued verbalization.

"Perhaps it will help to talk about your feelings."
"Where would you like to begin?"
"And then?"
"I follow what you're saying."

Placing the Event in Time or in Sequence

Nurse helps patient to clarify an event, situation, or happening in relationship to time.

"Was this before or after breakfast?"
"When did this happen?"
"Today is Monday. You had your fifth treatment this morning."

Making Observations

Nurse indicates awareness of change, notes effort patient has made, and verbalizes what is perceived. The comment contains no value judgment.

"You've changed your hair style."
"You've finished lacing the wallet."
"You keep rubbing your forehead; are you in discomfort?"

Encouraging Descriptions

Giving the patient the opportunity to verbalize his perceptions; to try to describe *how he feels* or *how he views* a situation.

"Try to describe how you felt."
"How do you believe it should have been done?"
"What's your opinion?"
"How do you feel about going home?"

Encouraging Comparisons

Nurse requests the patient to describe similarities and differences about thoughts, feelings, and situations, or to appraise the way his experiences have affected him.

"You said you were frightened when you first came to the hospital. How do you feel now?"
"How was this meeting different from yesterday's?"
"You say your feelings have changed. In what way?"

(continued)

Chart 5.1 (Cont.)
Therapeutic Communication Techniques

TECHNIQUE LABEL AND DESCRIPTION

EXAMPLES

Restating

Using different words to repeat the main idea the patient has expressed. (Another way of attempting to clarify the patient's communication.)

Patient: "I can't sleep. I stay awake all night."
Nurse: "You have difficulty sleeping."

Patient: "It takes great effort to talk to strangers."
Nurse: "You find it hard to talk with people you don't know."

Reflecting

Directing questions, feelings, and ideas back to the patient in an attempt to indicate to the patient that his point of view has value and that he has a right to express his feelings and thoughts.

Patient: "Do you think I should tell my husband?"
Nurse: "You seem unsure about telling your husband."

Patient: "That stupid jerk! How dare he talk that way to me? Who does he think he is?"
Nurse: You didn't like the way he spoke to you."

Giving Information

Nurse gives patient facts or specific information that is needed. Questions are answered simply and directly or when the nurse does not know, this is stated.

"The head nurses's name is Miss Grace Gordon."
"I do not know; Mrs. Day may have that information."
"No it is not unusual to have a headache after an ECT treatment."

Seeking Clarification

The nurse makes an effort to have the patient clarify comments that are vague, which have a meaning that is not understood, which have been spoken softly or quickly.

"I'm not sure what you mean."
"You spoke so softly I did not hear what you said."
"That thought I'm not able to follow."
"What do you mean when you say 'be a good patient'?"

Presenting Reality

When the nurse notices the patient is misrepresenting reality an effort is made to indicate that which is real.

"That's a stain on the blanket, it is not a bug."
"I see no other person in the room."
"The scream came from the program on the television."

Voicing Doubt

Expressing uncertainty about the reality of a patient's perception . . . but being careful not to contradict or belittle the patient's view.

"Can such actions be interpreted in that way only?"
"Are you saying that everyone is against you?"
"Are you sure you understood what Janice meant?"
"You *say* you are not upset . . . but you give the impression that all is not well."

(continued)

Chart 5.1 (Cont.)
Therapeutic Communication Techniques

TECHNIQUE LABEL AND DESCRIPTION	EXAMPLES
Consensual Validation A search for mutual understanding. The nurse tries to make certain that the words, ideas, concepts, or expressions being used during an interaction have essentially the same meaning for both participants.	"Tell me if my understanding is accurate. . . ." "Are you and I using the word 'friend' in the same way?" "Are you referring to the episode that happened yesterday?"
Verbalizing the Implied The nurse tries to put in more specific terms what the patient has hinted at or implied. It is an attempt to clarify what the patient has said implicitly but it *is not* an interpretation.	**Patient:** "There's no point in complaining." **Nurse:** "Are you saying no one listens?" <center>OR</center>**Nurse:** "Are you feeling discouraged?" **Patient:** "There's no use talking; it's a waste of time." **Nurse:** "Do you feel that no one will understand?"
Attempting to Translate into Feelings The nurse attempts to verbalize the feelings that are being expressed only indirectly by the patient, and watches for nonverbal cues that assist in making helpful "translations."	**Patient:** "It's like being on a merry-go-round." **Nurse:** "Are you saying you feel as if you're going nowhere?" **Patient:** "I'm just like an infant." **Nurse:** "Do you mean you feel helpless?"
Encouraging Fromulation of a Plan Nurse helps the patient to consider alternative ways and possibly more effective means for dealing with particular problems and situations.	"Can you think of another way you might be able to handle a situation like this?" "In what way can you make these visits less upsetting?" "Have you considered telling your mother directly that it annoys and irritates you?"

Adapted with permission of Macmillan Publishing Co., Inc. from Interacting with Patients *by Joyce Samhammer Hays and Kenneth H. Larson. Copyright © Macmillan Publishing Co., Inc., 1963.*

Chart 5.2
Nontherapeutic Communication Techniques

TECHNIQUE LABEL AND RATIONALE FOR NONUSE	EXAMPLES

Reassurance

This is an attempt to dispel a patient's anxiety by implying that there is no cause for worry or alarm or fear. It belittles, devaluates, or rejects the patient's feelings and communicates lack of understanding or empathy. Often it is more comforting to the nurse than it is helpful to the patient.

"Everything will be all right."
"Don't worry about it, you'll soon be OK."
"There's nothing to be afraid of. Relax, take it easy."
"You're coming along fine now, stop worrying."

Giving Approval

To state that what the patient is doing, feeling, or saying is "good" is to imply that the opposite is "bad." It often limits the patient's freedom to think, speak, or act in a way that will displease another. It can lead a patient to strive for praise rather than progress.

"That's good."
"I'm glad that you feel that way."
"Yes, I do approve of your decision."

Disapproving

Disapproval implies that the nurse has the right to pass judgment on the patient's thoughts, actions, and ideas. It implies too that the patient is expected to please the nurse.

"That's not a nice thing to say."
"You shouldn't do things like that."
"I'd rather you wouldn't. . . ."

Agreeing

Agreeing indicates that the patient is "right" rather than "wrong." It can deter the patient from forming his own opinions, drawing his own conclusions, or altering his position at a later point without seeing himself in error. It is important to distinguish agreement from consensual validation.

"Yes, indeed, I do agree with you."
"That's right."
"That was the right thing to do."
"You are so right."

Disagreeing

To disagree is to imply that the patient is "wrong" and places the nurse in opposition to the patient. The patient may feel it necessary to defend himself—defending ideas tends to strengthen them. Power struggles can then develop.

"I definitely disagree with you on. . . ."
"I don't believe that."
"That's wrong."

Rejecting

Cuts off therapeutic interaction, since the nurse refuses to consider or shows contempt for the patient's ideas or behavior. The nurse is likely to reject the kinds of behavior or ideas that are personally anxiety provoking.

"Don't talk that way!"
"I don't want to hear about. . . ."
"Let's not discuss. . . ."

(continued)

Chart 5.2 (Cont.)
Nontherapeutic Communication Techniques

TECHNIQUE LABEL AND RATIONALE FOR NONUSE	EXAMPLES

Advising

By telling a patient what he should think or how he ought to behave, the nurse implies she knows what is best for the patient and that he is not capable of any self-direction. Giving advice is different from giving information.

"If I were you I would. . . ."
"I think you should. . . ."
"The best thing for you to do is. . . ."
"Why don't you. . . ."

In general giving approval, disapproving, agreeing, disagreeing, rejecting, and advising imply that the nurse's personal opinion is important or relevant. Generally it is not! In addition such responses are nontherapeutic since they discourage a patient from expressing his own ideas, opinions, feelings, actions. They often result in the patient making reports to please or to avoid the displeasure of those in "authority" (nurse) regardless of how the patient thinks or feels.

Probing

Thoughtless, often irrelevant, prying questions which satisfy the nurses's curiosity rather than promoting the patient's well-being. Such questioning often resembles an interrogation rather than an interaction, tends to put the patient on the defensive, and frequently makes a patient feel that he is valued only for what information he reveals about himself. *Probing belongs in surgery,* not in interactions with patients.

"Why?"
"Why did you quit school when you were doing so well?"
"How old are you?"
"Why don't you ever talk to the other patients?"
"Why are you angry at your son?"
"Why do you feel that way?"

Challenging

Forces a patient to "prove" his point of view. The feelings of the patient go unrecognized. A patient's unrealistic ideas and/or perceptions will not be weakened by challenging comments—indeed they may be strengthened by the patient's efforts to prove his point of view.

"If you're dead, why is your heart beating?"
"How can you say your wife doesn't care when she. . . ."
"But surely you can't believe a doctor would do or prescribe something that would harm you."

Testing

Often done by nurses who believe they must convince the patient that he is "sick" and is need of help. Paradoxically, the nurse demands a patient have insight into his very lack of insight. Having a patient "admit" that he is in need of help meets the need of the nurse only.

"Don't you know what kind of a hospital this is?"
"You must know why you're here. People aren't admitted to a hospital unless they're sick and need help!"
"Do you still have the idea that. . . ?"

In general, the techniques labeled probing, challenging, and testing are hostile responses.

(continued)

Chart 5.2 (Cont.)
Nontherapeutic Communication Techniques

TECHNIQUE LABEL AND RATIONALE FOR NONUSE	EXAMPLES
Defending The nurse attempts to protect the person, place, or thing that the patient has criticized. The nurse implies that the patient has no right to express his negative feelings, opinions, or impressions. A patient's criticism may be unjust or unfounded, but the nurse's offering reasons or excuses does not change the patient's feelings.	"I'm sure Ms. Long had your best interest at heart." "Dr. Lee is a very busy man." "Ms. Adam always answers patients' lights promptly; if she didn't, she had a good reason." "Dr. Bart is one of the very best psychiatrists here." "This is the finest hospital in the city."
Requesting an Explanation Asking the patient to give a reason for his thoughts, feelings, and behavior places the patient in the position of having to justify his actions or verbal comments. Asking *why* is pointless, since the patient often does not know why, if he does know why, he may not wish to share this with you, and finally, knowing why does not mean that behavior or feelings will change. It is not unlike probing.	"Why do you do that?" "Why don't you want to go to the roof?" "Why are you always late for your appointments?" "Why do you ask the same question each time we talk?" "Why do you continue to smoke when you know it's bad for your health?"
Belittling Feelings Expressed Telling the patient that others have the same or bigger difficulties offers no comfort to a person experiencing his own misery. Lack of understanding or empathy is indicated by failure to acknowledge the feelings a patient says he has.	**Patient:** "Oh! I ache all over from ECT." **Nurse:** "You're lucky; Ms. Jay has terrible headaches too." **Patient:** "I wish I were dead, I've nothing to live for." **Nurse:** "How can you say that? You've a fine family."
Making Stereotyped Responses Meaningless clichés and trite expressions have little place in patient interactions. They communicate nothing except possibly a nurse's disinterest.	"It's for your own good." "Just do everything the doctor tells you and you'll be home in no time." "Keep your chin up."
Using Denial In essence the nurse indicates that the patient *should* feel differently. It closes discussion and fails to help the patient identify his difficulties.	**Patient:** "I'm nothing." **Nurse:** "Of course you're something. Everybody is someone." **Patient:** "I'm not getting any better." **Nurse:** "Of course you are."

(continued)

Chart 5.2 (Cont.)
Nontherapeutic Communication Techniques

TECHNIQUE LABEL AND RATIONALE FOR NONUSE	EXAMPLES
Interpreting	
Dangerous ground for anyone not trained as a psychoanalyst. Even this professional interprets rarely and with caution. It has no place in nurse–patient interactions.	"What you really mean is. . . ." "That means that. . . ." "Unconsciously you're saying. . . ."
Introducing an Unrelated Topic	
When the nurse changes the subject, the initiative for and direction of the conversation is taken away from the patient. It is a demonstration of the nurse's anxiety and/or insensitivity.	Patient: "I'm going home next week." Nurse: "How long have you been in the hospital?" Patient: "I hate being in the hospital." Nurse: "Are you expecting visitors today?"
Giving Literal Responses	
When the staff member responds to a figurative comment as though it were a statement of fact, the feelings the patient is trying to convey are ignored.	Patient: "I'm an Easter egg." Nurse: "What color?" Patient: "They're looking in my head with that TV." Nurse: "Change it to another channel."

Adapted with permission of Macmillan Publishing Co., Inc. from Interacting with Patients *by Joyce Samhammer Hays and Kenneth H. Larson. Copyright © Macmillan Publishing Co., Inc., 1963.*

Learning Theories

Many theories about the process have evolved which reflect the different interpretations of teaching–learning. Two major schools of thought exist today: behaviorism (stimulus–response conditioning) and the Gestalt field. Within behaviorism are found the classical and instrumental theories, while an example of Gestalt field is the cognitive field theory.

BEHAVIORISM

Behaviorism bases its learning theory on conditioning through stimulus–response. A stimulus is any factor or agent which produces a response of an observable action or behavior.

Classical Conditioning

In classical conditioning, learning takes place when an established stimulus known to produce a de-sired response is presented along with a new stimulus. The new stimulus is one that the teacher wants the learner to associate with the response. This association process is repeated until the desired response can be elicited without the original stimulus. No reinforcement or reward is provided in this kind of conditioning. An example of this type of stimulus–response conditioning can be seen in the following situation. An individual who cannot sleep is given a sleeping medication (stimulus) by the nurse. The medication produces the desired response, sleep. However, if for several evenings a back rub is given simultaneously with the sleep medication, according to classical conditioning theory, the individual will learn to associate a back rub with sleep, and eventually the original stimulus (sleep medication) will not be necessary to produce the desired sleep response.

Instrumental Conditioning

Instrumental conditioning incorporates a reinforcer or reward into the learning process. When a desired response to a stimulus is elicited, a reward which is meaningful to the learner is given. In behaviorism this reward is the partial or complete meeting of a basic need. The reward increases the probability that the desired response will be repeated. In this sense, the reward now serves as the stimulus for the desired behavior. The reverse situation is also true. If an undesirable behavior occurs, a negative reinforcement (denial of need fulfillment) will result in the decreased presence of the undesired response. An example of instrumental conditioning is the use of praise to reward a child cleaning his room. The praise, according to instrumental conditioning theory, acts as a reinforcer to the desired response (clean room), and the child learns to clean his room in expectation of praise.

Extinction of desired behaviors will occur if the reinforcer is withdrawn for a long period of time. Thus using the above-mentioned example, if praise is not occasionally given when the child's room is cleaned, the child will stop cleaning the room because he no longer expects the praise.

Instrumental behaviorists recognize two types of reinforcers, primary and secondary. Primary reinforcers are those which satisfy a basic physiologic need, while secondary reinforcers are those which satisfy higher-level needs.

Behaviorists view motivation as being produced by providing need satisfaction and not as something inherent within the individual. Thus the teacher, in order to motivate the learner, must identify and use a stimulus which produces the desired response rather than the learner generating his own motivation.

Complex Learning

Complex learning occurs when a series of simple learned behaviors are combined. Each singular behavior incorporates and builds on the previous learning. Operant conditioning, developed by Skinner, is a frequently used variation of this type of complex learning. Alcoholism, drug addiction, and behavioral disorders are often treated with this method.

GESTALT FIELD THEORIES

In contrast to behaviorism, the Gestalt field theories define learning as a problem-solving approach to discover new relationships or modify old ones. It is a conceptual theory of learning in which the learner first identifies patterns or sets of similar

concepts. The learner then recognizes the relationship between these concepts, thus developing insight into the nature of the problem. Finally, conclusions are drawn as to the appropriate response. As a result of learning, the individual may or may not overtly behave any differently, but his or her thought process will have been changed.

Gestalt field theories view learning as a relative process which depends, in part, on the individual's perception of self and the environment at any given point in time. Learning is continuously modified as the individual's situation changes. Basic to these theories is the relevance of the knowledge to the learner to achieve his goals. In this sense, Gestalt field theories are individualistic, since each person determines his own goals. The teacher facilitates learning by suggesting relationships and exploring the possible relevance of the information, but the learner must then evaluate the relevance in terms of his own goals.

An example of learning using Gestalt field theories is the nurse who wishes to teach an individual some aspect of health care. The nurse first looks at the principles of teaching—learning, the characteristics of the learner, and the nature of the subject to be taught. The nurse then determines the relevance of this information to the particular teaching—learning situation and finally determines the method and tools to be used to teach the subject matter. In turn, the learner in this situation will examine the subject matter presented in terms of personal goals and the relevance of this material in meeting those goals and will follow through on the information accordingly.

Successful goal achievement is seen as the major motivation in Gestalt field theories. Thus the teacher facilitates motivation by helping the learner see the relevance of the desired learning to goal achievement. It is the learner, therefore, who provides the motivation, while the teacher can only enhance or diminish it.

NURSING ASSESSMENT

In utilizing the teaching—learning process as an effective change strategy, the nurse needs to assess each learning situation. In this way the nurse can determine which theory or combination of theories will best suit the particular situation. The nurse can then modify the approach utilized, as well as decide on the appropriate motivation system.

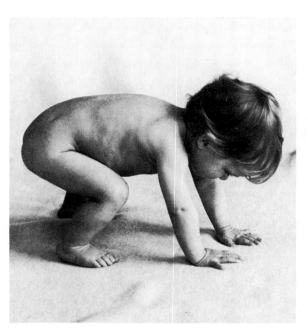 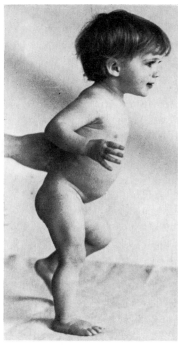 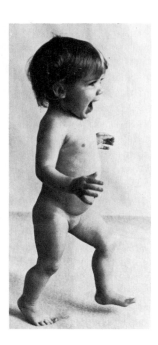

Illustration 5.1
When unique physical, physiological, and psychosocial abilities have developed appropriately within a child, he is ready to learn to walk. *(Photos © Gerry Cranham, from Photo Researchers, Inc.)*

Learner Demography

▶ **Learner demography** consists of the characteristics of the learner which influence the teaching–learning process. The characteristics of the learner determine the learning theories utilized, the method of approach, the setting, tools, and evaluation. Characteristics can be grouped according to level of growth and development, learning experiences, learner skills, and situational factors. Although each factor must be considered separately, the interdependence of factors creates a whole picture of the learner.

GROWTH AND DEVELOPMENT

The individual's level of growth and development plays a major role in guiding the teaching process. Each level has unique skills, capabilities, and characteristics that make methods and tools more or less appropriate for that group. In addition, there are critical periods throughout the life process which

provide the opportune time for learning skills. For example, each child in the late infancy period reaches a time when physical, physiologic, and psychosocial factors coalesce to make the "perfect" time for him or her to talk. If this critical point is missed, acquisition of this skill becomes more difficult. These critical periods are determined by such factors as physical ability, physiologic function, cultural pressure, and individual motivation. These factors may be equated with learner readiness. The type of information, the language used, the setting, and the basic manner of presentation will vary from level to level. (Illustration 5.1)

People in the upper levels usually have a wider scope of experience and knowledge from which to draw as well as more experience with the educational process. Educational experience should not be confused with formal education, since much of an individual's learning takes place outside the classroom. Frequently there is a correlation between age and level of growth and development; however, identifying the individual's age does not provide sufficient information about developmental skills and abilities.

Former Experience

As the individual develops, certain attitudes, values, and feelings toward the acquisition of knowledge are formulated. Previous learning experiences influence the individual's feelings about what information is important to be learned, how it should be learned, and the individual's role in the learning process. The individual's general level of knowledge is directly related to the type of educational experiences and the success with them that the individual has had. Based on these previous experiences, the individual may be able to identify what his or her learning needs are and the methods by which he or she best learns.

The nurse attempts to identify whether it is first-time learning or whether it is a relearning. First-time learning is often thought to be more easily accomplished, since it does not require the unlearning of previous patterns of behavior.

Motivation

The individual's present motivation is determined not only by attitudes, values about learning, and previous learning experiences, but also by the relevance of the information to be learned. Relevance is the importance of a subject to the individual and is affected by the person's level of growth and development and by his or her perception of personal needs and goals. If an individual sees little personal value in learning specific information, learning motivation will be low. Since individuals' perceptions of needs and goals differ, what is relevant to one person will not necessarily be relevant to someone else. Because the nurse-teacher views health information as relevant to the individual's well-being, he or she often assumes that the individual does also, without first identifying what the learner thinks is important.

Knowledge Base

Once previous learning experiences and the relevance of information have been identified, the nurse can then ascertain the individual's specific level of knowledge concerning the subject matter to be taught. This knowledge base serves as a foundation for future learning. Repetition of previously learned information or presentation of information which is too advanced decreases the individual's motivation and hinders the learning process.

The learner's cognitive, psychomotor, and communication skills greatly influence the learning process.

Cognitive Skills

Cognitive skills include the person's basic learning ability, attention span, ability to organize data, problem-solving skills, and powers of abstraction. These all work together to help the individual receive, interpret, analyze, and utilize the information which is being presented. All people are capable of learning, but the degree to which this learning occurs will vary from individual to individual. Therefore, accurate identification of the individual learner's cognitive capabilities increases the probability that learning will occur.

Psychomotor Skills

The individual's ability to translate learning into observable and purposeful behaviors is dependent on the learner's psychomotor skills. Identification of those capabilities and limitations aids the nurse and the learner to have realistic expectations of the outcome of the learning experience. The teaching–learning process with individuals who have limited psychomotor capabilities often requires creativity and imagination on the part of both the nurse and the individual to discover alternatives to traditional methods of acquiring and performing a skill. Failure to consider the psychomotor capabilities of the learner only serves to frustrate the efforts of both the individual and the nurse.

Ability to Use Language

Since the process of giving and receiving communication is an integral part of teaching–learning, the individual's skills in the use of language (both written and oral); ability to receive feedback; and ability to put thoughts, ideas, and feelings into meaningful language are important characteristics to consider. If there is no basis of communication, no part of the teaching–learning process can take place. Nonverbal communication is just as significant as verbal communication, since emotions, perceptions, and attitudes are often transmitted this way. Barriers and facilitators to communication must be recognized so that interference can be reduced and enhancers increased.

SITUATIONAL FACTORS

All of these learner skills are considered in relationship to the individual's level of growth and development, as well as certain situational factors. Culture, family and/or significant others, support systems, state of health, and availability of time and money are some major situational factors.

Culture

Cultural attitudes about what is appropriate to learn, who should teach, and who should learn, along with cultural mores and language use, can significantly alter the teaching–learning interaction and thus must be included in any consideration of learner characteristics.

Family and/or Significant Others

The family and/or significant others system can either facilitate or hinder the learner's participation in the process. The family and/or significant others may give support, reinforcement, and encouragement to the individual, as well as actively participate in the learning process. Or they may deter the learner's progress by ridicule, lack of interest, or absence from the process.

State of Health

The individual's state of health affects his or her cognitive skills, levels of energy, level of anxiety, psychomotor abilities, the relevance of information, and health care teaching needs. Individuals who are acutely ill rarely have the energy to focus on health learning. Distortions of body image (Chapter 22) as well as the grieving process (Chapter 25) are other aspects to be considered.

Time and Resources

The amount of time the individual has to invest in the process, the availability of money to spend on learning aids and equipment, and the existence of other resources complete the list of factors to be considered in learner demography. Realistic time schedules should be based on the time that is available and time requirements for the individual's learning process. When either too little or too much time is allotted, teacher and learner frustration occurs, and the effectiveness of the process is diminshed. While an abundance of materials exists for learning and carrying out of skills, all too often they are not evaluated in terms of teaching effectiveness and cost. While much of the equipment may make teaching and learning easier, in the long run the usefulness is outweighed by the cost. Again, ingenuity and creativity may produce equally beneficial tools and equipment. Often, when time, money, and expertise are not available, knowledge of community and personal resources available to the individual may be of great value.

Teacher Characteristics

A wide variety of teaching styles and approaches can be effective in facilitating the learning process. Each nurse develops a style with which he or she is most comfortable and effective. This requires time, practice, and evaluation to determine which behaviors facilitate the learning process and which hinder it. However, certain behaviors have been identified as enhancing learning.

KNOWLEDGEABILITY

Knowledge of the subject matter is one prerequisite for effective teaching. The nurse must have an understanding of the theories, principles, and skills related to the information to be taught. Since complete knowledge in all subjects is not possible for one person, the nurse may find that he or she is not the person with the most expertise in a particular area. Researching the information prior to undertaking the teaching and referring the individual to others with more knowledge are ways that the nurse can supplement the individual's learning.

CREATING COMFORTABILITY

The ability to create a give-and-take atmosphere where the learner does not feel intimidated or ridiculed is another important teacher asset. The climate that is set for the individual should be one in which questions can be asked and gaps in information and understanding acknowledged. The nurse helps to create a comfortable environment by using language understandable to the individual, setting aside enough time for the interaction, being sincerely interested in the individual and his or her learning needs, being open to suggestions, and collaborating with the individual throughout the plan. The nurse-teacher needs an understanding of therapeutic communication skills in order to ask questions in a nonthreatening manner, use therapeutic silence, and recognize when there are blocks to the communication process. (Illustration 5.2)

RECOGNIZING PLANNING NEEDS

The nurse needs to plan and organize the teaching–learning interaction so that goals can be accomplished in the least amount of time and with

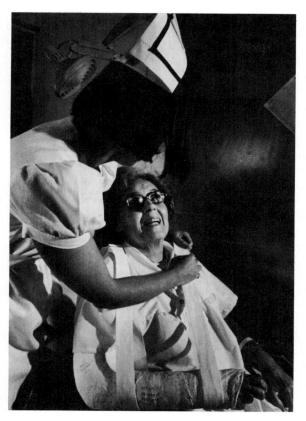

Illustration 5.2
To teach an individual about changes in her physical abilities and physiological functioning, the nurse creates a climate that encourages the individual to ask questions without feeling intimidated and with confidence that the nurse understands the condition. *(Photo by Ellis Herwig, from Stock, Boston)*

the least amount of effort for both the teacher and the learner. Planning also ensures that important subject matter is not omitted and that a logical sequence of presentation occurs. Planning and organization do not imply that every word is written down or that there is little flexibility in the carrying out of the plan. However, planning does allow the nurse to use opportunities for teaching when they arise. Whatever teaching is carried out utilizes the learner characteristics to personalize and individualize the process.

Goal Setting

Once the characteristics of the learner and his or her perception of personal learning needs in relation to the health care situation have been identified, the learner and the nurse collaborate, setting teaching–learning goals or objectives. Frequently, the individual's family and/or significant others are directly involved in the teaching–learning process. They may require information about the individual's health care needs and may also need to learn the same skills as the individual. Thus family and/or significant others may be included in the goal-setting process. Teaching–learning objectives include what measurable behavioral change will take place, the time frame in which it will occur, and the method by which it will be evaluated. Goals or objectives often represent a compromise between what the nurse and the individual each sees as necessary goals. They reflect the realistic abilities of both the nurse-teacher and the learner, as well as the time and setting limitations. Like other care goals devised with the individual, teacher–learner goals are first written as more general long-term goals, stating the learning that is to take place, and then as shorter-term goals enumerating the more specific steps in reaching the long-term goals.

When considering the time frame in which the goal can be achieved, time should be allowed for introduction of new information, assimilation of that information by the learner, and feedback and clarification. In the case of psychomotor skills, assimilation and feedback time allows for manual manipulation and practice of the skill. The time frame for goal achievement may range anywhere from a few minutes to several months, depending on the type of information being learned, the desired behavioral outcomes, and the learner characteristics. Evaluation is stated in the goal to provide a mutually agreed on means of determining the effectiveness of the teaching–learning process and to avoid haphazard or no evaluation at the end of the process. If consistent evaluation does not occur, it cannot be determined whether or not learning has actually taken place or where difficulties have arisen. (Chapter 9 has a further discussion of goal setting.)

An example of teacher–learner long- and short-term goals might look as follows:

- **Long-term goal:** Individual washes hands using aseptic technique before instilling eye drops within 2 weeks as shown by demonstrating technique three consecutive times.
- **Short-term goal:** Identifies scientific rationale for use of aseptic technique in handwashing before instilling eye drops within 4 days as evidenced by listing these principles when asked. Performs

handwashing using aseptic technique within 1 week as evidenced by three consecutive return demonstrations.

These goals would be integrated into a teaching–learning plan which includes the technique for instilling eye drops and any other identified learning needs related to the specific health care situation.

Methods and Tools

During the goal-setting process, the method by which the specific teaching–learning process will occur and the tools which will be used are established. A wide variety of methods are available, and the choice is based on the learner characteristics, the number of persons to be taught at one time, the information to be taught, the resources available, and an understanding of learning theory. Chart 5.3 outlines commonly used methods and their advantages and disadvantages. Often the best method and tools are those which combine the advantages of several modalities.

Settings

Although learning can take place in almost any setting, certain conditions make a location more conducive to the learning process. Environmental factors such as appropriate temperature, humidity, and ventilation provide a setting that is less distracting and more comfortable for the participants. Adequate nonglare lighting and comfortable seats and seating arrangements also promote a positive learning environment. The location chosen should be as free as possible from such distractions as interruptions from other people, ongoing procedures, and noise. Privacy allows both the teacher and the learner to speak more freely and possibly be more willing to take chances or to try out newly acquired skills.

All equipment and tools that will be needed for any teaching done should be assembled in advance and tested to make sure they are in working order. Tools and equipment used should be similar to those which the individual uses in the everyday situation. The setting is checked for availability of such things are electrical outlets, running water, and bathroom facilities. Settings outside the individual's room are evaluated for accessibility, particularly if the individual has difficulty in or uses special equipment for ambulation.

Evaluaton of Learning

Learning can be evaluated through use of many techniques. The technique chosen is carefully matched with the type of information being learned. For example, if the behavioral outcome of the learning experience is to be a psychomotor skill, such as installation of eye drops, the evaluation must include a demonstration by the learner of the ability to do so. Techniques which can be used for evaluation include pencil-and-paper tests, verbal identification of subject matter, role-playing demonstrations, return demonstrations, and integration of learned behavior into activities of daily living.

Good record keeping and communication with other members of the health team can provide for periodic reevaluation and reinforcement of learning. Since much information that is initially learned is forgotten with the passage of time unless reinforced, provision for follow-up is a necessary part of the teaching–learning process. Through written records and discharge plans, the nurse can alert other persons who will be following through on the individual's care to evaluate the learning that has been retained and to reinforce or supplement learning.

EVALUATING TEACHING

The nurse also needs to evaluate his or her effectiveness as a teacher. The nurse can do so by identifying the behavioral changes which have occurred in the individual and by ascertaining what changes could be made to facilitate the process. Peer evaluation and validation serve as a useful method for improving teaching techniques. The nurse may not always be able to recognize his or her own strengths and weaknesses, and a person not immediately involved in the situation may be able to do so. The individual also has input into the evaluation process. The individual can identify the degree to which and the process by which needs were met. Chart 5.4 summarizes some beliefs about learning.

GROUP PROCESS

Many times the nurse wants to bring about a change in more than one individual at a time or the nurse may be part of a group which is bringing about

Chart 5.3

Selected Teaching Methods

METHOD	ADVANTAGES	DISADVANTAGES
Lecture	Can be used to relay information to large numbers of people in least amount of time. Good for introduction to subject matter or general survey of subject.	Does not allow for individual participation or feedback. Cannot be used to teach specific psychomotor skills. Difficult to direct lecture to all levels of participants' abilities.
Lecture–discussion	Combines advantages of lecture with some participant feedback. Helps in clarification of information. Can be used with relatively large groups of people.	Cannot be used for psychomotor skills. Discussion must be limited according to group size and material to be presented within a given time. Level of participation is generally superficial and does not provide opportunity for individualization.
Discussion	Allows for participation of group members in subject matter. Helps in clarification of information and feelings and allows for a variety of input and sharing of information. Participants can be grouped according to learned characteristics.	Requires previous knowledge on subject. Cannot be used for large numbers of people. Requires organizational structure.
Panel	Presentation of wide variety of ideas by expert in subject matter. Useful in exploring controversial issues in which there are two or more positions on the issue. Can be used with large numbers of people.	Not useful in teaching psychomotor skills. Does not allow for individual participation from audience. Is not directed at all levels of partipant abilities.
Panel–discussion	Incorporates advantages of panel with advantages of discussion.	Same as for discussion and panel.
Role playing	Allows for expression of feelings, attitudes. Helps in identifying role behaviors. Can give opportunity for exploring empathetic behavior. Can assist individuals to acquire degree of comfort in difficult situations. Requires active participation.	Not effective with large groups. Can be time consuming. May not be suited for personalities of all types of learners.

(continued)

Chart 5.3 (cont.)
Selected Teaching Methods

METHOD	ADVANTAGES	DISADVANTAGES
Play therapy	A combination of role playing and demonstration–return demonstration. Allows for expression of attitudes, feelings, values. Allows for manipulation of equipment. Can be used to teach psychomotor skills. Effective teaching method for children. Can be individualized for level of growth and development. Useful for small groups or individuals.	Requires close supervision.
Demonstration	Allows relatively large group to observe use of equipment and procedure for carrying out activity. Useful when limited amount of equipment is available for use by individual. Often used in combination with lecture.	Does not allow for individual manipulation of equipment. Practice of psychomotor skills requires previous knowledge.
Demonstration– return demonstration	Incorporates advantages of demonstration with opportunity for individual manipulation of equipment and practice of skill. Many persons learn best by actually doing the skill.	Requires sufficient equipment for each individual and close supervision. Requires previous knowledge.
Multimedia	Takes advantage of wide variety of resources, such as programmed instruction, films, tapes, computer learning. Individual can proceed at own pace. Visual aids can be used with persons who cannot read. Can be used with large numbers at the same time. Teacher presence not required.	Requires equipment for use. Participant must be self-motivated. Unless prepared by teacher, may not cover desired subject matter completely or in customary manner. Does not allow for specific teacher–learner interaction.
Conversation	Excellent vehicle for ongoing teaching and reinforcement at individual's level of ability. May not be as threatening as formal teaching situation. Allows for introduction of sensitive subject matter. Teaching can be carried out concurrently with other care.	Cannot always be preplanned. May be carried out in setting where equipment is not available for follow-through.

Chart 5.4
Beliefs about Learning

New learning is based on previous learning.

Effective learning requires adequate identification of learner characteristics.

Learning is individual.

Learning requires practice and reinforcement of of the new skill.

Feedback is a necessary component of the learning process.

Motivation is a necessary component of learning.

All persons are capable of learning.

An ideal time exists for learning to take place.

change. Therefore, a knowledge of groups and the process by which they function is a valuable change strategy.

▶ A **group** is defined as a set of people having shared needs or goals. Groups exist to help individuals attain goals which would be unattainable otherwise. They provide a means for pooling such resources as ideas, expertise, and manpower to solve problems and satisfy needs. Dissemination of information can be achieved more rapidly to groups than to individuals when similar information has to be shared.

Groups can be effective change agents since the group often takes greater risks than individuals do. This occurs because responsibility is shared, and thus the consequences of risk taking are also shared. Group members provide support to each other in taking on these risks. However, when a group has a high sense of solidarity, it is more resistive to change initiated from within. Therefore, change, leadership, and communication skills are necessary for the nurse working with groups.

The nurse works with a wide variety of groups. They may range from a dyad (a two-person group), e.g., nurse–nurse, individual–nurse, and nurse–doctor, to a large, diverse population, e.g., community or professional organization. Within each of these groups the nurse may fulfill such different roles as member, advisor, leader, teacher, or learner.

Groups are systems with certain properties which are described in Chart 5.5. A change in one part, or property, of the system will result in a change in the rest of the system. By recognizing the relationships between these properties the nurse can work toward increasing or decreasing the properties in order to promote group effectiveness and satisfaction.

Types of Groups

Two major types of groups have been identified, primary and secondary. They may be examined in terms of structure and method of membership. The degree of contact the individual has with the group and the amount of influence the group has over each participant determines whether a group is primary or secondary.

▶ A **primary group** is a group whose members communicate with each other over a period of time in face-to-face interactions and have a high degree of influence over the behavior of individuals within the group. Families, work groups, and friendship cliques are examples of this type of group. Primary groups are characterized as having a high degree of cohesiveness, control, dependence, potency, stability, historicity, and viscosity. Norms are shared and the members become assimilated to a large extent. Permeability is low because of the strong sense of "oneness" that arises from the other group characteristics, thus making it difficult for outsiders to gain membership. Factors such as autonomy, flexibility, homogeneity, and hedonic tone depend on the structure, composition, and goals of a particular group. The nurse in providing care and in meeting the health needs of individuals works mainly with primary groups.

▶ A **secondary group** is a looser affiliation of people which may be short term, task oriented, or impersonal. "Task forces," ad hoc committes, and suprastructures are examples of secondary groups. Secondary groups generally have lower cohesiveness, dependence, potency, stability, historicity, and viscosity than primary groups. The degree of assimilation of the group is determined by the degree of shared norms, participation, and homogeneity. This, in turn, determines the degree of permeability, control, autonomy, and flexibility present within the group. Like primary groups, the structure, composition, and goals of each particular secondary group influences, to a large extent, its overall characteristics. The nurse deals with secondary groups within the context of the organization of the health care system and the profession.

Chart 5.5
Group Characteristics

CHARACTERISTIC	DEFINITION	CHARACTERISTIC	DEFINITION
Assimilation	The process of blending characteristics, values, attitudes, and beliefs among group members	Mores	The cherished values of groups
Autonomy	The amount of independence the group has from other groups	Norms	Expected, appropriate behavior of the group in accordance with its mores
Cohesiveness	The degree of solidarity or unity within the group; the attractiveness of the group to its members; a sense of "we-ness"	Participation	The amount of input into decision making and goal setting within the group
		Permeability	The degree of access to membership in the group by outsiders
Control	The amount of influence the group has over its members	Polarization	The movement toward a common goal by group members
Dependence	The reliance members have on the group for meeting their needs	Position	The status or rank the member has within the group
		Potency	The amount of importance the group has for its members
Flexibility	The degree of structure of the group	Role	The function one has within a group
Hedonic tone	The general feeling of pleasantness or unpleasantness of group membership	Size	The number of members within a group; ranges from two to infinity
Historicity	The sense of meaningful past or continuity felt by the group	Stability	The degree of permanence of the group
Homogeneity	The degree of likeness or similarity of characteristics, values, attitudes, and beliefs of group members	Viscosity	The degree to which a group functions as a single unit

FORMAL AND INFORMAL STRUCTURES

The structural system by which the group operates designates it as either formal or informal. **Informal groups** have much spontaneous interpersonal behavior with few written rules and regulations. However, there are usually a strong code of ethics and a set of unwritten laws. The informal group does not depend on structure for its existence, but on interpersonal interactions. This type of structure is characteristic of the primary group.

In contrast, the **formal group** has stated rules and regulations which result in imposed norms. These groups usually exist to carry out a task or goal rather than to meet the needs of the group members. Interpersonal interactions among the group as a whole may be limited; however, informal subgroups may form.

METHODS OF ATTAINING MEMBERSHIP

The method of gaining membership into the group can be either ascribed or assigned. **Ascribed groups** are groups whose members have voluntarily chosen to be members. The degree of choice involved varies from joining because of interest, e.g., camera club, to joining because of a need imposed by circumstances, e.g., a union. Ascribed groups may be primary, secondary, formal, or informal. The influence an ascribed group has depends on the other properties present in the group, such as hedonic tone, shared norms, control, or flexibility.

Assigned groups are those into which the members are born or involuntarily drafted. Sex, race, age, religion, the armed forces, and prison are examples of assigned groups. These groups have almost no permability, whereas the ascribed group has some degree of permeability. Regardless of the influence the assigned group has over the individual, no choice about membership in the group exists.

Group Dynamics

The nurse, in order to facilitate primary group interactions and to bring about change, studies the dynamics of the group. **Group dynamics** are the constantly changing interaction patterns, movements, and processes present within the group. Analysis of the group's properties, the roles the members play, the status or position of persons within the group, the degree of conformity to group mores, the goals, and the methods the group uses to reach goals are all important factors in assessing group dynamics. Some factors that the nurse looks at in analyzing group dynamics follow:[1]

- What are the rules this group operates by?
- Are group task and maintenance functions being served?
- What causes confusion in this group?
- What prevents/aids reaching group goals?
- What leads to conflict in this group?
- How are conflicts resolved in this group?
- What is the leadership pattern? Is leadership shared?
- What is the communication pattern in this group?
- What enhances/cuts off communication?
- How sensitive is one group member to another's needs?
- How does the group react to a new member?
- How does a new member react to the group?
- How are group decisions made?
- How does the group get its members to conform?
- When do silences occur? What kind of silences are they?
- What themes emerge in the group?
- Who relieves tension? Why?
- Who in the group:
    clarifies
    validates
    summarizes/evaluates
    restates
    gives/gets information
    expresses group feeling
    monopolizes
    encourages
    elaborates
    initiates
    gives opinions
    blocks
    mediates, etc.
- What phase of development is the group in?
- Are goals mutually shared?
- What is the level of group satisfaction?
- Does the group evaluate itself in terms of goal setting and process?

ASCERTAINING BEHAVIORS

Within each group there are certain interaction patterns which can either facilitate or inhibit the ability of the group to move toward achievement of goals, group satisfaction, cohesiveness, and stability. These interaction patterns can be seen in terms of the behavior exhibited by the group and the roles they assume. Figure 5.9 illustrates types of behaviors manifested by group members. If the behavior exhibited by group members helps the group to move ahead with its goals or is related to the activities needed for goal achievement, the behavior is often termed *task functions* of the group. Behaviors such as initiating, clarifying, or elaborating are included here. However, if the behaviors exhibited are designed to maintain the continuity, cohesion, and stability of the group, they are termed *maintenance and building functions* of the group. Included here are such behaviors as accepting, mediating, encouraging, and relieving tension. Those behaviors which do not enhance group solidarity or effectiveness but are aimed at the personal gratification of individual participants are called *individual functions* of the group. Such behaviors as disagreement, attention getting, withdrawal, and aggression are individual function behaviors.

The Sociogram

One method of ascertaining these roles, as well as overall interaction patterns of the group, is the sociogram. A sociogram is a diagram of the interactions of group members. The individuals in the group are represented by symbols, and arrows are drawn showing who is speaking to whom and the nature of the interaction, e.g., positive, negative, or neutral. Figure 5.10 illustrates a form of this technique. Using interaction analysis, the nurse can objectively observe and analyze the dynamics within a group and identify areas of strength and weakness.

PHASES OF GROUP DEVELOPMENT

The type of interaction pattern and the roles assumed by group members may vary according to the stage of development of the group. When groups first form, there is an *initiation phase* during which members attempt to become familiar with others, gain acceptance by other members of the group, determine

Figure 5.9

Group member behaviors. *(From Robert F. Bales,* Interaction Process Analysis. *University of Chicago Press, Chicago, Illinois, 1974. Copyright © Robert F. Bales)*

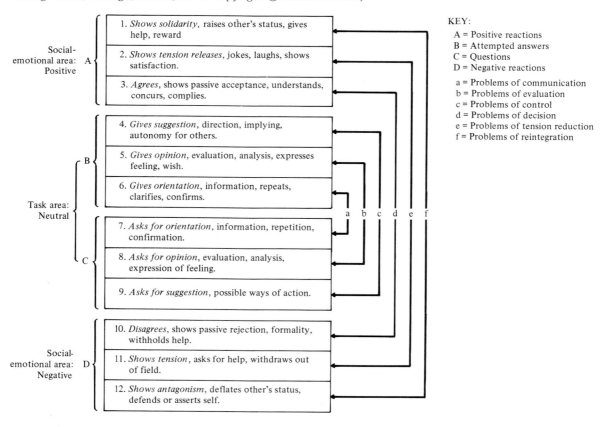

KEY:

A = Positive reactions
B = Attempted answers
C = Questions
D = Negative reactions

a = Problems of communication
b = Problems of evaluation
c = Problems of control
d = Problems of decision
e = Problems of tension reduction
f = Problems of reintegration

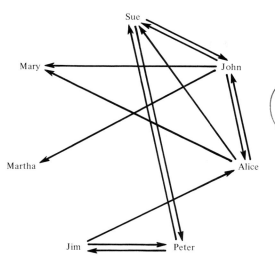

Figure 5.10

Example of an interaction sociogram (direction of arrow indicates the direction of flow of verbal communication)

the relevance of the group to their needs, and establish a format for proceeding and a position within the group. Testing behaviors, group task behaviors, and individual behaviors predominate at this stage.

Once group members become relatively comfortable with each other the group enters its *functional phase*. Here group goals are established, and movement toward their accomplishment takes place. Assimilation of group members occurs in this stage, and cohesiveness, conformity, stability, viscosity, and similar properties increase. Maintenance and building functions, as well as the task functions of the group, are in evidence at this stage, while individual behavior roles are less obvious.

The *dissolution phase* occurs when group goals have been accomplished, the members no longer see a need for the group, or group cohesiveness and assimilation have not been established. In a task-oriented group, this phase is anticipated and preplanned. The degree of relief or anxiety felt at the dissolution will depend on the meaning the group had for its members, the hedonic tone of the group, and the degree of assimilation.

Nursing Assessment

The nurse looks to see what stage the group is in to determine how to best help group members to satisfactorily move through these stages. By identifying problem areas, factors which are hindering or helping movement, positive and negative interaction patterns, and the degree of group properties, the

nurse can assist the group to achieve its goals with maximum satisfaction.

LEADERSHIP

▶ **Leadership** is the facilitation of change through creative direction, motivation, and guidance of others toward achieving mutually accepted goals. Effective leadership is necessary, since change requires the organized participation and cooperation of all persons involved in the process.

The nurse uses leadership in a variety of interactional situations. When working with individuals in the care situation, the nurse utilizes leadership skills to promote achievement of mutually accepted goals between the individual and the nurse. At the same time the nurse uses these skills with the individual's family and/or significant others, the nursing team, and the health care team to help provide an integrated, safe system of care. In addition, the nurse utilizes leadership skills within the health care system, the profession, and the society to improve health care and to advance the nursing profession.

Leadership is a dynamic interaction between the leader and those with whom the leader is working. According to Yura, Ozimek, and Walsh,[2] effective leadership is a combination of decision making, relating, influencing, and facilitating. (Illustration 5.3)

Decision making involves the ability to assess the situation and to determine probable and possible methods for changing the situation and the approaches for implementing the chosen method. Knowledge, experience, and a sensitivity to the dynamics of a system are all prerequisites to the decision-making process.

Relating is the ongoing use of effective communication skills to bring about the desired change with minimal dissension and dissatisfaction. This requires an understanding of the communication process, the facilitators and barriers to communication, principles of motivation, and the interaction behaviors of people involved in change.

Influencing other people through the selective use of power is another important factor in the leadership process. Without an ability to utilize power, the desired change will be limited in scope and duration.

Facilitating is the use of actions which help bring about a change in the most efficient and effective

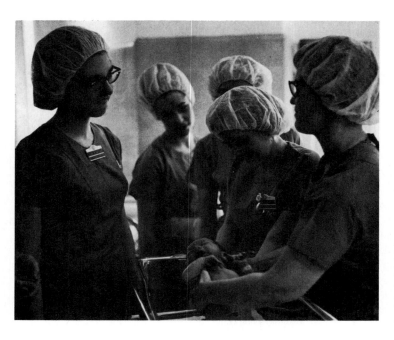

Illustration 5.3
Leadership skills are utilized within the nursing profession itself to improve health care. Here, a teacher of nursing creatively brings about change by facilitating the participation of students in the learning process. *(Photo by Roger Malloch, © Magnum Photos, Inc.)*

manner. Facilitation occurs through use of interpersonal skills, knowledge, experience, and leadership and change principles.

Leadership Styles

Three general leadership styles have been identified: autocratic, democratic (supportive), and laissez faire.

AUTOCRATIC LEADERSHIP

A leadership style that is autocratic is one in which the leader makes decisions for the group with little or no consultation with the group. Underlying this style is the basic assumption that the group is incapable of making its own decisions and needs to be externally controlled to work satisfactorily. Decisions made by the leader are not subject to question by the group and are usually nonnegotiable. In addition, the implementation process is usually closely supervised by the leader or a few carefully chosen representatives. The power of this type of leader usually lies in a recognized reward and punishment system. This system is derived from a knowledge of what motivates the group.

While autocratic leadership has negative connotations (e.g., dictatorship) and frequently results in group dissatisfaction, it can be very effective when decisions must be made rapidly, when situations are disorganized or chaotic, and when members of the group do not want to participate in the decision-making process.

Autocratic leadership ceases to be effective when the reward and punishment system is not strong enough to control the behavior of the group. When the group gains enough power to override the leader's decisions or the group wishes to become involved in the decision-making process or collaborative knowledge of the group is necessary to bring about the desired change, the autocratic style may become inefficient and nonfunctional.

DEMOCRATIC LEADERSHIP

Democratic or supportive leadership involves a recognition of the ability of the group to make decisions and implement change. The basic premise with this style is that the group is capable of making meaningful decisions and is internally motivated to carry out the change. The leader utilizing this style consults with the group and considers the impact of the change before making decisions. Responsibility is delegated at all levels of participation, and it is assumed that all members are interested in meeting the group's goals; thus they do not need to be constantly "watched over."

Many studies have shown that the democratic

method increases the productivity and satisfaction of the group. This is true only if the group values independence and rejects authoritarianism. Thus while democratic leadership style is generally viewed as the most effective method of leadership and has positive connotations (e.g., facilitatory guides), it requires time for consultation with the group and a willingness on the part of the group and the leader to collaborate on decisions and mutually shared goals.

The reward and punishment system within the democratic style of leadership is based on the belief that group members are self-motivated to reach common goals. Thus the rewards are the satisfactory meeting of goals. However, this does not negate the use of other types of reward systems.

LAISSEZ FAIRE LEADERSHIP

The third leadership style is that of laissez faire. With this style the leader is nondirective and participates only when requested. The belief that underlies this method is that the group seeks out its own level of participation and direction and will be self-regulating.

Laissez faire leadership is effective with groups in which the individuals have separate and distinct areas of expertise, responsibilities, and tasks. The leader functions as a consultant and resource person to the group members. This type of leadership style is reinforced by the group members' need for autonomy. The leadership position is maintained as long as the group recognizes the leader's expertise. However, when group decisions have to be made, this style of leadership becomes inefficient.

A BLEND OF STYLES

These three styles of leadership are not often seen in a pure form, but rather in a selective combination depending on the situation and the personalities and needs of the leader and the group. Perhaps the ideal leadership style is one in which the leader can blend the styles according to the circumstance. Thus when emergency decisions must be made rapidly, the leader takes the responsibility for doing so; when time is available and the situation is appropriate, the leader collaborates with group members to make decisions; and when the situation requires autonomous functioning, the leader steps back to give group members the opportunity to function independently.

The appropriateness of any one leadership style is determined by the setting, group composition, types of situations encountered, and interaction patterns of the group. Changes in any or all of these factors will require a reassessment of the style being used and its effectiveness.

Therefore, effective leaders are able to accurately assess the effects of their behavior on others, the effects of the behavior of others on themselves, the interactions of the system in which they are working, and the needs and goals of the group members, and leaders are sensitive to the forces which are acting for and against change. The leader must then be able to utilize this assessment and flexibly modify his or her behavior according to these perceptions. The effective leader plans and organizes the activities of the group. This helps to facilitate meeting group goals by preventing a breakdown in communication, duplication of effort, and confusion, and it provides predictability for the group.

Stimulating Motivation

Motivation is an essential ingredient of successful leadership. Motivation is the desire to carry out some activity or behavior pattern. While the leader cannot provide motivation, the leader can provide an environment which stimulates it. The leader, therefore, identifies those factors which motivate (motivators) the individual or group.

NEED FULFILLMENT

Maslow's hierarchy of needs (Chapter 3) provides a useful framework for creating an environment which stimulates motivation. Maslow states that a need or the desire to continue meeting a need serves as a motivator. These needs may occur at any level of the hierarchy.

Generally, when physiologic needs are not met, the fulfillment of these needs becomes the prime motivator. In the care situation, the individual may have an interference in the meeting of such basic physiologic needs as oxygen, circulation, sexuality, or movement. Therefore, meeting these needs will be the primary motivator for all their behavior. On the other hand, these same physiologic needs can be effective motivators for care givers when individuals are denied fulfillment of such basic needs as sleep, rest, and food, or when continuing fulfillment of these needs is threatened, as with loss of income to buy food.

When the physiologic needs are met, the next level of needs—safety and security—takes on priority. At this point, factors such as basic physiologic and psychologic safety, predictability, familiarity, and protection of perceived personal welfare become prime motivators.

The next level of the hierarchy, the need for love and affection, can be interpreted on two levels: one as the need for an intimate relationship with another person or persons and the other as the need for belonging to a group. A threat to fulfilling these social needs, such as fear of ostracism from the peer group, is the inducement for action at this point.

The ego-sustaining needs of esteem—i.e., privacy, approval, respect, and positive reinforcement from the environment—are the primary motivators at the next level in the hierarchy. A deficiency in any of these areas will produce feelings of inferiority or helplessness with compensatory responses such as discouragement, hostility, or depression.

The final group of motivators within Maslow's model are those related to satisfaction. Interferences with becoming what one feels oneself best suited for or with fulfilling life goals fit within this category.

By identifying the level of the individual's or group's needs and recognizing the specific factors that are acting as motivators, the nurse can plan effective motivation techniques. The specific techniques will vary according to the setting, situation, and ability to meet these needs through other sources. This approach to motivation can be as readily used with the individual with whom the nurse is working as with members of the health care team. It should be recognized, however, that a fully satisfied need no longer acts as a motivator unless there is a threat to its continued fulfillment.

A CONDUCIVE ENVIRONMENT

In addition to identifying motivators at different levels of the need hierarchy, Maslow identified environmental preconditions to motivation. An environment can be created which enhances motivation at levels in the hierarchy. This milieu is one in which the person feels that he is free to voice his opinion, perform within his abilities, seek out new information and learning, and defend himself against threats to his ego. Motivation is further facilitated when the environment further provides a feeling of justice, honesty, and organization.

TASK AND RELATIONSHIP ORIENTATIONS

Other assessment factors the nurse utilizes to motivate people are *task orientation* and *relationship orientation*. If a person feels his abilities and talents can be best utilized in carrying out activities, he will be most readily motivated when the goals are task oriented. On the other hand, if he perceives his strengths to be best suited in forming interpersonal relationships, the person will be primarily motivated in relationship-oriented situations. Thus once the nurse assesses the orientation of the person, the situation can be presented in an appropriate manner. Again, it should be recognized that these factors are as applicable to the care situation as to the work, professional, or societal situation.

Leadership Evaluation

The nurse can evaluate the effectiveness of his or her leadership skills by examining such factors as the satisfaction of all participants in the change process, the degree of desired change, the efficiency of goal achievements, and, in a work situation, the turnover of personnel. Examining these factors provides for the scrutiny of all the basic components of leadership.

POWER

Power is the influence one has over others within a reward system to bring about a change. It is not necessarily a negative concept denoting domination, control, or coercion of others.

Actual and Designated Power

Two basic types of power exist: actual and designated. **Actual power** is the visible influence one realistically has over others. **Designated power** is the supposed power given to a person by a recognized authority source such as society or an administrative body. Designated power may also be actual power, although this is not frequently the case.

In order to effectuate change, it is necessary for the nurse to possess power and also to recognize

---

Chart 5.6
Sources of Power

SOURCE	EXAMPLE	SOURCE	EXAMPLE
Corporeal Ability to threaten life or well-being	Imprisonment, beating, execution, degradation, threatening	Associative Person related or affiliated by friendship, blood, or bureaucracy to actual power source	"Right-hand man," a vice president, president's wife, friend, any type of power source, advocate
Reward and Punishment Ability to provide or withhold a desired motivation	Salary, promotion, discharge, getting well, visitors, "special privileges," ego reinforcers, praise, friendship, food, vacation	Charismatic Possession of power through personal attributes	Any idol, role model, an emulated person
Authoritative or Expert Possession of needed information or skills	Clinical specialist, teacher, surgeon, anyone who can do something the best	Divine Possession of power by designation of a religious or of cultural sanction	Kings, priests, rabbis, ministers, medicine men, geniuses
		Representative Attainment of power through election by a group. The group voluntarily gives powers to the individual for a span of time and group can take it away.	Class president, committee chairperson, team leader

power structures within the working situation. When assessing actual power, the nurse should not assume that it lies with the designated or appointed leader, but look to see to whom people turn for advice and guidance, who determines the overall mood of the group, and who sets the day-to-day routine within the setting. The person who influences these factors will most likely be the person with the actual power. Change will occur more rapidly and efficiently and be more permanent if the individuals who are seeking to bring about change consult and recruit as an active participant the person with actual power. Otherwise, the person with the actual power may very effectively sabotage the person with designated power.

Sources of Power

Power can come from a variety of sources. Chart 5.6 lists power sources and some examples. The technique used to acquire power will be dependent upon the personalities of the leader and the group, the setting, the situation, and the needs of the individuals involved.

Enhancing Power

Certain strategies can enhance the leader's use of power.

ANALYSIS OF THE SYSTEM

Analysis of the system the person is working in is one of the first steps to using power effectively. Basic to this analysis are such factors as the table of organization, the bureaucractic structure, the people with designated and actual power, the goals of the system, the usual way of doing things within the system, and the reward system. This analysis is carried out in terms of what changes the leader wants to make and how the leader wants to bring these changes about. The leader determines whether what is wanted is solely to increase productivity or group satisfaction or whether the leader desires a combination of both, since different types of power are more effective for different goals.

PLANNING FOR CHANGE

The leader then takes the information gathered from the analysis to establish goals for change and to plan the methods and approaches to be utilized. The leader determines the realistic time frame within which the change will occur. The time frame will depend on the resources available, the goals of the group, and the urgency of the situation. It is often useful at this time for the leader to share plans with other people who have actual power and to utilize their resources and input for reaching the goals.

INCLUDING THE GROUP

Once the leader has a framework for reaching the goals and a support system of other power people, it is necessary to share plans with all members of the group who will be affected, gather their input, and modify the leader's basic plan according to their input. Ensuring that the group sees the value and relevance of the change is a component of this collaboration. The leader must be honest and open with the group as to what the plans are for meeting the goals, who will be involved, and the time within which the plan will take place. If this is not done, the leader's credibility will soon be decreased and the power base eroded. This collaboration increases the group's sense of security and predictability and thus makes the group feel that the leader has its best interests in mind. (Illustration 5.4)

CONTINUING EVALUATION

Once plans for meeting the goals have been put into action, the leader constantly evaluates the process and be willing to modify or even abandon plans in the best interests of the group. In order to maintain power, the leader must look at both the movement toward goal achievement and group satisfaction.

Increasing Sphere of Influence

Specific power techniques can be used to increase one's sphere of influence no matter what the setting or situation.

EYE CONTACT

Maintaining eye contact when in confrontation situations is interpreted in the American culture as indicating that the person has awareness of, control over, and conviction about the situation. This

Illustration 5.4
To insure that group members see the value of a planned change, it is important that the nurse in the position of leadership openly share the plan with each group member. *(Photo © Leonard Speier, 1979)*

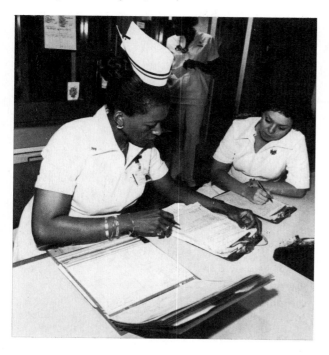

technique can be practiced and acquired by anyone. In addition, eye contact can indicate a real interest in the other individual.

CONTROLLED TONE OF VOICE

The tone of voice the individual uses contributes to an assumption of power by others. A controlled, calm, low, clear, and nonhesitant speech pattern usually carries more influence than one which is emotionally wrought and hesitant. A tone which is low requires that other people listen more carefully if they are to hear what is said. Screaming and yelling are usually ignored or results in hostile reactions from the recipients.

BODY POSITIONING

Different body positions have different connotations for power. Standing over another person looking down on him gives the person who is standing a power advantage. However, the person with power may choose to use the reverse technique and force the other individual to stand while he is sitting. The basic principle behind this technique is that the power person can structure the situation to prevent the other person from being on the same plane with him, since being on the same plane implies equality.

MAINTAINING CONTINUITY

Maintaining a continuity of demands with a regular evaluation or checkup system is another effective power technique. If individuals know that when demands are made of them they will be expected to comply and that a meaningful reward and punishment system will be operative, they are more likely to follow through on assignments. The effective user of power never promises or threatens anything without the power to back it up. Occasionally it may be necessary to demonstrate one's "power" through the use of reward and punishment.

EFFECTIVE USE OF OBJECTS AND SPACE

Physical objects can be used to demonstrate power. Desks, tables, credentials, or any other object which denotes power within the system the individual is working in can be used in this way. Often the fact that the system allows an individual to use these power objects is sufficient to impart power.

Individuals can also utilize territory, location, and space to their advantage when exerting power. Requiring that someone come to the leader (to his or her "own territory") automatically implies that a person has the power to influence the other person's movements. This is based on the premise that people are more comfortable and in control in their own space. However, again, the reverse can be true. The power person, by going into the other person's "territory" implies having the right and authority to come and go as he or she chooses.

Utilizing Power

The effective leader learns to utilize power, not for personal "grandeur and glory," but to facilitate the movement of the group toward mutually established goals. The techniques and strategies used will depend on the outcomes desired, the leader's own interpersonal style and abilities, the setting, and the situation.

MANAGEMENT

Often the concepts of leadership and management are ► confused. In contrast to leadership, **management** is the systematic organization and administration of institutionally set goals through delegated authority. Management is indigenous to an institutional setting or bureaucratic structure, whereas leadership can be found in any setting where people are working toward common goals.

Managers are usually selected by the organization to carry out its policies, procedures, and goals. The manager's role is to keep the system running smoothly and efficiently. Thus effective management will in and of itself not create change, but can provide the vehicle for transmitting change throughout an institutional setting. The manager initially gets power from the organization by virtue of the position and the authority that goes with it. However, the manager may gain actual power through use of various power techniques and strategies.

Facets of a Bureaucracy

The structure within which the manager most often works is a bureaucracy. A **bureaucracy** is a formalized organization of people which has as its aim maximum productivity. The product may be a car, the election of a candidate, or the provision of health care. A bureaucracy is composed of several facets, namely, the division of labor, delegation of authority, formalized channels of communication, and coordination.

DIVISION OF LABOR

The assignment of tasks according to specialization or expertise is the division of labor. Each person contributes special skills to create the desired finished product. Therefore, such positions as director of nursing, nursing supervisor, head nurse, staff nurse, and nurse's aid are created.

HIERARCHY OF AUTHORITY

Concomitant with the division of labor is a hierarchy of authority. A hierarchy is a graded order of power. The bureaucratic structure is usually pictured as a pyramid (Fig. 5.11). The individual or group of individuals with the most power is at the apex of the structure. This person(s) wields the greatest power and decides the policies, rules, and goals of the organization. Moving down the pyramid, each succeeding lower level is less autonomous in decision making and policy setting and has less power.

CHANNELS OF COMMUNICATION

Within the hierarchical structure there are formalized channels of communication. There is a vertical channel through which the highest level gives messages to the next highest level and so forth down to the base of the organizational structure. In turn, communication from the base moves upward. The communication in both directions may be selective as to how much information moves to the next level. Vertical communication is usually in written form, as with a memo or requisition.

Horizontal channels of communication are those which exist within any one level. These communications are usually among peers of equal rank and thus are often less formal in nature. Messages may be either verbal or written.

Within the bureaucratic structure, failure to use the appropriate channels of communication can result in either the messages being ignored or the communicator being punished in some way. For example, if a staff member complains to a supervisor without first going to the head nurse, the staff member may be told to see the head nurse first or chastized for not understanding how the system works or even labeled as a troublemaker. However, when channels of communication are followed but the message is stopped and ignored at the next level, the initiator of the message can bypass that first level and move to the one above it.

COORDINATION

The final aspect of a bureaucracy, coordination, is the presence of a reward and punishment system and a written set of rules and procedures for how things are to be carried out. This facet of a bureaucracy provides the framework for and continuity of the other bureaucratic properties.

The Manager

The manager is an integral part of the bureaucratic structure, since he or she is responsible for the or-

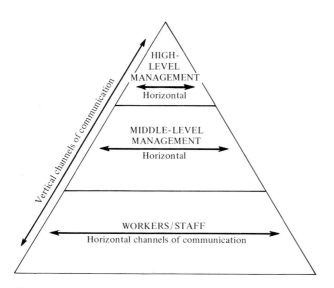

Figure 5.11
Hierarchy of authority with vertical and horizontal channels of communication.

ganization and coordination of any subordinate level. Thus, skills which promote the manager's ability to accomplish tasks are necessary if the manager is to be effective. The manager needs to assess the strengths and weaknesses of the staff and assign responsibilities and delegate authority according to this assessment. The manager must also be able to match personnel, time, equipment, and resources to devise a realistic schedule for meeting the organization's goals. Next, the manager must be able to supervise and evaluate the performance of the personnel under the manager's sphere of authority. He or she checks to see whether delegated responsibilities are carried out in the most efficient and effective manner and, if not, the manager modifies assignments and gives rewards and punishments accordingly.

Finally, the manager acts as a liaison between subordinates and the next higher level by suggesting changes and carrying messages. To do this the manager must be aware of the specific bureaucratic structure and the procedures, rules, and regulations of the organization.

Effective management, like effective leadership, can be carried out in a variety of ways. The manager may use an autocratic or "iron-hand" style or a supportive one. A laissez faire style is not compatible with efficient management. The same variables will determine the management style as determine leadership style.

PSYCHOMOTOR SKILLS

Psychomotor skills are an integral part of providing direct nursing care to individuals in order to bring about a positive change in their health state. ▶ **Psychomotor skills** are those learned processes requiring manual dexterity and practice. They are based on scientific principles and are the translation of thought into action. Competency in psychomotor skills serves to create a change in the individual's state of health and also serves as a role model for other health workers.

Foundation in Theory and Scientific Principles

These skills are developed on a sound foundation of theory and scientific principles which guide their use in the health care situation. The acquisition of

psychomotor skills begins with recognition of the outcome which is desired in a particular situation. Next, the nurse identifies the actions necessary to achieve the desired outcome. From there, the theories and principles which underlie these actions are determined, and appropriate behaviors stemming from them are selected. This implies that psychomotor skills are not rote reactions which are automatically used in a ritualized fashion, but are thought-out responses tailored to the given situation.

While specific actions and principles can be generalized and transferred from situation to situation, each time the nurse uses a particular psychomotor skill, professional judgment is required to determine what modifications are needed in the situation, the appropriateness of the action, and the possible consequences. In this way, any activity the nurse carries out is purposeful and individualized for one person and a unique situation.

It is the recognition of the general principles that need to be followed which serves as the basis for skill practice and equipment manipulation. The nurse can gain competency in psychomotor skills by repeated analysis of situations that can be generalized for basic principles, by manipulation of equipment frequently utilized in carrying out the skills, and by practice in using the equipment in various situations.

Psychomotor skills are performed to gather information about the individual's state of health, to prevent and treat the sequelae of illness, and to meet those health care needs which the individual cannot meet alone. Skills which are carried out competently ensure the individual's safety, decrease his or her level of anxiety, help develop a trust relationship between the nurse and the individual, and serve as an example for other health care workers to follow. As the nurse's scope of professional experiences and knowledge increases, the nurse develops a wider range of skills from which to choose and a greater sense of security in performing them.

NURSING RESEARCH

The research process is a valuable change strategy. Traditionally, nurses have neither actively engaged in research nor applied its findings in their clinical practice. Research is the systematic process of testing theories, validating assumptions, generating new information, and discovering new relationships. These findings can provide the basis for implementing change in nursing intervention, improving delivery of health care, supplying new insights into human behavior and its relationship to nursing care, and improving interactions between and among health care staff and individuals in their care. In addition, research can provide the means for developing a unique body of nursing knowledge. Chart 5.7 defines some commonly used terms in research.

Approaches to Research

Many types of research are currently being used to explore different aspects of knowledge and relationships. Chart 5.8 briefly describes these types of research and their uses. The approach that an individual researcher chooses depends on the subject to be studied, the perspective from which it is viewed, the researcher's skills, and the resources available.

Two broad categories can be identified: *descriptive research* and *experimental research*. Descriptive research attempts to describe phenomena as they exist or have existed in relationship to one another, while experimental research sets up tests under carefully controlled conditions to discover new relationships.

Steps in the Research Process

Regardless of the type of approach used, certain basic steps are followed in the research process.

PROBLEM IDENTIFICATION

The first step is identification of the problem. Here the researcher identifies areas where there are gaps in knowledge or unresolved controversies. This

---

Chart 5.7
Definitions Commonly Used in Research

Causation—the process of determining what factor(s) most probably brought out (caused) or effected other factor(s) (effect).

Concept—a word or term which represents an abstraction that is observable, e.g., height.

Construct—a word or term developed by the researcher to describe unobservable concepts or a category of concepts, e.g., motivation.

Correlation—the degree of relation between two or more factors.

Control group—a comparison group of subjects who are treated the same as the test group except they received no treatment.

Population—all the subjects in the "universe" who possess a trait or characteristic which is to be studied.

Randomization—the process of selecting subjects from a population by chance.

Reliability—the dependability or accuracy of a tool or data; +1.00 reliability means research results are exactly the same; 0.00 reliability means there is no similarity whatsoever.

Sample—the subjects chosen from a population who are actually studied.

Statistical significance—the percentage of

phenomena occurring as a result of chance or a test error; e.g., level of significance of 0.05 means that 5 times out of 100 the phenomena occur by chance.

Statistics—the mathematical methods used to analyze data.

Theory—a set of concepts or constructs purposed to explain observable phenomena.

Treatment—any tests, experiments, or actions used on a group of subjects in order to study the resultant effects.

Validity—the degree to which a test or tool measures what it states it measure.

Variable—a value or characteristic which can be isolated and studied.

Independent variable—the probable causative factor; can be manipulated to observe how changes in it influence outcomes.

Dependent variable—the probable effect or result of interaction between independent variables.

Intervening—unmeasurable factors which influence the interaction between variables.

Variance—the degree of dispersion or scattering from the expected norm.

general problem gives the researcher direction for the research process.

GOAL SETTING

The researcher then states the purpose of the research, which sets the goals for the study.

LITERATURE REVIEW

Next, an initial review of the literature is done to discover what knowledge already exists pertaining to the problem. This review of the literature may reveal an existing theory base from which the research can be conducted.

DEFINITION OF STUDY SUBJECTS

The fourth step is the delineation of the population to be studied and the definition of what factors are to be studied. Delineation of the population includes the specific requirements and characteristics of the study subjects. These criteria are based on the in-

formation gathered in the initial review of the literature. Factors are defined specifically as to the meaning they will have within the process and how they will be measured.

DEVELOPING THE SPECIFIC PROBLEM

Once the above-mentioned steps have been accomplished, the problem is specifically identified and stated in the form of a question. The literature is now reviewed a second time with a focus on the specific problem. Hypotheses are then formulated which predict the relationship between the factors to be studied. These relationships are stated in a manner which forecasts the direction of the outcomes. These hypotheses are what will actually be tested in the research process. Determination of the research design, the methodology, and the tools to be used comes next. This tells the researcher exactly how the research project and data collection will be carried out. Once the manner of carrying out the research has been determined, the method for analyzing the data is decided on. The researcher selects the statistical or analytical techniques to be used to inter-

---

Chart 5.8
Types of Research

TYPE	DESCRIPTION AND USES
Historical	Study and interpretation of past events—including people, behaviors, and relationships—to determine effects on present-day phenomena. Cannot be controlled by research.
Survey	Process of obtaining facts and data about a certain subject or subject area through use of questionnaires, polls, and review of related literature; useful in obtaining data base or profile; does not give causal information.
Case study	Analysis of one or more occurrences of a phenomenon for causation and interrelationships; can be either retrospective or ongoing.
Observational field study	The observation of ongoing phenomena or their natural settings; useful in identifying areas for future study and for gathering specific information, but not identifying causation.
Laboratory experimentation	Study of relationships in highly controlled environments where the researcher creates the situation and combines interrelated factors in new ways to discover causality; the researcher determines the situation and the procedures to be followed. Used for generating new knowledge and identifying the effects of a particular treatment.
Field experimentation	Similar to laboratory experimentation except that the testing occurs in a less controlled, more natural setting; provides less control over influencing factors; used for generating new knowledge and identifying the effects of a particular treatment.

pret the data collected. This step completes the preparatory phase of the research process.

IMPLEMENTATION AND INTERPRETATION

The researcher can now select the sample of subjects to be studied. The sample is a proportion of all cases (population) demonstrating the quality to be studied. Sample size can be determined statistically. The method for selecting the subjects is also determined at this point. The methodology is now put into action and the data collected. When all the data have been collected, they are analyzed according to the predetermined techniques. From the analyses, conclusions are drawn, interpretations made, and the hypotheses either supported or disproved. Finally, recommendations for further studies are proposed. These recommendations recognize inadequacies of the present research and identify new relationships which have been brought to light during the process.

The steps of the research process are summarized below:

Recognition and identification of a problem
Statement of purpose
Initial review of the literature
Delineation of population and definition of factors
Specific problem statement
Second review of the literature
Statement of hypothesis
Determination of research design methodology and tools
Selection of statistical or analytical techniques
Selection of sample
Implementation of research design and methodology (selection of data)
Analysis of data
Statement of conclusions and interpretation
Recommendation for further study

Levels of Participation

The nurse can participate in the research process on several levels.

INDEPENDENT STUDY

The nurse can institute and carry out an independent research project. This usually requires specialized education in research methodology. However, small informal research projects are possible without extensive educational preparation. In fact, many nurses, by use of their observational skills, carry out informal research without even realizing it. For example, the nurse who notes that the healing rate of pressure sores is better in one group of individuals than another and then identifies the factor(s) which differ in the two groups can be said to be engaging in a form of research. Oftentimes nurses tend to underestimate the value of this type of research and do not document it or follow through. (Illustration 5.5)

COLLABORATION

Collaboration on research projects that have been instituted by others is another way in which the nurse can take part in the research process. The nurse may act as an observer for the researcher, be a subject of a study, or assist the researcher in creating the type of controlled environment which aids the research. Research, particularly clinical research, requires the cooperation of all those in the environment if it is to be meaningful. Thus while not always an active participant, the nurse may greatly contribute to the success of a study by exhibiting supportive attitudes and behaviors.

Illustration 5.5
Conducting independent research projects in the clinical area is one level of nursing research carried out to improve the quality of health care. *(Photo ©Leonard Speier, 1979)*

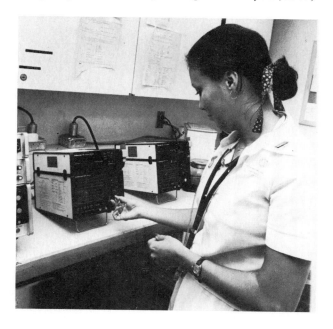

READING ABOUT RESEARCH

One way all nurses can participate in the research process is by becoming critical consumers. To do this the nurse must first be aware of and read the research which is available in nursing. Many nursing journals report research findings in a variety of areas which have significance for nurses and nursing. All too often these are passed over in favor of the more familiar type of article.

EVALUATING RESEARCH PROJECTS

Next, the nurse must evaluate the research study to determine its quality and applicability. Evaluation factors the nurse looks at include the clarity with which steps of the process are stated, the soundness of the theoretical framework, the depth of literature review, the adequacy of sample size, the specificity of delineations and definitions, the logic of conclusions, and the biases and qualifications of the researcher. Research evaluation skills are developed with practice. First attempts may seem difficult and meaningless, but repeated exposure to the process is not only exciting but also produces much up-to-date information which will expand the nurse's professional repertoire.

PUTTING RESEARCH INTO PRACTICE

Finally, the nurse can apply pertinent findings to practice. It is through this application to practice that the nurse can provide options for care and create change. Research becomes only an academic practice when findings remain on the library shelf. The nurse can validate care given and not rely on untested assumptions and past practices. It is only when nurses can generate new knowledge and base their care on it that change can be created and nursing can come into its own as a profession.

NOTES

1. Adapted from Carolyn Chambers Clark, *Nursing Concepts and Processes*. Albany, Delmar, 1977, pp. 460–461.
2. Helen Yura, Dorothy Ozimek, and Mary B. Walsh, *Nursing Leadership*. New York, Appleton, 1976, p. 94.

SELECTED REFERENCES

Armiger, Sister Bernadette. "Ethics of Nursing Research: Profile, Principles, Perspective." *Nursing Research*, 26:330, September-October, 1977.

Ashley, Jo Ann. "About Power in Nursing." *Nursing Outlook*, 21:637, October, 1973.

Bakdash, Diane. "Becoming an Assertive Nurse." *American Journal of Nursing*, 78:1710, October, 1978.

Bales, Robert F. *Interaction Process Analysis*. Chicago, University of Chicago Press, 1951.

Battan, Joe D. "Face to Face Communication." *Nursing Digest*, 1:89, Spring, 1977.

Benoliel, Jeanne Quint. "The Interaction Between Theory and Research." *Nursing Outlook*, 25:108, February, 1977.

Berlo, David. *The Process of Communication*. New York, Holt, Rinehart and Winston, 1960.

Berne, Eric. *The Structure and Dynamics of Organizations and Groups*. Philadelphia, Lippincott, 1963.

Bigge, Morris L. *Learning Theories for Teachers*, 2nd ed. New York, Harper & Row, 1971.

Bloom, Robert S. "Stating Educational Objectives in Behavioral Terms." *Nursing Forum*, 14(1):30, 1975.

Bowman, Rosemary A. and Culpepper, Rebecca. "Power: Rx for Change." *American Journal of Nursing*, 74:1054, June, 1974.

Clark, Carolyn Chambers. *Nursing Concepts and Processes*. New York, Delmar, 1977.

"Communication with Young Children" (A Special Feature). *American Journal of Nursing*, 77:1960, December, 1977.

Connell, Edwina A. "What Kind of Delegator Are You?" *Nursing 78*, 8:105, October, 1978.

Cospor, Bonnie, "How Well Do Patients Understand Hospital Jargon?" *American Journal of Nursing*, 77:1932, December, 1977.

Crawford, C. and Palm, M. "Can I Take My Teddy Bear?" *American Journal of Nursing*, 73:286, February, 1973.

Creighton, Helen. "Legal Concerns of Nursing Research." *Nursing Research*, 26:337, September-October, 1977.

Devito, Joseph A. *The Interpersonal Communication Book*. New York, Harper & Row, 1976.

Diers, Donna. "A Different Kind of Energy: Nurse Power." *Nursing Outlook*, 26:51, January, 1978.

Donnelley, Gloria. "The Assertive Nurse." *Nursing 78*, 8:65, January, 1978.

Eaton, Sharon, Davis, Grace L., and Benner, Patricia E. "Discussion Stoppers in Teaching." *Nursing Outlook*, 25:578, September, 1977.

Egolf, Donald B. and Chester, Sondra L. "Speechless Messages." *Nursing Digest*, 4:26, March-April, 1976.

Ellis, Henry C. *The Transfer of Learning*. New York, Macmillan, 1965.

Fox, David L. *Fundamentals of Research in Nursing*, 3rd ed. New York, Appleton, 1976.

Fuhrer, Lois M. and Bernstein, Ronne. "Making Patient

Education a Part of Patient Care." *American Journal of Nursing,* 76:1798, November, 1976.

Garant, Carol. "The Process of Effecting Change in Nursing." *Nursing Forum,* 17(2):152, 1978.

Giffin, Kim and Patton, Bobby R. *Fundamentals of Interpersonal Communication,* 2nd ed. New York, Harper & Row, 1976.

Gortner, Susan R. and Nahm, Helen. "An Overview of Nursing Research in the United States." *Nursing Research,* 26:10, January-February, 1977.

Guinée, Kathleen. *Teaching and Learning in Nursing.* New York, Macmillan, 1978.

Hays, Joyce S. and Larson, Kenneth. *Interacting With Patients.* New York, Macmillan, 1963.

Herth, Kaye. "Beyond the Curtain of Silence." *American Journal of Nursing,* 74:1060, June, 1974.

Jacox, Ada and Prescott, Ruth. "Determining a Study's Relevance for Clinical Practice." *American Journal of Nursing.* 78:1882, November, 1978.

Jones, Patricia and Oertal, William. "Developing Patient Teaching Objectives and Techniques: A Self Instructional Program." *Nurse Education,* 11:3, September-October, 1977.

Johnson, Walter L. "Research Programs of the National League for Nursing." *Nursing Research,* 26:172, May-June, 1977.

Kohut, Sussane A. "Guidelines for Using Interpreters." *Nursing Digest,* 4:55, January-February, 1976.

Kramer, Marlene and Schmalenberg, Claudia. "Constructive Feedback." *Nursing 77,* 7:102, November, 1977.

Kretzer, Joan B. "What Does Your Patient Need to Know?" *Nursing 77,* 7:82, December, 1977.

Krieger, Dolores. "Therapeutic Touch: The Imprimatur of Nursing." *American Journal of Nursing,* 75:734, May, 1975.

Kron, Thora. *The Management of Patient Care,* 4th ed. Philadelphia, Saunders, 1976.

———. "How to Become a Better Leader." *Nursing 76,* 6:67, October, 1976.

Larson, Margaret and Williams, Reg. "How to Become a Better Group Leader." *Nursing 78,* 8:65, August, 1978.

Lasswell, Harold. "The Structure and Function of Communication in Society," in *The Communication of Ideas,* Lyman Bryson, ed. New York, Harper & Row, 1948.

Leonard, Ann M. "Role Imagery: A Delicate Balance." *Journal of Nursing Education,* 17:42, March, 1978.

Lelettier, Marian. "You Can Change Nursing Practice." *Nursing 77,* 7:65, March, 1977.

Levin, Lowell S. "Patient Education and Self-Care: How Do They Differ?" *Nursing Outlook,* 26:170, March, 1978.

Luft, Joseph. *Group Processes.* Palo Alto, California, National Press Books, 1970.

Lynch, James J. "The Simple Act of Touching." *Nursing 78,* 8:32, June, 1978.

MacDonald, Malcom. "How Do Men and Women Students Rate in Empathy." *American Journal of Nursing,* 77:998, June, 1977.

Mager, Robert. *Preparing Instructional Objectives.* Palo Alto, California, Fearon, 1962.

Mager, Robert and Pipe, Peter. "You Really Oughta Wanna . . . or How Not to Motivate People." *Nursing 76,* 6:65, August, 1976.

McGreevy, Abigal and VanHeukelen, Judy. "Crying: The Neglected Dimension." *Nursing Digest,* 1:61, Fall, 1977.

Miller, Jean R. and Messenger, Susan R. "Obstacles to Applying Research Findings." *American Journal of Nursing,* 78:632, April, 1978.

Mitchell, Ann C. "Barriers to Therapeutic Communication With Black Clients." *Nursing Outlook,* 26:109, February, 1978.

Moniz, Donna. "Putting Assertiveness Techniques into Practice." *American Journal of Nursing,* 78:1713, October, 1978.

"Nursing Research: Reflection of Values." *Nursing Research,* 26:4, January-February, 1977.

Orlando, Ida Jean. *The Dynamic Nurse-Patient Relationship.* New York, Putnam, 1961.

Peplau, Hildegarde E. *Interpersonal Relations in Nursing.* New York, Putnam, 1952.

Pugh, Elizabeth. "Dynamics of Teaching—Learning Interaction." *Nursing Forum,* 15(1):47, 1976.

Redman, Barbara. "Curriculum in Patient Education." *American Journal of Nursing,* 78:1363, August, 1978.

———. "Guidelines for Quality of Care in Patient Education." *Nursing Digest,* 4:25, Fall, 1976.

———. *The Process of Patient Teaching in Nursing,* 3rd ed. St. Louis, Mosby, 1976.

Riley-Kesler, Arlene. "Pitfalls to Avoid in Interviewing Out-Patients." *Nursing 77,* 7:70, September, 1977.

Sampson, Edward and Marthas, Marya S. *Group Process for the Health Professions.* New York, Wiley, 1977.

See, Elizabeth M. "The ANA and Research in Nursing." *Nursing Research,* 26:165, May-June, 1977.

Schwier, Mildred E. and Gardella, Frances A. "Planning, Orienting and Preparing for a New Kind of Nurse Leadership." *Nursing Outlook,* 18:42, May, 1970.

Shannon, Claude E. and Weaver, Warren. *The Mathematical Theory of Communication.* Urbana, Ill., University of Illinois Press, 1949.

Shipley, Robert. "Applying Learning Theory to Nursing Practice." *Nursing Forum,* 16(1):83, 1977.

Sloboda, Sharon. "Understanding Patient Behavior." *Nursing 77,* 7:74, September, 1977.

Smith, Dorothy M. "Writing Objectives as a Nursing Practice Skill." *American Journal of Nursing,* 71:319, February, 1971.

Smoyak, Shirley A. "Is Practice Responding to Research." *American Journal of Nursing,* 76:1146, July, 1976.

UNIT II
The Nursing Process

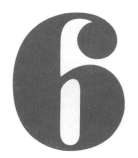

Undoubtedly we have no questions to ask which are unanswerable. We must trust the perfection of the creation so far as to believe that whatever curiosity the order of things has awakened in our minds, the order of things can satisfy.
—Ralph Waldo Emerson, Nature

INTRODUCTION TO THE NURSING PROCESS

The nursing process is a tool for effecting change and is applicable in a wide variety of settings. It is a specialized form of problem solving which has been adapted to the needs of nursing.

PROBLEM SOLVING

Problem solving is used in everyday life, often without conscious awareness, to make decisions about courses of action. When to eat, when to go to sleep, and what to wear all involve problem solving. For example, when a person wants to cross a street at a busy intersection, he or she uses all the steps of problem solving rapidly and without actual recognition of having used them. First, one realizes that one has to cross the street. Then one notices such things as the pattern of traffic flow, the absence or presence of a traffic light, the movement of pedestrians across the street, the weather conditions, and one recalls one's previous street-crossing experience. One then realizes the street is heavily trafficked and potentially dangerous.

With that information the person can look more

specifically at the situation: namely, that it is rush hour; the traffic is slow moving; many people are attempting to cross at the same time; the weather is clear; it is twilight; the person is tired after a day of classes; there is a traffic light which changes every two minutes; and the street is four lanes wide with a divider in between. The person decides to wait until the light turns green before starting across. When the light changes, the person crosses, thus carrying out the plan. Arriving safely at the other side of the street, the person decides that he or she has successfully handled the situation.

The problem-solving steps utilized in the situation were:

1 Recognition of a problem—the street had to be crossed.
2 General survey of the problem—noting the traffic flow, the light, etc.
3 Identification of the specific problem—crossing a heavily trafficked and potentially dangerous street.
4 Data collection related to the specific problem—evening rush hour, being tired, etc.
5 Statement of hypothesis—it would be possible to cross safely when the light turned green.

6 Testing the hypothesis—crossing on the green light.

7 Analysis and evaluation—having crossed safely, the plan worked, and the person adds this experience to previous experiences of street crossing.

▶   Thus **problem solving** is the step-by-step process of inquiry for determining choices of action. This method forms the basis for the scientific method, the various types of research, and the nursing process. Effective problem solving requires critical thinking and is greatly enhanced by creativity.

Critical Thinking

▶ **Critical thinking** is a logical pattern of thought based on knowledge, experience, problem-solving ability, and reasoning. Critical thinking allows for the ordering of information and the selection of relevant information. It enables the individual to make decisions in an efficient and effective manner, to analyze relationships, to conceptualize, and to make reasoned judgments. One is not magically endowed with the ability to think critically. It is a skill which is developed and refined throughout life. Young children have a limited ability to think critically. Lack of knowledge and experience as well as nervous system immaturity have much to do with it.

As developing individuals, we are exposed to new situations which we attempt to deal with mainly through trial and error. As a result, we build up a set of experiences and skills which can be incorporated into our thinking. We continue to gain new knowledge, which increases our options. We then can select from and organize these experiences, pieces of information, and skills to further increase our frames of reference. As these ideas are tested, they are modified and expanded, and the process continues.

Creativity

▶ **Creativity,** which is the generation of new patterns of thought and actions, allows the individual to utilize the ideas drawn from critical thinking in original ways. Sutterly and Donnelly state that "it is the ability to productively and compatibly combine the logical and the illogical that is the mark of the creative person."[1] Creativity implies a freedom from automatically accepting what is and the ability to seek alternative options or solutions to problems.

Their Role Together

Problem solving, critical thinking, and creativity are used to bring about change. The use of these processes can effect change by allowing the individual to visualize clearly all available information, to analyze the relationships between groups of information, and to see a variety of options which can be individualized and modified to the specific situation. In this way, innovative methods of dealing with situations can be utilized to bring about change, be it a changed idea or health state.

NURSING PROCESS

▶ **The nursing process** as a modification of the problem-solving method is a systematic method for organizing the change process within the nursing context. It helps the nurse to make a positive difference in the individual's ability to meet his or her daily health needs. Like problem solving, the nursing process is composed of a series of phases. They are assessment, planning, intervention, and evaluation.

Phases of the Process

ASSESSMENT

▶   **Assessment** is the collection, organization, and analysis of information relevant to the person's health status at that point in time. It includes the initial recognition of an existing or potential negative health behavior; collection of available general information and impressions; identification of the specific negative health behavior; and collection of all available data specific to the negative health behavior. Data are usually classified in two categories:
▶ subjective and objective. **Subjective data** are not directly observable or measurable by persons other than the person to whom the data relate. It is that which the individual tells another as perceived by himself. Subjective data are synonymous with
▶ **symptoms** when they reflect the health state. **Objec-**
▶ **tive data** are observable and measurable by people
▶ other than the individual himself. The word **sign** is used to denote these kinds of data. An example of a

subjective datum (symptom) is an individual's complaint of itching along the backs of his legs. The objective datum (sign) is the observation of a circumscribed papular rash, 6 by 4 inches (15×10 cm) bilaterally along the posterior thighs. On occasion some symptoms presented by the individual may be observable by others. Those symptoms may be termed objective. Throughout the phase of assessment the nurse simultaneously organizes data and analyzes the relevancy of the incoming information (input).

▶ Assessment culminates in a **nursing diagnosis,** which is a statement of an existing or potential negative health behavior related to those factors which influence this response. It is analogous to the hypothesis step of the problem-solving method, as it associates the negative health behavior with the conditions that most likely account for its occurrence.

Nursing diagnoses, like hypotheses, are statements of the relationship between the negative health behavior and the factors influencing it.

Nursing diagnoses provide a focus for intervention, or direction for a plan. They are specific and based on sound data.

PLANNING

▶ The next phase in the nursing process, **planning,** is creating an organized course of action designed to change the negative health response to a more positive one.

▶ A first step in planning is to set viable, obtainable, individual-centered goals. A **goal** is an aim or objective for action and provides a framework on which the plan is developed.

The next step in the planning phase is to organize a blueprint designed to meet individual-centered goals in the most effective and efficient manner. Goal setting and planning are a collaborative effort on the part of the individual, family and/or significant others, nurse, and other health team members to effect change.

INTERVENTION

▶ **Intervention** is the action phase of the nursing process. It is seen as those nursing actions the professional nurse *initiates* in giving direct care and not merely the implementation or passive carrying out of her plan of care. Actions that the nurse independently initiates are based on her nursing expertise, her assessment of the care situation, and those dependent activities which evolve from the medical regimen. Both the planning and intervention phases are similar to the stage of hypothesis testing in the problem-solving method.

EVALUATION

▶ **Evaluation,** the final step of the nursing process, involves ongoing measurement of the process of change and its outcomes. Although considered the last phase of the nursing process, evaluation should be occurring throughout all the phases so that appropriate revisions can be made as needed.

Interrelationship of Phases

In learning to use the nursing process, the learner may see it as artificial and fragmented. However, one must deal with the parts first to understand the whole. It is not until the parts have been synthesized that one can see the interdependent, cyclical nature of the whole process.

The successful use of the nursing process greatly relies on the complementarity and interrelationships of all the phases. For example, without an adequate data base and accurate analysis of the health behavior, nursing diagnoses will be incomplete and nonspecific. Vague or poorly stated nursing diagnoses result in goals which do not direct the desired change, and plans are haphazard and often fruitless. As a result, evaluations made from poorly stated nursing diagnoses cannot be based on measurable outcomes. Evaluation becomes a herculean task, since there is no documentation as to what may or may not have caused the changes or which phase was inadequately developed.

Each phase, as well as the process as a whole, is continuously evaluated, updated, and modified. The nursing process is a dynamic and creative process which must reflect the constantly changing nature of the health situation. No situation is static; therefore, constant assessment, diagnosis, planning, intervention, and evaluation are necessary to make a positive difference in the individual's health state.

The nursing process provides an excellent method for bringing about health changes, as it is a systematic approach which requires critical thinking and allows for the development of individual creativity. The use of the nursing process provides an opportunity for independent thought and action on the part of the nurse. It is a framework for care but in no way limits the chance for exploring different modes of care. Successful use of the nursing process depends on collaboration among the individual, the family and/or significant others, the nurse, and other health team members. Channels of communication must be open to allow for the free flow of thoughts, ideas, and feelings. Organizing the nursing process will help to assure that care efforts stay within the context of the health care situation. This speeds the change in health behavior and aids in avoiding false starts and dead-end approaches. The frustrations of both the nurse and the individual are thereby decreased. This, in turn, frees the energies of both for involvement in the care process.

The critical thinking necessary in the nursing process helps the nurse to select appropriately from the many variables present in the health care situation and then to make valid judgments which will minimize error and enhance nursing care. Critical thinking assists the nurse in synthesizing knowledge learned from one situation and, in turn, transferring it to other care situations. This results in an increased repertoire of care behaviors for the nurse.

Creativity, when added to critical thinking, enables the nurse to devise new care options and expand on already existing ones, using them in new and challenging ways. These skills ultimately provide not only for quality nursing care, but also for the growth of nursing as a vital and learned profession based on much more than rote following of physicians' orders and the carrying out of tasks. Chart 6.1 compares the nursing process and problem solving.

Versatility of the Nursing Process

The use of the nursing process is not limited to any one time, place, or circumstance. Rather it is a tool that is applicable to a diversity of settings. It is useful in the community *and* in institutions, with groups *and* with individuals, in health promotion and teaching *and* in variations from the well state, with infants *and* with elderly persons, and in critical care *and* in long-term care. Through continued and concentrated use of the nursing process, skill and ease are developed in employing the process.

Chart 6.1
Comparison of Nursing Process and Problem Solving

STEPS INVOLVED

Problem solving	Nursing Process
Recognition of the problem	Identification of interference with health care needs
General survey of problem	
Identification of specific problem	Assessment
Data collection	
Hypothesis	Nursing diagnosis
Testing of hypothesis	Planning and intervention
Analysis and evaluation	Evaluation

RECORDING AND THE NURSING PROCESS

Transmission of information obtained within the health situation is a major part of the effective use of the nursing process. A variety of health team members contribute to the provision of care, and it is vital that all participants be well informed regarding the delivery of health care. Oral transmission of information, while appropriate to some situations, can be incomplete, distorted, or inaccurate. And it provides no pertinent point of reference for any changes that may be taking place. One need only remember the child's game of Gossip to recognize that these difficulties occur. Written documentation of information obtained, orders written, care given, teaching done, and evaluations made provides many advantages for both the individual and the health care team.

Written records are a channel of communication among health care workers to keep each other informed as to their actions and findings, thus increasing the quality of care. Written records help in preventing duplication of efforts, sharing new knowledge, guiding care, and giving a more complete view of the individual's situation. Information which is shared increases the quality of care provided. Care is enhanced when duplication of efforts is avoided and everyone can see what changes are or are not occurring. Through the use of written records, care is not random or haphazard, and the chances of making an error are reduced. In addition, providing care that is individualized for a person and his or her needs is facilitated by his or her specific profile being available to all. (Illustration 6.1)

Continuity of care can be achieved through written records. Accessibility of information allows for the integration of efforts among health team members. In this way, the care provided is a follow-through of preceding actions and not only a series of isolated events.

Written records can be used as an evaluative tool. One or many records can be reviewed to determine the quality of care given. This review may be done by consulting agencies or the health team members themselves, and recommendations for improved care can then be made.

The record can later be used to provide a base line of information in other health situations. The knowledge base of the health professions can be increased through written records. The record provides statistics that may be studied, case histories, and information about the effectiveness of treatment modalities.

Finally, the written record is a legal document which can be introduced into a court of law as a record of the type and quality of care given or omitted. Therefore, the record should reflect care accurately and concisely.

The Chart

▶ The individual's health care record is called a **chart.** The composition and format of the individual's chart will vary according to the type of health care setting and from agency to agency or even from unit to unit. However, the chart will typically contain the following:

1 Record of admission—an account of what brought the individual to the health care setting and how he entered.
2 Personal data sheet—the vital statistics of the individual such as name, address, age, occupation, next of kin.
3 Consent forms—permission slips for carrying out procedures.

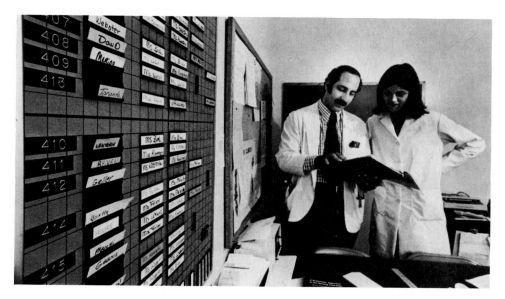

Illustration 6.1
Written documentation of an individual's care is an essential aspect of providing quality care.
(Photo by Ellis Herwig, from Stock, Boston)

4   Nursing history—previous health histories; relevant personal habits, e.g., drug consumption, smoking, bowel habits, eating pattern; attitudes toward previous health care; allergies; family health history.

5   Medical history—physician's record of previous diseases, their patterns and treatment; family medical history; allergies; social habits.

6   Physical examination findings—a system-by-system physical examination report.

7   Progress sheets—day-by-day reports by various members of the health team concerning changes in the individual's health state, treatments given, and plans for care.

8   Laboratory and procedure data sheets—reports of laboratory test values, diagnostic test results, surgical process reports, and pathology reports.

9   Flow sheets—a concise record of measurable data over a period of time, e.g., blood pressure, temperature, pulse, respiration, diabetic urine testing, wound drainage.

10 Physician's orders—treatments prescribed by the physician.

11 Medication record—a complete record of any medication ordered: the drug name, date ordered and given, times and method of administration, dosage and persons administering.

12 Discharge planning record—the plan for discharge and follow-up care, including health teaching.

13 Utilization review sheet—a form used in hospitals and related facilities for determining the appropriateness of the type and length of hospitalization.

Approaches to Recording

Several types of formats exist for the written record of health care. The diversity of these formats results from the different approaches used in delivery of health care.

THE TRADITIONAL APPROACH

In the traditional approach, each health care professional functions in a parallel, complementary manner. As a result, the health care record is composed of distinct sections for each group. Thus physicians record their findings, plans, and evaluations in such sections as medical history and examination, physician's progress notes, and doctor's orders. Nurses record in a section labeled nurses' notes, entering their observations, plans, interventions, and evaluations. Other health-related professionals record their findings in a similar fashion. (Illustration 6.2)

Nurses' notes written from this approach are logs of events taking place during a specific time period. The time period varies. For example, it is from event to event in critical care situations; hour to hour in subacute settings; shift to shift in convalescent areas; and month to month or longer in long-term care facilities or community health agencies.

When the time span between records is short, e.g., every 15 minutes or half hour, the notes focus on specific events occurring within that time span. Figure 6.1 exemplifies this approach. When the time span between recordings is longer, e.g., every shift, the notes center on a summary of events occurring during that time period. Figure 6.2 shows this recording method.

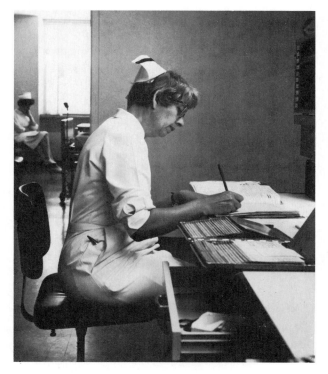

Illustration 6.2
With many health team members contributing to an individual's care, continuity of care is facilitated by careful recording in the individual's chart and, in turn, careful analysis of its contents. *(Photo by Hugh Rogers, from Monkmeyer Press Photo Service)*

THE BROOKLYN HOSPITAL

NURSES' PROGRESS NOTES

SHEET NUMBER 1

Short-term notes

ADMISSION NOTES

DATE: ______ TIME: ______ AM PM MODE OF ARRIVAL ______

ALLERGIES: ______

PHYSICIANS NOTIFIED: 1- ______ at ______ AM PM 2- ______ at ______ AM PM

VITAL SIGNS

B.P. ______ PULSE ______ WT. ______

TEMP. ______ RESP. ______ HT. ______

LABORATORY SPECIMENS

CBC: ☐ SENT ☐ COMPLETED URINE: ☐ SENT ☐ COMPLETED

NURSES OBSERVATIONS (PLEASE INDICATE BELOW)

DATE	TIME	NOTES
6/20/80	6:00PM	Short of breath even when lying quietly in bed. Respirations 28, regular and
		hollow; skin color ashen. Profuse diaphoresis present, pajamas changed x 2 in
		last half hour. Face pinched, fists clenched with neck and shoulder muscles
		contracted. Moving about in bed. Blood pressure 190/110, pulse 90, regular
		and full. Physician notified. Head of bed elevated and oxygen 7 liters by
		nasal cannula started. Dawn Kilts, R.N.
	6:30PM	Seen by Dr. McCarren. Blood for serum enzymes drawn, Stat EKG done. 10 mg
		Valium IM administered for anxiety. Explanations of procedures and medica-
		tions given. Request to call wife carried out. Sat with for 5 minutes. Left
		lying quietly in bed. States "Maybe I can sleep now." Dawn Kilts, R.N.

Figure 6.1
Short-term nurse's notes *(Nurse's note form courtesy of The Brooklyn Hospital)*

THE PROBLEM-ORIENTED RECORD

In the late 1960s, Dr. Lawrence L. Weed focused attention on the problem-oriented system of health care delivery.[2] Within this system all health professionals function in a horizontal, integrated way. Therefore, the health care record (*P*roblem *O*riented *R*ecord, POR) integrates all groups within one frame of reference.

The problem-oriented system focuses on the needs of the individual himself, not on the actions of the health care worker. This method uses the problem-solving and nursing process approaches as its basis. The major components of the record are (1) collected data and observations to form a data base, (2) analysis of the data which translates into a list of problems, (3) a plan for solving those problems, and (4) a report in the progress notes of the interventions, changes in health state, and evaluations. Flow sheets supplement the progress notes.

Each group of health care professionals collects data related to its own area of expertise. All data collected are placed in a centralized section of the record. It is updated or modified throughout the care sequence by any member of the health team. From this data base problems relevant to the individual's health are compiled and given a sequential number. The problem list reflects all the individual's needs,

THE BROOKLYN HOSPITAL

NURSES' PROGRESS NOTES

SHEET NUMBER 1

Long-term notes

ADMISSION NOTES

DATE: ______ TIME: ______ AM PM MODE OF ARRIVAL ______

ALLERGIES: ______

PHYSICIANS NOTIFIED: 1- ______ at ______ AM PM 2- ______ at ______ AM PM

VITAL SIGNS

B.P. ______ PULSE ______ WT. ______

TEMP. ______ RESP. ______ HT. ______

LABORATORY SPECIMENS

CBC: ☐ SENT ☐ COMPLETED URINE: ☐ SENT ☐ COMPLETED

NURSES OBSERVATIONS (PLEASE INDICATE BELOW)

DATE	TIME	NOTES
6/20/80	11:00PM-	Awake at 2AM to urinate; stated "This is the first time I've been awake all
	7:00AM	night." Slept rest of night as evidenced by snoring, respirations and
		relaxed state. Dawn Kilts, R.N.

Figure 6.2
Long-term nurse's notes. *(Courtesy of The Brooklyn Hospital)*

both past and present, such as nursing, medical, and social service needs. The list directs the health care workers in formulating a plan of care. As with the data base and problem list, the plan of care represents the input of the entire health team. Interventions, changes in health state, and evaluations are recorded as they relate to the problem and in order of occurrence by whomever is involved in the process at that time. For example, one might see an entry by the social workers followed by an entry by the nurse, followed by the physician's or the respiratory therapist's, related to one specific problem. Figure 6.3 and Chart 6.2 illustrate the components the problem-oriented record system.

Many benefits derive from this system, for the individual, the nurse, and all health team members. Primarily, it is individual centered, focusing on what the individual's health needs are and how to solve them. Care is integrated and individualized. This method also encourages more open communication and sharing of information and helps to avoid duplication of efforts and services.

SOAPIE

One problem-oriented method of charting is the **Subjective and Objective data, Analysis, Plan, Intervention, and Evaluation** (SOAPIE) method. Using this approach, charting entries are made only when there is pertinent information related to the problems. First, the problem is stated, and then subjective (S)

Chart 6.2
Reflection of a Problem-Oriented System in a Problem-Oriented Record

PROBLEM-ORIENTED SYSTEM	PROBLEM-ORIENTED RECORD
I. OBSERVATION (defined Data Base) Subjective Objective	A. Family Data Base B. Patient Data Base Subjective Objective Assessment
II. ASSESSMENT Interpretations (All possible meanings) Rule in/out (Validation process) Identification of health problems	C. Problem List Active Problems At Risk Problems Inactive Problems
III. PLANNING Set priorities among problems Consider all possible plans for solution Consider probabilities of success of various plans (In establishing probabilities examples of factors considered are: Soundness of theory, patient's values, beliefs, and abilities, family and community resources, compatibility of plan with other health care providers' plans such as MD, MSW, etc. Establish details of selected plan Establish criteria for measuring effectiveness of plan (Expected Outcomes)	D. Plan Plan and Expected Outcomes Physicians' Orders Plans of Other Providers
IV. INTERVENTION	E. Progress Notes S
V. EVALUATION Relative to established criteria (Expected Outcomes)	O A
VI. PLAN REVISION	P
VII. SCHEDULED TOTAL REASSESSMENT Data for reassessment gathered using defined data base to guide systematic observation	D. (Above) A, B, C, etc., as needed (above)

From: Elaine J. Matthis, "Nursing Process: Development and Application," in *Problem Oriented Systems of Patient Care.* (New York: National League for Nursing, 1974), p. 16.

and objective (O) data relating to the specific problem are written. After this, an analysis (A) of the data is given. This analysis is a conclusion or judgment drawn directly from the data concerning the problem. The plan (P) for solving this particular problem is then presented. Interventions (I) done to carry out the plan are recorded, and evaluations (E) of the changes that did or did not occur as a result of the interventions are stated. Figure 6.4 gives an example of the SOAPIE method.

Chart 6.2 summarizes the realtionship between the problem-oriented care approach and the problem-oriented record.

General Guidelines for Effective Recording

No matter what form of charting is used, certain guidelines apply to basic effective recording. Notes should give a clear, accurate, and objective descrip-

DATA BASE

Routine data:

- Historical
  Medical history
  Nursing history
- Physiological
  General physical
  Daily function
- Laboratory

PROBLEM LIST

- Index to patient's record
- Problems dated and added as new ones appear
- Potential problems commonly associated with any major problems are often not listed on the primary problem list, but are dealt with in the plans.

SUMMARY OF DATA BASE FOR PATIENT A:

Alaskan Indian male, 26 years old; policeman in small community

One of ten brothers, parents deceased; high school education, unmarried

Transferred to teaching hospital 5 days after acute subarachnoid hemorrhage. Onset of SAH while on patrol with partner. Sudden, severe headache, seizure, loss of consciousness. Blood in spinal fluid with opening pressure of 350 mm H_2O

No previous serious illnesses.

PROBLEM LIST xxxx Medical Center		A. 000-0000-00	
Date	Problem	Identified (initials)	Resolved
7/5/75	#1 SAH 2° ruptured aneurysm right MCA	M.D.	
7/9/75	#2 Fear of job loss	R.N.	

Figure 6.3

Components of the problem-oriented record system. *(From: Judith B. Walker, Geraldine P. Pardee, and Doris M. Molbo,* Dynamics of Problem Oriented Approaches: Patient Care and Documentation. *Philadelphia, Lippincott, 1976)*

tion of the behavior and changes which are occurring at that particular time. Terms that label, clichés, judgmental statements, or catch-all terms do not convey a clear, accurate picture of behaviors. For example, the term "ate well" does not describe what criteria are being used for the kind and amount of food or for the manner in which the food was eaten. In addition, there are no indications of any changes which may have occurred in the eating pattern. A much clearer and more informative notation might be "Entire breakfast of 1 slice buttered toast, 1 scrambled egg, and 1 cup coffee with milk eaten by self. Stopped to rest between bites. Appeared to take greater interest in food today than yesterday. States, 'It is good to have my appetite back to normal.'"

Notations are focused on the individual and his

capabilities, limitations, and reactions to care received. Relevant data that contribute to the total picture and possible sequelae are included. Wordiness does not make for better notes; therefore, words that do not give any new or pertinent information about the individual or the care situation are omitted. However, in trying to be brief and concise, important information that is not directly related to the situation but that may be indicative of new or potential change should not be excluded.

Since written records are a form of communication as well as legal documents, entries should be legible and made in ink to avoid misinterpretations. Errors in charting are clearly labeled. Abbreviations that are not commonly used or that are of one's own

PLAN

- Noted in record in initial progress note for each problem

- In institutions using Kardexes, the Kardex can be utilized to summarize and communicate care required and to tie down responsibility and accountability. Physician's orders are included in relation to the problem for which they are ordered

PROGRESS NOTES

- Initial plans for each problem
- Progress notes for each problem
- Summaries of flow sheets (recurrent data for each problem)
- Problem-oriented summaries:
  used for long term care, referral, discharge

PROGRESS NOTE PLAN

Date	Problem-oriented Progress Notes
7/5/75	#1 SAH 2° ruptured aneurysm Physician evaluation and medical plan of care included here; nurses' implementation of plan illustrated on Kardex below
7/9/75	#2 New problems: Fear of job loss S — Several times commented, "I sure hope I don't lose my job over this." Didn't recall discussing concern with anyone. O — Dr. X has talked with employer and told Mr. A this. Mr. A said he was glad to hear this. Commented about job concerns several times afterward, however. A — Objective danger of job loss resolved. However, he is still concerned about effect of illness on job. Anxiety about job could be detrimental to him at this time. P — Goal: decrease anxiety about job 1. allow him to discuss his concerns

PROGRESS NOTES (including summary of flow sheet data)

Date	Progress-oriented Progress Notes
7/9/75 1500 hrs.	Nurses' 8 hour summary: #1 SAH: Observations: LOC: alert but drowsy; easily awakened; oriented x3; talked about impending surgery and desire to have done with it. Motor: symmetrical. plantar reflex now flexor; left arm stiff and painful from restraint. Eyes: PERLA; EOM intact. Vital signs: Temp. −37° 38° C; BP fluctuated 146/92-154/102; P −68-80; R −24-40. Assessment: condition continues stable with improved motor and LOC; L = arm showing disuse problems Plan: continue frequent observations; passive ROM to restrained limbs Q 4 hr. #2 Fear of job loss.......................

KARDEX CARE PLAN

Date	Problem	Approaches	Sig.
7/5/75	#1 SAH 2° ruptured aneurysm Goal: Prevent re-rupture Plan: 1) Aneurysm precautions *2) Restrict fluids free fluid allowance special mouth care Q 4th Goal: prevent ventriculostomy infection Plan: 1) Bacitracin 5cc in buretrol *Q 12 hr. after draining buretrol 2) Observe for fluctuations in CSF level in tubing (patency of tube)	 900cc dietary 900cc nursing unit 400cc days 300cc p.m. 200cc night	R.N.
7/9/75	#2 Fear of job loss Goal:.		

Room	Name	Diagnosis	Physician
	Mr. A	SAH	Dr. X

*these portions of plan indicate nursing implementation of physician orders (plan): for example, fluid order might read: restrict fluids to 1800 cc per 24 hours

FLOW SHEET

Time	Date 7/9/75 A. 000-0000-00							
	BP	P	R	T	Pupils	In	Out	Comments
8A	154/96	68	28	37²	PERLA	120 60 40	200	Alert; oriented x3
10A	148/90	92	36	37²				Sleeping, restless
12A	152/96	80	24	37⁴	PERLA	150 110 90		Concerned re job

THE BROOKLYN HOSPITAL

NURSES' PROGRESS NOTES

SHEET NUMBER 1

Soapie

ADMISSION NOTES

DATE: _____ TIME: _____ AM PM   MODE OF ARRIVAL _____

ALLERGIES: _____

PHYSICIANS NOTIFIED: 1- _____ at _____ AM PM   2- _____ at _____ AM PM

VITAL SIGNS	LABORATORY SPECIMENS

B.P. _____ PULSE _____ WT. _____   CBC: ☐ SENT   URINE: ☐ SENT

TEMP. _____ RESP. _____ HT. _____   ☐ COMPLETED   ☐ COMPLETED

NURSES OBSERVATIONS (PLEASE INDICATE BELOW)

DATE	TIME	NOTES
6/20/80	4:20PM	Problem: Obesity
		S: States she would like to lose 25 pounds. Usual pattern of eating: skips
		breakfast, has midmorning snack of danish and coffee, lunch usually
		consists of "hero"-type sandwich, french fried potatoes, ice cream sundae or cake and a diet soft drink; usually snacks on cookies or potato
		chips before dinner; dinner-meat, potatoes, bread, vegetable, dessert, and
		coffee; frequently has late-night snacks such as a sandwich or buttered
		popcorn. Likes fried foods and carbohydrates, dislikes most fruits and
		vegetables. Likes to watch sports events. Says she has "tried to lose
		weight a million times."
		O: Weight, 190 pounds. Height, 5'11". Activity level-sedentary. Knows
		basic four, meaning of calories. Income allows for purchase of
		protein. Talked with dietician and was given 1800-calorie diet. No
		history of cardiovascular or renal disease. Medical clearance for diet.
		A: Obesity related to high calorie intake and limited exercise. Limited
		motivation for weight loss related to food preferences and previous
		diet failures.
		P: 1. Discuss self-help organizations such as Weight Watchers
		2. Assist to plan sample menus within the 1800-calorie diet
		3. Explore possible reasons for overeating
		4. Assist to set up a weight loss program
		5. Assist to set up an exercise schedule
		6. Refer to local YWCA for increased activity
		7. Schedule return visit to clinic in 2 weeks
		I: As above
		E: Appeared willing to investigate Weight Watchers. Stated that sample menus
		were not "as bad" as she expected, and she felt they could be worked into her
		daily schedule. Seemed reluctant to change exercise pattern at this time.
		Life-long eating habits and social patterns encourage her overeating. She is
		going to attempt to lose 5 pounds before next clinic visit. Esther Brill, R.N.

Figure 6.4

An example of the SOAPIE method of charting. (Courtesy of The Brooklyn Hospital)

invention can add to misinterpretation and cause errors. Every notation also includes the date and time of entry and the name and title of the person writing it.

The following list contains abbreviations commonly used in records concerning the health care situation:

- **a.c. (ante cibum)** — before eating
- **ad lib. (ad libitum)** — as desired
- **alt. hor. (alternis horis)** — every other hour
- **alt. noc. (alternis nocte)** — every other night
- **b.i.d.** — twice a day
- **BP (B/P)** — blood pressure
- **C** — centigrade
- **c̄ (cum)** — with
- **cc** — cubic centimeter
- **CC** — chief complaint
- **cm** — centimeter
- **CNS** — central nervous system
- **c/o** — complains of
- **CSF** — cerebrospinal fluid
- **/d** — per day
- **ENT** — ear, nose, and throat
- **F** — Fahrenheit
- **GI** — gastrointestinal
- **Gm (gm)** — gram
- **gr.** — grain
- **gtt (gutta)** — drop
- **H. (hora)** — hour
- **h.s. hora somni** — hour of sleep, at bedtime
- **hx.** — history
- **IM** — intramuscular
- **IV** — intravenous
- **kg** — kilogram
- **L** — liter
- **mEq.** — milliequivalent
- **mg** — milligram
- **ml** — milliliter
- **mm** — millimeter
- **noc. (nocte)** — night
- **NPO (nihil per ora)** — nothing by mouth
- **O.D. (oculus dexter)** — right eye
- **O.S. (oculus sinister)** — left eye
- **oz.** — ounce
- **P** — pulse
- **p.c. (post cibum)** — after meals
- **per** — through or by
- **p.r.n. (pro re nata)** — as needed

- **p.o. (per ora)** — by mouth
- **qd (quaque die)** — daily, every day
- **Q.h. (quaque hora)** — every hour
- **Q2h (quaque 2 hora)** — every 2 hours
- **Q4h (quaque 4 hora)** — every 4 hours
- **q.i.d. (quatuorindie)** — four times a day
- **q.s. (quantum sufficit)** — a sufficient quantity, as much as may be needed
- **R** — respiration
- **Rx. (recipe)** — prescription
- **s̄ (sine)** — without
- **s.c.** — subcutaneous
- **s.o.b.** — short of breath
- **s.o.s. (si opus sit)** — if necessary
- **stat. (statim)** — immediately
- **sx.** — symptom
- **T.** — temperature
- **tab.** — tablet
- **t.i.d.** — three times a day
- **tinct.** — tincture
- **Tx** — treatment
- **ung. (unguent)** — ointment
- **V.S. (V/S)** — vital signs
- **X** — times, multiplied
- **♂** — male
- **♀** — female

NOTES

1. Doris Cook Sutterley and Gloria Ferrara Donnelly, *Perspectives in Human Development.* Philadelphia, Lippincott, 1973, p. 251.
2. Lawrence L. Weed, *Medical Records, Medical Education and Patient Care.* Cleveland, The Press of Case Western Reserve, 1969.

SELECTED REFERENCES

Archer, Claude and Swearingen, Delores. "Application of Benjamin Franklin's Decision-Making Model to the Clinical Setting." *Nursing Forum,* 14(34):319, 1977.
Bailey, June and Claus, Karen. *Decision Making in Nursing.* St. Louis, Mosby, 1975.

Becknell, Eileen Pearlman and Smith, Dorothy M. *System of Nursing Practise.* Philadelphia, Davis, 1975.

Brainerd, Susan and LaMonica, Elaine. "A Creative Approach to Individualized Nursing Care." *Nursing Forum,* 14(2):188, 1975.

Fredette, Shiela. "Problem Solving with a Difficult Patient." *American Journal of Nursing,* 77:622, April, 1977.

———. "The Art of Applying Theory to Practise." *American Journal of Nursing,* 74:856, May, 1974.

Hansen, Marilyn. "Make Your Charting the 'Topic-of-the-Day'." *Nursing 76,* 6:74, May, 1976.

Johnson, Mae and Davis, Mary Lou C. *Problem Solving in Nursing Practise.* Dubuque, Iowa, Brown Foundation of Nursing Series, William C. Brown, 1970.

Miller, Benjamin and Keene, Claire. *Encyclopedia and Dictionary of Medicine, Nursing and Allied Health.* Philadelphia, Saunders, 1978.

Rosenow, Ann M. "Helping Practitioner Students Put Concepts Into Action." *Nursing Outlook,* 25:446, July, 1977.

Schaeffer, Jeannette. "The Interrelatedness of Decision Making and the Nursing Process." *American Journal of Nursing,* 74:1852, October, 1974.

Sundeen, Sandra, Wiscerz Stuart, Gail, DeSalvo-Rankin, Elizabeth and Parrino Cohen, Sylvia. *Nurse-Client Interaction: Implementing the Nursing Process.* St. Louis, Mosby, 1976.

Visiting Nurse Association, Burlington, Vt. *The Problem Oriented System in a Home Health Agency—A Training Manual.* New York, National League for Nursing, 1975.

Woody, Mary and Mallison, Mary. "The Problem Oriented System for Patient Care." *American Journal of Nursing,* 73:1168, July, 1973.

Yura, Helen and Walsh, Mary. *Human Needs and the Nursing Process.* New York, Appleton, 1978.

———. *The Nursing Process—Assessment, Planning, Intervention, Evaluation,* 2nd ed. New York, Appleton, 1978.

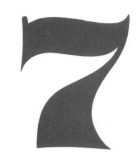

Obviously, a man's judgment cannot be better than the information on which it is based. . . .
—Arthur Hays Sulzberger

ASSESSMENT

The complexity of human beings and their interactions with their environment is reflected in the vast array of information that may be obtained about a single human situation. In the assessment phase of the nursing process the nurse selects, organizes, and analyzes information from the data which is applicable to the person's health status at a specific time. He or she looks at the relevance of incoming data and weeds out information that is not pertinent to the present situation. Assessment is not merely a random gathering of facts, but a purposeful process designed to provide a foundation on which to build nursing diagnoses, plans, interventions, and evaluations that will help change negative health behaviors to more positive ones. Therefore, nursing care is only as good as the assessment from which it is drawn.

PROCESS OF ASSESSMENT

In assessing, the nurse is like an investigative reporter who is sifting through superficial and often irrelevant findings to unearth the facts which will expose the real story. The nurse uses as sources the individual's thoughts, feelings, perceptions of the present situation, the nursing history, and the medical history. Testimony is provided by the individual directly, his or her level of growth and development, basic needs, family and/or significant others, the health team members, diagnostic tests, and written references.

Subjective and Objective Data

Basically, two categories of information are presented by this assessment—subjective and objective. To gather objective data, the nurse looks at the general environment, using observational skills, and then proceeds to do a cephalocaudal examination of the individual. At times the nurse will want to break down these general areas into more specific parts, for example, when measuring the individual's blood pressure or checking the temperature of the room. Collection of the objective data also includes the analysis of references such as the chart, textbooks, research studies, and conferences. The chart gives the past and present sequence of events for this individual, his or her actual behaviors, a record of therapies and interventions, and conclusions of the health team. References such as textbooks, research studies, and conferences provide the nurse with a point of reference, a knowledge base of expected behaviors, sequence of events, and outcomes of interventions.

Subjective data are collected through interviewing the individual and his or her family/significant others, verbal and nonverbal communication, team conferences, and inferences drawn from observation of behavior.

Both subjective and objective assessments of the nurse are guided, on the one hand, by the individual's level of growth and development, communication skills, basic health care needs, especially those threatened by the present situation, and health state, culture, and interaction patterns; and, on the other hand, assessments are guided by the use of all the nurse's senses, knowledge base, critical thinking skills, prior experiences, and culture and interaction patterns.

▶ The information the nurse has gathered is in the form of raw data. **Raw data** are the descriptions of objective and subjective information without analysis or interpretation. For these data to be useful the nurse must make inferences about their meanings and relationships to the individual's health state. In order to do this, the nurse simultaneously organizes and analyzes the incoming data.

Organization and Analysis of Data

The nurse first collects data and then organizes it into meaningful units. The process of organization takes place by identifying commonalities among the data. Therefore, information that is similar is grouped, such as all information related to the individual's ability to communicate or to ambulate. The categories that result from this grouping can then be examined for existing or potential threats to the person's ability to meet personal basic health care needs and thus affect his or her health state. Recognition of these threats can be facilitated by comparing the data in terms of abilities versus disabilities, capabilities versus limitations, strengths versus weaknesses, comfort versus discomfort, or expected behaviors versus actual behaviors. Chart 7.1 outlines examples of these comparisons.

Much information, though informative and interesting, is disregarded at this point since it does not relate to the present health care situation. It may be utilized at a later time or prove valuable if shared with another member of the health team within whose area of expertise it falls. People unfamiliar with assessing often have difficulty discriminating between relevant and irrelevant information. Oftentimes, asking the question "How does this information relate to a particular health situation or health care need assessment and what inferences can be made from this information?" helps to clarify the placement of data.

The nurse then searches for more information that will pertain to the threats she has identified. The same techniques are used, but the focus of the data collection is now specific. Thus if the nurse recognizes that an individual's comfort needs are being compromised by abdominal pain, the nurse looks at all available sources of information relevant to this pain. The chart, the individual's diagnosis, history of previous pain, what the person says about the pain, factors which increase or decrease the pain, reactions to the pain, ways of dealing with it, medical therapies prescribed for the pain, and research studies on pain are just some of the specific data the nurse might collect.

Assessment Factors

Regardless of the situation being assessed, the nurse collects information within the context of certain areas. These areas include the following:

- Vital statistics—identifying data such as age, sex, height, weight, and occupation
- Attitudes of the family and/or significant others—toward health care and present health state
- Personal preferences—concerning carrying out activities of daily living, personnel, scheduling
- Cultural factors—those social, ethnic, and spiritual factors which have a bearing on meeting health care needs
- Family and/or significant others interaction patterns—including structure, roles assumed, and supports
- Level of growth and development—effects of level of growth and development on health care needs
- Learning capacity—intellectual abilities and skills and motivation
- Socioeconomic factors—living environment, social pattern, and income

```
Chart 7.1
Comparison of Information
_____

COMPARISON        EXAMPLE

Ability           Ambulates without
                  assistance

Disability        Paralysis of left leg

Capability        Long-term recall of
                  information

Limitation        Short attention span

Strength          Family unit which
                  supports individual's
                  health choices

Weakness          Unemployed

Comfort           Free of pain

Discomfort        Complains of pain in
                  abdomen when
                  walking

Expected          No shortness of breath
                  when walking

Actual            Shortness of breath
                  when walks one block
```

```
Chart 7.2
Basic Health Needs and Subgroupings
_____

  I. Awareness needs
     A. Need for communication
     B. Sensory needs

 II. Safety needs
     A. Body kinetics
     B. Asepsis
     C. Environmental safety
     D. Chemical safety
     E. Psychosocial safety

III. Energy needs
     A. Intake of oxygen
     B. Transport and utilization of oxygen
        and removal of waste products
     C. Nutrition needs: intake
     D. Elimination needs: output
     E. Fluid and electrolyte needs

 IV. Security and esteem needs
     A. Body aesthetic needs
     B. Sleep and comfort needs
     C. Sexuality needs
     D. Grieving and loss
```

- Personal habits—smoking, drug taking, eating, exercise, etc., including frequency and amounts
- Previous experience with health care setting, personnel, and treatments
- Medical diagnosis and regimen—the physician's diagnosis(es) and plan of therapy
- Relationship of medical diagnosis(es) and regimen to nursing care
- Expected behaviors—what the individual is presenting
- Direction of desired change
- Available resources—support system present in the environment
- Influence of the environment on present health state
- Ways the individual is dealing with present health situation
- Communication skills and how the individual communicates needs

The nurse is now ready to identify negative health behaviors and analyze them for the factors that relate or contribute to these behaviors in order to form the nursing diagnosis (see Chap. 8). This same process is utilized for assessing all basic health care needs. Chart 7.2 lists the basic health care needs and their subgroupings. The nurse's assessment skills, the individual's diagnostic tests, and medical diagnoses provide the nurse with information from which to form the nursing diagnoses and subsequent plan of care.

ASSESSMENT TOOLS

The collection of data, both objective and subjective, requires that the nurse be proficient in many psychomotor and communication skills. These skills, like any others, are acquired and refined through repeated use in a variety of settings. The skills discussed here include observation, interviewing, history taking, and psychosocial and psychomotor evaluations.

Observation

▶ **Observation,** a basic tool for assessing information and behavior, is the use of all the senses to identify and categorize stimuli in the environment. Frequently, observation is thought to be only visual. However, one observes through the use of touch in order to identify shape, consistency, texture, temperature, and moisture; smell; hearing; and taste.

The process of observation begins with the presence of a stimuli which is received by a sense organ or group of sense organs. The sense organ picks up the stimuli and the afferent nerves transmit the stimulation through various pathways to higher centers in the brain. In the brain the stimuli are perceived, interpreted, and analyzed. It is at this point that the stimuli are actually identified and characterized. Finally, the efferent nerves transmit a message to the appropriate site for response.

Identifying and characterizing stimuli in the environment are influenced by empiricism, intuition,
▶ and reasoning. **Empiricism** is the use of facts and experiences as the basis for the interpretation and
▶ analysis of data, while **intuition** is one's perception of the meaning of an event or set of stimuli without any specific knowledge or facts about it. Intuition is based on the synthesis of previous knowledge and experi-
▶ ence to create a new insight into a situation. **Reasoning** is the use of inductive and/or deductive thinking to draw conclusions from a given set of stimuli or in-
▶ formation. **Inductive reasoning** is the drawing of
▶ generalized conclusions from specific data, and **deductive reasoning,** on the other hand, is the drawing of specific conclusions from general theories or principles. For example, a sound is produced by a door slamming. A person's ears receive the sound waves. The stimulation is transmitted to the auditory centers in the brain where it is identified and categorized as the sound of a slamming door and analyzed within the context of its occurrence. As a result of the analysis and interpretation a response is produced, such as calling out, "Who's there?" This process, while generally applicable for the reception and interpretation of stimuli, does not hold true for basic reflex reactions.

Several factors are necessary for the successful use of observation. First, sensory organs and afferent and efferent nerve tracts must be intact and functioning. Next, perceptual ability cannot be impaired as it may be in a person with brain damage or someone who uses certain categories of drugs or a person with a psychiatric disorder. Third, the individual has to have a knowledge and experience base on which to make an interpretation. Finally, the person must have the functional ability to respond.

OBSERVATION, A CONSCIOUS, PURPOSEFUL PROCESS

Observation is an ongoing process combining empirical, intuitive, and rational inferences, which more often than not occurs unconsciously. However, the nurse, to make best use of observation, must be consciously aware of the need to observe and consciously focus attention on what is to be observed. The ability to concentrate on what is being observed is enhanced by alertness, openness, and attentiveness. Therefore, interest in what he or she is observing plays an important part in the effectiveness of the process.

When assessing the individual or his or her behavior, observation should be planned, purposeful, and directed. This does not imply rigidity of action, but the focusing prevents distraction and incomplete observation. As the nurse observes, simultaneous reassessment and evaluation are occurring to determine whether the focus of the nurse's observation should be changed. Observation can be facilitated by first surveying the total environment to place subsequent observations in context. Then, the nurse zeros in on the specific event to observe it in detail and, finally, looks again at the whole picture to place the observation in context once more.

Since a large part of observation is interpretation analysis, it must be remembered that previous experiences, culture, and rigidity of thought can impart false or misleading connotations or values to the stimuli received. Thus if laughter is always equated with happiness by the observer, then situations when laughter is not motivated by happiness can be misinterpreted and inaccurate assessments made.

Observation can also be ineffective when the observer has preset ideas about what he or she will find. In this case the nurse may unconsciously select those stimuli which substantiate preformed ideas and overlook stimuli which would give a truer picture of the situation.

Once observations have been made, they can be

grouped with other data which pertain to the health situation. Then conclusions and judgments can be made as to the relevance of the observations and what further steps need to be taken. Observations are recorded in objective, descriptive terms rather than as subjective, interpretive conclusions.

Observation is rarely done in isolation, but rather in conjunction with other assessment and intervention skills such as interviewing. (Illustration 7.1)

Interviewing

▶ **Interviewing** is a communication skill in which the nurse explores thoughts, feelings, and perceptions of the individual; gathers and gives information; and clarifies goals. It is the major communication skill used in assessment. Interviewing incorporates the basic principles of communication discussed in Chapters 5 and 12 and is purposive, planned, and goal directed.

Illustration 7.1
Nursing assessment provides the foundation for the nursing process. Here, the nurse interviews *and* observes an individual, both important methods of assessing a person's health state. *(Photo by Ken Heyman)*

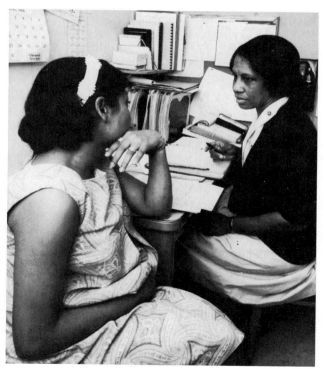

In attempting to collect objective and subjective data which are relevant to the health care needs of the individual, the nurse plans which areas to assess, the method to use, the setting in which the interview will take place, and the time to be allocated. By planning the direction of the interview, the nurse decides which general questions will best elicit the information desired and how most effectively to open the discussion. In part, the direction that is chosen will determine the approach the nurse will use and the type of questions asked.

THE DIRECTIVE APPROACH

If the nurse wishes to obtain straight factual information, the directive approach is used. In this type of approach, the nurse has a set of questions in mind, or even a written form in hand, such as a nursing history. The interview is usually opened by the nurse with a statement of the information that is being sought and the direction the interview will be taking. However, the direction of the interaction can change when and if the individual demonstrates a desire, whether expressed or not, to talk about an area which is not within the plan but for which there is a need. In this type of interaction, in-depth exploration of thoughts, feelings, and questions arising from the discussion is at a minimum. Verbal or written questionnaires are examples of this type of interview.

THE NONDIRECTIVE APPROACH

In contrast is the nondirective approach which focuses on exploration of the thoughts and feelings of the individual. This approach does not imply that the nurse does not guide the movement and direction of discussion. This type of interview usually opens with some general discussion and gradually moves to the focus point. In other words, it moves from the periphery to the center. This approach facilitates expression of thoughts and feelings, since it is usually nonthreatening and allows the individual to control the flow of discussion. The nurse directs the interview as common threads which keep appearing and need to be discussed are recognized, when situations or statements seem unclear, when the individual has difficulty expressing himself, and when the nurse feels the discussion is ready to move ahead.

A "COMBINED" TECHNIQUE

Most effective interviews are a combination of these two approaches. The directive approach is used to help open the interview and focus on the area for discussion. The nondirective approach is used to facilitate the expression of the thoughts, feelings, questions, and perceptions of the individual that are an outgrowth of the interview.

Questions which are asked can be either open or close ended. **Open-ended questions** encourage the individual to pursue his reactions in some detail. For example, "Tell me about the reactions your family had to your surgery" is an open-ended question. On the other hand, a **close-ended question** is one which requires only a single word or a short phrase as a response. "Did your family have any reactions to your surgery?" is an example of a close-ended question. Both types have a place in the nursing interview. There are times when a simple yes or no or a brief response is most appropriate. This is particularly true when the nurse is trying to collect vital statistics such as name, age, sex, and occupation. At other times, more detail and spontaneity of discussion fit the situation best.

Interview Conditions

The time the nurse sets aside for the interview is determined by the type of interview that is planned and the area of discussion. The time should be adequate enough to meet the purposes of the interview without interruptions that would necessitate starting and stopping the interview several times. A sufficient amount of time allows for continuity of thought and expression, a chance to develop rapport, and opportunity for the absorption of material discussed, and room for a relaxed, unhurried approach.

The atmosphere that is created for the interview should be conducive to the free exchange of information. Privacy, comfort, and freedom from distraction help achieve this atmosphere.

Interviewing can be done in conjunction with psychomotor skills. In fact, this is often the most natural time for such interactions to take place, for they do not appear contrived, and the interview can be directly placed within the care context.

Interviewing can be facilitated through the use of language and terminology the individual can understand and which is consistent with the individual's level of knowledge and stage of growth and develop-

ment. Medical terms, health jargon, and abbreviations often bewilder the individual and decrease communication. For example, rather than asking an individual how his ecchymotic area is resolving, the question can be more clearly and naturally asked as, "Is your black and blue mark going away?"

When taking a nursing history, the nurse finds out what terms the person uses for activities of daily living, for example bowel movements or eating. This is particularly true for children, who may have a private language for bodily activities and objects.

The nurse often uses phrases which may have negative connotations to the individual. Such questions as, "I understand you have been complaining of pain?" may evoke a defensive response from the individual. While the nurse simply means that the individual is experiencing pain, the individual may think that the nurse is saying he is being troublesome. Therefore, any expressions which may have mixed messages or confusing connotations are avoided.

Judgmental statements or actions can also hinder effective communication. The nurse's realization and acceptance that the individual may have a value or belief system that is different from the nurse's will help prevent the nurse from contradicting or cutting off discussion by judging it.

Allowing time for the individual to think and respond is necessary for the expression of thoughts, feelings, and values. Interrupting responses may make the person feel his responses are inappropriate or unimportant. Jumping in during silences may not give the individual time to organize or clarify his or her thoughts before speaking. Silences, though often anxiety provoking, can be a useful interviewing tool.

FEELING AT EASE

When first learning interviewing skills, the nurse sometimes feels that questioning an individual may be an invasion of privacy. However, if the interaction is planned for the purpose of helping the individual with his or her health care needs, then any information sought is not prying. When individuals are given the purpose behind a question, and understand it, and the tone in which it is asked is nonthreatening, neither the nurse nor the individual being interviewed needs be uncomfortable. Questions which do not pertain to meeting health care needs are not asked. Ultimately, it is remembered that the individual does have the right to refuse to answer questions or reveal any thoughts or feelings. However, many people who seem uncomfortable in revealing information may do so more easily once a feeling of trust and rapport has been established and the purpose of the interview explained.

PROCESS RECORDING

A useful method for analyzing the therapeutic and nontherapeutic aspects of an interview is **process recording**. In a process recording the nurse records all verbal and nonverbal interchanges between herself and the individual being interviewed. The nurse later identifies the development, movement, and direction of the interaction. In this way the nurse can recognize possible strengths in technique which enhanced the communication or what changes in technique should be made.

ACHIEVING EFFECTIVENESS

With practice each nurse finds a unique, comfortable style of interviewing which consistently gets the desired results. This effectiveness is often related not to an orthodoxy of approach, but to the sincere and sensitive nature of the nurse's interactions.

The Nursing History

The **nursing history** is obtained by using a specialized form for collecting nursing data. When completed, it provides the nurse with information about the individual's usual pattern of activities of daily living, perceptions of his or her illness and hospitalization, the family/significant others' structure and roles, economic supports, culture, social pattern, personal preferences, and chief complaints. The nursing history is usually taken on admission to the health care system and updated as necessary. It presents a base line of information used by the nurse in developing an assessment of the individual's health state.

The nursing history differs from the medical history in that it deals with the individual's responses to changes in his health status and patterns of living. The medical history, on the other hand, focuses on the sequence of events of the individual's present illness, contributing factors, and his illness—wellness history. Together the nursing and medical histories give a complete picture of the individual and his health care needs.

There are many types of nursing history forms. They range from questionnaires the individual fills out by checking appropriate responses to an unstructured interview, the results of which are then recorded. The ideal is a combination of open- and close-ended questions combined to give straight factual data as well as to explore thoughts, feelings, attitudes, and values. Chart 7.3 gives an example of one type of nursing history form.

Psychosocial Assessment

Several psychosocial areas need to be assessed to plan care which is based on the individual's competencies, abilities, and supports. Careful assessment of the individual's actual level of growth and development provides a basis of comparison with the expected behaviors at that level of growth and development. Chronological age cannot be automatically assumed to be representative of the actual level of growth and development. Hospitalization, anxiety, illness, changes in activity patterns, and individual differences may bring about variations from the expected. These variations may either be a movement to a higher level of growth and development or utilization of behaviors that were anxiety reducing at an earlier level. For example, a young adolescent faced with a severe illness may demonstrate an ability to make mature decisions relevant to the changes induced by the illness and follow through on those decisions. On the other hand, the school-age child, when hospitalized, may revert to the use of baby talk to express his needs.

Knowledge of expected behaviors such as psychomotor skills, language development, cognitive skills, psychosocial interaction patterns, physiological and physical development, play patterns, and body image development provide criteria for assessment. Most individuals, particularly adolescents and younger children, will demonstrate patterns of behavior which move across the strict lines of developmental stages. However, most people will have a pattern of behavior that predominates.

The composition and interaction patterns of the family and/or significant others and the support system which they provide for the individual are other necessary assessment areas. The role that the individual has within the structure of the family and/or significant others is examined to determine the effects his present health state has on his ability to fulfill that role. Any changes that take place are considered in re-

(continued on p. 140)

Chart 7.3

Assessment Data Collection Sheet

Student: _____   Date: _____

Patient: _____ Sex: _____ Marital status: _____ Admission date: _____

Culture: _____ Allergies: _____

Age: _____

Current health history: _____

Past health history: _____

PHYSICAL CHARACTERISTICS

Height: _____ Weight: _____ Body makeup: _____

Skin: Color: _____ Turgor: _____ Bruises: _____

           Discolorations: _____ Cyanosis: _____

           State of hydration: _____ Other: _____

Eyes: Sclera: _____ Pupils: _____

           Secretions/drainage: _____

           Vision: _____ Glasses/contact lens: _____

POSITION/ALIGNMENT

Position: Prone _____ Sims _____ Dorsal Recumbent _____ Lithotomy _____

            Supine _____ Fowlers _____ Semi-Fowlers _____ Other _____

Alignment: Appropriate _____ Inappropriate _____

MENTAL ACUITY

Oriented _____ Coherent _____ Appropriately responsive _____ Other _____

Disoriented _____ Incoherent _____ Inappropriately responsive _____

SENSORY/MOTOR RESTRICTIONS

Amputation _____ Deformity _____ Paresis _____ Paralysis _____ Fracture _____

Gait _____ Hearing disorder _____ Speech disorder_____ Other _____

EMOTIONAL STATUS

     Term   Description of behavior

Euphoric _____

Depressed _____

Apprehensive _____

Angry/hostile _____

Other _____

MEDICALLY IMPOSED RESTRICTIONS

CBR_____ BR-BRP _____OOB-Chair _____ Restricted ambulation _____

OTHER HEALTH BEHAVIORS

Fatigue _____ Restlessness _____Weakness _____ Insomnia _____Coughing _____

Dyspnea _____ Dizziness _____ Pain _____Others _____

(continued)

Chart 7.3 (Cont.)
Assessment Data Collection Sheet

ENVIRONMENT

Room Temperature: Comfortable _____ Uncomfortable _____
Lighting: Adequate _____ Inadequate _____
Access to needed items: Callbell _____ Personal items _____
Presence or absence of roommate _____

SAFETY

Violations of Medical Aseptic Techniques *(Describe):* _____
_____
_____

Violations of Safety Measures *(Describe):* _____
_____
_____

ACTIVITIES OF DAILY LIVING

Ability to perform the following tasks: Exercising _____
Bathing _____ Dressing _____
Feeding _____ Transferring _____
Other _____

GROWTH AND DEVELOPMENT (ERICKSON)

Chronological Age: _____ Developmental task for age: _____
_____
_____

Presenting behaviors: _____
_____
_____

Adaptations: _____
_____
_____

Sociocultural influences: _____
_____
_____

HIERARCHY OF NEEDS (MASLOW)

Based on data collected identify needs which are not being adequately met.
Physiologic _____ Security/survival _____ Self-respect _____
Belongingness–love–affection _____ Knowledge and understanding _____
Self-fulfillment _____ Aesthetics _____
What evidence do you have to support your statement?
_____
_____
_____

What resources are available to help the client meet his or her needs?
_____
_____
_____

(continued)

Chart 7.3 (Cont.)
Assessment Data Collection Sheet

COMMUNICATION

Influencing Factors:	Factors influencing communication

Mental alertness: _____

State of consciousness: _____

Culture: _____

Speech/language barriers: _____

Environmental distractions: _____

Level of growth and development: _____

Anxiety level: _____

State of health: _____

Therapeutic regimes: _____

Other: _____

Techniques: Techniques to promote effective communication

Comfortable environment: _____

Provisions for privacy: _____

Using broad openings: _____

Therapeutic use of silence: _____

Using reflective techniques: _____

Seeking clarification: _____

Attentive listening: _____

Verbalizing/noting observations: _____

Communicating concern/interest: _____

Therapeutic skills employed by nurse *(List)* _____

_____

_____

_____

Therapeutic skills observed by nurse *(List)* _____

_____

_____

_____

Verbal: Characteristics

Voice pitch: _____

Rapidity of speech: _____

Clarity of speech: _____

Verbal responses: Appropriate _____ Inappropriate _____

Extent of interaction: _____

Maintenance of content focus: _____

Nonverbal: Types *(Hays and Larson)*

Sign language: _____

Action language: _____

_____

Object language: _____

_____

Significant aspects of nonverbal communication observed *(Hays and Larson):* _____

_____

_____

Resources: What resources are available to promote effective communication? _____

_____

_____

(continued)

Chart 7.3 (Cont.)
Assessment Data Collection Sheet

SENSORY PERCEPTION

Influencing   Factors which affect the client's sensory perception
Factors: Mental alertness: _____
              State of consciousness: _____
              Environmental stimuli: _____
              State of sensory organs: _____
              Level of growth and development: _____
              Sleep: _____
              State of health: _____
              Psychosocial—cultural: _____
              Therapeutic regimes: _____
              Others: _____
Stimuli: Environmental
              Sources of stimuli: _____
              _____
              _____
              _____
              _____

              Which of the above stimuli appeared meaningful to the client? _____
              _____

              Which of the above stimuli appeared to lack meaning for the client? _____
              _____

              What presenting behaviors suggested the need for alteration in quantity and quality of stimuli? __
              _____
              _____

              Intervention measures designed to alter environmental stimuli: _____
              _____

              Intervention measures designed to alter the individual's response to environmental stimuli: _____
              _____
              _____

ASEPSIS

Medical   Techniques employed by nurse/Appropriate handling of:
Asepsis: Hands: _____
              Contaminated linens: _____

              Contaminated disposable items: _____

              Contaminated nondisposables: _____

              Body discharge/drainage items: _____

              Disinfection techniques employed:
              Concurrent: _____
              _____

(continued)

Chart 7.3 (Cont.)
Assessment Data Collection Sheet

Terminal: _____

Isolation Precautions:
Type:
Strict _____ Reverse _____ Respiratory _____ Enteric _____
Discharge _____ Blood _____ Wound/skin _____ Other _____
Measures for implementing precautions:
Gown _____ Glove _____ Mask _____ Linen _____ Clothing _____
Needles/syringes _____ Eating utensils _____
B-P apparatus _____ Other _____
Special safety precautions observed by nurse:
_____
_____
_____

Surgical Asepsis:
Techniques employed by nurse/Appropriate handling of:
Sterile objects: _____
Sterile fields: _____
Sterile solutions: _____
Sterile gloves: _____

Wound Care:
Characteristics of wound and drainage:
Affected part: _____
Type of wound: _____
Appearance and size of wound: _____
Type and color of drainage: _____
Amount of drainage: _____
State of surrounding skin: _____
Factors affecting healing:
Nutrition: _____
Circulation: _____
Infectious processes: Systemic _____
Local _____
Care of wound:
Frequency of care: _____
Cleansing solution: _____ Amount: _____
Type of dressing: _____
Equipment/supplies needed: _____
Care of surrounding skin: _____
Other: _____
Aseptic technique (medical/surgical) employed by nurse:
_____
_____
_____

Influence of wound on:
Mobility/kinetics: _____
Comfort: _____
What resources are available to help the client meet his need for aseptic safety? _____
_____
_____
_____

(continued)

Chart 7.3 (Cont.)
Assessment Data Collection Sheet

BODY KINETICS

Exercises: Type:
Active _____Passive _____Resistive _____
Active resistive _____Other: _____
Joint movement:
Flexion: _____
Extension: _____
Dorsiflexion: _____
Internal rotation: _____
External rotation: _____
Plantar-Palmar flexion: _____
Factors influencing functional capacity of muscles:
Strength: _____
Endurance: _____
Atony: _____Atrophy: _____
Contractures: _____Hypotonia: _____
State of health: _____
Others: _____
Influence of state of health on body kinetics—positions and alignment:
Prone: _____Sims: _____
Supine: _____
Semi-Fowlers: _____Fowlers: _____
Dorsal recumbent: _____
Other: _____
Alignment: _____

Transfer: Type of transfer activity:
Transfer technique: _____
Mental alertness/responsiveness: _____

Physical capabilities/limitations: _____

Safety of equipment: Aseptic _____
Mechanical _____
Assistive devices needed:
Cane _____Walker _____Crutch _____Brace _____Lift _____
Splints _____Trapeze _____Safety belts _____
Artificial limb _____Side rails _____Restraints _____
Others: _____
Equilibrium prior to transfer:
Dangling: _____
Subjective observations: _____

Objective observations: _____

(continued)

Chart 7.3 (Cont.)
Assessment Data Collection Sheet

Body
Mechanics: Body mechanics techniques employed by nurse:
_____
_____
_____
_____

What resources are available to assist the client with body kinetics? _____
_____

BODY AESTHETICS

Skin Care: Type of care:
Bath: _____
Provisions for privacy: _____
Provisions for comfort: _____
Client's ability to assist: _____
_____

Emollients/deodorants used: _____
Care to intertriginous areas: _____
Inspection of skin:
Reddened areas: _____ Decubiti: _____
Dryness: _____ Cracks/breaks: _____
Rashes: _____ Other: _____
Medical aseptic techniques employed:
_____
_____
_____

Mouth Care: Inspection and care of teeth and mucous membranes:
Teeth: _____ Brushed? _____
Gums: _____ Massaged? _____
Tongue: _____ Cleaned? _____
Mucous membrane: _____
Lips: _____ Lubricated? _____
Dentures: _____ Care: _____

Mouthwash: _____ Other: _____
Nails: Inspection and care:
Appearance: _____ Cuticles: _____
Peeling/breaks: _____ Cleaned? _____
Footcare: Inspection and care
Skin: _____
Interdigital areas: _____
Emollients used: _____
Soaks _____ Powder _____ Cotton _____ Dried _____
Influencing   Factors influencing body aesthetics:
Factors: Physical limitations: _____
Medical restrictions: _____
Psychosocial factors: _____
State of health: _____
Self-esteem: _____
Interest: _____

(continued)

Chart 7.3 (Cont.)
Assessment Data Collection Sheet

Other: _____

What is your rationale for the type of care administered? _____

_____
_____

What resources are available to assist the client with aesthetic needs? _____

_____
_____

OXYGENATION–CIRCULATION

Respirations: Characteristics:
    Rate: _____ Polypnea: _____
    Depth: Shallow _____ Deep _____ Hyperpnea _____
    Nature: Eupnea _____ Dyspnea _____ Stertorous _____
          Orthopnea _____ Other _____
    Factors/stressors influencing respirations:
    Emotional: _____
    Activity: _____
    Positioning/alignment: _____
    State of health: _____
    Other: _____
    Respiratory secretions:
    Type: _____ Color: _____
    Consistency: _____ Odor: _____
    Other: _____
    Intervention measures to facilitate adaptation (Oxygen-carbon dioxide exchange):
    Coughing exercises: _____
    Breathing exercises: _____
    Oxygen therapy: type _____ liters/min _____
    IPPB: coughing following treatment—NP _____ P _____
    Tracheotomy: _____
    Other: _____
Pulse: Characteristics: _____
    Rate/min _____ Tachycardia _____ Bradycardia _____
    Rhythm: Regular _____ Intermittent _____
    Volume: Bounding _____ Feeble–thready _____
    Site: Temporal _____ Carotid _____ Radial _____ AR _____
        Pedal _____ Femoral _____ Apical _____ Facial _____
    Factors/stressors influencing pulse rate:
    Emotional: _____
    Activity: _____
    Temperature and blood pressure: _____
    State of health: _____
    Other: _____
Temperature: Characteristics:
    Reading: _____ Hypothermia _____ Hyperthermia _____
    Site obtained: _____
    Variation from established pattern: _____

    Factors/stressors influencing temperature:
    Emotional: _____

(continued)

Chart 7.3 (Cont.)
Assessment Data Collection Sheet

Level of activity: _____

State of health: _____

Environmental temperature: _____

Intervention measures to facilitate adaptation:

(Temperature regulation):

Sponge bath: _____ Frequency _____ Other _____

Restricted activity: _____

Increased fluid intake: _____

Other: _____

Circulation: Blood pressure: _____ Systolic _____ Diastolic _____

Skin–mucous membrane inspection: Blanching _____

      Ecchymosis _____ Petechiae _____ Cyanosis _____

      Nailbed color _____ Other _____

Factors/stressors influencing circulation:

Activity–exercise: _____

Temperature: _____

Electrolyte balance: _____

State of health: _____

Other: _____

Intervention measures to facilitate adaption (circulation):

Application of heat and cold: Type _____

    Body part _____ Frequency _____

    Length of time _____

    Aseptic precautions _____

    Thermal precautions _____

Active exercise/ambulation: _____

Buerger-Allen _____ Teds _____ Ace bandages _____

Laboratory Values:	Test	Expected range	Presenting value
	Hct	_____	_____
	Hgb	_____	_____
	RBC	_____	_____
	CBC-diff.	_____	_____
	P_{CO_2}	_____	_____
	P_{O_2}	_____	_____
	BUN	_____	_____

FLUID AND ELECTROLYTES

Intake: Oral: Type _____ Amount/24 hr _____

        IV: Type _____ Amount/24 hr _____

           Amt. in bottle at start of tour _____

           gtts/min _____ cc/hr _____

           Electrolytes added _____

           Patency of tube _____

           Amt. in bottle at end of tour _____

           Phlebitis _____ Infiltration _____

Factors/stressors influencing fluid/electrolyte intake:

Amount of fluid intake: _____

(continued)

Chart 7.3 (Cont.)
Assessment Data Collection Sheet

Amount of food intake: _____

Environmental temperature: _____

Body temperature: _____

Elimination patterns: _____

Nausea/vomiting: _____

Other: _____

Laboratory Values:	Test	Expected range	Presenting value
	Na^+	_____	_____
	K^+	_____	_____
	Ca	_____	_____
	Mg	_____	_____
	Cl	_____	_____
	HCO_3	_____	_____
	HPO_4	_____	_____
	pH	_____	_____
	BUN	_____	_____

Output: Urinary:

Frequency _____ Amount/24 hr _____

Appearance _____ Color _____ Odor _____

Concentration _____ S-G _____ S-A _____

Blood _____ Other _____

Other: _____

Factors/stressors influencing fluid/electrolyte output:

Intake: _____

Stress/emotional status: _____

Diet: _____

Diuresis: _____ Electrolytes: _____

Other: _____

Intervention measures to facilitate adaptation (fluid/electrolyte output):

Diuretics: Type _____ Amount _____

Foley catheters: amount in bag at start of tour _____

    Amount in bag at end of tour _____

    Patency of tube _____

Gomco suction: pressure setting _____

    Patency of tube _____

    Replacement fluid _____

    Amount in bottle at start of tour _____

    Amount in bottle at end of tour _____

Other: _____

Gastrointestinal:

Frequency_____ Amount/24 hr _____

Appearance _____ Color _____ Odor _____

Consistency _____

Factors/stressors influencing GI output:

Diet: _____

Exercise/activity: _____

Stress/emotional status: _____

Medications: _____

(continued)

Chart 7.3 (Cont.)
Assessment Data Collection Sheet

Elimination habits: _____
State of health: _____
Other: _____
Intervention measures to facilitate adaptation:
(GI output)
Cathartics/laxatives: Type _____ Amount _____ Results _____
Enemas/irrigations: Type _____ Amount _____ Results _____
Dietary modifications: _____
Colostomy: Type _____ Psychosocial–culture factors/stressors _____

Rectal tube: Frequency _____ Results _____
What resources are available to assist the client with meeting fluid and electrolyte needs? _____

NUTRITION

Intake: Characteristics:
Pattern: _____
Adequacy: _____
Level of knowledge: _____
Psycho-social–cultural factors/stressors: _____

Other: _____
Factors/stressors influencing intake:
State of health: _____
Dietary restrictions: _____
Activity/exercise: _____
Dietary supplements: _____
Medications: Type _____ Frequency/amount _____ Results _____
Level of nutritional independence/dependence: _____
Emotional: _____
Other: _____

Laboratory Values:	Test	Expected range	Presenting range
	Upper GI	_____	_____
	Series	_____	_____
	Barium enema	_____	_____
	Gallbladder series	_____	_____
	Stool for:		
	Occult blood	_____	_____
	Parasites	_____	_____
	Other	_____	_____
	FBS	_____	_____
	Other:	_____	_____
		_____	_____
		_____	_____
		_____	_____

Intervention measures to facilitate adaptation (nutrition):
Nutrition teaching: _____

(continued)

Chart 7.3 (Cont.)
Assessment Data Collection Sheet

Assistance with feeding: _____
IV therapy: type: _____ amount: _____
Calories: _____
Feeding tube: type _____ formula: _____
Frequency: _____ amount: _____
Hyperalimentation: formula _____ frequency _____
Amount _____
Other: _____
What resources are available to assist the client with meeting nutrition needs? _____

SEXUALITY

Characteristics:
Pattern of expression: _____
Mode of expression: _____
Level of knowledge: _____
Psychosocial–cultural factors/stressors: _____
Variations from established pattern: _____
Other: _____
Factors/stressors influencing sexuality:
State of health: _____
Emotional: _____
Privacy: _____
Medications: _____
Level of growth and development: _____
Other: _____
Intervention measures to facilitate adaptation:
(Sexuality):
Sexuality teaching: _____
Counseling: _____
Environmental supports: _____
Other: _____

What resources are available to assist the client with meeting sexuality needs? _____

PHYSICAL ASSESSMENT

System:	Findings:
_____	_____
_____	_____
_____	_____
_____	_____

Used with permission of Uda Grant and Dorothy Booker, 1979.

lation to their effects on the whole system. The availability of family and significant others in terms of location, time, support, and resources is also an important assessment area. All these factors are assessed, not to be labeled as bad or good, but to provide the basis for planning any modifications that may be necessary in meeting the individual's health care needs. It is the family/significant others structure from which the individual comes and to which he or she will most likely return.

Much of this information is obtained through interviewing the individual and his or her family/significant others and through observing their interactions. As with any other assessment area, judgments and assumptions cannot be made based on one's own values and expectations. The existence of family members does not necessarily mean that they are the significant others in the individual's life or that they should be available and provide support. Significant others may range from intimate long-term friends to seemingly casual acquaintances to pets; and their supports may be obvious only to the individual.

Psychomotor Skills

Many psychomotor skills such as blood pressure or other vital sign measurements or neurologic checks are used in assessment but are discussed in more appropriate chapters subsequently.

PHYSICAL ASSESSMENT

In recent years more and more nurses have been gathering objective data through the physical examination. Findings made through physical examination assist the nurse in assessing the need for specific nursing care and in evaluating the effects of nursing care on the individual. The nurse does not use the exam to diagnose illness as does the physician when the physician carries out the physical examination. However, the tools the nurse uses and the procedures that the nurse follows are the same as those employed by the physician.

The most efficient approach for the physical examination is to begin with a general survey of the individual and then proceed in a cephalocaudal system-by-system examination. This approach gives the nurse an overview of the individual and often provides clues to areas that may need special attention. The orderly progression from head to toe ensures that no significant findings are missed. Throughout the physical examination the nurse will be interviewing the individual to discover feelings of discomfort, changes, and questions the individual might have. Also, the nurse will be explaining the examination procedure. Findings, whether expected or not, and variances should be recorded.

The general survey includes noting the overall appearance of the individual: appropriateness of dress, cleanliness, overall nutritional state (obese, thin, well nourished), hydration state, and apparent state of health and age. Skin, hair, and nails are assessed for texture, color, and pattern. Any odors should also be noted. Body structure is observed for bilateral symmetry, stature, and proportion. Gross neuromuscular coordination is another factor assessed: gait, coordination of movements, extraneous movements, posture, and use of extremities. The presence of supportive, prosthetic, or corrective devices are noted. Reports of any area of pain, discomfort, or disability are recorded and kept in mind for more specific examination.

The individual's appropriateness of mood, affect, and response are part of the general survey. Communication skills, speech pattern, and ability to answer questions and give a history are also considered.

The nurse proceeds to the cephalocaudal examination using the methods of inspection/observation, palpation, percussion, and auscultation.

All the physical examination skills require considerable practice for the examiner to acquire proficiency. It is often beneficial to begin practice on individuals who fall within the expected ranges and then proceed to individuals with notable variations. This gives the examiner a basis for comparison of the expected and actual findings.

The specific examinations of body systems are described in the subsequent chapters pertaining to the health care need being discussed.

Inspection

▶ **Inspection** is the visualization and observation of the individual's body. When inspecting the individual's body surface, proper lighting is an important factor in preventing distortion of findings. Natural sunlight is the best light; however, any nonfluorescent illumination will do. (Illustration 7.2)

Comparisons are made between expected and actual findings. Variations from the expected such as swelling, discoloration, eruption, discontinuity, scarring, and alterations in size, shape, and symmetry are described as well as expected findings. Height and weight are measured as are any changes in surface appearance such as rashes, wounds, or swollen parts.

Any extraneous and audible sounds made during breathing, speaking, or moving are assessed. These and other observations are assessed in detail as the examination progresses.

Equipment used for inspection includes the otoscope to examine the structure and integrity of the ear canal; a tuning fork to test hearing acuity; the ophthalmascope to view the internal parts of the eye and blood vessels; a flashlight to trigger reactions of the pupil; specula to examine the nose, vaginal canal, cervix, and rectum; and a tape measure to measure masses, lesions, or body parts.

Palpation

▶ **Palpation** is the use of touch to determine the temperature, texture, size, shape, movement, and location of skin surfaces, organs, or masses and to feel pulsations. The fingers, palms, or backs of the hands are used, depending on the type of palpation being done.

When palpating areas of the body which are bilateral, one side of the body is compared with the other for symmetry. During palpation, attempts are made to relax the individual so that muscle tension does not interfere with obtaining accurate information. Chart 7.4 outlines the characteristics of nodes or masses.

Percussion

When one surface taps or strikes another, a sound vibration is produced which will reflect the density of the underlying surfaces. This tapping is known as ▶ **percussion.** The vibration is both heard and felt by the examiner. During the physical examination, the middle finger of one hand is lightly placed on the area to be percussed and is lightly tapped at the base of the distal phalanx by the tip of the middle finger of the other hand. These tappings should be quick and rebounding to prevent interference with vibration, and movement should be initiated from the wrist

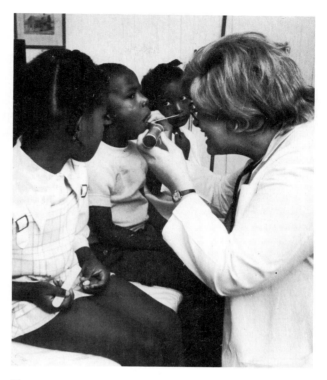

Illustration 7.2
A nurse inspects the mouths of students for cleanliness, oral deformities, and dental caries, as well as for indications of systemic disease. An additional hand light is used to insure adequate vision. (*Photo by Paul Conklin, from Monkmeyer Press Photo Service*)

(Illustration 7.3). The more dense the area percussed, the higher, less discernible, and shorter lived will be ▶ the sound. The reverse is also true. **Tympany** is the sound which is produced when closed air-filled cavities ▶ are percussed, e.g., the stomach. **Hyperresonance** is produced in an area where either the amount of air has increased or the amount of tissue has decreased in relationship or both. Air-filled cavities such as the lung ▶ and thorax produce **resonance** when percussed. ▶ **Dullness** occurs in tissues that are relatively dense such as the kidney, spleen, and liver. When the area is completely solid, as with muscle tissue, the sound ▶ produced is **flatness.**

Percussion is used to determine the borders of various organs, to detect collection of fluid or air in body organs, to discover fibrous formations in tissue, and to explore tissue tenderness. Percussion is also used to elicit tendon reflexes at the elbow, wrist, knee, and ankle. This type of percussion can be done

Chart 7.4

Characteristics Assessed in Examination of Lymph Nodes or Masses

Location	Be specific in describing the site. Use imaginary body lines or axes and bony prominences to relate findings. Draw pictures where appropriate.
Size	Define the volume in centimeters in three dimensions of length, width, and thickness. State the total volume. Describe the shape lucidly (round, cylindrical); if irregular, draw pictures.
Surface characteristics	Describe accurately as smooth, nodular, irregular.
Consistency	Describe as hard, firm, soft, resilient, spongy, cystic.
Symmetry	Used as a comparison of paired structures.
Fixation, mobility	Describe exact mobile parameters in centimeters. If mass is fixed in position, identify whether fixation is to underlying or overlying tissue.
Tenderness	Describe whether present without stimulation or elicited by palpation or movement. Indicate whether direct, referred, or rebound.
Erythema	Describe extent of color change if present.
Heat	Describe extent if present.
Pulsatile nature	Describe pulsations when they are usually not palpable at this locus. Auscultate all pulsating masses for *bruits*.
Increased vascularity	Describe prominence of overlying veins or cyanosis of the area
Transillumination	If pathologic structure is in an anatomical area that can be transilluminated such as the scrotum, describe the results of the procedure.

From: Lois Malasanos, Violet Barkauskas, Muriel Moss and Kathryn Stoltenberg-Allen. *Health Assessment,* (St. Louis: Mosby Company, 1977, p. 167).

by using the ulnar aspect of the hand or a percussion hammer.

Auscultation

Listening with the aid of a stethoscope for sounds made by the body is called **auscultation.** Auscultation is used to listen to sounds emanating from the flow of blood through the heart and blood vessels and the flow of air through the respiratory tree and gastrointestinal tract. The diaphragm head of the stethoscope is used to hear high- and midrange-frequency sounds such as abdominal, breath, or heart sounds; and the bell head is used for low-frequency sounds such as heart murmurs. (Illustration 7.4)

DIAGNOSTIC TESTS

A source of meaningful objective data is diagnostic tests. They provide information as to the individual's actual physiologic and physical status to allow comparison with the expected values. While these test results assist the physician to diagnose and treat the individual's illness, they provide the nurse with valuable guides to what may be expected in the individual's behavior and what care should be planned. For example, if the individual has a low hemoglobin level (anemia), the nurse can anticipate that the individual will fatigue easily; therefore, care activities will have to be geared toward energy preservation.

Diagnostic tests frequently include hematologic studies, urinalyses, radiographic studies, scans, elec-

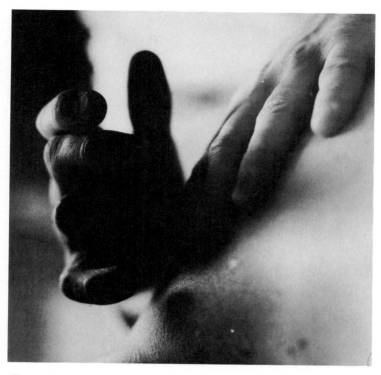

Illustration 7.3
Palpation. *(Photo © Mottke Weissman, from Photo Researchers, Inc.)*

trocardiograms, specimen analyses, and biopsies. Hematologic studies assay the constituents of the blood. These specimens are commonly taken from the venous circulation. Urinalyses test the components of the urine and often reflect renal function, metabolism, and catabolism. The electrocardiogram measures the electrical impulses generated by the heart muscle. Radiographic studies are comparative examinations of radiopaque (dense areas which absorb rays) and radiolucent (less dense areas which do not absorb rays) structures. They take the form of simple gross or microscopic visualizations of tissues such as bone or visualization after the introduction of a radiopaque dye. In scanning, an organ-specific radioactive element is given, either by mouth or intravenously, and detectors are used to record the movement of the isotope in the tissue. Specimen analyses are the microscopic and chemical studies of body cells, fluids, and excreta. In biopsies, body tissue is removed through surgery, scraping or aspiration and analyzed for cellular composition and distribution.

These tests often engender anxiety and fear in the individual undergoing them and in the family and/or significant others. These reactions may be the result of fear of the test itself, concern about the outcome, or apprehension over possible side effects or after effects of the test. No matter how routine a diagnostic test may seem to the nurse, it is not an everyday experience for the individual undergoing it or for the family and/or significant others. Each procedure is explained in terms the individual and the family and/or significant others can understand, and questions concerning it are answered honestly. This reduces fear of the unknown and helps prevent acute anxiety reactions during the procedure which will interfere with testing. Cooperation is usually increased as a result of appropriate explanations.

The role the individual will play during the procedure is also explained. For example, if the individual is to lie still or hold a particular position for the test, pretest instructions will allay anxiety and increase cooperation. The equipment that is used and the set-

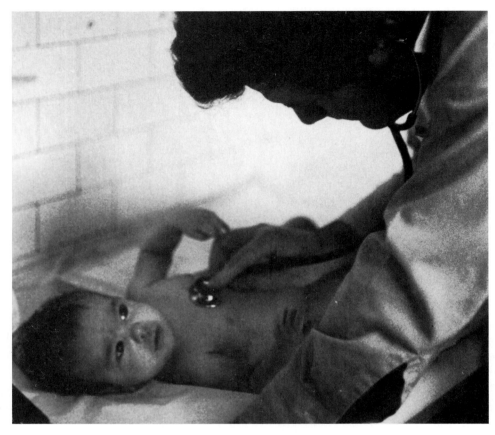

Illustration 7.4

Auscultation. A nurse uses a stethoscope to listen to an infant's heart sounds. *(Photo © Jan Lukas, 1979, from Photo Researchers, Inc.)*

ting for testing is also discussed to help the individual anticipate what will happen to him.

Any specific posttest care, e.g., bed rest, is explained both before and after the test. This may alleviate any fears that the individual and the family and/or significant others have that the individual is receiving special care because "something went wrong." It also increases posttest cooperation.

All diagnostic tests are basically invasive processes. The individual may fear disruption of his or her body pattern, which could result in a distortion of self-image. People often seem to have exaggerated or atypical anxiety responses to seemingly painless or "simple" procedures. The individuals themselves may not even understand their reactions. These reactions, however, may be a total body response to the invasion of body boundaries.

Specific diagnostic tests and pertinent nursing care are discussed in the subsequent appropriate chapters.

MEDICAL DIAGNOSIS AND PHYSICIAN'S ORDERS

Based on the physical examination, diagnostic tests, and previous knowledge, the physician makes a diagnosis of the individual's pathologic condition. In many cases the data may be insufficient for the physician to make a definitive diagnosis, so the impressions of probable or possible pathologies are stated for further investigation.

Actual or tentative diagnoses provide the nurse

with further data. Medical diagnoses expand his or her knowledge base as to the disease process and its effect and possible sequelae. The nurse also utilizes this information in order to recognize and anticipate therapies that will be ordered, possible negative health behaviors the individual may demonstrate, and what teaching the individual will require.

The physician's orders, like the medical diagnosis, provide information for the nurse. They state those functions the physician has delegated to the nurse. These dependent and collaborative nursing activities provide some of the basis for her plan of care. The nurse's knowledge of the expected outcomes of the therapies ordered helps in anticipating the probable health behaviors for which the nurse will plan nursing actions that will best support the individual throughout the therapeutic regimen.

ASSESSMENT—AN ONGOING PROCESS

Assessment, no matter how thorough, is never complete, since the individual and his environment are constantly changing. Also, the investigative nature of data collection will often uncover gaps in data which will have to be filled in if accurate nursing diagnoses are to be made. Thus nursing assessment is a continual process of collection, organization, and analysis of data, and of evaluation and reassessment.

Figure 7.1 shows examples of assessment (pages 146–51).

SELECTED REFERENCES

Baer, Ellen D., McGowan, Madeline, and McGivern, Diane. "Taking a Health History." *American Journal of Nursing,* 77:1190, July, 1977.

Batten, J. D. "Face to Face Communication." *Nursing Digest,* 1:89, Spring, 1977.

Bates, Barbara. *A Guide to Physical Examination.* Philadelphia, Lippincott, 1974.

Bayer, Mary. "Community Diagnosis—Through Sense, Sight and Sound." *Nursing Outlook,* 21:712, November, 1973.

Byers, Virginia. *Nursing Observation,* 3rd ed. Dubuque, Iowa: William C. Brown, 1977.

Chinn, Peggy L. *Child Health Maintenance Concepts in Family-Centered Care,* 2nd ed. St. Louis, Mosby, 1979.

——— and Leitch, Cynthia J. *Child Health Maintenance: A Guide to Clinical Assessment,* 2nd ed. 1979.

Frances, Gloria and Munjas, Barbara. *Manual of Social Pscychologic Assessment.* New York, Appleton, 1976.

Crawford, C. and Palm, M. "Can I Take My Teddy Bear." *American Journal of Nursing,* 73:236, February, 1974.

Eggland, Ellen. "How to Take a Meaningful History." *Nursing 77,* 8:77, July, 1977.

Fowler, Marsha. "Behold the Great Right Toe." *American Journal of Nursing,* 74:1817, October, 1974.

Malasanos, Louis, Barkauskas, Violet, Moss, Muriel and Stoltenberg-Allen, Kathryn. *Health Assessment.* St. Louis, Mosby, 1977.

Malloy, Jan. "Taking Exception to Problem-Oriented Nursing Care." *American Journal of Nursing.* 76:582, April, 1976.

Mezey, Mathy, Rauckhorst, Louise, and Stokes, Shirlee A. "The Health History of the Aged Person." *Journal of Gerontology,* 3:47, May-June, 1977.

Murphy, Rev. John B. "Recognizing Your Patients Spiritual Needs." *Nursing 77,* 7:64, December, 1977.

National League for Nursing. *Problem-Oriented Systems of Patient Care.* New York, National League for Nursing, 1974.

"Patient Assessment: Taking a Patient's History (Programmed Instruction)." *American Journal of Nursing,* 74:293, February, 1974.

Riley-Kesler, Arlene. "Pitfalls to Avoid in Interviewing Outpatients." *Nursing 77,* 7:70, September, 1970.

Sana, Josephine M. and Judge, Richard D. *Physical Appraisal Methods in Nursing Practise.* Boston, Little, Brown, 1975.

Snyder, Joyce C. and Wilson, Margo F. "Elements of a Psychologic Assessment." *American Journal of Nursing,* 77:235, February, 1977.

Walter, Judith, Pardee, Geraldine, and Molbo, Doris, eds. *Dynamics of Problem-Oriented Approaches: Patient Care and Documentation.* Philadelphia, Lippincontt, 1976.

Wolff, Helen and Erickson, Roberta. "The Assessment Man." *Nursing Outlook,* 25:103, February, 1977.

Figure 7.1
An example of a completed assessment data collection sheet. (Adapted with permission from initial assessment by Victoria Reilly, Fundamentals of Nursing student, Long Island University, Department of Nursing)

ASSESSMENT DATA COLLECTION SHEET

Student: _Victoria Reilly_   Date: _3/12/79_

Patient: _Lydia Stone_   Sex: _F_   Marital Status: _Widow_   Admission Date: _3/10/79_

Culture: _American Black, Protestant_   Allergies: _none_

Current Health History: _Chronic brain syndrome, hip & knee contractures bilaterally, atherosclerosis, dehydration, unresponsive to stimuli, agitated_

Past Health History: _Cerebral vascular accident, chronic anemia, chronic brain syndrome. Transferred from nursing home to hospital as a result of lack of response to stimuli. No previous history available. Pt. unable to relate history. No known significant others._

PHYSICAL CHARACTERISTICS

Height: _5'4"_   Weight: _130 lbs_   Body Make-up: _medium frame_

Skin: Color: _Ebony_   Turgor: _Slight tenting_   Bruises: _no_

Discolorations: _no_   Cyanosis: _no_

State of Hydration: _Skin mucous membranes dry, no edema, skin cracked on feet, dime sized reddened areas on both heels_   Other: _____

Eyes: Sclera: _clear_   Pupils: _PERLA_

Secretions/drainage: _none_

Vision: _cannot be assessed at present_   Glasses/contact lens: _none_

POSITION/ALIGNMENT

Position: Prone _____ Sims _____ Dorsal Recumbent _✓_ Lithotomy _____

Supine _____ Fowlers _____ Semi-fowlers _____ Other _____

Alignment: Appropriate _____ Inappropriate _left hip internally rotated & left knee pressed against right knee, foot drop_

146

MENTAL ACUITY

Oriented _____ Coherent _____ Appropriately responsive _____ Other _____

Disoriented ___✓___ Incoherent ___✓___ Inappropriately responsive _____

oriented X1, repeats non word syllables, mumbles, answers to questions do not follow logical thought process

SENSORY/MOTOR RESTRICTIONS

Amputation _____ Deformity ___✓___ Paresis _____ Paralysis _____ Fracture ___✓___

Gait _____ Hearing disorder _____ Speech disorder ___✓___ Other _____

hip & knee contractures bilaterally, foot drop, on complete bedrest has aphasia other- sensory restriction, perceptual deprivation - inability to apply meaning to stimuli

EMOTIONAL STATUS

TERM   DESCRIPTION OF BEHAVIOR

Euphoric ___✓___ *laughed @ no apparent stimuli*

Depressed _____

Apprehensive _____ *watched every move. at times would relax & return smile, clutched bed clothes*

Angry/hostile _____ *attempted to hit when bed clothes were removed*

Other _____

MEDICALLY IMPOSED RESTRICTIONS

CBR ___✓___ BR – BRP _____ OOB – Chair _____ Restricted ambulation _____

Posey restraints ordered PRN

OTHER HEALTH BEHAVIORS

Fatigue ___✓___ Restlessness _____ Weakness _____ Insomnia _____ Coughing _____

Dyspnea _____ Dizziness _____ Pain _____ Other _____

although she was alert & awake in my presence, fell asleep as soon as I left the room

ENVIRONMENT

Room temperature: Comfortable *but draft from window* _____ Uncomfortable _____

Lighting: Adequate *blinds open, room light on* _____ Inadequate _____

Access to needed items: Callbell _____ Personal items _____ *available but she did not seem to be aware of their presence or use*

Presence or absence of roommate: *two bedded room, student with other individual, roommate: 21 year old with frequent visitors, OOB as desired spends much of time in solarium*

U. Grant D. Booker 2/26/79

(continued)

Figure 7.1 (Cont.)

SAFETY

Violations of Medical Aseptic Techniques (*Describe*)

incontinent of urine & feces-this provides an ideal place for organisms to grow & can cause tissue breakdown-found with dried fecal matter

on perineum

Violations of Safety Measures (*Describe*)

found with side rail down, no postural supports to maintain alignment

ACTIVITIES OF DAILY LIVING

Ability to perform the following tasks: Exercising   *limited-can turn from side to side*

Bathing   *none*   Dressing   *none*

Feeding   *none*   Transferring   *none*

Other   *Can perform no ADL without complete or partial assistance*

GROWTH AND DEVELOPMENT (*Erickson*)

Chronological age   *79*   Developmental Task for Age: *Integrity vs despair stage when individual attempts to maintain ego integrity in face of*

role loss, chronic illness, loss of significant others

Presenting behaviors: *because of individual's disorientation, aphasia & lack of appropriate response it is difficult to say wehther or not she has been*

successful in meeting developmental task, one would have had to assess this from previous history or significant others which are unavailable

Adaptations: *previous adaptation cannot be determined because of above mentioned factors, on day of admission, poseys necessary all day, now only*

at night - fewer reports of hitting

Socio-cultural Influences: *cannot be assessed at present - however - no known significant others to provide supports, has been institutionalized for*

six years

148

HIERARCHY OF NEEDS (Maslow)

Based on data collected identify needs which are not being adequately met.

Physiological ✓_____ Security/survival _____ Self Respect ✓_____

Belongingness-love-affection ✓_____ Knowledge and Understanding ✓_____

Self-fulfillment ✓_____ Aesthetics ✓_____

What evidence do you have to support your statement? _Because of physiological & cognitive impairments she does not seem to understand why or what the nurses are doing for her. This may increase her apprehension & uncooperativeness. Although the environment is providing for her survival needs she does not act as if she feels secure. According to Maslow to meet self fulfillment needs one has to have an accurate perception of reality which she does not give evidence of having. It is difficult to assess the degree to which her needs are being met because of her present condition. I am not certain that her self respect needs are not being met but she did show signs of modesty & because of her incontinence she may have lost some self respect. I could not adequately assess this but I saw no signs from her non verbal communication to this effect._

What resources are available to help the client meet his/her needs? _patient responds favorably to touch, smiles, soft voice, time spent with her by personnel, bedside physical therapy, visiting volunteers, continuity of care_

COMMUNICATION

INFLUENCING FACTORS: _Factors Influencing Communication_

Mental alertness: _alert but disoriented_

State of consciousness: _alert but doesn't respond appropriately at all times_

Culture: _not known_

Speech/language barriers: _aphasia, mumbles_

Environment distractions: _upon looking back may have been too much going on - possible sensory overload_

Level of growth & development: _can't be determined at present_

Anxiety level: _not known_

State of health: _aphasia, cognitive dysfunction & perceptual deprivation improve communication ability_

Therapeutic regimes: _↑d hydration, ↑d exercise, ↑ oxygenation_

Other: _soft voice, explanations increase cooperation_

UG/DB 2/26/79

(continued)

149

Figure 7.1 (Cont.)

TECHNIQUES: *Techniques to Promote Effective Communication*

Comfortable environment: _unhurried activity, maintain privacy, repetition of explanations, time to respond_

Provisions for privacy: _pulled curtains during bath_

Using broad openings: _not therapeutic for this individual at this time needs specific structured interactions_

Therapeutic use of silence: _____

Using reflective techniques: _____

Seeking clarification: _attempted to clarify, repeat, speak more slowly, attempted to associate actions with words_

Attentive listening: _allowed time for her speaking_

Verbalizing/noting observations: _validated facial expressions & gestures_

Communicating concern/interest: _did things in unhurried manner, used tongue frequently, accepted behavior, verbalizations_

Therapeutic Skills Employed by Nurse (List) _listening, touch, smiling, unhurried actions low, calm tone of voice, met basic physiologic needs carried on conversation appropriate to level of growth & development & state of health, oriented her to time & place, used positive reinforcement of appropriate behavior_

Therapeutic Skills Observed by Nurse (List) _head nurse entered room – introduced self & oriented individual #3. Physician stroked patients arm while examining_

VERBAL: *Characteristics*

Voice pitch: _low_

Rapidity of speech: _rapid_

Clarity of speech: _words slurred together_

Verbal responses: Appropriate _____ Inappropriate _at times_

Extent of interaction: _carried on conversation with individual responding frequently altho not always appropriately_

Maintenance of content focus: _attention span extremely short, essentially individual unable to communicate verbally_

150

NONVERBAL: *Types (Hays & Larson)*

Sign language: _nodding, eye contact, smiling_

Action language: _attempting to pull up covers, held on to my hands, attempted to hit when approached rapidly_

Object language: _individual unable to arrange own belongings, had food hoarded in pillow case_

Significant Aspects of Non-verbal Communication Observed (Hays & Larson)

major appropriate mode of communication for patient

RESOURCES: What resources are available to promote effective communication?

continuity of care by staff - use of same staff to provide care, initially structured repetitive activities, orientation x3

stable environmental setting, acquisition of personal belongings from nursing home, correlation of sounds & gestures used by

patient to meanings, encourage verbalization, use of magazines to increase verbalization & attention span

NOTES:

UG/DB 2/26/79

151

The power to guess the unseen from the seen, to trace the implications of things, to judge the whole piece by the pattern. . . .

—Henry James

NURSING DIAGNOSIS

IDENTIFYING ELEMENTS OF THE NURSING DIAGNOSIS

Once data have been collected, organized, and analyzed, a picture of the individual's existing or potential negative health behavior emerges. A **negative health behavior** is any pattern of observable responses which indicates an inability to meet a health care need. For example, using Figure 6.5, information gained from the collection and organization of data reveals that this individual has basically two negative health behaviors: overeating and limited motivation for weight loss. These two behaviors are interrelated and both refer to the same group of health care needs. While both are similar, they are not the same, as they reflect different aspects of the data collected and lead to different plans for nursing care. In many instances negative health behaviors may not be so directly related. However, no matter how divergent the behaviors, there is an overall interaction among them as they relate to the whole person, since a change in any part of the human system results in a change in the whole system.

The negative health behaviors are then analyzed for the factors that contribute to their occurrence.

The nursing diagnoses that are finally formulated show relationships between an identified negative health behavior and the factor(s) which are most likely contributing to its occurrence.

To recognize the factors that are most likely contributing to the negative health behavior, it is first necessary to identify all possible factors which may account for the behavior. This is done by the nurse's sifting through all collected data. A broad knowledge base and previous experience will expand the nurse's ability to recognize choices. When reviewing the data, the nurse groups similar negative health behaviors (there may be many) which relate to the same health care need or group of needs.

When grouping data, analysis also helps to show the relationship between seemingly dissimilar negative health behaviors which are, in fact, related to the same health care need. Often the same set of circumstances directly influences many body subsystems, resulting in apparently divergent negative health behaviors. For example, the individual on long-term bedrest may develop respiratory difficulty, constipation, or loss of muscle tone. These negative health behaviors appear to belong to different categories of health care needs; however, inactivity is the major contributing factor for them all.

Once the contributing factor has been identified, the nurse analyzes it for specificity. This means that the contributing factor has been taken to its least common denominator so that the factor cannot be further broken down into units which could by themselves account for the negative health behaviors. Therefore, terms such as immobility, loss of appetite, or anxiety are not specific enough, since each one can be broken down into components which could contribute to the negative health behavior. The least common denominator is not a medical diagnosis or disease or a factor that cannot be altered through nursing intervention. Thus contributing factors such as pneumonia, deafness, or economics are not appropriate in a nursing diagnosis.

NURSING DIAGNOSIS DEFINED

Nursing diagnoses are statements of probable relationships between an identified negative health behavior and the factor(s) most likely contributing to its occurrence. Like hypotheses, they are statements of probable relationships whose validity is tested through evaluating the effectiveness of the nursing intervention that is directed at changing the negative health behavior by alleviating the contributing factors. When interventions have not produced the predicted change, evaluation may show that the contributing factors were not related to the negative health behavior.

Several factors influence the formulation of nursing diagnoses. The complexity and urgency of the situation helps determine the number of nursing diagnoses appropriate for a situation, the specificity of the contributing factors, and the priority of the diagnoses. The nurse's previous experience and knowledge aid in the identification of the negative health behavior, the contributing factors, and the relationship between them. The more information and experience the nurse has, the more versatile he or she becomes in formulating accurate, useful nursing diagnoses. The degree to which the individual follows the expected course of events in his behavioral response to health situations greatly influences the ability of the nurse to predict the individual's pattern of responses and thus formulate potential nursing diagnoses. Nursing diagnoses are only as good as the as-

sessment on which they are based. Therefore, an incomplete or inaccurate data base will lead to less reliable nursing diagnoses.

TYPES OF NURSING DIAGNOSES

Nursing diagnoses can be categorized as immediate, foreseeable or possible. **Immediate nursing diagnoses** are based directly on behaviors the person is presently exhibiting and for which there are verifiable data. **Forseeable nursing** diagnoses are statements of behavior having a high probability based on the person's previous health responses, the nurse's prior experiences, and the usual sequelae of events for similar occurrences, but which are not presently manifested. **Possible nursing diagnoses** include statements of behavior that have been known to occur in similar circumstances but for which there is not presently an adequate data base.

Immediate nursing diagnoses can be considered actual, while foreseeable and possible nursing diagnoses can be considered potential. An example of an immediate nursing diagnosis is obesity related to high caloric intake and limited exercise, a forseeable nursing diagnosis is potential for decubitus ulcer on sacrum related to decreased blood supply to area from long periods of sitting; a possible nursing diagnosis is possible sensory deprivation related to decreased stimulation during isolation precautions.

PURPOSES OF NURSING DIAGNOSES

Nursing diagnoses written in this way provide a direction for care. A nursing diagnosis is the fulcrum between the assessment that has been made and the planning and intervention being carried out. It not only enables the nurse to see the negative health behavior to be changed but also provides a focus for the method of change. If the nursing diagnosis has been appropriately and accurately stated the nurse can bring about the desired change by alleviating the contributing factors.

Care that is organized around the individual's

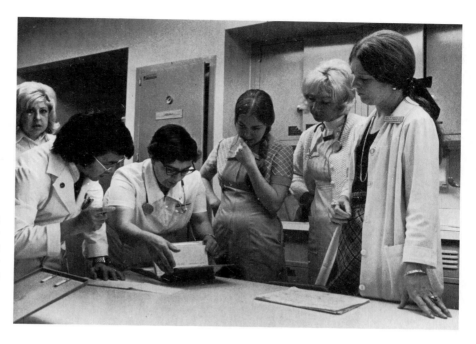

Illustration 8.1
In reviewing data, health team members assist the nurse to analyze an individual's negative health behaviors. From that analysis, nursing diagnoses are set forth and intervention planned. *(Photo by Suzanne Wu, from Jeroboam)*

presenting behavior rather than isolated data is less fragmented and goal oriented rather than task oriented. Thus, care is more comprehensive and individualized and recognizes the interrelationships within the total person. (Illustration 8.1)

Stating the specific negative health behavior enables the nurse to measure the direction and quantity of change that ensues. Pinpointing the contributing factor(s) that the nurse has determined as the basis for the negative health behavior assists the nurse in evaluating the effectiveness of the methods utilized to bring about the change and the appropriateness of the contributing factors that were selected.

Validation for the use of the nursing process is facilitated by the nursing diagnosis. The nursing diagnosis documents the critical thinking, problem solving, and analytic processes the nurse has utilized to formulate a plan of care, which is scientifically based. Therefore, care is not random or hit and miss. Furthermore, the nursing diagnosis gives evidence of the need for time to be spent with the individual and his family and/or significant others, and in team conferences; the need for equipment and staff; and the need for the nurse's activities in assessing, planning, intervening, and evaluating.

Through compilation, evaluation, and validation of nursing diagnoses a compendium of diagnoses can be developed which will add to the unique body of nursing knowledge. Care is improved and the profes-

sion is benefited by having a common language and a sharing of thought since this compendium would be common to all.

DIFFERENTIATION BETWEEN NURSING AND MEDICAL DIAGNOSES

A nursing diagnosis is not to be confused with a medical diagnosis. Medical diagnoses deal with disease, while nursing diagnoses deal with the human responses to changes in health status. These two types of diagnoses are not in conflict with each other as they evolve from distinct areas of expertise and are both aimed at helping the individual through differing but complementary methods. There is an overlapping of much of the data used to make both a nursing and a medical diagnosis—for example, the principles of anatomy and physiology, psychology and chemistry. However, the interpretation of the data will differ, thus resulting in the different diagnoses.

Comparable diagnoses generated from the same set of data may appear as "viral pneumonia" (a medical diagnosis) and as "difficulty breathing in a recumbent position related to increased mucus production" (a nursing diagnosis).

Medical diagnoses are usually written as statements of pathophysiologic processes or illness. Since these diagnoses have evolved through the years from symptoms and therapies, a plan of care is usually implied with these statements. Through assembling a compendium of nursing diagnoses, nursing is attempting to create the same uniformity of methodology.

ACTUAL AND POTENTIAL DIAGNOSES

Many actual and potential nursing diagnoses can be derived from each nursing assessment. As previously discussed, the exact number will be dependent on the scope and depth of assessment, the priorities of the care situation, the setting, the time available and the nurse's knowledge and skills. An example of an actual nursing diagnosis derived from the assessment in the previous chapter could be:

- Decreased ability to communicate verbally related to disorientation.

A potential nursing diagnosis could be:

- A potential for loneliness related to an absence of significant others in the immediate environment.

Part Two gives additional examples of actual and potential nursing diagnoses as they relate to specific basic health care needs. Part Three illustrates a more comprehensive set of nursing diagnoses based on an in-depth nursing assessment.

SELECTED REFERENCES

Aspinall, Mary Jo. "Nursing Diagnosis—The Weak Link." *Nursing Outlook,* 24:433, July, 1976.

Bircher, Andrea U. "On the Development and Classification of Nursing Diagnoses." *Nursing Forum,* 13:10, 1974.

Brown, Martha M. "The Epidemiologic Approach to the Study of Clinical Nursing Diagnoses." *Nursing Forum,* 13:346, 1974.

Gebbie, Kristine M. and Lavin, Mary Ann, eds. *Classification of Nursing Diagnoses: Proceedings of the First National Conference.* St. Louis, Mosby, 1975.

Gordon, Marjorie. "Nursing Diagnosis and the Diagnostic Process." *American Journal of Nursing,* 76:1298, August, 1976.

———. "Classification of Nursing Diagnosis." *The Journal of the New York State Nurses Association,* 19:5, 1978.

Mundinger, Mary O. and Jauron, Grace D. "Developing a Nursing Diagnosis. *Nursing Outlook,* 23:94, February, 1975.

In the long run men hit only what they aim at.
—Henry David Thoreau, Walden

9

PLANNING

Effective change is created when nursing intervention evolves from a plan based on the assessment of the individual's health care needs and scientific reasoning and collaboration with the individual, his family and/or significant others and the health care team. Planning serves to make a positive change in the direction of the individual's health responses in the most organized, efficient, and effective manner. Through goal setting, provision of options, identifying alternative approaches of care, and scheduling of time, energy, personnel, and equipment, the nurse produces a plan which can bring about the desired changes. The several steps involved in devising a plan are goal setting, formulating a blueprint to achieve the goals, and communicating the plan to others.

GOAL SETTING

Goals are derived from nursing diagnoses that are based on a sound nursing assessment of the individual's actual health state. This process determines how broadly or specifically the goals are stated. Nursing diagnoses delineate the negative health behaviors to be changed, and the **goals** are statements of the specific changes to be planned. Goals may be directed toward treating an existing condition, preventing a more negative health state, or both. Like nursing diagnoses, goals are written in behavioral terms so changes in the individual can be measured. Goals state the criteria for what observable behavior will occur as a result of the change and the time frame within which it will occur.

Goals reflect the behaviors to be observed in the individual, not the activities to be carried out by the nurse. Thus goals are individual centered, not nurse centered. Goals are written in language which is precise and specific so all who are involved in the individual's care understand their meaning and intent. Goals are individualized for a particular person and should not be so global in scope that they become "catchalls." For instance, "increased fluid intake" gives very little information to the reader. However, "increased intake of fluid of choice to 8 ounces every hour while awake" gives the health care team information as to what negative health behavior of the individual is to be changed, the method for changing it, and the criteria by which the change can be measured.

Factors Influencing Goals

In setting meaningful goals, the nurse considers the capabilities, limitations, and preferences of the individual. Nursing assessment factors such as physiologic state, endurance, interaction patterns, level of growth and development, and conditions which affect the individual's environment are important determinants in goal setting. External factors such as the care setting and the availability of personnel, equipment, and time are other components of the goal-setting process. To complete the preparation for the setting of obtainable and realistic goals, interactions are initiated between the individual, his family and/or significant others, and relevant health team members in order to incorporate all their potential for changing the direction of the individual's health state.

These components (the individual's environment, certain external factors, and interpersonal interaction) are interdependent, and therefore, all three are necessary considerations in the setting of successful goals. For example, nursing assessment of the individual may indicate that to prevent an increase in the diameter of his *decubitus ulcer* (pressure sore), the individual needs to be turned every hour around the clock since he or she is incapable of doing so alone. But the necessary manpower to carry this out may not be available during certain hours of the day, and the individual may not want to be awakened every hour while asleep. Therefore, while the goal, "prevention of increase in diameter of decubitus ulcer by turning every hour" may be physiologically preferable, other important factors make this goal unrealistic, and thus unattainable.

Scope of Goals

Goals that the nurse sets fall within the realm and expertise of the nursing team and are not activities carried out by other health team members. However, collaboration among the individual, his family and/or significant others, the nurse, and other health team members is vital to the success of the plan. Goals should be complementary with the goals of the individual, the family and/or significant others, and other health team members and not conflict with their plans for care. No matter how well formulated, goals which do not have input from all concerned are doomed to failure. Since the goals center around the individual's behavior, the nurse cannot plan in isola-

tion or impose her will on the individual and the family and/or significant others. For example, the nurse is assisting to limit an individual's sodium intake severely by not adding salt in food preparation. The nurse's assessment, however, has revealed that he is Jewish and follows the Orthodox tenets of his religion, which include the soaking of all meats in salt solution. The nurse, therefore, discards that particular goal and works with the individual to find alternate goals which meet the individual's health needs as well as his preferences. This approach not only includes collaboration with the individual, but also indicates the nurse's flexibility in goal setting.

Types of Goals

Individualizing the goals establishes their range and priority. Goals may be immediate, intermediate, and long range. **Long-range goals** are future-oriented objectives toward which all other goals are directed. They represent the general health change that is ultimately desired. The time span set for their achievement may vary greatly. It is not the length of time involved which makes a goal long range, but the progressive building on previous goals.

Goals which are **intermediate range** are transitional steps from the specific to the general. They are more future oriented than immediate but are not the final health behavior change desired.

Immediate-range goals are present-oriented objectives which must be accomplished before successive intermediate and long-range goals can be accomplished. These goals are often directed at the basic human needs, although any level need may be included in an immediate goal. They require no prior goal setting to be met, but usually have many complementary goals. They are specifically stated behaviors, which need to occur to bring about the desired general health change. As with intermediate and long-range goals, it is not the amount of time designated for the achievement of this type of goal which makes it immediate range, but rather that it must be accomplished before succeeding goals can be met.

Long-range goals are established first. From these goals the intermediate and then the immediate range goals are derived. This progression allows for building on levels of achievement and helps to insure that the goals are purposeful and directed. For example, if the nursing assessment has indicated that "ambulating in room without assistance 5 days after surgery" is an obtainable, realistic, long-term goal, then the intermediate goal of "ambulating in room with assistance 3 days after surgery" might be developed. This is followed by a set of immediate goals such as "dangling legs over side of bed for 15 minutes evening of surgery" and "ambulating to chair with assistance 1 day postoperatively."

Priority of Goals

The establishment of priorities is an important factor in goal setting. The goals of the highest priority are those aimed at changing threats to basic survival. Maslow's hierarchy of needs (Chap. 5) provides a guideline for determining priorities of care. Once the basic physiologic needs have been met, priorities are determined through collaboration with the individual and his family and/or significant others. What is a priority to the nurse may not be a priority for the individual. Assessment data provide information about priority needs of the individual.

Unless the individual sees a goal as relevant to himself, he will not be an active participant in meeting it. Open discussion between the nurse and the individual about each other's goals avoids conflict and allows for the compromise and cooperation necessary to achieve both sets of goals. Explanation of the variety of options available enables an individual to increase his or her choices and make informed decisions. The ultimate decisions for health care rest with the individual and the family and/or significant others.

ORGANIZING A PLAN

Organization of the nursing care plan focuses on devising an efficient, effective method for reaching goals, thereby making a positive change in the health status of the individual. The state of the individual's internal and external environment determines the plan of choice, but alternative plans are kept in mind if changes become necessary. The nurse uses his or her knowledge, experience, and repertoire of professional responses in identifying alternative approaches. These approaches are in turn discussed with the individual and the family and/or significant others so that the most appropriate course of action for the individual's care can be chosen. In this way,

the person and the family and/or significant others are truly active, informed participants. Consultation with the other members of the health team takes advantage of their knowledge and resources and helps to ensure their cooperation in carrying out the plan. For instance, if the nurse plans to use a mechanical lift to transfer an individual who is afraid of the lift, then an alternative plan of using a three-person lift can be employed instead. (Illustration 9.1)

Scheduling

Scheduling the sequence of care is based on priority of needs, availability of personnel, equipment, time, and the preferences of the individual. The individual whose health state i.e., nutrition, integument, level of consciousness, and mobility, requires that he or she be turned every 2 hours must have a schedule of hours to be turned and devices and personnel to assist with the turning integrated into the plan for meeting this person's other health needs.

It is rare in the care situation that the nurse will care for a single individual. Therefore, it can be both practical and beneficial for the nurse to plan to carry out appropriate group activities such as exercise classes and nutrition teaching. This not only makes efficient use of the nurse's time and energy, but also allows the individuals to share experiences and to assist one another.

The plan must be as concise and detailed as possible to include the who, what, where, when, and how of the care, as well as the preferences of the individual. In this way, care can be individualized, continuity is maintained, and care improved and made more efficient, since every person reading the plan will have a complete and comparable picture of the care to be given.

Ordering the Plan

Once the priorities have been established and the details of the plan determined, a useful way for the nurse to organize care is to group interventions into those which she "must do," "should do," and "would like to do." The "must do" activities are those which are essential to the individual's health, comfort, and general well-being. The "should do" activities are those which the nurse feels will augment the effectiveness of his or her care but which are not vital to the individual's state of health. Finally, the

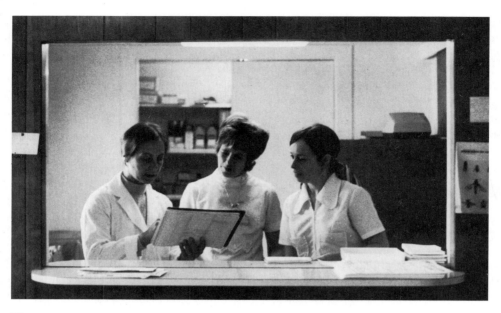

Illustration 9.1

In planning for an individual's health care needs, collaboration among health team members will promote effective change. *(Photo © Peter Arnold, from Erika)*

"would like to do" activities are those which can be eliminated when time and personnel are limited without compromising safety and effectiveness of care. These groupings are different for each care situation, as a "must do" in one case may be a "should do" in another. Grouping interventions in this way helps to overcome the overwhelming feeling of pressure and stress when the nurse is faced with a multifaceted care situation or multiple assignments.

Because of the constant nature of change, no plan can take into account all circumstances. Therefore, the strict adherence to any one plan leads to frustration of both the nurse and the individual and to the inadequate provision of effective personalized care.

COLLABORATIVE PLANNING ACTIVITIES

The nurse is most often the coordinator of health care. Since the nurse spends the most time with individuals, sees them in all phases of health, has round-the-clock input, comes in contact the most with the family and/or significant others, and is pivotal in care activities, the nurse is the most likely choice for this role.

As the coordinator of care, the nurse needs to plan for the full participation of all health team members. Collaboration is facilitated when all team members share common philosophies and goals of care. This sharing is expedited and new ideas generated through frequent health care team meetings which include the individual and the family and/or significant others. Information is shared during these meetings through effective recording and verbal communication and when there is mutual respect of each member for the contributions of all the others.

Team conferences are planned on a regular basis when the greatest number of people involved are available. Tape recordings can be made of these conferences so absent members concerned can refer to the proceedings and share their input. Ideas generated in this way are incorporated into the plan of care.

PLANNING FOR DELEGATION OF ACTIVITIES

The nurse may intervene directly with the individual and indirectly through supervision of those to whom he or she has delegated activities. The nurse delegates care activities to other nurses and ancillary personnel.

Chart 9.1
Nursing Goals and Plan

NURSING DIAGNOSIS	GOAL	PLAN
Decreased ability to communicate verbally related to disorientation.	**Short Range** Orientation 3 times in week	1. Present time and place information when providing care 2. Place large calendar within sight 3. Place clock within sight 4. When OOB in chair place near window 5. Discuss current events 6. Identify meals, e.g., breakfast, lunch, dinner 7. Provide stimuli to all senses 8. Keep number of personnel caring for individual to a minimum 9. Meet physiologic needs as outlined in plan for other nursing diagnoses
	Intermediate Increased appropriate verbalization as evidenced by accurate and reality-based responses to stimuli within 2 weeks	1. As above 2. Positively comment on and reinforce appropriate verbalizations 3. Accept but do not validate inappropriate responses 4. Without arguing with individual, provide reality 5. Give individual time to express complete thoughts 6. Ask simple questions using simple terminology which is appropriate to level of growth and development related to activities of daily living 7. Take to dayroom BID 8. Introduce to other people in dayroom 9. Provide time and opportunity to carry out own activities of daily living within capabilities 10. Ask other personnel to visit individual
	Long Range Initiates appropriate interactions verbally Sustains verbal interactions	1. As above 2. Provide opportunity to initiate interactions through use of open-ended questions 3. Relay information on plan and progress to nursing home personnel 4. Reinforce progress with individual

Delegation of activity is based on matching the needs of the individual with the expertise of the nursing team member, the laws regarding nursing activities, and the policies of the health care facility.

When supervising personnel who have been delegated activities, the nurse may be accountable for their acts of omission and commission and is also accountable to the individual for the quality of health care he or she receives. Thus the nurse plans the teaching and guiding of the nursing team, the collation and synthesis of their reports on the direction of change in the individual's health state, and the evaluation of the entire process of defining and meeting health care needs.

Through collaborative goal setting and organization of the care plan which includes the individual, the family and/or significant others, the nurse, and the other health team members, the interventions which follow from the plan are best directed to meet the health care needs of the individual.

Chart 9.1 gives an example of the goals and plan devised for the actual nursing diagnosis stated in Chapter 8.

SELECTED REFERENCES

Bayer, Mary and Brandner, Patty. "Nurse/Patient Peer Practice." *American Journal of Nursing,* 77:86, January, 1977.

Little, Dolares and Carneveli, Doris. *Nursing Care Planning,* 2nd ed. Philadelphia, Lippincott, 1976.

McClosky, Joanne C. "The Nursing Care Plan: Past, Present and Uncertain Future—A Review of the Literature." *Nursing Forum,* 15:364, 1975.

Rivers, R. E. "Priorities According to Need." *Nursing Outlook,* 26:404, July 1978.

Smith, Dorothy M. "Writing Objectives as a Nursing Practice Skill." *American Journal of Nursing,* 71:319, February, 1971.

Wiley, Loy. "The ABC's of Time Management." *Nursing 78,* 8:105, September, 1978.

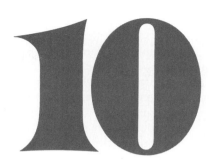

So much one man can do, that does both act and know.

—Andrew Marvell

INTERVENTION

Once the goals have been set and the plan devised, the action phase of the nursing process begins. Intervention is based directly on the plan which is aimed at changing negative behaviors to more positive ones. As with the plan, intervention is not merely a set of tasks to be completed, but a means of most effectively helping to meet the individual's health needs.

DYNAMICS OF INTERVENTION

Individuals are complex, dynamic, unique beings who are constantly changing. As they change, their health needs necessarily change also. Since goals are a means to an end, not the end in themselves, the nurse takes into account the nature of human beings when intervening. Therefore, the intervention phase of the nursing process is not a stagnant, rote following of a rigid plan, but rather a tool for creative change.

Throughout intervention the nurse is constantly reassessing the situation for any modification which needs to take place. As the individual's level of wellness increases or decreases, priorities of care may

rapidly or subtly alter. The implementation of one seemingly small nursing action may be sufficient to necessitate a major revision in the plan and thus in the intervention. For example, the nurse has planned to spend 15 minutes to begin teaching a diabetic person how to self-administer insulin. In starting, the nurse recognizes that the individual is very much worried about his wife's not calling him at the usual time. Realizing that anxiety blocks learning, the nurse spends that time helping him contact his wife. In this situation, the nurse's versatility has allowed for effective intervention to meet the needs of the individual at that time, although the original and subsequent plans had to be revised.

The ability to recognize that it is often necessary to alter original plans and institute a new one is an important factor in promoting flexibility in intervention to meet the health needs of the individual most effectively. Critical thinking skills allow for rapid assessment and modification. When new actions need to be substituted for previously planned ones, the nurse's knowledge, experience, and repertoire of professional responses facilitate flexibility. If, initially, the nurse's plan adequately included options and anticipated modifications, this "switching of gears" is easier.

INTERVENTION SKILLS

The execution of the intervention phase requires the utilization of all the nurse's change skills. Intervention is often thought of as the use of only the psychomotor skills. However, communication, teaching–learning, leadership, management, and group process skills are equally necessary to create a change in the health state of the individual.

The type of change skill which predominates during intervention depends on the individual's ability to meet his own needs at that point in time. When the individual's basic physiologic needs are severely threatened, the nurse concentrates on those psychomotor activities which will best meet these needs and support and restore vital function.

If security, love, and self-esteem needs are the ones most threatened, then the emphasis is placed on interaction skills, while at other times the individual's health state will demand an equal combination of all types of intervention skills. However, the focus on one type of skill does not exclude all the others. Nursing actions are balanced so that care is directed at meeting the health needs of the total person. (Illustration 10.1)

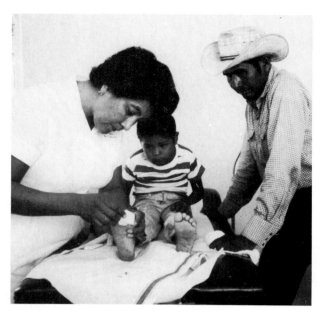

Illustration 10.1
During intervention, as during the other phases of the nursing process, the nurse takes into account the unique nature of human beings in order to effectively meet an individual's health needs. Here, a Native American youngster is treated by a nurse on an Arizona reservation. *(Photo by Paul Conklin, from Monkmeyer)*

SCIENTIFIC PRINCIPLES AND INTERVENTION

All nursing interventions, whether independent, dependent, or collaborative, are based on scientific principles. This foundation for nursing provides the nurse with a broad scope of knowledge on which to base critical thinking and from which to select interventions. This knowledge base is extrapolated from the liberal arts, including the natural sciences, the fine arts, and the social sciences, and allows the nurse to develop multifaceted insights and judgments into the holistic nature of human behavior. Through synthesis the nurse can then transfer pertinent information to the identification and treatment of health-related behaviors.

Care that is built on scientific principles is logical, defensible, and safe. Since there are many ways to achieve any one care goal, recognition of underlying principles assists the nurse in choosing the one method which best fits the situation at hand. In addition, understanding the probability of the outcome of specific interactions allows the nurse to anticipate the nature and direction of change.

COLLABORATIVE INTERVENTION

Any type of intervention is a collaborative effort of the individual, family and/or significant others, nurse and other members of the health team.

The Nurse and the Individual

The nurse works with the individual to supplement those areas of function where disabilities, weaknesses, limitations, and discomfort impede the individual's ability to meet his or her own health goals. The nurse also works with the individual to support those abilities, strengths, capabilities, and comforts that are sufficient to fulfill his or her own needs satisfactorily and to meet personal health goals. As the individual's level of wellness and independence increase, the nurse's supplemental actions decrease while supportive functions increase. When the individual's level of wellness and independence decrease, the reverse is true. For example, when an individual in an acute phase of illness is unable to feed, bathe, or even turn alone, the nurse carries out these activities. As the individual recovers his or her ability to do these things, the nurse concurrently relinquishes the responsibilities. However, the nurse then works with the individual to promote and support these capabilities. Assisting the individual to conserve energy by pacing and teaching methods of self-care are just some of the ways the nurse gives support.

The Health Care Team and the Individual

Collaborative interventions that include all health team members and the individual provide for continuity of care. Through each member contributing his or her expertise to complement one another's action, care is focused on the individual, and there is an optimum utilization of time, energy, and personnel. In this way, health team members are less apt to lay claim to one area of intervention while ignoring the overall health care picture. Care is not divided or segmented; rather each member builds on and substantiates all efforts to provide integrated interventions that enhance the care situation.

For example, the individual scheduled for physical therapy twice a day to strengthen muscles weakened by illness interacts not only with the physical therapist, but also with the nurse, the dietitian, and physician. With collaboration, an exercise program is developed which accounts for the changes in dietary needs, the energy levels of the individual, follow-through in nursing care, correlation of physician's orders, and scheduling of the individual's daily activities. Thus the individual's caloric intake is increased to provide for energy expenditure and support muscle growth; frequent rest periods are planned throughout the day; nursing care builds on and utilizes newly acquired abilities; a mild pain medication (analgesic) is ordered for joint pain; and other energy expending therapies are not scheduled just prior to or after exercise.

In addition, an atmosphere of cooperation and interchange of information is created so the individual's preferences are complied with; progress or lack of progress is shared; reactions to care are assessed; and modifications are made in interventions.

The Family and/or Significant Others and the Health Team

When the family and/or significant others are active participants in the health care regimen, the full circle of collaboration is completed. This collaboration helps to meet the needs of the individual, the family and/or significant others, and the health care team. It recognizes the reciprocal roles and interdependence between the individual and the family and/or significant others and provides more complete care than the health team can by itself. The involvement of the family and/or significant others in providing health care prevents the usurping of their ties and supports. It also allows health team members to utilize their time and energy more efficiently and effectively.

The family and/or significant others can be involved, with guidance from the nurse, in all areas of care such as feeding, bathing, and ambulating. Their inclusion in teaching health promotion and maintenance increases the cooperation of both the individual and the family and/or significant others, ensures continuity of care in the home setting, promotes understanding of the individual's abilities and limitations, and helps the individual and family and/or significant others to feel in control of the situation.

Following is an excerpt from a nurse's notes that pertains to the interventions for the sample plan:

DAY 1
2 P.M. Active assistive range of motion exercises done to all extremities. Full range of motion in upper extremities. No change in hip movement. Did not wince when feet dorsiflexed to 45° angle. Asked, "When is lunch?" Informed lunch was an hour ago by time on clock and asked if she were hungry. No response elicited but drank 4 ounces orange juice. Transferred to chair by window with no distress noted. Shown buds on trees. Left with magazine.

Douglas Edwards, R. N.

SELECTED REFERENCES

Carlson, Carolyn and Blackwell, Betty, eds. *Behavioral Concepts and Nursing Intervention,* 2nd ed. Philadelphia, Lippincott, 1978.
Nordmark, Madelyn and Rohweder, Anne. *Scientific Foundations of Nursing.* Philadelphia, Lippincott, 1975.

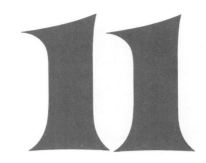

The best laid plans of mice and men often go astray.
—Robert Burns

EVALUATION

Evaluation of the individual's health care needs focuses on the direction of the change in the person's health state. All the factors which contribute to the individual's health state must be evaluated to provide a comprehensive picture of not only the degree of change, but also the process by which it has occurred. Since the individual simultaneously receives care from many health team members, the goals and care of those groups must be examined to see whether they complement or conflict with each other. The health care setting (the environment in which the individual receives health care services) must also be considered. Nursing care is therefore looked at in the context of the total care regimen.

CRITERIA

▶ **Evaluation** is a continuous and ongoing process which takes place throughout all phases of the nursing process, as well as at the completion of the care situation. Whenever possible, it is important to decide the criteria for evaluation prior to initiating any

action which is to be evaluated, such as degree of ability to perform a task. When the general goals for the overall care process as well as the specific individual-centered goals are stated in behavioral terms, the evaluation process is simplified and made easier since the evaluation criteria (the expected behaviors) are built in. When evaluation is not based upon pre-established criteria, significant factors are overlooked and the evaluation can be unconsciously manipulated to reflect the desired results. For example, before the nurse makes her assessment, he or she has in mind the general areas which he or she will be examining to determine the individual health care needs and their effects on the total care process.

The criteria for evaluation includes not only what changes occurred but also whether the direction of change was the predicted one, what phase of the nursing process went right and what phase went wrong and the process by which the change took place. The purpose of evaluation is not to lay blame on any individual or chain of events but to determine what modifications can be made within the system to improve the effectiveness and efficiency of care. The method of evaluation is not as important as the recognition of which factors are the significant ones to be examined.

General criteria for evaluating changes in the individual's health state include:

- How do the physiologic, psychosocial, and environmental changes relate to the individual's ability to meet health care needs?
- Have the changes in one system affected the other systems?
- Has the presenting behavior moved closer to the expected?
- What is the direction of change towards independence in meeting health care needs?
- What are the factors which account for the changes?
- What skills have been acquired by the individual and the family and/or significant others in utilizing equipment, performing exercises, communicating needs, etc.?
- What are the changes in attitude of the individual and the family and/or significant others toward changes in the individuals health state?
- What are the changes in knowledge about the health state?
- Have there been changes in personal habits?
- What are the changes in abilities, capabilities, comfort, safety, etc.?
- What are the changes in coping with increased/decreased stress?
- Can the person function safely in the existing environment?
- What environmental changes need to be made? Have they been made?
- Have the health care needs of the individual changed?

The actual factors that are evaluated will depend on the individual and the particular situation. Evaluation, like assessment, is not merely the answering of a series of questions with a yes or no, but an objective description and analysis of the process that is occurring.

EVALUATION OF NURSING PROCESS

The nursing process is evaluated for its effectiveness as a problem-solving technique in meeting the health care needs of the individual. As with other care evaluations, each phase should be evaluated as it is occurring and the total process examined when it is completed.

General criteria for evaluating the nursing process include:

- Was the assessment complete? Appropriate?
- Were the nursing diagnoses complete? Appropriate?
- Were the goals set behaviorally? Appropriately?
- Were the goals met?
- Were all participants (individual, health team members, family and/or significant others) satisfied with the manner in which the goals were met?
- What was the degree of participation of health team members, individual, family and/or significant others?
- Was the planning complete? Appropriate?
- What changes were necessary in planning and intervention?
- Was the intervention safe? Efficient? Effective?
- Did evaluation take place throughout all steps?
- What modifications in care are needed?
- Were all steps of the nursing process communicated effectively? To whom?

EVALUATION OF THE NURSING TEAM

The nursing team's ability to set and reach health care goals and to create a conducive health care environment is another aspect of care to be evaluated. The nurse may be called on to evaluate the nursing team or participate in the group's evaluation of itself.

General criteria for evaluating the effectiveness of the nursing team include:

- Were the individual's needs matched with the capabilities of personnel?
- Did each nursing team member understand the assignment and have the skills necessary to carry it out?
- What teaching was necessary?
- What changes in ability resulted?

- Was the time available adequate to carry out activities? Personnel? Equipment?
- What modifications are still necessary?
- Was there continuous, effective communication among nursing team members?
- What were the reactions of the individuals receiving care to the care given?
- What were the reactions of the personnel to assignments?
- Were there shared philosophies and goals of care among team members?
- Did the group work as a cohesive team?
- What ideas were generated by team conferences?
- How were these ideas incorporated into nursing care?
- Was the care given safe? Efficient? Effective?
- What modifications are necessary to ensure quality care?
- Were people available to nursing team members for guidance and supervision?
- Were resources available for updating skills and knowledge?

EVALUATION OF CARE

Other types of evaluation the nurse is involved in include examinations of the quality of care within the particular health care setting and the utilization of the total health care given in that setting. The nursing audit is the current method used to evaluate nursing care. It is a peer evaluation system where health care records and situations are reviewed retrospectively for safe practice, uniformity of methodology, follow-through of care, outcomes of care, discharge planning, teaching done, and adequacy of staffing. It is based on criteria established by the health care facility and the professional community. These audits enable the nursing staff to identify areas of strengths and weaknesses and to focus on specific aspects of care which need to be modified in a specific nursing unit or department or in the entire agency. Based on these audits, inservice education programs are developed, goals for care established, plans for change instituted, and further evaluation carried out. The actual format and methodology for carrying out nursing audits will vary from institution to institution.

(See the references at the end of this chapter for detailed descriptions of nursing audits.)

Health care professionals from all disciplines participate in similar audits to evaluate the availability and distribution of health care, the effectiveness and efficiency of care, and the appropriateness of the utilization of facilities and staff. These audits are used to enact changes which will increase the quality of the facility, personnel, and care given.

SELF-EVALUATION

Perhaps the most important area of evaluation is self-evaluation, which is carried out as systematically and routinely as other types of evaluation. When this process is criterion-based, the nurse who is hypercritical of her mistakes or who avoids examining her ineffective actions is guided to a realistic appraisal of her behavior.

General criteria for self-evaluation include:

- Was my level of knowledge adequate? Complete? Current?
- Were my judgments based on accurate assessment of the situation?
- Were my thought processes organized?
- Were my skills effective? Current?
- What were my reactions to the care situation and how did they influence others?
- What learning took place?
- What activities were most satisfying?
- What activities could be done differently?
- What resources were available for assistance?
- What peer support was available?
- What were my expectations of the care situation?
- What were the relationships between the expectations and the reality of the care situation?
- What are my methods for coping with change and stress?
- Do these methods work for me?
- What are my goals for professional development?
- What steps are necessary for me to realize these goals?
- Did I use my creativity in providing care and coping with the resulting stresses?

SUMMARY

The culmination of all evaluation is the synthesis of knowledge gained. From each care situation are drawn those behaviors that the nurse wishes to add to a personal repertoire of professional responses. The nurse avoids those behaviors evidenced in care situations that were ineffective in providing care. In this way modifications of care result and information learned is transferred from situation to situation. Over time, synthesis of evaluations results in a wide variety of experiences and knowledge from which the nurse can draw.

One type of evaluation is the discharge summary. Following is an excerpt from the evaluation of an individual's level of orientation in the sample situation.

ORIENTATION:

Self: continues to be oriented to self. Responds appropriately to name and states first and last names when asked. Is now aware of age and accurately states she is a widow with no children.

Place: appropriately names hospital, unit, and room. States she is returning to nursing home; however, does not remember location. Frequently confuses it with previous address.

Time: maintains time orientation when frequently referred to clock and calendar. Exhibits disorientation if awakened during night. Regains orientation when presented with location and time.

SELECTED REFERENCES

Decker, Frances, Stevens, Linda, Vancini, Margaret, and Wedeking, Lorene. "Using Patient Outcomes to Evaluate Community Health Nursing." *Nursing Outlook,* 27:278, April, 1979.

Gold, Harold, Jackson, Marjorie, Sachs, Barbara, and Van Meter, Marjie J. "Peer Review—A Working Experiment." *Nursing Outlook,* 21:634, October, 1973.

Mayers, Marlene G., Norby, Ronald B., and Watson, Annita B. *Qualtiy Assurance for Patient Care.* New York, Appleton, 1977.

Moore, Karen, "What Nurses Learn from Nursing Audit." *Nursing Outlook,* 27:254, April, 1979.

Phaneuf, Marie. *The Nursing Audit: Self Regulation in Nursing Practice.* New York, Appleton, 1976.

Ramphal, Marjorie. "Peer Review." *American Journal of Nursing,* 74:63, January, 1974.

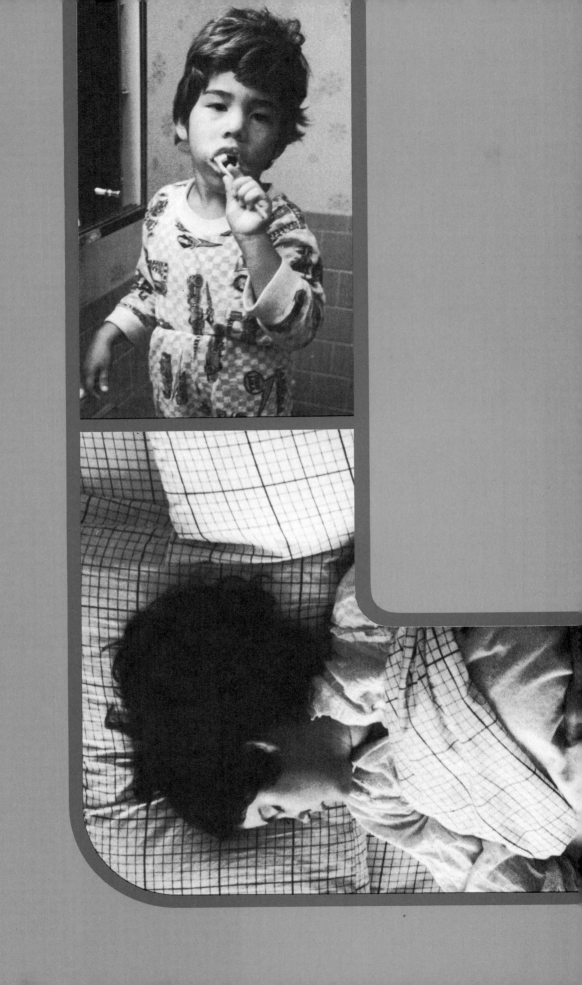

Health Care Needs

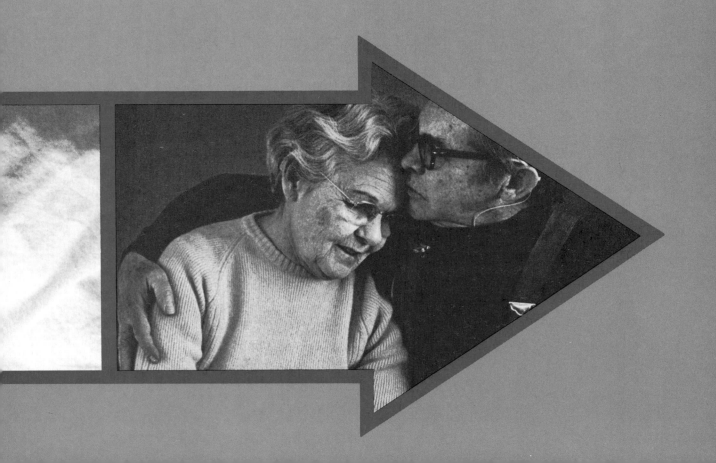

This part is a presentation of the theoretical and practical application of the nursing process to help create a change in the individual's health status. Utilizing the process of growth and development, related scientific principles, knowledge of anatomy and physiology, and a human needs approach, a foundation for nursing practice is built. Significant racial, cultural, and ethnic variations are highlighted as they bear on the individualizing of nursing care. Related psychomotor skills are presented in a step-by-step manner, along with the rationale for each step. The multidimensional approach pulls together information from many sources and allows the beginning student to see a more complete picture of the individual in order to assess more completely his or her needs, plan for intervention, and predict nursing care outcomes. In addition, this approach is one which can be applied to any theoretical framework.

Freud, Erikson, Piaget, Havighurst, and Peck are the main theorists drawn on for a discussion of growth and development. Needs are explored in terms of the implications that the behaviors found at each level of growth and development have on nursing care.

Scientific principles from the physical, natural, and behavioral sciences are outlined as a guide for the student in understanding the rationale for his or her care and a help in selecting the most appropriate strategies of care.

Diagrams of related anatomy and physiology are given at the beginning of each chapter to stress the physiologic basis of nursing care and to provide a ready review and integration of anatomy and physiology principles into the nursing care given. Where applicable the differences in anatomy and physiology at various levels of growth and development are reviewed.

A human needs approach presents a comprehensive look at the requirements essential for life and provides a relatively easy way for the student to establish priorities of care. It is straightforward and versatile in its application to a variety of theories.

This part consists of five units. The first deals with awareness needs, i.e., communication and sensory input and output. Awareness needs are those which enable the individual to receive stimuli, perceive, interpret, and react to and with his or her environment. These needs are basic to an understanding of the modes of interaction that the individual utilizes in meeting and imparting his or her other needs.

The second unit includes the safety needs arising in the areas of body kinetics, asepsis, environment, and chemicals. Safety needs are those needs which relate to the security and protection of the individual within the home and health care environments.

The third unit deals with the energy needs of oxygenation, circulation, intake and output, and fluid and electrolyte balance. This unit deals with those requirements of the individual for energy uptake, transport, utilization, and removal of byproducts.

The fourth unit deals with the self-esteem needs of body image, aethetics, sleep and comfort, sexuality, and grieving and loss.

The final unit deals with the surgical process and its effects on the ability to meet basic needs. Self-esteem needs relate to the individual's view of self through body image, body aesthetics, and comfort and the ability to deal with self and his or her environment.

Most chapters use the following format:

Scientific Principles	Goal setting
Introduction	Nursing care plan
Assessment	Intervention
Growth and development	Psychomotor skills
Assessment factors	Evaluation
Physical assessment	Medications to Review
Diagnostic tests	Diets to Review
Nursing Diagnosis	Charting and Recording Factors
Planning	Teaching—Learning Factors

Clinical applications are given in selected chapters to provide additional knowledge in specific situations.

The use of this format provides a comprehensive approach to care as it relates to a specific need.

The first two parts of this book have given the knowledge base and methodology necessary for the use of the nursing process in helping individuals to meet their health care needs. Part III gives an indepth and real situation using the nursing process as a whole to bring together the strands of change, human needs, growth and development, communication, and teaching—learning.

No health care need takes place in isolation. Rather, it occurs within the context of the individual's total physical, physiologic, and psychosocial status. Therefore, a comprehensive view of the assessment, nursing diagnoses, planning, intervention, and evaluation of an actual care situation is presented to aid in the synthesis of the nursing process.

One of the primary goals of nursing is to make a positive difference in the ability of the individual to meet his or her daily health care needs through the process of change. Thus we now focus on specific behavioral changes, scheduling, and activities which can be utilized to bring about the desired positive change in the individual's health state.

The dynamics of care are continuously changing in any health care setting, and selected goals and plans may not work for that particular situation. As a result the evaluation section in this Part indicates areas of necessary reassessment and modification of plans. However, without the original specificity of assessment, nursing diagnosis, goals and plans, evaluation takes place in a vacuum and does not reflect the actual changing aspects of the individual's health state.

UNIT III
Awareness Needs

"Then you should say what you mean," the
March hare went on.

"I do," Alice hastily replied; *"at least—at
least I mean what I say—that's the same thing,
you know."*

"Not the same thing a bit!" said the Hatter.
*"Why you might just as well say that 'I see what
I eat' is the same thing as 'I eat what I see!'"*
Lewis Carroll—Alice's Adventures in Wonderland

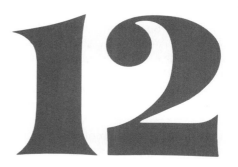

COMMUNICATION NEEDS

PRINCIPLES RELATED TO COMMUNICATION NEEDS

Communication is a dynamic process.

Each individual's communication pattern is unique.

All behavior is a form of communication.

Communication is influenced by the individual's
level of growth and development, culture, interaction style, cognitive abilities, level of anxiety, and
state of health.

Language is the use of symbols to represent
thoughts, ideas, and objects in one's internal and
external environments.

Communication is enhanced when individual
differences are recognized and incorporated into
interactions.

Stereotypes, biases, and assumptions can hinder
communication.

Honesty, trust, and recognition of individual differences facilitate communication.

Cognitive dissonance arises when an interaction
creates tension.

An increase in level of anxiety decreases perception.

Lower levels of anxiety are necessary for survival.

Communication is the means by which we share our humanity. Human emotions, thoughts, ideas, and needs are communicated in a variety of ways. Sounds, language, touch, signs, and movements are just a few ways in which individuals communicate. Without communication interactions would not be possible, and survival would be threatened. Communication patterns are developed and refined throughout the life process and rely on feedback from the environment to develop into meaningful tools. The nurse is in constant contact with individuals who are attempting through one method or another to communicate their basic needs. Thus it is necessary for the nurse to be able to assess the individual's level and methods of communication, to develop his or her own repertoire of communication skills, and to intervene to facilitate the individual's expression of needs to his or her environment.

ASSESSMENT

Language Development

Language development is an important factor to consider when assessing the individual's ability to meet communication needs. Language is the use of symbols to represent thoughts, ideas, and objects in one's internal and external environments. Language can be expressed orally, in writing, or through movement. If language development is interfered with, the individual loses a major mode for self-expression. Language development can be disturbed through structural defects which prevent speech and purposeful movements, through cognitive disabilities which impair the ability to translate symbols into meaningful units, and psychosocial deprivation which limits the individual's experiences with the use of symbols.

Language development begins at birth. The infant makes a variety of sounds and gestures which are received and interpreted by persons in the environment. Some of these are positively reinforced by significant others and fed back more consistently to the child than others. Through this process the infant and young child attach meaning to certain sounds and movements and attempt to duplicate those which are meaningful to them. As the child's interaction with the environment increases and greater exposure to different people, objects, and events occurs, more

meaningful symbols are added, and the child's repertoire for expressing needs expands. As development continues, the child's use of symbols moves from the very concrete to the more abstract, and symbols take on many forms. For example, a spoken word can be expressed as a picture, a written word, or movement. This use of language continues to develop as the child, and later the adult, increases his or her field and scope of interaction. Chart 12.1 outlines the development of language throughout the life process.

The nurse assesses the appropriateness of the individual's language skills for the individual's level of growth and development and the adequacy of those skills for meeting that person's communication needs. Many times one aspect of language development lags behind others, but the individual may have developed another facet to such a level that his or her communication needs are being met. For example, the young child who has limited oral proficiency may have an intricate gesturing and movement skill which conveys messages very clearly. However, this compensatory system may have limited applicability if persons outside the family unit are unable to interpret it. In addition, the nurse attempts to determine what factors may be interfering with the development of language. (See Illustration 12.1)

Nursing assessment related to language development includes descriptions of:

- presenting language skills
- expected language skills
- relationship of level of growth and development to language skills
- adequacy of language skills
- areas of language deficiency
- areas of language compensation
- major mode of communication
- possible interferences with language development

Cultural Influences

Culture is a great influence on the individual's choice of language, predominant mode, the symbolic meaning, and the situations in which specific forms of language are used. The actual language which is spoken is determined by the cultural reference group of the individual. The dialect—which includes the intonation of words, slang words, and the pronunciation of sounds—will vary from one subcultural group to

Chart 12.1
Language Development throughout the Life Process

LEVEL	CHARACTERISTICS
Infant	Newborn's cries are automatic and have no specific meaning. As the infant grows, cries become differentiated and related to internal and external feelings of discomfort. Around 3 months of age, recognizes significant mothering person with smiles. Enjoys making sounds—cooing, babbling. At around 5 months begins to entertain self through verbalization of vowels and other sounds. At around 8 months, sounds are imitative. Begins to put sounds together; responds to symbolic meaning of some words, such as "no." At around 10 months, says "mama" and "dada" appropriately; begins to imitate nonverbal communication of others. At around 1 year, vocabulary increases to 5 or 6 words. Uses private language to express needs. According to Piaget, time of sensorimotor cognitive development.
Toddler	Vocabulary progressively increases up to 900 words at end of toddlerhood; symbolic use of nonverbal behaviors; connects symbols of different modes, e.g., words with pictures, gestures, objects. In Piaget's view, begins to have more symbolic thought processes. (Continues through preschool age.)
Preschooler	Vocabulary increases to more than 2000 words during this period. Begins to apply grammatical rules to language.
Schoolage child	Can use all adult forms of speech patterns; learns to read and write. Vocabulary continues to increase. Continues to develop use of symbolism and nonverbal communications.
Adolescent	Begins to use abstractions. Development of subgroup language.
Adulthood	Has a full range of language skills; use of abstractions and logic.

another, as well as be geographically determined. For example, at times the midwesterner with a characteristic twang may not seem to be speaking the same language as the southerner with a pronounced drawl. In the United States, where the first language of many groups may not be English, it is not uncommon to hear two languages intermingled or the words of one culture assimilated into the vocabulary of the general population.

guage, with little or no emphasis on the written or movement aspects. If an individual from this culture develops an interference with the speech process, he or she may be more handicapped than individuals from cultures that use another mode or a variety of modes. This occurs because the individual may not have developed a skill in communication through writing or movement. In addition, other persons in the individual's culture may not be able to understand these modes even if they are developed.

MODES OF COMMUNICATION

Some cultures use one mode of communication more than other modes. For example, a culture may rely predominantly on the oral component of lan-

SYMBOLIC MEANINGS

Each culture designates a primary (denotation) and secondary (connotation) meaning to words and movements. For example, moving one's head up and

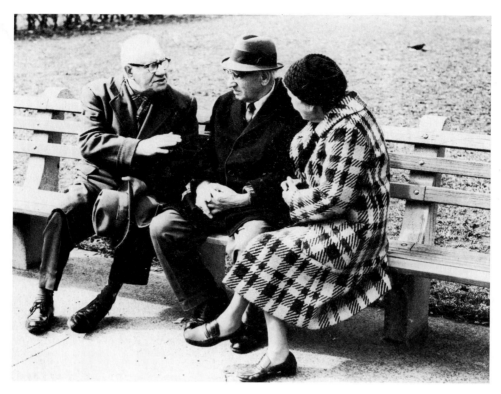

Illustration 12.1
Gesturing and movement often convey messages very clearly. *(Photo © Joel Gordon, 1978)*

down in a vertical direction signifies yes or agreement in some cultures, while in other cultures, such as the East Indian, this movement signifies no or disagreement. Some cultures have many words for a concept or construct, while others may have no words or symbols for these things. For example, the Eskimo language has many words to describe snow, while English has only one word. Since language reflects the conceptualization process of the people who use it, transcultural communication becomes difficult. Conceptual sets do not match. For example, the Navaho do not have a concept of the future and thus are unable to communicate effectively with individuals from future-oriented cultures. Since it is impossible to become well versed in all the cultural variations or the symbolic meanings of language, the nurse in caring for individuals needs to assess carefully the meanings they are applying to language. Time orientation and the physical distance people take when interacting are two of the major communication areas in which cultural differences appear.

LANGUAGE FORM IN VARYING SITUATIONS

The ways in which words, symbols, gestures, and movements are used in various situations are also determined culturally. Most cultures have "rules" about interactions between different age groups, sexes, social classes, and people from other cultures. For example, a young woman or girl from some cultures is not allowed to speak to or look directly at an elder. In other cultures, young children are allowed to say or do what they choose without any adult restrictions. Another instance of this is found in cultures in which even middle-aged adults will not interact with others before first receiving permission from the older designated leaders of the group.

Many misunderstandings arise and negative labelings occur as a result of transcultural distortions in communication. The nurse, therefore, needs to be aware of his or her own cultural patterns and how they influence interactions with others as well as how the individual's cultural patterns influence the individual's ability to communicate with the nurse and the health care system.

Nursing assessment of cultural influences on communication includes descriptions of:

- the actual language(s) used
- the meanings of intonations, pronunciations, and slang phrases
- major mode(s) of communication
- cultural connotations and denotations of words and symbols
- cultural time orientation
- cultural distancing patterns
- cultural interaction "rules"
- cultural attitudes toward communication
- areas of cultural difference in communication patterns among nurse, staff, and individual

Level of Anxiety

The level of anxiety greatly influences how individuals perceive what is being communicated and their ability to communicate. Anxiety is not necessarily destructive to the individual; in fact, low levels of anxiety are necessary for the individual's survival. Without anxiety the individual would not be able to perceive and deal with threats to safety and security. Situations which are anxiety producing to one person may not be so for another. Thus the nurse does not automatically assume that a given situation is or is not anxiety producing.

As the level of anxiety increases, the individual's ability to perceive environmental stimuli alters. While a mild anxiety motivates the individual and helps him or her to focus on what is occurring, more severe anxiety lessens these abilities and eventually causes a distortion of perception. Since communication involves the reception and interpretation of messages and feedback from the environment, changes in anxiety levels will directly influence the communication process. Incoming messages may be distorted, disregarded, or interrupted. Likewise, outgoing communication can be inappropriate, exaggerated, or diminished.

When the individual experiences anxiety, physical, physiologic, and psychosocial mechanisms are activated which result in an increased feeling of ten-

sion, disorganization, dread, and autonomic nervous system activation. The degree to which these signs and symptoms are manifested depends on the level of anxiety. With mild or moderate anxiety, the individual feels vaguely tense and has feelings of low-grade, generalized discomfort. The person perceives situations as being not quite right but is not overwhelmed by the anxiety.

The individual may be restless, have a decreased attention span, appear preoccupied, feel irritable, and be categorized as "nervous" or "upset." Changes in sleep and eating patterns may occur. The individual may have difficulty falling asleep, may wake frequently, or sleep more than usual. Food intake may either increase or decrease depending on the individual's usual mode of coping with anxiety-provoking situations. Feelings of nausea and "butterflies in the stomach," headache, malaise, and muscular tension all can accompany mild and moderate anxiety. With these levels of anxiety the individual is able to use his or her usual coping mechanisms to reduce tension and reorganize thought processes. The nurse identifies which behaviors are coping behaviors and assists the individual in using those behaviors which decrease the anxiety.

Severe anxiety, however, results in feelings of disorganization and an overwhelming sense of threat or doom. The stress reaction is activated with all its attendant signs and symptoms. The individual may not be able to cope with the situation and crisis is precipitated. The person may have a severe loss of appetite (anorexia), extreme changes in sleep and waking patterns, illogical thought patterns, and behavioral changes such as aggressiveness, suspicion, hysteria, or withdrawal. The individual's ability to accurately perceive environmental stimuli may be drastically reduced. Learning is impaired and any information received or transmitted at this time may be distorted. Psychosomatic illness may result from severe anxiety. (Chart 12.2)

While any situation can result in anxiety for one individual or another, entry into the health care system, especially hospitalization, is generally accepted to be anxiety producing. Fear of the unknown; changes in lifestyle and roles; threats to privacy, independence, and body image; pain; and unfamiliar and unpredictable people and surroundings all contribute to increases in anxiety.

In the health care situation, interferences with communication can result in serious consequences. For example, the individual who is being taught

Chart 12.2
Response Categorization to Anxiety Levels

LEVEL OF ANXIETY	PHYSIOLOGIC	COGNITIVE	BEHAVIORAL AND EMOTIONAL
Minimal	Relaxation response: ↓ Pulse ↓ Respirations ↓ O$_2$ consumption Pupillary constriction ↓ Muscle tension ↓ Blood pressure	States of altered awareness: Daydreaming Yoga Relaxation Biofeedback Transcendental meditation Some stages of sleep Emotional and cognitive activity minimal. Focus typically on single mental image.	Disregard for environmental stimuli; no attempt to deal with external stimuli. No verbal interaction. Muscles relaxed; passive movement easy.
Mild (+)	Muscle tension at minimum; passive control of interaction between psychologic processes and muscular activity.	Perceptual field broad: Ability to take in multiple stimuli. Passive awareness of environment.	Feelings of safety and comfort. Behavior primarily automatic; carrying out well-known habits and skills, noncompetitive games and pastimes. Solitary activities. Facial muscles appear relaxed. Voice calm.
Moderate (++)	Increased tension that is tolerable, even pleasurable. Maximum conscious interaction between mind, body, and emotions. Attention focus: sees, hears, and grasps fewer stimuli than +1 anxiety. ↑ Alertness	Perceptual field narrowed: Ability to solve problems at all levels, optimal level for learning. Can attend to specifics if directed to do so.	Feelings of challenge and the need to handle the situation at hand. Competitive games; carrying out less familiar skills and habits, learning new skills. Voice denotes concern and interest with environment.

(continued)

about medications may be told to take one drop every 4 hours but may "hear" 4 drops every hour because his or her anxiety level is so high. The anxiety the individual is experiencing does not have to be directly related to the health care situation to interfere with health care communication. The nurse's level of anxiety may also interfere with communication.

The coping behaviors the individual uses to deal with anxiety also affect the communication process. Different coping behaviors can increase or decrease the effectiveness of messages given or received. For instance, the individual who uses denial will not hear

Chart 12.2 (cont.)
Response Categorization to Anxiety Levels

LEVEL OF ANXIETY	PHYSIOLOGIC	COGNITIVE	BEHAVIORAL AND EMOTIONAL
Severe (+++)	Survival response (fight or flight). Sympathetic nervous system activation: ↑ Epinephrine ↑ BP, P, R Skin vasoconstriction ↑ Body temperature Diaphoresis Dry mouth Urinary urgency Loss of appetite: ↓ Blood to digestive system ↑ Glucose production by liver Sensory changes: ↓ Hearing perception Pain perception lessened Pupils dilated; vision fixed Muscles tense, rigid (may be fixed)	Perceptual field greatly reduced: Time sense distorted. Selective inattention operates: stimuli threatening to self-system and biologic integrity or expectations may be filtered out. Dissociating tendency: events and/or feelings are denied existence in awareness. Selective enhancement operates: focus on one particular or many scattered details. Problem-solving difficult.	Feelings of increasing threat; need to respond to situation is heightened. Personal space is extended. Physical activity may increase with decreasing organization and purposefulness (pacing, wringing of hands, running away, freezing on the spot, trembling, stammering, fidgeting). May feel nauseated. May experience "cold sweat." Anxiety easily increased with new stimuli such as noise or people approaching patient. Verbalization typically rapid and/or characterized by blocking. Flight behavior may be manifested psychologically with withdrawal, denial, depression, somatization.
Panic (++++)	Continued physiologic arousal. Eventual release of sympathetic discharge: Blood returns to major organs (individual may appear pale). May be hypotensive. Ability to respond to pain, noise, external stimuli at minimum. Motor coordination poor. ↓ Blood flow to skeletal muscles.	Perceptual field closed, may be distorted: Thoughts are random; logical thinking impaired. Details may be "blown up" or the speed of scattering increased. Unable to solve problems; new stimuli tend to overload mental functioning.	Feelings of anger, helplessness emerge; may be experienced as rage, dread, awe, terror. Individual may strike out physically or verbally or may withdraw. Behavior may be primitive: crying, biting, flailing, curling up. Physical activity increasingly disorganized. Voice pitch higher, louder; flow of words rapid; sometimes may experience blocking of speech. Facial expression of terror, grimacing.

From: Longo and Williams. *Clinical Practice in Psychosocial Nursing: Assessment and Intervention*, New York, Appleton-Century-Crofts, 1978, p. 95.

any communication related to the area being denied. On the other hand, the individual who focuses on all information related to an anxiety-provoking area may not be able to get enough information on this area.

During the communication process, a state of tension often develops in the individual as a result of the interaction. The cause of the tension is not clear to the individual; however, the perception of tension is. This is known as the process of **cognitive dissonance**. When cognitive dissonance exists, the individual sets out to lessen his or her perception of tension. These efforts are usually concentrated on alleviation of the state of tension and not on alleviation of the cause. Thus the individual may act inappropriately or aggravate the situation that originally created the tension. If the behavior is coincidentally successful in reducing the tension state, it will be reinforced and will be used again whenever a similar situation rises.

Previous experiences the individual has had, therefore, influence the way the individual enters into the communication process. Positive and negative reinforcements in the past, the degree of satisfaction with previous experience, and the success of previous interactions affect the individual's willingness to engage actively in communication and help to determine the mode of interaction the individual will use. For example, the individual who has found crying to be a useful way of coping with tension and receiving assistance may repeatedly use this behavior in many situations, whether it is appropriate or not.

Situations in which the individual will actively participate are also greatly influenced by previous experiences. If the individual has found one-to-one situations highly satisfactory and group interactions less satisfying, that individual will have a greater tendency to seek out the former and to avoid the latter. Therefore, the individual's expectations of interactions are assessed to provide a basis for the optimum type of interaction and to find areas requiring intervention to facilitate the communication process. The nurse also assesses his or her own expectations for interaction in various situations to determine areas of strengths which can be readily utilized to enhance communication and areas needing further development and refinement. For example, the nurse who has not been able to deal effectively with individuals who use crying as a coping behavior may react negatively when encountering this behavior. An interference with communication can then result, since the in-

teraction is not satisfactory to either side and cognitive dissonance occurs.

Nursing assessment related to level of anxiety and the communication process includes descriptions of:

- level of anxiety
- manifestations of anxiety
- factors contributing to level of anxiety
- relationship between level of anxiety and communication
- degree of tension created by interaction process
- degree of cognitive dissonance
- previous experiences with interactions
- types of interaction which are satisfying or dissatisfying
- influence of nurse's interaction patterns on communication

Interaction Style

An individual's communication style is affected by a variety of factors, including the individual's cognitive abilities, personal interaction patterns, attitudes, and level of knowledge. Interaction style is the way in which the individual characteristically engages in the communication process. The individual may be aggressive, assertive, hostile, reticent, docile, or loquacious in daily interactions. The basic interaction pattern is the one the individual usually continues. However, changes in the individual's internal and external environment may exaggerate or alter the usual style.

The individual's unique makeup, in addition to previously mentioned factors, contributes to interaction style. Frequently, those interaction behaviors which have met the individual's needs are reinforced and repeated. Recognition of the interaction styles and the factors which contribute to them assist the nurse in determining the most effective manner of communicating with individuals. Assumptions are not made about an individual's skills, knowledge, interest, or abilities on the basis of his or her interaction style.

Nursing assessment related to interaction styles includes descriptions of:

- type of interaction style
- relationship to cognitive ability, attitudes, and level of knowledge

- influence of culture, level of growth and development, and level of anxiety
- effectiveness of interaction style on expressing self and meeting needs
- factors which alter the usual interaction style

Nonverbal Communication

Since the individual is always communicating, whether speaking or not, the nurse needs to be attuned to nonverbal cues and how they affect the communication process. Such cues as gesturing, posturing, facial expressions, use of touch, distancing, manner of dress, personal care patterns, and giving gifts impart valuable information as to the message the individual is communicating or receiving.

GESTURES

Gestures are culturally and societally determined and must be interpreted in light of the meaning the individual gives to them. A gesture that is hostile or aggressive to one person may not be so to another. Many people use a great deal of gesturing as an adjunct to their verbal communication, while others use little at all. Frequently, connotations are attributed to certain styles of gesturing. For example, the individual who waves his or her arms rapidly while speaking may be labeled highly emotional when the waving is only a part of the usual method of communication. Thus gestures are assessed in terms of the context in which they are found rather than automatically assigned a meaning.

POSTURE AND EXPRESSION

The posture the individual assumes also has an assigned connotation which can interfere with the communication process. Similarly, facial expressions are other nonverbal cues to the individual's feelings and attitudes. Like gesturing and posturing, these can be deceptive and reflect habits or be purposefully manipulated in an attempt to control the interaction.

TOUCH

Individuals vary in their manner of touching other individuals and their reactions to touch from others. Within the health care situation, intimate touch of relative strangers is a frequent occurrence. The automatic right of the nurse to touch the individual within the context of the health care system should not be assumed; rather the nurse ascertains the individual's reactions to touch so that interventions can be modified to stay within the parameters acceptable to the individual. Each individual has "rules" governing the use of touch. Factors such as the age of the individual who is touching and being touched, the sex, situation, and need for touch all directly influence the individual's reaction to touch. (Illustration 12.2)

DISTANCING

The distance which the individual places between self and others and the degree of threat felt when this territory is invaded also affect the communication. These behaviors are similarly influenced by the situation, the culture, the age, degree of intimacy of the situation, and the familiarity with the people. **Proxemics** is the term used to describe these distancing patterns. Eight ranges of distances which Americans commonly use in different situations have been identified, and these are outlined in Chart 12.3.

Within the health care situation, the intimate zone is commonly used for intervention, with little or no opportunity to develop the relationship which is usually associated with the use of this zone. As a result, the individual may feel resentful or intruded on and react negatively to the situation. In an attempt to delineate their own territory and prevent outsiders from invading their personal space, individuals often use furniture and personal objects to set up barriers. The nurse assesses the individual's use of territory and the effects of invading it on the communication process.

PERSONAL APPEARANCE

The individual's manner of dress and personal care activities may either facilitate or hinder the communication process. If the individual's habits of dress and personal care are not consistent with the cultural and societal expectations for a given setting, biases, stereotypes, and assumptions are brought into play and affect the communication process. The re-

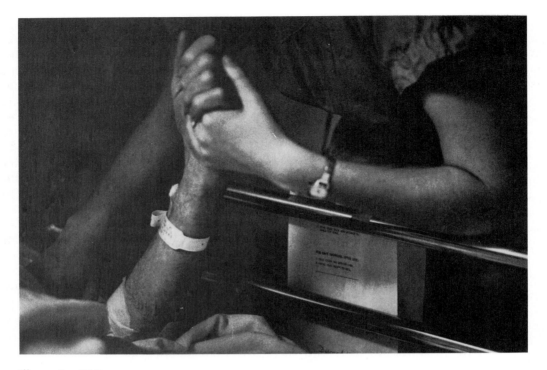

Illustration 12.2
Touch is a meaningful form of communication. *(Photo © Sherry Suris, from Photo Researchers, Inc.)*

verse is also true as to the individual's reactions to the dress and personal appearance of the nurse and of other health care workers. If the responses are negative, the quality and quantity of communication is usually decreased. Therefore, assessment of the relationship between the individual's or nurse's manner of dress and personal appearance and the communication process is necessary to facilitate communication.

GIFT GIVING

Gift giving may be a form of bargaining or attention getting. Some individuals believe that they cannot accept services or concern from others without giving something in return. Others may see giving a gift as a payment for individualized, competent care without which care will be withheld. Still others simply view this as a sign of appreciation. Whenever a nurse is offered a present, its acceptance is deter-

mined by the meaning of the gift to the individual giving it and the circumstances under which it occurs.

Nursing assessment related to nonverbal communication includes descriptions of:

- gestures
- meaning of gestures
- posturing
- meaning of posturing
- facial expressions
- meaning of facial expressions
- use of touch (individual, family and/or significant others, nurse)
- reactions to touch
- meanings of touch
- use of distancing
- meanings of distancing
- responses to changes in usual distancing patterns
- manner of dress
- meaning of dress

Chart 12.3
Common Distancing Ranges

RANGE	COMMUNICATION
Very close (3–6 in.)	Soft whisper; top secret
Close (8–12 in.)	Audible whisper; very confidential
Near (12–20 in.)	Indoors, soft voice; outdoors, full voice; confidential
Neutral (20–36 in.)	Soft voice, low volume; personal subject matter
Neutral (4½–5 ft)	Full voice; information of nonpersonal matter
Public distance (5½–8 ft)	Full voice with slight overloudness; public information for others to hear
Across the room (8–20 ft)	Loud voice; talking to a group
Stretching the limits of distance	20–24 ft indoors; up to 100 ft outdoors; hailing distance, departures

From: Edward Hall. The Silent Language. *New York, Doubleday & Company, Inc. 1959, pp. 163–164.*

- personal appearance
- meaning of personal appearance
- relationship of nonverbal cues to communication process

State of Health

The individual's level of wellness influences the energy available for communication, the types of communication needed, and the ability to receive and send communication. Individuals in negative health states may not have the energy or ability to participate verbally in the communication process. Instead, they may rely on nonverbal messages to communicate their needs. The individual's sensory process (Chap. 13) greatly affects his or her ability to receive, interpret, and respond to messages from the environment.

The nurse therefore assesses how the present state of health influences the individual's capacity for self-expression and communication of health care needs. The existing pathology may interfere with communication by distorting reception, decreasing the individual's ability to focus on the meanings of interactions in the internal and external environments, and altering the way the individual responds to situations and events.

A negative state of health in the individual increases his or her level of anxiety, brings coping behaviors into action, changes the individual's usual interaction style, and refocuses his or her areas of interest. In addition, illness can restrict the individual's scope of interaction and bring the individual in contact with many unfamiliar people. By recognizing the alterations in the communication process which result from changes in the individual's ability to relate to others in his or her usual style and mode, the nurse can more effectively intervene to meet the individual's communication needs.

Nursing assessment related to state of health and its effects on the communication process includes descriptions of:

- state of health
- needs interfered with by health state
- communication requirements resulting from changes in health state
- amount of energy available for communication
- ways of communicating needs
- communication interferences related to health state

NURSING DIAGNOSIS

A 19-year-old woman, Ms. Dunne, is visited by the community health nurse for a follow-up visit 2 weeks after delivering her first baby. The nurse assesses Ms. Dunne's presenting behaviors and finds information pertaining to this individual's communication needs as outlined in the nursing assessment on pp. 190–192.

ASSESSMENT FACTOR	EXPECTED BEHAVIOR	PRESENTING BEHAVIOR
Language development	See Chart 12.1.	Frequently uses slang. Expresses feelings and ideas clearly, but often switches from one subject to another. Uses common lay terms to describe birthing process and physiologic functions.
Major modes of communication	—	Characterizes self as "a real talker." Uses many gestures. Changes facial expression to accent conversation. States, "I never was much of a reader."
Areas of language deficiency	—	None noted.
Primary language	—	English
Culture	—	Irish-American background, third generation. Catholic. Married to 21-year-old man of similar background.
Cultural connotations and denotations of words and symbols	—	Unable to determine on initial visit.
Cultural time orientation		Speaks about present with some reference to near future.
Cultural interaction "rules"	—	"It seems strange to talk to a man about babies and things like that." "My husband never wants to discuss bringing up the baby. He says that's for women to talk about."
Cultural attitudes toward communication	—	"My mother says I musta kissed the Blarney Stone since all I do is talk."
Level of anxiety	—	Moderate level as evidenced by short attention span, jumping from subject to subject, fidgeting in chair. Frequently mentions fears about adequacy of care she is giving baby, and the change in her husband since the baby was born.

(continued)

ASSESSMENT FACTOR	EXPECTED BEHAVIOR	PRESENTING BEHAVIOR
Factors contributing to level of anxiety	—	States, "I haven't got a good night's sleep since I came home from the hospital." "My mother and mother-in-law keep calling all the time to tell what I'm doing wrong." "My husband never seems to want to talk to me anymore. He says all I can talk about is that baby." "A baby is sure a lot more work than I ever expected." "All my friends are out having a good time and earning money, and I'm stuck here in the house."
Relationship between level of anxiety and communication	—	Concern over child care interfering with communication process with husband. Anxiety interfering with ability to focus on interaction process. Anxiety over adequacy as mother interfering with interactions with mother and mother-in-law.
Previous experiences with interactions	—	"It sure is a lot easier talking just to you than it was in that dumb mother's class with a whole bunch of strangers." "I never thought it would be so easy to talk to a man about all these things."
Type of interaction style	—	Loquacious, outgoing. Unable to assess style with others. States, "I guess sometimes I talk so much that nobody listens to what I say."
Effectiveness of interaction style on expressing self and meeting needs	—	Unable to fully assess on one visit. However, initial impression is that individual is concerned with interferences in communication with husband, mother, and mother-in-law, and that some interactional tension exists with these people.

(continued)

ASSESSMENT FACTOR	EXPECTED BEHAVIOR	PRESENTING BEHAVIOR
Factors which alter usual interaction style	—	Fatigue. New role as mother. Limited interactions with usual group of friends. States, "We used to go out dancing with our gang at least once a week; now we never go out."
Gestures	—	Gestures with hands frequently to point out and complete statement.
Facial expressions	—	Uses appropriately to accentuate speech.
Use of touch	—	Holds baby gently and deftly. Caresses baby's face and hands.
Reactions to touch	—	Chuckles when baby grasps her finger and snuggles up to her.
Manner of dress and personal appearance	—	Hair neatly combed and pulled back in a barrette. Dressed in clean jeans and t-shirt. Baby dressed in clean stretch suit; baby freshly bathed, has pink ribbon on small tuft of hair.

Resulting nursing diagnoses in the situation of Ms. Dunne may include:

- increased level of anxiety related to changes in interaction patterns
- changes in interaction patterns related to inexperience with new role
- decreased tolerance to stress related to fatigue
- possible interferences with ability to express feelings and needs related to interaction style

PLANNING

Understanding the individual's communication needs and actual and potential interferences with his or her ability to meet those needs helps the nurse to plan care that is focused on working with and directed at the person. Plans to meet communication needs must be tailored to the individual so as to create an environment conducive to open and free self-expression and in which the least amount of tension is generated. The interaction process which is produced is particularly important, since much of the nurse's ability to intervene effectively with all health care needs will depend on the quality and quantity of communication which exists.

The plan for one of the nursing diagnoses listed above in the situation of Ms. Dunne might look like the plan on page 193.

NURSING DIAGNOSIS	GOAL	PLAN
Changes in interaction patterns related to inexperience with new role	1. Increased ease with new mothering role within 2 weeks as evidenced by positive statements about mothering abilities.	1. Review care of infant. 2. Reinforce strengths. 3. Point out positive mothering behaviors demonstrated. 4. Supplement areas in which gaps in knowledge exist. 5. Discuss behaviors Ms. Dunne considers positive and negative mothering behaviors. 6. Compare perceived positive behaviors with actual. 7. Explore ways to modify perceived negative behaviors. 8. Schedule revisit in 2 weeks.
	2. Resumption of interaction patterns with friends within 2 weeks.	1. Explore relationship between decreased social interaction and feelings of stress. 2. Explore other ways of keeping in contact with friends, e.g., telephoning.
	3. Increased conversations with husband within 2 weeks as evidenced by subjective reports.	1. As above for Goals 1, 2, and 3. 2. Explore perceptions of reasons for husband's avoidance of conversation. 3. Discuss reasons for her need to discuss baby all the time. 4. Explore possible topics of conversation other than baby. 5. Discuss ways to increase husband's role in parenting process. 6. Schedule next visit when husband is at home.
	4. Increased ability to assert self with mother and mother-in-law within 2 weeks, as evidenced by subjective reports.	1. As above for Goals, 1, 2, and 3. 2. Explore feelings about mother's and mother-in-law's reactions. 3. Discuss possible ways of dealing with statements which create cognitive dissonance. 4. Role-playing conversations. 5. Explore assertive behaviors which Ms. Dunne sees as negative and positive. 6. Discuss ways of introducing assertive behaviors identified.

INTERVENTION

Therapeutic Relationship

The development of a therapeutic relationship between the individual and the nurse involves five steps: the contact phase, contract phase, associative phase, working phase, and termination phase. The **therapeutic relationship** is a dynamic, collaborative process established to assist the individual in meeting health care needs. The relationship takes into account the environment, its resources, the individual's level of growth and development, the individual's support system, his or her specific needs at the time, and the nurse's repertoire of professional responses. The time frame in which it occurs can be several hours or several months, depending on the setting and the needs of the individual.

Characteristics of a Therapeutic Relationship

Although similarities exist among different therapeutic relationships, each relationship is unique, since it is individualized to focus on a specific person and that person's needs. The goals of the interaction are those which develop from this individualized focus. Since each relationship is unique, the nurse must use a variety of approaches and techniques rather than rely on a standardized or automatic approach to every interaction. Thus empathy is an important component of the therapeutic relationship.

EMPATHY

Empathy is the ability to share another person's feelings to the extent that one can actually put oneself in another's place. Sympathy, on the other hand, is a feeling for the individual without a real sense of understanding what the person is experiencing. Through the empathetic process the nurse is able to plan and implement care which is based on the individual's feelings, thoughts, and needs, not on assumptions about people in general. An empathetic interaction allows the nurse to work *with* rather than *on* or *at* the individual.

One way of developing empathetic behaviors is for the nurse to simulate the individual's actual situation. For example, the nurse can attempt to carry out a series of activities of daily living while using a wheelchair or describe what one sees or feels when lying in bed for several hours "being taken care of" by others. This role playing helps the nurse to develop insight into the enormous strength individuals need in facing their health care situation and the restrictions or limitations that result from it. (Illustration 12.3)

SELF-AWARENESS

To develop a therapeutic relationship, the nurse needs to assess realistically his or her own capabilities, limitations, biases, and assumptions and to look honestly at how these influence the nurse's ability to intervene effectively. For example, topics the nurse is uncomfortable in pursuing or types of individuals that the nurse avoids or limits contact with, need to be identified so that the nurse can work to prevent their affecting the therapeutic relationship. The nurse needs to help the individual to become more self-aware so that situations can be dealt with honestly and realistically. Honesty is necessary for the development of a trust relationship, since the individual depends on the nurse to provide accurate information and not to avoid issues that the nurse finds uncomfortable. Charged areas of information giving can be dealt with honestly if feelings are recognized and considered within the context of the given situation. Honesty does not imply simply giving straightforward facts, but the exploration of the true meaning of questions and the absence of a hidden agenda.

Illustration 12.3
Empathy is a vital element in any thereapeutic relationship. The importance of being able to share the feelings of others, or to empathize, is especially evident to the nurse when communicating with a dying individual. *(Photo courtesy of Connecticut Hospice Inc., New Haven, Connecticut)*

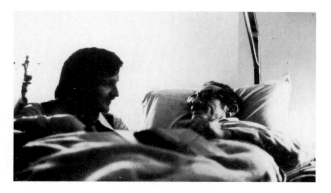

SECURITY

Relationships in which the individual feels a sense of safety and security are fostered by the nurse's carrying out interventions competently, maintaining confidentiality, not making promises that cannot be kept, following through on those promises that the nurse does make, being available, and collaborating on all goals, plans, and interventions. If it is clear that the nurse will intercede to protect the individual from threats in the environment, he or she will be able to trust the nurse and engage in a meaningful interaction. Recognizing the individual's validity as a human being and treating the person with dignity and respect is a basic prerequisite for the establishment of a therapeutic relationship.

Phases of a Therapeutic Relationship

CONTACT PHASE

The first phase in establishing the therapeutic relationship, the contact phase, involves the initial assessment of the individual. Through interviewing (Chap. 7), the nurse gathers information about the individual's needs, thoughts, feelings, and perceptions. The nurse and the individual are strangers at this time and there is much "feeling out" and testing on the part of both nurse and individual. The "feeling out" process is influenced by previous experiences with the health care system, the individual's perceptions of what is happening, and expectations of the outcome of the interactions as well as the individual's level of growth and development, cultural values, and level of anxiety. At this time the nurse attempts to clarify the individual's perceptions and needs and to attain a base line of information on which to plan the progress of the interaction.

CONTRACT PHASE

During the contract phase, the nurse and the individual negotiate the goals and the expected outcomes of the interaction. This is done by each one's clarifying his or her role within the interaction and sharing expectations about each other and the health care system. In most cases, the contract will not be a formal written one but, rather, a framework for the succeeding relationship. This contract is renegotiated throughout the span of the interaction as needs and abilities change. In some circumstances the first contract may involve the nurse's meeting most of the individual's needs with a plan for the individual to assume more and more of his or her own care as the ability to do so increases. At other times the individual may be carrying out his or her own health care activities with the nurse acting as a guide or resource person.

The nature of the contract depends very much on the abilities, needs, and expectations of the individual at that particular point in time. Establishing a contract allows both the nurse and the individual to know what the mutual expectations are and enables them to predict outcomes and follow-through on the plan. The nurse does not allow his or her biases to dictate what the contract should be, but formulates the contract on the basis of what is. For example, the individual may initially appear capable of carrying out all of the health care activities but, in spite of this, expect the nurse to do so and not relinquish the right to be taken care of by the nurse. Unless the nurse realizes that the individual's dependency needs may outweigh independence needs at this time, a conflict may arise and a mutually unsatisfactory contract be established. This phase is the planning phase of the nursing process and requires ongoing assessment and formulation of nursing diagnoses.

ASSOCIATIVE PHASE

Once the individual and the nurse have established the goals and desired outcomes of the relationship and have begun to trust one another, the associative phase begins. This phase is a transition period during which the nurse and individual become familiar with each other, and a degree of predictability develops. This is accomplished through carrying out of the contract, increased interaction time, and a realization that health care needs are being met.

WORKING PHASE

The fourth phase, the working phase, is the time when goals are being actively met through intervention measures. At this time the individual may be moving toward independence in meeting health care needs. Through use of change strategies the nurse is helping to make a positive difference in the individual's health state. Assessment, planning, and renegotiation of the contract continue throughout this time. This period may extend for many months, particularly in community settings.

TERMINATION PHASE

The termination of the relationship occurs when the individual leaves the specific health care system. This phase actually begins during the initial contact when plans are made for discharge. There are elements of planning and evaluation in this phase as the nurse plans and reinforces the learning and skills the individual needs to function at an optimum level of wellness and evaluates how the goals and desired outcomes were achieved. In addition, the nurse and individual attempt to anticipate future needs and plan for follow-up care and utilization of available resources.

In the actual final phase of the relationship, separation anxiety frequently occurs on the part of both the nurse and the individual. The nurse may be concerned about the individual's ability to meet his or her own needs, and the individual may worry about

functioning independently. A sense of loss is expected whenever a relationship which was therapeutic is dissolved for whatever reason. However, preplanning and anticipation of this allow both participants to deal with these feelings. This separation process is further complicated by the desire of both the individual and the nurse to achieve goals and thus terminate the relationship (Chart 12.4).

Promotion and Support of Language Development

One means of meeting communication needs is by promoting and supporting language development. Through the use of terms which are appropriate to the situation and to the individual's level of growth and development, cognitive abilities, and level of knowledge, the nurse can teach the proper names of things and improve the individual's ability to communicate with a wider scope of people.

By promoting a therapeutic environment, the nurse can assist the individual in expanding and refining modes of communication. Through use of role playing, play therapy, multimedia, and group interac-

---

Chart 12.4

Continuum of Therapeutic Intimacy

THERAPEUTIC INTIMACY DEPENDS ON:	SUPERFICIALITY ───► INTIMACY				
Focus of conversation	Focuses on people or events not personally known to nurse and patient.	Focuses on people or events known to either nurse or patient.	Focuses on people or events known to both patient and nurse.	Focuses on patient's concerns and self-disclosures or on nurse's concerns re patient.	Focuses on mutually shared aspects and concerns of therapeutic relationship.
Pertinence of topic	Topic is not pertinent or important to nurse or patient.		Topic is important to nurse or patient.		Topic is of concern and importance to both nurse and patient.
Time orientation	Past or future orientation that does not clarify or relate to present time.			Focus on present time; any discussion of people or events that helps to clarify the present.	
Relationship of experiences to topic	Abstractions and vague reports of events or interactions; no supportive, illustrative examples; sense of uninvolvement.			Sense of involvement in interaction or event; supported with specific, concrete examples and observations; recognition that distortion occurs with indirect knowledge.	
Use of feelings	Sharing of feelings is avoided and is considered disruptive and meaningless; indirect reflection of feelings is common: generalizations, judgments, intellectualizations about events and people.			Sharing of feelings is considered beneficial; feelings are considered natural and acceptable by nurse and patient; initially, feelings are shared from patient to nurse, but as therapeutic relationship develops the nurse shares feelings re present time and therapeutic relationship.	
Recognition of individual worth and autonomy	Lack of acknowledgment of individual worth and autonomy; patient or nurse may strive to convince the other to be like him/her; to do as he/she does.			Fundamental integrity and worth of individual as acknowledged; respect for personal autonomy. This concept is valued by nurse and patient.	

LEGEND:

- - - - = All variables are not simultaneously at the same point on the continuum.
───── = All variables are simultaneously at the same point on the continuum.

From: Longo and Williams: *Clinical Practice in Psychosocial Nursing: Assessment and Intervention*, Appleton, New York, 1978.

tions, the nurse gives the individual opportunities to become familiar with and practice new modes of and approaches to communication. The nurse also serves as a role model for language and communication development. The nurse's everyday use of a variety of techniques is frequently imitated by the individual.

When structural or physiologic disturbances interfere with language development, the nurse assists the individual in finding compensatory techniques and in removing underlying pathologies. When psychosocial interferences are impeding language development, the nurse, through counseling and referral of family and/or significant others to appropriate resources, can aid in decreasing these interferences.

Cultural Considerations

The nurse can promote effective communication by working within the context of the individual's cultural frame of reference. Recognition of cultural differences in language use, time orientation, distancing, and health care preferences allows the nurse to choose the interventions which will best meet the individual's needs in a personalized manner.

It is frequently necessary for the nurse to use other resource persons, interpreters, for example, to ensure that communication is understood clearly and precisely. When working with individuals from cultures which are unfamiliar to the nurse, the nurse will need to consult with persons knowledgeable about the culture and its implications for nursing care. Nonetheless when working with individuals from other cultures, general assumptions are not made, since many people do not follow cultural expectation or have assimilated characteristics from other cultures.

Altering Levels of Anxiety

Through the use of verbal and nonverbal communication skills, the nurse can help reduce the individual's level of anxiety to manageable levels. The nurse's exact approach will be determined by the individual's specific level of anxiety and how the individual is manifesting it. The nurse recognizes that behavior such as aggression, withdrawal, crying, and suspicion are examples of coping mechanisms which the individual is using to deal with anxiety and not a direct reflection of the individual's feelings toward the

nurse. This recognition helps the nurse to decrease his or her own anxiety as well as that of the individual. By recognizing the contribution of his or her own anxiety, the nurse can modify the approaches taken so as to minimize the interfering effects of that anxiety.

Certain general techniques can assist the nurse in intervening to help the person reduce the level of anxiety. Clear and concise explanations of all techniques and procedures assist the individual in predicting what will happen and allow the individual an opportunity to plan behaviors. By collaborating with the individual during each step of the care process, the nurse not only prepares the individual for what is coming, but also gives the individual control over the situation.

Care which is carried out in a competent, trustworthy manner and is aimed at meeting the individual's needs for safety and security also lowers anxiety. The nurse can help the individual explore the relationships between his or her anxiety and the factors which increase or decrease it. Providing the time and creating an open atmosphere for the free expression of feelings, identifying with the individual methods for coping with anxiety, and implementing actions which will help to lower it are other techniques which help reduce anxiety. When severe anxiety precipitates a crisis, intervention (Chap. 25) is necessary to enable the individual to function effectively once again.

Release of tension through physical and diversional activities that are appropriate to the limitations of the individual's health state also release anxiety, as well as deal with some of the disturbances produced by the anxiety. Any physical or physiologic manifestations are dealt with symptomatically. For example, if the individual is perspiring perfusely, such activities as bathing and changing clothing and linen increase the individual's level of comfort. Increased comfort levels frequently help to decrease anxiety. In addition, interventions aimed at reducing any pain the individual is experiencing help to alter anxiety levels, since pain is a frequent contributor and potentiator of anxiety (Chap. 23).

Relaxation techniques such as breathing exercises, meditation, and yoga are useful adjuncts to any intervention whose purpose is relief of anxiety. When anxiety is overwhelming, medications such as tranquilizers may be useful in helping the individual deal with the anxiety or the symptoms produced by it. However, medication should not be used to the exclusion of other anxiety-reducing interventions.

Since the nurse recognizes the role that the family and/or significant others play in reducing or increasing the individual's level of anxiety, the nurse incorporates these persons into the total care process. Many of the same interventions are utilized with the family and/or significant others as with the individual. Their input often provides much valuable information that can be utilized in meeting the individual's communication needs. The individual often is coming from and returning to the family and/or significant other system.

The interactions discussed in this chapter must be considered as part of the individual's overall communication needs if the individual is to reach his or her optimum level of functioning.

EVALUATION

Evaluation for meeting communication needs focuses on the direction of change in the person's ability to meet these needs and the effectiveness of intervention. Evaluation of communication needs also considers the effects of communication skills on the individual's ability to meet all other health care needs.

Specific criteria for evaluating whether communication needs are being met include:

- How do physiologic changes relate to changes in meeting communication needs? Psychologic changes? Environmental changes?
- Has the presenting communication pattern moved closer to the expected?
- What are the changes in the degree of interference with communication needs?
- What are the changes in coping with interferences with communication—by the individual? by family and/or significant others?
- What are the changes in knowledge about the communication process?
- What skills have been acquired in meeting communication needs, e.g., alternate modes of communication?
- What is the direction of change in the individual's ability to meet communication needs?
- What are the changes in attitude toward the communication process (by individual? by family and/or significant others?)
- What are the changes in level of anxiety and language development?

- What is the nature of the therapeutic relationship that has developed?
- What are the changes in the barriers to the development of the therapeutic relationship?
- What are the changes in the facilitators to the development of the therapeutic relationship?
- What are the changes in the ways needs are communicated?

RECORDING AND TEACHING–LEARNING ACTIVITIES

Teaching–Learning Topics

- rationale for the therapeutic regime
- methods to match capabilities with limitations
- ways to structure the environment to enhance the communication process
- ways to modify language skills to meet communication needs
- methods to reduce anxiety
- methods to increase language development
- ways in which to deal with cultural differences in communication
- factors which affect communication process
- resources available

Charting

Using appropriate terminology related to communication needs, objectively describe such factors as:

- objective base-line data on language development, interaction style, cultural influences, level of anxiety, nonverbal communication, state of health
- objective and subjective data on changes in the individual's ability to meet communication need
- subjective data on the communication process
- attitudes toward communication
- responses to interventions which promote meeting the need
- schedule and methods of care
- teaching carried out
- contract established
- discharge planning done

■ family and/or significant others' interactions and responses

Update Kardex on changes in goals and plans for meeting communication needs.

SELECTED REFERENCES

Babcock, Dorothy. "Transactional Analysis." *American Journal of Nursing,* 76:1152, July, 1976.

"Communicating With Patients" (Special Feature). *American Journal of Nursing,* 79:1074, June, 1979.

"Communicating with Young Children" (Special Section). *American Journal of Nursing,* 77:1960, December, 1977.

Cosper, Bonnie. "How Well Do Patients Understand Hospital Jargon?" *American Journal of Nursing,* 77:1932, January, 1977.

Goodykoontz, Lynne. "Touch: Attitudes and Practice." *Nursing Forum,* 18(1):4, 1979.

Green, Karen. "Being Tough With Tony Was the Kindest Thing We Could Do." *Nursing 78,* 8:36, October, 1978.

Hardy, Mary Kniep and Burkhardt, Margaret. "Nursing the Navajo." *American Journal of Nursing,* 77:95, January, 1977.

Hein, Eleanor and Leavitt, Maribelle. "Providing Emotional Support to Patients." *Nursing 77,* 7:38, May, 1977.

James, Sybil. "When Your Patient is West Indian." *American Journal of Nursing,* 78:1908, November, 1978.

Kreiger, Dolores. "Therapeutic Touch: The Imprimatur of Nursing." *American Journal of Nursing,* 75:784, May, 1975.

Loesch, Larry and Loesch, Nancy. "What Do You Say After You Say 'MM-Hmm.' " *American Journal of Nursing,* 75:807, May, 1975.

Lynch, James. "The Simple Act of Touch." *Nursing 78,* 8:32, June, 1978.

Mooney, Judith. "Attachment-Separation in the Nurse-Patient Relationship." *Nursing Forum,* 15(3):259, 1976.

Moritz, Derry Ann. "Understanding Anger." *American Journal of Nursing,* 78:81, January, 1978.

Primeaux, Martha. "Caring for the American Indian Patient." *American Journal of Nursing,* 77:91, January, 1977.

"Programmed Instruction: Helping Depressed Patients in General Nursing Practice." *American Journal of Nursing,* 77:1007, June, 1977.

Riley-Kesler, Arlene. "Pitfalls to Avoid in Interviewing Outpatients." *Nursing 77,* 7:70, September, 1977.

Shubin, Seymour. "Familiarity: Therapeutic? Harmful? When?" *Nursing 76,* 6:18, November, 1976.

Sloboda, Sharon. "Understanding Patient Behavior." *Nursing 77,* 7:74, September, 1977.

Snyder, Joyce and Wilson, Margo. "Elements of a Psychosocial Assessment." *American Journal of Nursing,* 77:235, February, 1977.

Stillman, Margot. "Territoriality and Personal Space." *American Journal of Nursing,* 78:1670, October, 1978.

"Therapeutic Touch" (Special Feature). *American Journal of Nursing,* 79:660, May, 1979.

Truesdell, Sandra and Wood, Tom. "Communication: Key to Efficient Patient Care." *Nursing 77,* 7:52, August, 1977.

Ujhely, Gertrude. "Touch: Reflections and Perceptions." *Nursing Forum,* 18(1):18, 1979.

Walke, Mary Anne Kelly. "When a Patient Needs to Unburden His Feelings." *American Journal of Nursing,* 77:1164, July, 1977.

Wisser, Susan Hiscoe. "When the Walls Listened." *American Journal of Nursing,* 78:1016, June, 1978.

The elimination of environmental stimuli leads not to Nirvana, but first to a vegetable-like existence and soon to a disintegration of personality.
— *René Dubos,* Man Adapting

13

SENSORY NEEDS

PRINCIPLES RELATED TO SENSORY NEEDS

Continuous meaningful stimuli from the environment is necessary for survival.

Any stimulus which is repetitious and unchanging becomes meaningless to the individual (white noise).

Stimuli from the environment are received through the sense organs: the eyes, ears, nose, mouth, skin, and viscera.

The sensory process involves reception of a stimulus, perception and interpretation, transmission, and response.

Perception requires proper reception and translation of stimuli into units meaningful to the individual.

The body responds to reception of all stimuli in both observable and nonobservable behaviors.

The meaning of stimuli is individual.

The characteristics of a stimulus, in part, determine its meaning.

Intact receptors, afferent pathways, efferent pathways, and effector sites are necessary for the total utilization of the sensory process.

Behavioral alterations occur whenever there is an interruption in the sensory process.

The central nervous system coordinates all higher level cognitive, physical and motor activities.

The autonomic nervous system, along with the hormonal system integrates vital functioning of the body.

Sensory deficits result in alterations in body image.

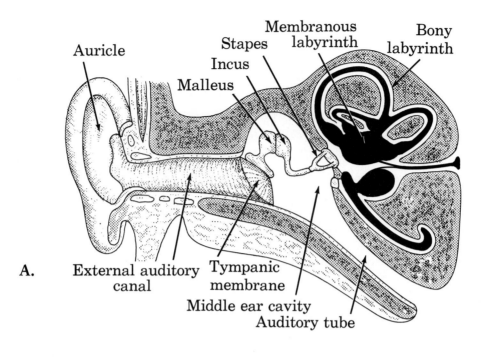

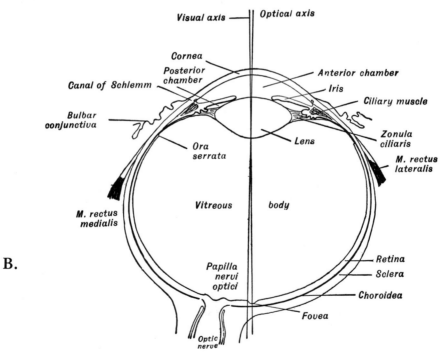

Figure 13.1
A. The external, middle, and internal portion of the ear. **B.** The eyeball and the optic (second cranial) nerve. The two vertical axes, visual and optical, depict the lines of visual accomodation. *(Courtesy of Helen Dawson,* Basic Human Anatomy, *2nd ed., Appleton New York, 1974)*

Individuals need to receive and integrate stimuli from the environment in order to successfully respond to the complexity of ever-changing input. This is the **sensory process.** The sense organs controlling sight, hearing, smell, taste, and touch are the receivers of the multiplicity of stimuli from the external environment, while the neurologic system, in conjunction with the hormonal system, regulates and coordinates the reaction of the individual to the environmental stimuli. In addition, the individual's cognitive and perceptual abilities influence the degree to which the individual can interpret the stimuli correctly, thus bringing together the reception of input with the appropriate response. At any given time, individuals are bombarded with sound waves, light waves, odors, tastes, and changes in temperature and pressure, which require them to modify their internal environments and behaviors in order to maintain the integrity of body subsystems as well as protect them from potentially harmful stimuli. Changes in the sense organs, neurologic system, hormonal system, cognition, perception, or the type and intensity of stimuli alter the individual's ability to meet sensory needs. The nurse's recognition of sensory needs and the implications of actual and potential interferences with them assists the nurse in creating an environment which maximizes the individual's abilities and safety and helps the nurse to teach the individual to compensate for sensory losses. (Fig. 13.1)

ASSESSMENT

Nursing assessment of the individual's sensory needs is directed at ascertaining the individual's level of functioning for each component of the sensory process. The sensory process begins with a stimulus that is meaningful to the individual and the reception of that stimulus by a sense organ. The stimulus is then perceived and interpreted by the neurohormonal system. In the case of reflex action, this part of the process occurs at a lower level of neurologic function (e.g., at local synapses), while other types of stimuli are perceived and interpreted at higher levels (e.g., the *cerebrum*).

As a result of perception and interpretation, a message is sent along efferent pathways to the appropriate effector site, where some type of behavior occurs. This behavior may be an observable action, such as focusing attention on a conversation, or a covert one such as storing information for later use.

Receptors

In assessing the sensory receptors, the nurse looks at the structure and patency of the organ, the nerve supply to and from the organ, and the individual's level of growth and development. The sensory receptors for external stimuli are the eyes, ears, nose, mouth, skin, and deep tissues. The eyes have electromagnetic receptors which are sensitive to light waves; the ears have mechanoreceptors for receiving sound waves and establishing equilibrium; the nose and mouth have chemoreceptors for smell and taste; the skin has thermoreceptors which are stimulated by heat and cold, mechanoreceptors which respond to changes in pressure, and nociceptors which are activated by pain (Chap. 23); and the deep tissues have mechanoreceptors and nociceptors which react to deep pressure, changes in skin tension, and pain.

STRUCTURE AND FUNCTION

The nurse, through physical assessment, determines the integrity of structure and function of these receptors. General observation and interviewing gives the nurse indications as to possible sensory interferences. Often the structure of a receptor may be intact but function may be impaired by factors such as accumulation of mucous secretions, foreign bodies, or superimposed pathologic conditions. Until these interferences are removed, the function of a receptor cannot be fully or accurately assessed.

The individual's response to stimuli is assessed through observable behaviors such as the individual's focusing on sounds, objects, and smells. Lack of appropriate response does not necessarily imply an interference with the receptor's structure or function, but may indicate an interference with some other components of the sensory process.

NERVE SUPPLY

Damage to the nervous supply of a receptor results in the loss or distortion of stimuli with resulting behavioral changes. Because of compensation, the individual may appear, on superficial observation, to be functioning as usual. With careful history taking, in-

Chart 13.1
Major Developmental Changes in Reception

DEVELOPMENTAL LEVEL	RECEPTIVE RESPONSE
Neonate	*Sight*—Uncoordinated movements of eyes; pupils react to light with total body response; difficult to evaluate actual visual ability.
	Hearing—Reacts to sound at approximately 90 decibels with total body response. Internal ear difficult to visualize because of small size.
	Taste—Sweet-sour discrimination (prefers sweet). No association of food with taste.
	Smell—Reacts to strong odors. No association.
	Touch—Responds with total body movement to all types of tactile stimulation.
Infant	*Sight*—Develops binocular vision. Depth perception begins. Vision 20/100. Farsighted. Has voluntary eye movements. Can accommodate. Differentiates colors.
	Hearing—Begins to differentiate sounds. Responds to sound by turning head instead of moving whole body.
	Taste and smell—Begins to associate.
	Touch—Associates tactile stimulation with specific body part.
Toddler through young adult	Fine discriminations continue to develop and cognitive associations increase and play a major role in reception and response. Adult levels reached in schoolage period.
Middle-aged adult	*Sight*—Acuity and accommodation begin to decline; more farsighted; color discrimination decreases, especially blue end of spectrum.
	Hearing—Acuity begins to decline.
Older adult	*Sight*—Continued visual decline; lens thicker, less elastic, and less transparent. Farsightedness increases. Vision improved by increased illumination and corrective lens. Pupils smaller. Color discrimination continues to decline.
	Hearing—Some loss of hearing, especially high tones. Degeneration of organ of Corti—more loss in men than in women. Inability to select specific sound when many sounds present *(masking)*.
	Taste—Decrease in number of taste buds.
	Touch—Tactile sensitivity and sense of vibration decrease.

terviewing, and physical assessment, the nurse can often detect these changes. Gradual losses in nervous supply are compensated for more readily than abrupt losses are, since the individual becomes accustomed to the change and modifies his or her behavior accordingly.

LEVEL OF GROWTH AND DEVELOPMENT

The individual's level of growth and development influences both the ability to receive stimuli and the manner of response to the stimuli. In part, this is related to developmental changes in the structure and function of the receptors themselves and of the neurologic system. Chart 13.1 describes some of the major changes in reception at various levels of growth and development. Generally, reception is less well defined in infancy because of structural and functional immaturity and less well defined in old age because of structural and functional degeneration.

Neurologic development parallels receptor development. As myelination of nerves proceeds (in a cephalocaudal fashion) the receptors become more discriminating in the reception of incoming stimuli. Also, as the neurologic system matures, the response to stimuli changes from a generalized, total-body response to a local effector-site response. For example, the neonate reacts to loud noises by rapidly moving the whole body, while the schoolage child reacts by turning the head toward the direction of the sound.

Nursing assessment related to reception of stimuli includes descriptions of:

- response to receptor stimulation
- general appearance of receptor
- subjective statements related to reception
- history of changes in reception
- duration of change
- factors related to changes in reception (e.g., trauma, infection)
- relationship of level of growth and development to reception

Perception and Interpretation

Perception and interpretation include the recognition of the stimulus, differentiation among stimuli, and the association of a stimulus with previous or other present stimuli. These are complex processes which integrate the physical, physiologic, and cognitive aspects of the individual.

Physically, the efferent nerve pathways and the central nervous system, particularly the cerebral cortex, must be intact to allow the stimulus to be transmitted for perception and interpretation. The individual's level of growth and development helps determine the degree of myelinization of nerves and thus influences the conduction of impulses along nerve pathways.

Physiologically, the appropriate chemical environment must be maintained for nervous system function. Adequate blood supply provides oxygen and nutrients for metabolism, while removing waste products. Cerebrospinal fluid acts to protect the central nervous system, as well as to supply some nutrients. In addition, transmission of impulses at synaptic junctions requires appropriate amounts of acetylcholine and the catecholamines.

The individual's cognitive processes of memory, organizational abilities, abstract reasoning, recall, level of knowledge, attention span, and orientation play a major role in the individual's ability to assign meaning to stimuli.

The perception and interpretation of a stimulus is greatly influenced by the characteristics of the stimulus itself, the relevancy of the stimulus to the individual, the context in which the stimulus occurs, the individual's past experience or familiarity with the stimulus, the individual's attitudes and values, general state of mind, and level of wellness. These factors are interdependent and often cannot be isolated one from another.

CHARACTERISTICS OF THE STIMULI

The duration, intensity, and type of stimuli affect the individual's interpretation of the stimuli and the meanings that the individual may attach to them. The clarity and presence or absence of conflicting stimuli help determine the amount of energy the individual has to focus on the stimulus. A single, clear stimulus requires less attention than a muffled, ambiguous one.

RELEVANCY

The importance (meaning) of the stimulus to the individual helps determine the speed and willingness with which the individual will respond to it. For example, a mother will quickly check when she hears her own child crying but may not even notice the cry of another child. Directly related to this is the context in which the stimulus is delivered. A particular stimulus under one set of circumstances may not evoke the same response as the same stimulus under different circumstances. Using the example mentioned above, if the mother is responsible for the care of both children, she may respond equally to both their cries. Her past experience and familiarity with the stimulus also alter the way in which she responds. If she knows from experience that a certain pitch in the cry signifies pain, she may be quicker to react than if she recognizes the cry as that of an overtired, sleepy child.

ATTITUDES AND CULTURE

The attitudes, values, and culture of the individual may directly influence the meaning or interpretation that the individual assigns to a stimulus. The way in which a person has learned to interpret or respond to stimuli throughout life is dependent on the way in which people around the individual, the family and/or significant others, cultural subgroup, and peers have traditionally perceived and interpreted the stimuli. The cultural and family and/or significant-others group from which the individual comes greatly influence the types of stimuli with which the individual has come in contact and the attitudes and values the individual has derived from these exposures. These in turn influence the way in which the person responds. For example, some cultural groups do not perceive pain as significant unless the individual is totally unable to carry out usual activities. Thus an individual from one of these cultures may not attach any importance to pain until it is completely debilitating.

PRESENT STATE OF MIND

The individual's state of mind, including level of anxiety and preoccupation with other stimuli, may either potentiate or decrease the perception and interpretation of stimuli. Anxiety usually results on a focusing of attention and energy on the event or events which are related to that anxiety. If a given stimulus is a precipitating factor in the individual's anxiety, the individual may become hypersensitive to the stimulus. On the other hand, if the stimulus is not directly connected with the anxiety, the individual may not have energy to direct attention to the stimulus. In addition, high levels of anxiety tend to cause a distortion in the perceptual and interpretative process.

When individuals are preoccupied with other events, activities, or cognitive processes, their perception and interpretation of stimuli may be affected. Their attention span on the stimuli may be decreased, resulting in a lack of sufficient attention to the stimuli for accurate perception and interpretation. For example, the toddler who is caught up with play may

not place significance on the stimulus to urinate and consequently wets his or her pants.

LEVEL OF WELLNESS

The individual's overall level of wellness may also alter perception and interpretation of stimuli. Pathologies, drugs, debilitation, pain, state of nutrition, and fatigue are some of the influencing factors. Disease processes which affect the central nervous system have a direct influence on perception and interpretation, while those illnesses which reduce the supply of oxygen to the tissues, particularly the brain, or increase the amount of waste products in the blood and tissues will indirectly, but significantly, affect stimuli perception and interpretation. Drugs can also directly or indirectly affect perception and interpretation. For example, central nervous-system depressants or stimulants can either heighten or reduce the individual's ability to deal with stimuli. Other drugs, like insulin, aid metabolism and can assist with supplying the brain with sufficient nutrients.

Debilitation may affect the perceptual and interpretative processes by reducing the amount of energy available to focus on stimuli and by decreasing the ability of the individual to come in contact with a variety of stimuli. In addition, the debilitated persons may be preoccupied with and anxious about their states of health and thus focus on certain stimuli while ignoring others. Pain affects perception and interpretation in a similar fashion. The individual may place more significance on other stimuli if the individual feels those stimuli contribute to increasing or decreasing the pain while ignoring those stimuli which do not seem to have a connection with the pain. General health factors such as nutrition and level of rest also influence an individual's perception of a given stimulus.

NURSING ASSESSMENT

The nurse assesses the individual's perceptual and interpretive processes through indirect means. The individual's behavior gives many clues to perception and interpretation of stimuli. Once the level of receptor function has been established, the appropriateness of the individual's behavior in response to stimuli is assessed.

Appropriateness of Emotions

Keeping in mind the influence of the previously discussed factors, the nurse observes whether the individual has the appropriate emotional affect for the given stimulus. For example, does the individual cry when the situation usually calls for laughter and vice versa? The activities the individual engages in are assessed for logical sequencing and appropriate use of common objects. The individual and family and/or significant others should be questioned as to changes in perception and interpretation of stimuli. Often the individual may not be aware of these changes, but those around the individual may provide useful information.

Cognition

The individual's cognitive processes are also assessed. Memory, both long- and short-term, is tested. Long-term memory can be checked by asking the individual to recall events or dates from the past. This information must be validated for accuracy from existing records or family and/or significant others. Short-term memory can be ascertained by having the individual repeat a sentence or series of digits. Speech pattern and thought sequences give the nurse some indication of the individual's organizational abilities. Abstract reasoning may be explored by asking the person to explain common proverbs or having the individual make analogies between words or thoughts.

Orientation

Orientation to self, place, and time is a major area of assessment for the nurse. *Orientation times three* is the term used to describe these three factors in the specific order listed above. *Orientation times two* means the individual is oriented to self and place but not to time; *orientation times one* means the individual is only oriented to self.

The nurse checks for self-orientation by asking the person his or her name. It is not sufficient to call the person's name and receive an affirmative response, since disoriented persons may be responding to the sound rather than the meaning.

Place orientation can be assessed both directly and indirectly. Directly, the nurse asks the individual to state specifically the individual's location. The nurse can indirectly assess place orientation by listening to the content and appropriateness of the person's conversation. For example, if the individual talks about being in the hospital or clinic and refers to the personnel by appropriate title, the person is said to be oriented to place.

Time orientation can be determined by asking the individual the year, season, month, day, date, and time of day. This, too, may be ascertained indirectly by listening to the conversation of the individual. It should be noted that many hospitalized or home-bound individuals, because of the monotony of stimuli and routine and the lack of calendars and clocks, may not know the exact time or date.

Obstacles in Assessment

Blocks in associative or communication skills may interfere with the individual's ability of self-expression and thus with the nurse's ability to assess perception and interpretation. Blocks such as apraxia, agnosia, and aphasia are commonly encountered in persons with neurologic pathologies. **Apraxia** is the inability to recognize previously known, common stimuli by use of the senses. For example, the individual who cannot recognize the sound of a crying baby may be apraxic. **Agnosia** is the inability to use familiar objects in a purposeful and appropriate manner. For instance, a person may pick up a toothbrush and toothpaste and be able to recognize the objects but not how to use them. **Aphasia** is the inability to understand and/or use written or spoken communication.

Nursing assessment of perception and interpretation of stimuli includes descriptions of:

- interferences with neural pathways
- related physiologic factors
- cognitive processes (e.g., abstract reasoning, memory, recall, orientation)
- characteristics of stimulus
- relevancy of stimulus
- context of stimulus
- past experience and familiarity with the stimulus
- attitudes and values related to the stimulus
- general state of mind (level of anxiety, preoccupation)
- level of wellness (e.g., drugs, pathologies)
- appropriateness of behavior

Behavioral Response to Stimuli

While the individual's behavioral responses are assessed as indications of the functioning of the other parts of the sensory process, these responses are also assessed as a distinct component.

INTERFERENCES IN THE SENSORY PROCESS

Intact, functional efferent nervous pathways and effector sites are necessary for transmission of messages for action which result from perception and interpretation. In addition, musculoskeletal integrity is necessary for carrying out the responses. Any interference with these subsystems alters a person's ability to respond appropriately. Through physical assessment the nurse looks at the function of these subsystems.

The nurse also observes the individual's behavior to see if it is safe and appropriate to the stimulus and level of growth and development, and whether the individual has successfully compensated for interferences with receptors or perception and interpretation.

HAZARDOUS BEHAVIOR

Loss of receptor function, distortions in perception and interpretation, and interferences with response mechanisms can manifest themselves in behavior which is actually or potentially dangerous to

---

Chart 13.2
Major Safety Hazards Resulting from Sensory Interference

SENSORY ALTERATION	HAZARD	IMPLICATIONS
Decreased vision	Difficulty in distinguishing objects in the environment.	Bumping into and tripping over objects, difficulty recognizing people, difficulty manipulating equipment.
	Difficulty in reading labels, signs.	Taking wrong medication, difficulty in finding places, things or in following written instructions.
	Altered depth perception.	Falling downstairs, difficulty crossing streets.
Loss of vision	Inability to use sight to carry out activities of daily living.	Must use other senses to compensate for loss.
Decreased hearing	Sounds muffled, indistinguishable.	Difficulty in understanding conversation.
	May not be able to recognize the direction of sound source.	Difficulty in picking up environmental warnings such as horns honking, people shouting.
	May not distinguish variations in sound.	Inability to focus on direction of warnings.
	Certain sound ranges may be present while others lost, thereby making it difficult to recognize the alterations in sound.	May lose sound from environment without realizing or accepting loss. Inappropriate responses to name, or sounds; may appear as disorientation.
Loss of hearing	Inability to use hearing to carry out activities of daily living.	Must use other senses to compensate for loss.
Altered equilibrium	Inability to distinguish place in space. Dizziness Nausea Lack of coordination	Difficulty in maneuvering.

(continued)

the individual. When reception is interfered with, the individual receives inaccurate or decreased stimulation from the environment. That individual may fail to compensate for the change and act in a potentially unsafe way. Chart 13.2 outlines examples of the major safety hazards resulting from interferences with the sensory process. The nurse assesses for these losses and identifies potential and actual hazards that the individual may encounter. The nurse notes the degree and range of the loss and whether it is **bilateral** (on both sides of the body) or **unilateral** (on one side of the body only).

Chart 13.2 (Cont.)
Major Safety Hazards Resulting from Sensory Interference

SENSORY ALTERATION	HAZARD	IMPLICATIONS
Alterations in smell	Inability to smell noxious odors.	May not be alert to dangerous odors such as smoke, gas fumes.
	Decrease in taste.	Decreased enjoyment of food. Decreased ability to distinguish noxious foods.
Alterations in taste	Inability to distinguish among various tastes.	Decreased enjoyment of food. Decreased ability to distinguish noxious foods.
Alteration in pressure sense	Inability to distinguish changes in weight of objects. Inability to distinguish changes in force of objects.	Injury to skin and body parts without recognition of injury. Decreased recognition of objects that bind such as braces, tight clothing, and dressing.
	Inability to distinguish texture.	Banging into objects without realization of degree of impact.
Alterations in temperature sense	Decreased ability to distinguish heat and cold.	Burns or frostbite as result of exposure to hot or cold objects without realization of temperature of object.
Alterations in neuromuscular coordination:		
Paresis (muscle weakness)	Inability to carry own weight. Inability to hold objects securely.	Stumbling, falling, dropping.
Paralysis (loss of muscle function)	Inability to bear weight on affected body part. Inability to perform activities of daily living with affected body part.	Supports needed for walking, such as braces, crutches, walkers. Tissue injury, incontinence, skills need to be relearned or performed by others.
Ataxia (uncoordinated muscle movement)	Unsteady gait. Uncoordinated gross motor movements.	Loss of balance when walking, bumping into objects, dropping things; difficulty in carrying out purposeful activities.
Tremors	Difficulty in carrying out minute motor functions.	Spilling, lack of clarity in writing, speech.

APPROPRIATENESS OF BEHAVIOR

The nurse observes if the response is appropriate in degree; in other words, does the individual under- or overreact and does the response match the stimulus that initiated it? For example, the person who says "I'm fine" in response to the statement, "Good morning," is not making the expected response for the given stimulus. Inappropriate behaviors both endanger the individual's safety and limit the individual's ability to communicate effectively with the environment.

Level of Consciousness

One way the nurse can determine the appropriateness of the individual's response to a stimulus is
▶ to assess the individual's level of consciousness. **Level of consciousness** is the individual's ability to respond to external stimuli. It differs from orientation since it involves the gross neurologic response to stimuli rather than the appropriateness of the response. There are five levels of consciousness: aware (alert), drowsy (lethargy), stupor, semicoma, and coma.

Aware. Awareness (alertness) is the ability to respond to all stimuli without difficulty. The person readily awakens from sleep when aroused with a gentle touch or noise.

Drowsy. Drowsiness (lethargy) is said to be present when responses are slow or delayed. The individual appears groggy and frequently falls asleep at inappropriate times. The individual can still be aroused, but when awakened, responses are dulled.

Stupor. In stupor, the individual requires a greater degree of stimulation to arouse. For example, shaking the person firmly may be necessary. When the individual does respond, both physical and cognitive reactions are decreased and are inappropriate to the amount of stimuli evoking them.

Semicomatose. A semicomatose state is one in which the individual does not respond to usual environmental stimuli such as sound, light, and gentle touch, but can be minimally aroused by painful stimulation. Stimulation of the pain reflex can be accomplished by firmly pinching the individual, firmly pressing the thumbnail along the sides of the bridge of the nose, and by squeezing the Achilles tendon. These testing techniques are not used unless there is evidence of decreased consciousness. (Illustration 13.1)

Coma. Coma exists when the individual does not consistently respond to any stimuli. Basic reflexes may be depressed or absent. Eye movements may be uncoordinated and pupils may not respond to light.

APPROPRIATENESS OF BEHAVIOR FOR LEVEL OF GROWTH AND DEVELOPMENT

Behaviors that are appropriate for one level of growth and development are not necessarily appropriate for another level. For example, it is perfectly acceptable for the young toddler to eat all his foods with his hands and spill food on himself and the furniture; however, in our society, this is not acceptable behavior for the young adult. Thus the nurse must examine behavior in terms of both the individual's expected and actual levels of growth and development, and should identify the differences between these findings. The nurse attempts to determine factors that contribute to the differences in the actual and expected responses for the given stimulus.

COMPENSATORY BEHAVIOR

When interferences with the sensory process are relatively slow in onset, many individuals are able to

Illustration 13.1
In assessing an individual's gross neurological response to stimuli, the nurse is assessing the level of consciousness. One indication of coma, the fifth level of consciousness, is when an individual's pupils do not respond to light. *(Photo © Leonard Speier, 1979)*

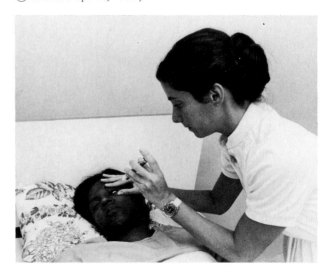

compensate for these losses. The individual may not always be aware that either the loss or the resulting compensation has taken place. For example, the person with a decrease in hearing may turn toward the sound source and focus on it, may begin to turn up the volume of the television and radio, or even begin to lipread in order to compensate for the hearing deficiency, without realizing these changes in behavior or their cause. Family and/or significant others may often provide information about these kinds of compensatory changes. At other times, the individual may be aware of sensory deficiencies and "build" compensatory mechanisms into responses. For example, the older person who is aware of a decrease in visual acuity may put higher wattage light bulbs into reading lamps. The nurse assesses the type of compensatory behavior as well as the effectiveness of this behavior. Not all compensatory behavior promotes wellness. For instance, if the individual, as a solution to sensory loss, withdraws from social interaction, he or she may indeed be compensating for the loss, but not in a healthful manner. The individual's perceptions and interpretation of the deficit and its compensations are explored to determine the individual's recognition and level of knowledge and understanding of them.

AFFECT

▶ The individual's affect is also observed. **Affect** is the emotional content of behavior. When emotions are extreme and change rapidly, the individual's af-
▶ fect is said to be **labile.** Moods which the individual
▶ displays such as **apathy** (lack of interest), **euphoria** (inappropriate feeling of well-being), depression, and anxiety are identified and examined in relationship to the appropriateness of the situation. Although these emotional states may be indicative of many things, they may result from interferences with cerebral function and, as such, should be assessed in the context of the sensory process.

Nursing assessment of behavioral responses includes descriptions of:

- relationship of behavioral response to stimuli
- appropriateness of response (e.g., to stimulus; level of growth and development)
- relationship of response to safety
- compensatory mechanisms

- recognition of compensatory mechanisms (by individual, family and/or significant others)
- duration of loss and compensatory mechanisms
- adequacy of compensatory mechanisms
- actual and/or potential environmental hazards
- characteristics of loss
- level of consciousness
- affect

Stimuli

The type and quality of stimuli which are present in the individual's environment are another facet in the assessment of the sensory process. The ability of the individual to utilize his or her sensory process is altered if the individual is not exposed to meaningful stimuli and to change in intensity and pattern. The section on perception and interpretation (pages 205–207) discusses the characteristics of stimuli which provide meaning to the individual and affect how the individual will respond to them. The intensity of stimuli refers to its strength and degree. Words such as *loud, soft, bright, dull, intense,* and *severe* refer to the intensity of a stimulus. The rhythm and form of the stimulus constitutes its patterns. Terms such as *unchanging, monotonous, varied,* and *inconsistent* describe pattern. Intensity and pattern together help contribute to the meaning a stimulus has for the individual. For example, a stimulus which is significant to an individual but continues at the same intensity and pattern over a period of time will lose its meaning to the individual and no longer provide stimulation.

Many behaviors which seem to be caused by interferences with reception or perception and interpretation are actually the result of alterations in meaningful stimuli. Such behaviors as decreased attention
▶ span, poor judgment, **hallucinations** (subjective activation of the senses without objective external stimuli), paranoia, aggression, nightmares, interferences in communication, and activation of the stress response are some examples of responses to alteration in meaningful stimuli. Alterations in meaningful
▶ stimuli are termed **sensory deprivation.**

SENSORY DEPRIVATION

Six categories of sensory deprivation can be identified. The first type is an absolute reduction or absence of stimuli in the external environment, and is also termed sensory deprivation. While, in the everyday world, there is rarely a total absense of stimuli, there are many situations which produce a reduction in stimuli. Individuals whose environment lacks changes in intensity, pattern, and meaning are susceptible to this type of deprivation. Reduction in environmental stimuli range from the frequently occurring situation of the bedridden institutionalized person to the extreme circumstance of the prisoner in solitary confinement. Although this type of sensory deprivation can produce negative health behaviors, there are times when it is therapeutically desired. For example, the neurologically impaired individual, the psychotic person, or the toxic pregnant woman, who is hypersensitive to stimuli, may be placed in an environment which has decreased auditory, visual, and tactile stimulation until the condition resolves.

RECEPTION DEPRIVATION

▶ A second type of sensory deprivation, **reception deprivation,** occurs when the receptor organs are impaired and either partial or complete loss of sensations results. In this situation the stimuli in the environment are unchanged but the individual is unable to receive them, and thus there is a decrease in meaningful stimuli by which the individual can interpret the environment.

PERCEPTUAL DEPRIVATION

Closely related to reception deprivation, and ▶ often a result of it, is perceptual deprivation. **Perceptual deprivation** exists when the individual is unable to recognize and interpret stimuli from the external environment. This may result from drug therapy, particularly central nervous system depressants, any type of cerebral brain dysfunction, or psychiatric states, especially thought disorders.

CONFINEMENT DEPRIVATION

Confinement deprivation, a fourth type, is seen when individuals are separated from significant others and familiar objects. This type of deprivation is basically a social process which results from decreased interactions with meaningful stimuli. The loss of familiar objects decreases the individual's ability to orient himself or herself to place. The individual

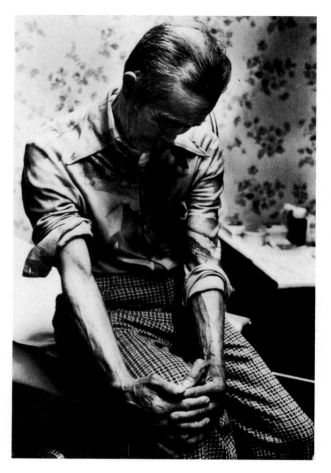

Illustration 13.2
Depression is an emotion experienced by all people, in varying degrees. It has many causes, ranging from sensory deprivation to interferences with cerebral function. *(Photo © Emilio Mercado/Jeroboam)*

hospitalized for long periods of time, the person who lives in a single-room-occupancy setting, or the homebound individual are particularly prone to confinement deprivation. (Illustration 13.2)

IMMOBILITY DEPRIVATION

▶ **Immobility deprivation** is a predominantly physiologic phenomenon which results from a decrease in physical movement and activity. The individual on strict bed rest, in a body cast or traction, in a weak or debilitated condition, or in a paralyzed state has decreased muscular, skeletal, and neurologic stimulation and thus does not have the opportunity to interact or respond to physical stimuli. (Chapter 14 has a more complete discussion of immobility.)

SENSORY OVERLOAD

▶ **Sensory overload,** the sixth category of sensory deprivation, may not appear to belong with the other types of deficits, since it involves an increase in the amount of environmental stimuli. However, since there is a multisensory bombardment by stimuli in the environment, the increase in pattern and intensity of these stimuli becomes meaningless. Therefore, the individual cannot appropriately perceive and interpret them. Any situation which produces increases in sound, sight, taste, smell, or touch may produce sensory overload. Everyday circumstances such as a crowded, noisy party can percipitate sensory overload. In the health care situation, a typical example of this occurs in any type of intensive care unit where many machines are buzzing, the lights are continuously on, and many persons are present.

RELATIONSHIP OF DEPRIVATIONS

Any type of sensory deprivation can exist by itself or in combination with other types. Often the presence of one sensory deficit will increase the likelihood that others will follow. For example, the elderly person with a decrease in auditory and visual acuity may develop reception deprivation and even perceptual deprivation. This, in turn, can lead to the individual's decreasing interaction with others, resulting in confinement deprivation. The situation is further aggravated if the individual enters a long-term care facility and is separated not only from family and/or significant others, but also from familiar objects and possessions.

Nursing assessment of sensory stimulation includes descriptions of:

- characteristics of stimuli (e.g., intensity pattern, duration, type)
- meaning of stimuli to individual
- behaviors present related to sensory deprivation
- type of sensory deprivation present
- factors contributing to sensory deprivation

Physical Assessment

The total neurologic assessment of the individual consists of cranial nerve, reflex, and sensation testing, as well as testing for muscle strength and tone and for balance and coordination. In addition, cerebral function is assessed with tests for level of consciousness and orientation (discussed in the previous section).

CRANIAL NERVE TESTING

Testing cranial-nerve function gives the nurse information about the status of the receptor organs and cerebral integrity. A combination of observation and palpation is used to test these nerves. In the overall nursing assessment of the neurologic system, all 12 cranial nerves are tested, but more commonly the nurse looks at specific cranial-nerve function as it relates to the individual's needs at a particular point in time. For example, the oculomotor, trochlear, and abducens nerves are frequently tested to evaluate intracranial pressure. Chart 13.3 outlines the tests for cranial-nerve function. See Figure 13.2 and 13.3.

REFLEXES

The nurse can obtain further data about the individual's neurologic status through reflex testing. The reflex arc gives information about the reception of a stimulus, its afferent transmission, its reception, and translation at the anterior horn cell, efferent transmission, and the ability of the effector site to respond. Therefore, the presence or absence of a reflex does not specifically pinpoint the area of disturbance but helps to give a more complete picture of neurologic functioning. Reflexes can be divided into those of infancy, which disappear during the first years of life, and those which can be elicited throughout life. Charts 13.4 and 13.5 describes the major reflexes.

Reflexes which are found throughout life are of two types—deep and superficial. Deep reflexes test the contractability of underlying muscles by stretching the tendon or tapping the bony prominence which lie over them. In contrast, superficial reflex testing assesses the contractibility of muscles lying close to the skin surface. Both types of reflexes indicate the function of anterior horn cells at various levels of the spinal cord as well as the other components of the reflex

Chart 13.3
Tests for Cranial Nerve Function

CRANIAL NERVE	FUNCTION	TEST	EXPECTED RESULTS	POINTS TO NOTE
Olfactory	Smell	Equipment: containers with odoriferous substances such as cloves, onions, coffee, or tobacco. Procedure: Individual closes eyes and substance is passed under the nose. The individual is asked to identify the smell.	Individual can identify odor.	Any substance used must have an odor familiar to the individual. This nerve may be difficult to test in cases where the individual is not able to verbalize well; in such cases, sharp, noxious odors such as spirits of ammonia are used to obtain an avoidance reaction.
Optic	Visual acuity	Equipment: Snellen chart or any printed matter. Procedure: With Snellen chart, the individual is placed 20 ft from chart and covers one eye and reads the smallest, but still distinct, line from the chart. Repeats procedure with other eye. Printed matter—the individual is asked to read a line from print.	Individual range varies greatly, but the nurse notes what line can be read at 20 ft. Notation is also made of the manner in which the line is read, e.g., 20/40 smoothly (the individual can therefore read with ease a line of print at a distance of 20 ft which most people can read at a distance of 40 ft). Notation is made of ease of reading and distance print is held away from eyes.	Symbols must be used that the individual can recognize. Nerve function difficult to assess if person cannot verbalize. If individual wears corrective lenses, the test should be done with and without them. These tests examine gross acuity and are not for the purpose of fitting for corrective lenses.
	Field of vision	Equipment: pencil, pen, or any similar object.	Individual will see object in all quadrants of each eye at same distance as examiner with predetermined "normal" peripheral vision.	Extended index finger may be used as point of reference.

Cranial Nerve	Function	Procedure	Normal Findings	Comments
	Field of vision (cont.)	Procedure: Examiner and individual are seated facing one another at the same eye level, separated by approximately 3 ft. Individual covers one eye, while the examiner covers his own opposite. The individual looks straight at the examiner's uncovered eye. With object in hand, the examiner extends arm full length and moves object through each visual quadrant (see Fig. 13.2). The procedure is repeated with other eye.		
Oculomotor	Muscle control of eyelid; constriction of pupil; superior, inferior, and medial control of eye movements	*Gross eye movement* Individual follows examiner's finger as the examiner slowly moves it through all possible visual angles (see Fig. 13.2). The nurse observes for quivering movements of the eyes (nystagmus), lid drooping (ptosis), as well as range of eye movements.	Can move eyes up and down, laterally, and medially.	These three nerves are commonly tested as a group, since they control the overall coordination of eye movements. Mild nystagmus can be expected in extreme lateral field. Toys and bright objects can be used to test infants and children.
Trochlear	Controls inferior and lateral movement of eye			
Abducens	Controls lateral eye movement	*Pupillary reaction* Equipment: penlight, pencil. Procedure: In a darkened room. The nurse compares the size, shape, and equality of the individual's pupils. The nurse checks the pupillary light reflex by flashing a concentrated beam of light first into one eye and then the other.	Pupils should be equal in size and shape and react to light equally.	Wide variations will be found in the size and shape of the pupils. The size, shape, and pupillary reaction can be assessed on any individual, but gross eye movement and accommodation testing require the individual's cooperation.

(continued)

Chart 13.3 (Cont.)
Tests for Cranial Nerve Function

CRANIAL NERVE	FUNCTION	TEST	EXPECTED RESULTS	POINTS TO NOTE
		The beam of light is brought from the side to the nose. The nurse observes for direct and consensual constriction of the pupils The pupils are then tested for the pupillary accommodation reflex. The examiner holds an object at the same level as the individual's nose at a distance of 3 ft and slowly moves the object up to the individual's nose.	Pupils should equally constrict as individual focuses on an object as it moves closer to the eye.	Direct constriction is the decrease in the size of the pupils into which the light is flashed. Consensual constriction is the concurrent, but less obvious, decrease in the size of the pupil in the eye which has not received the light flash. When expected results are found, it is commonly noted, as PERLA (Pupils Equal, Reacting to Light and Accommodating).
Trigeminal	Controls sensation of the face and mucous membrane of the nose and mouth. Controls the corneal reflex, the movement of the masseter, temporal, maxillary, and mandibular muscles	*Sensation testing* Equipment: pin, test tube filled with cold water, test tube filled with hot water, cotton. Procedure: The individual closes the eyes and the examiner touches the skin of the individual's face with a wisp of cotton in a zigzag fashion from forehead to chin. Same procedure is followed for heat and cold. Varying temperatures used. Procedure again repeated with light pin prick.	Can identify touch equally on both sides of forehead, cheeks, chin. Can identify differences in temperature equally on both sides of face. Can identify pain equally on both sides of face.	Difficult to evaluate in person who cannot verbalize. Avoid stabbing or scratching individual.
		Corneal reflex testing Equipment: small piece of cotton	Individual should blink when cornea is lightly stroked.	Conjunctiva should not be touched.

Nerve	Function	Procedure	Expected Findings	Considerations
		Procedure: The examiner lightly strokes the cornea of each eye with small piece of cotton.		If blink reflex has already been established, this test may be omitted.
		Muscle movement testing Procedure: The individual is asked to clench jaws tightly. The examiner then attempts to open jaws by pulling down on the chin. The muscles of the jaws are palpated for equality and tension.	Can clench jaws and resist opening them. Muscles should be equal in tension and size.	Individual is told to resist efforts to open jaws. Examiner's effort should be firm but not painful.
		The individual is then asked to open and close mouth, and the nurse observes for any difficulty in movement or lateral deviation.	Should be able to open and close mouth smoothly without any lateral deviation.	Trigeminal nerve should not be tested in presence of acute phase of trigeminal neuralgia (hyperirritability and inflammation of trigeminal nerve).
		Maxillary reflex Equipment: reflex hammer Procedure: The examiner lightly taps the center of the individual's chin while individual holds mouth slightly opened.	Mouth should quickly and abruptly close with tap.	
Facial	Muscle control of the face, eyelids, and mouth and the bilateral sensations of sweet and sour taste on the anterior portion of the tongue	*Muscle control* Procedure: The nurse asks the individual to frown, grimace, smile, wrinkle forehead, raise forehead, and manipulate mouth.	Should be able to move all parts of the face symmetrically.	Individual must be cooperative in order to carry out testing. Nurse notes any weakness, asymmetry, or drooping.
		Testing eyelids Procedure: Individual tightly closes eyelids while the examiner attempts to open them by firmly pulling upward on the superior portion of the eyelid.	Should be able to keep both eyelids equally closed against pressure.	Avoid injury to eyelids and avoid pressure on eyeball.

(continued)

Chart 13.3 (Cont.)
Tests for Cranial Nerve Function

CRANIAL NERVE	FUNCTION	TEST	EXPECTED RESULTS	POINTS TO NOTE
		Testing anterior tongue taste Equipment: A few grains of sugar and salt. Procedure: Individual protrudes tongue while the nurse drops a small amount of sugar first on one side, then on other on the tip of the tongue. Repeat with salt.	Individual should be able to recognize sweet and sour tastes equally on both sides of anterior tongue.	Tongue must remain protruded throughout the examination to prevent movement of substance to posterior taste buds. Individual should be given water to rinse mouth between sugar and salt tests.
Acoustic Cochlear branch	Hearing	*Test for gross sounds* Procedure: Individual closes one ear with finger. The nurse stands approximately 2 ft from unoccluded ear and softly whispers numbers. Individual is asked to repeat back numbers. Test is repeated with increasingly louder whispers to test range. Repeat with opposite ear.	Identify sounds at all ranges.	Adequate occlusion of the ear not being tested is necessary to prevent compensation.
		Test for air and bone Conduction (Rinne Test) Procedure: The individual is seated. The examiner strikes tuning fork on own knuckle and places base of the tuning fork on the mastoid process until individual no longer hears sound; then fork is moved so that prongs of fork are	Hears air conduction longer than bone conduction.	Tuning fork with a frequency of 500–1000 cycles should be used. Placement of tuning fork on mastoid process tests for bone conduction of sound, while placement in front of ear canal tests for air conduction. Individual is taught signal to indicate when sounds are no longer

Nerve/Branch	Function	Procedure	Normal Findings	Special Considerations
		in front of ear canal. Individual signals when sound is no longer heard. *Test for lateralization (Weber Test)* Equipment: tuning fork Procedure: Individual is seated. Nurse strikes tuning fork on knuckle and places the base on center top of individual's head or center of individual's forehead.	Sensation of sound should be equal on both sides.	heard. Time span can be measured by use of second hand on watch. Individual with a deficit in air conduction of sound will have a greater sensation of vibration on the affected side because environmental noise is not being conducted on that side.
Vestibular branch	Equilibrium	Not regularly tested in routine exam. Complaints of dizziness, nausea, or loss of balance may indicate an interference with this branch of the acoustic nerve, and individual should be referred to an otologist.		
Glossopharyngeal	Taste in posterior tongue. Sensory innervation of pharynx, soft palate, tonsils, and surrounding tissues.	Equipment and procedure is the same as facial nerve test. However, substances are placed on posterior tongue.	Can identify sweet and sour taste bilaterally.	Cranial nerves IX, XX are tested as a group because they have similar actions.
Vagus	Motor innervation of pharynx, larynx, soft palate. (In addition, vagus nerve supplies innervation to heart, lungs, aortic body, and abdominal viscera. However, these functions are not tested during the neurologic exam.)	*Gag reflex test* Equipment: tongue depressor or applicator stick. Procedure: lightly touch posterior tongue *Palatal reflex test* Equipment: tongue depressor or applicator stick. Procedure: the nurse quickly touches each side of the uvula.	Gags. The touched side of the uvula rises.	Avoid prolonged or forceful touch as person may vomit.

(continued)

Chart 13.3 (Cont.)
Tests for Cranial Nerve Function

CRANIAL NERVE	FUNCTION	TEST	EXPECTED RESULTS	POINTS TO NOTE
Vagus (cont.)		The vagus alone is also tested by asking individual to speak and swallow. With penlight and tongue depressor, examiner observes movement of soft palate and uvula when individual says "ah."	Swallows. Speaks clearly without any hoarseness. Symmetrical movement of soft palate and uvula.	Tongue depressor should not touch pharynx as this will produce gagging and/or vomiting.
Accessory	Innervates the trapezius and sternocleidomastoid muscles	Procedure: Nurse asks individual to shrug shoulders and tighten neck and shoulder muscles. Nurse palpates both sides of trapezius and sternocleidomastoid muscles for tension and symmetry.	Shrugs shoulder. Shoulders raised bilaterally. Muscle tension equal bilaterally.	
Hypoglossal	Controls muscles of tongue	Procedure: Nurse asks individual to protrude tongue and move it in all directions. *Test for strength of tongue muscles* Equipment: tongue depressor. Procedure: Individual protrudes tongue. Nurse places tongue depressor firmly against one side of tongue and asks individual to try to push it away. Repeat on other side.	Tongue can be moved in all directions. No deviation when protruded. Can resist pressure of tongue blade equally on both sides.	

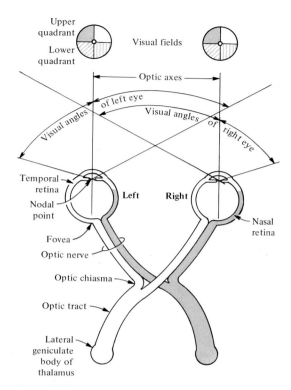

Figure 13.2
Visual quadrants and fields.

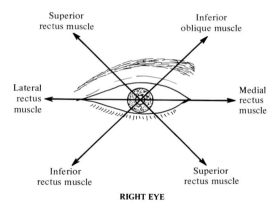

RIGHT EYE

Figure 13.3
Expected extra-ocular movements.

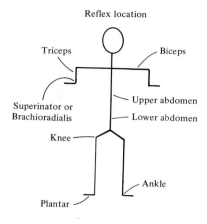

Reflex description:
0 = Absent
+ = Diminished, hypoactive
++ = Expected
+++ = Brisker than expected, hyperactive
++++ = Very brisk, hyperactive

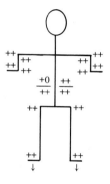

Figure 13.4
Reflex assessment—the deep and superficial reflexes may be tested to assess the functioning of a reflex arc. Above, symbolic descriptions are given of the contractibility of muscles in the various reflex locations, as are the proper body locations for testing.

arc. The presence and strength of reflex is noted by a 0–4 scale. Zero denotes an absence of the reflex; 1, present but diminished response; 2, expected response; 3, mildly hyperactive response; and 4, hyperactive response. Figure 13.4 shows the schema widely used for these notations.

SENSATIONS

The physical assessment for neurologic functioning continues with the nurse identifying the individual's ability to perceive primary sensations. Heat, cold, touch, pain, and vibration are the sensations tested. In addition, the individual's subjective reactions and behavior in response to these sensations are assessed in order to validate the test findings.

Since different areas of the body are innervated

Chart 13.4
Reflexes of Infancy*

REFLEX	EXPECTED RESPONSE	METHOD OF TESTING	EXPECTED AGE OF DISAPPEARANCE	POINTS TO NOTE
Rooting	Infant turns head toward stimulus and searches for stimulus with mouth.	Examiner lightly strokes infant's cheek in the same plane with the side of the mouth. Repeat with other side.	When awake, 3–4 months When asleep, 9–12 months	Reflex should be present at birth. Absence indicates serious CNS pathology.
Sucking	Infant sucks object strongly with equal pressure bilaterally.	The examiner places a clean object, such as a nipple, in the infant's mouth so that it touches the palate. Once infant has begun to suck, examiner withdraws object, noting degree of resistance.	12–16 months	If sucking reflex is present, it is generally implied that gag and swallow reflexes are intact. However, if the infant indicates any difficulty in swallowing, this should be tested separately (Chap. 19).
Moro response	Infant abruptly extends arms, spreading fingers. Legs may extend simultaneously to a lesser degree. Arms and legs then adduct. All movements should be bilaterally symmetrical.	With the infant lying on his back, the examiner raises the infant's head and shoulders 3–4 inches above the trunk and lower extremities and quickly lets the head and shoulders fall.	4 months	Arm movements may resemble a hugging or embracing motion. In performing this test the infant is protected from hitting any surfaces. Absence of reflex or asymmetricality indicate CNS pathology, and/or structural defects.
Startle	Infants blinks bilaterally and Moro response is elicited.	With infant in back-lying position the examiner produces a loud noise by clapping hands or banging objects together. Test is repeated on both sides.	Blinking at loud noises is a lifelong reflex. Moro response should disappear by 4 months.	In addition to testing reflex action, this test gives information on infant's gross hearing ability. Absence of blinking may indicate an interference with hearing.

Reflex	Procedure	Expected Age	Comments
Tonic neck	Infant's head turns in one direction while arm and leg on same side extend and opposite arm and leg flex (also known as fencing position).	With infant in back-lying position, the examiner turns infant's head to one side. Repeat on opposite side.	May or may not be present at birth but appears by 1–2 months and disappears at approximately 6 months. Can remain until approximately 2 years.	May be totally or partially absent without neurologic impairment. This reflex must be considered within the context of the total neurologic exam.
Grasping (palmar)	Infant firmly grasps object to the degree that infant can be raised to a sitting position.	Examiner places object, usually forefingers, in both palms of infant and attempts to raise infant to sitting position, noting degree and symmetry of grasp.	4 months	Infant should be protected from falling backward. Eliciting sucking response may enhance this reflex. Grasp strength is greater when infant's hand is flexed.
Dancing	Feet move in a walking, dancing, or running motion.	Infant is suspended in an upright position with soles of feet lightly touching a surface.	3–4 months	Usually not tested before 4 days of age.
Babinski	Spreading of the toes in an upward direction.	The outer lateral aspect of the sole of the infant's foot is gently stroked with a pointed object such as thumbnail or applicator stick.	1½–2 years	Absence or presence up to 2 years is expected. However, after 2 years, the presence of this reflex is indicative of neurologic impairment.

*These reflexes test cephalocaudal and proximodistal myelination and maturation of the nervous system. These reflexes may be absent or incomplete in the premature neonate or may remain past the expected age.

Chart 13.5
Reflexes Present Throughout Life

REFLEX	CORD SEGMENT STIMULATED	METHOD OF TESTING	EXPECTED RESPONSE
Deep		Firm tap with reflex hammer on †:	
Biceps	C5, 6	Biceps tendon when forearm is supinated and elbow flexed.	Biceps muscle contracts.
Brachioradialis	C5, 6	Styloid process of radius when forearm is supinated.	Elbow flexes and forearm pronates.
Triceps	C6, 7, 8	Triceps tendon above olecranal when elbow is flexed with forearm placed across forearm.	Elbow extends.
Patellar	L2, 3, 4	Patellar tendon with individual sitting on edge of sitting surface with legs dangling outside.	Knee extends.
Achilles	S1, 2	Achilles tendon with person in same position as patellar reflex testing.	Plantar flexion of the foot.
Superficial		With firm pressure, stroke with sharp, but non-traumatizing object such as tongue blade or handle end of reflex hammer†:	
Upper abdominal	T7, 8, 9	Upward and outward from the umbilicus.	Umbilicus shifts toward point of stimulus.
Lower abdominal	T11, 12	Downward and outward from the umbilicus.	Umbilicus moves in a downward direction.
Cremasteric	T12, L1	Upper inner aspect of the thigh.	Testicle on the same side (ipsilateral) of stimulation rises.
Plantar	S1, 2	Lateral dorsum of the foot.	Toes flex.
Gluteal	L4–S3	Gluteal area.	Skin contracts in gluteal area.

†Reflexes are tested bilaterally.

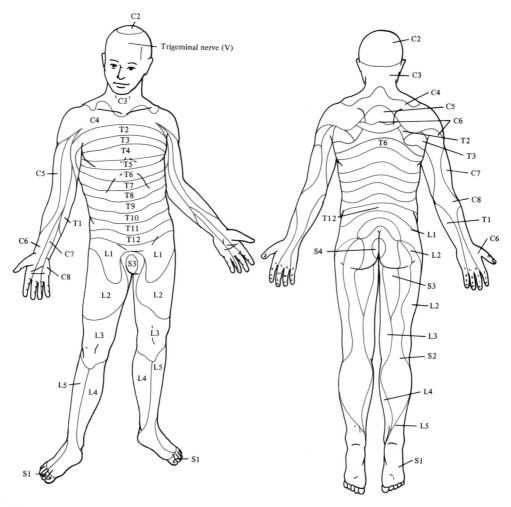

Figure 13.5
Dermatomes—anterior and posterior views of the body showing what areas (dermatomes) are innervated by various spinal cord segments. C refers to cervical segments; T, thoracic; L, lumbar; and S, sacral.

by different spinal cord segments, testing for sensation proceeds cephalocaudally in a zigzag fashion with the individual's eyes closed. This ensures complete examination of these areas of innervation. The thoroughness of the examination depends on the individual's presenting signs and symptoms. If the person has no indication of neurologic impairment, a random spot check of sensations can be done. The zones of innervation (**dermatomes**) have been mapped out (Fig. 13.5). Thus if a loss of sensation is felt in the thumb and forefinger, an interference with reception and transmission of nervous impulses to and/or from the sixth cervical cord segment is suspected.

The equipment used for testing sensations includes one test tube filled with hot water and one test tube filled with ice water to assess temperature sensation; a pin to test superficial pain; a tongue blade to test touch sensation; and a tuning fork to assess vibratory sensation. The temperature of the test tubes is reevaluated by the nurse throughout the exam to ensure the proper temperature. Findings can be recorded on a sketch similar to Figure 13.2.

In addition to testing primary sensations, the discriminatory and position sensations are also assessed. They include deep pain, position, localization, two-point discrimination, extinction, and discrimination. Chart 13.6 describes these tests.

Chart 13.6
Testing for Discrimination and Position

SENSATION	METHOD OF TESTING	EXPECTED RESPONSE
Deep pain	Examiner pinches individual's Achilles tendon firmly. The examiner notes the degree of reaction.	Individual reports sharp pain (either through posturing or verbalization).
Position	While the individual's eyes are closed, the examiner moves the individual's fingers and toes into different positions and asks individual to report their location.	Individual can identify the location of body part in space.
Localization	While the individual's eyes are closed, the examiner randomly touches parts of the body and asks the person to identify areas touched.	Individual identifies area of body being touched.
Two-Point discrimination	While the individual's eyes are closed, the examiner, using pointed objects, such as pins, touches various areas of the body with a random mixture of two pins at different distances apart and one pin. The examiner notes the individual's ability to differentiate between the touch of one pin and two pins, and the least amount of distance for discriminating between the two points.	The individual differentiates one-point touch from two-point touch and can discriminate two-point touch with a minimal distance of 2–3 mm on fingerpads. (Different parts of the body have differing minimal distances.)
Extinction	While the individual's eyes are closed, the examiner touches two different parts of the individual's body at the same time and asks the individual to identify where touched.	Individual recognizes being touched on two different body parts at the same time.
Discrimination Part A: stereognostic	While the individual's eyes are closed, the examiner places common objects, such as a pin or coins, into the individual's hand; the individual is asked to identify the object after feeling it.	The individual recognizes familiar objects which are placed in the hand.
Part B: graphesthetic	While the individual's eyes are closed, the examiner uses a finger to draw a number or letter on the palm of the individual's hand and asks the individual to identify the figure drawn.	The individual recognizes a number or letter drawn on the palm of the hand.

MUSCLE STRENGTH AND TONE

The status of effector sites is, in part, assessed through testing the strength of major muscle groups. General muscle strength and tone are assessed by observing the individual walking, sitting, standing, and carrying out activities. The individual's weight-bearing abilities, coordination, symmetry of movement, and agility are observed.

Strength

Muscle strength itself is tested by putting all joints through a full range of motion with and without resistance (Chap. 14). Any objective signs of muscle weakness, paresis or loss of muscle function or any subjective reports of either are noted. The biceps and quadriceps muscle groups and the gastrocnemius and soleus muscles are measured for bilateral comparisons.

Tone

In checking muscle tone, the nurse observes for any involuntary movements. The individual is observed both when carrying out deliberate and purposeful activities, such as writing or picking up an object, and when at rest. The nurse looks for any signs of *flaccidity* (muscle limpness), *rigidity* (muscle stiffness), and *spasticity* (increased muscle tension). Any *tremors* (involuntary trembling or shaking) or *tics* (involuntary spasms or twitching) are also noted. Noted, too, is whether these occur during purposeful activities (intentional) or at rest (nonintentional).

COORDINATION AND BALANCE

The cerebellar functions of coordination and balance are tested by asking the individual to perform a series of integrated muscular tasks. Activities which can be used are attempting to walk a straight line in a heel-to-toe fashion; touching forefinger to nose with eyes open and closed; or touching the thumb with each finger in rapid succession. Notation is made of any tremors, ataxic movements, loss of balance, or inability to carry out the task. Any interferences with afferent or efferent pathways without cerebellar impairment can affect the individual's performance of these tasks.

SPECIAL SENSES

The receptor organs of sight, hearing, and smell are assessed individually for structure and for any evidence of irritation or inflammation.

The Eyes

The eyes are observed for symmetry, shape, and position.

External Eye.　The external eye and surrounding structures are examined first. The eyebrows are inspected for distribution of hair and the condition of the underlying skin. The ability to move the eyebrows is controlled by the facial nerve and is discussed in the section on cranial-nerve testing.

The eyelids are examined for structure, continuity, color, skinfolds, and edema. Racial differences may account for differences in eyelid skin folds; for example, Oriental people often have inner epicanthal folds. Such differences are expected findings rather than signs of pathologic process, as might be the case with people of other racial backgrounds. The eyelids should not be swollen, inflamed, or have masses or lesions. The eyelashes should grow outward, rather than inward, and the distribution of lashes should be even.

The lacrimal apparatus is then inspected and palpated. The lacrimal gland and sac are examined for swelling. The sac is palpated for obstruction by pressing the medial canthus with the forefinger. If there is a backflow (regurgitation) of lacrimal secretions (tears) onto the eye, a blockage of the lacrimal duct is suspected.

The lower conjunctiva and sclera of the eye are examined by the nurse asking the individual to look up while the nurse pulls the lower eyelid down with the thumb. The conjunctiva is inspected for color, swelling, and masses. It is expected to be pink, smooth, and without swelling or masses. The sclera is examined for color and vascularity. The sclera is expected to be white. However, the periphery of the sclera is frequently yellowish and may contain dark flecks, especially in highly pigmented individuals.

The upper palpebral conjunctiva is inspected by everting the upper eyelid. This is done as gently as possible and requires the cooperation and relaxation of the individual being examined. As with any procedure, the process is thoroughly explained to the individual before beginning. An applicator stick is necessary for the performance of this procedure. The individual is asked to look downward while keeping the eyes open. The nurse takes hold of the upper eyelashes and gently pulls the lid downward. The nurse then places the applicator stick at the upper border of the tarsal plate (at least 1 cm above the margin of the lid) and pushes the stick downward on the lid while continuing to hold the eyelash. This will result in the eyelid everting. Pressure must not be put on the eyeball during the procedure. The nurse secures the lid against the brow of the eye (below the eye brow) and slides the applicator stick out. The nurse now examines the upper conjunctiva for color, continuity, and masses. (This procedure is also used to search for foreign bodies in the eye.) After inspection, the nurse returns the eyelid to its original position by again taking hold of the eyelashes, pulling them slightly forward, and asking the individual to look up and then blink.

The cornea and lens are inspected next for clarity and translucency. The nurse shines a penlight at a slanted angle toward the eye. The cornea and lens are expected to be clear and translucent. The iris of the eye is examined for color markings and distinctness. The color and markings of the iris will vary but it is expected to be clearly circumscribed. Examination of the pupil is discussed in the section on cranial-nerve testing.

Internal Eye.   After examination of the external eye and its surrounding structure is complete, ophthalmoscopic examination of the retinal structure is done. As with any other equipment, manipulation and familiarity with the use of the ophthalmoscope are necessary before attempting this procedure. This procedure is carried out in a darkened room with the nurse and the individual sitting at the same eye level. The individual is instructed to focus on a distant object over the nurse's shoulder. The nurse holds the ophthalmoscope in the right hand against his or her own right eye to examine the individual's right eye. While examining the retinal structures, the nurse and the ophthalmoscope function as a unit to ensure vision of the structures. The nurse adjusts, as necessary, the setting of the lens to ensure clarity. The nurse steadies the individual's head with the free hand.

Starting from a distance of 12–15 inches (30–37.5 cm) the nurse shines the light into the individual's pupil and looks for the red reflex. The red reflex is the interaction of the light with the fundus of the eye and is seen as a circular reddish-orange area. Any opacities in the lens and cornea appear as darkened

areas distorting the reddish circle. Once the red reflex is located, the examiner moves, as a unit, closer to the individual's eye. As the examiner moves closer, the optic disc can be identified. The optic disc appears as a distinct yellowish oval or circle. If the disc cannot be readily located, the nurse should follow a blood vessel as it increases in size. This should bring the examiner to the optic disc. The optic disc is inspected for distinction, color, shape, and physiologic cup (a pale area of depression).

The retinal vessels are then examined for continuity, size, tortuosity, and shape. Vessels are expected to be continuous, smooth, and to decrease in size as the examiner moves away from the optic disc. Arterioles appear light red and thinner than the dark red veins. The areas where the arterioles and veins cross should not be indented. The entire periphery of the retinal structures is examined by having the individual move the eyes in all directions.

The examination of the retinal structures concludes with the examination of the central point of vision, the macula. The macula is located temporal to the optic disc and appears as a dark area. The darker the pigmentation of the individual, the darker the macula will appear. To examine the macula, the nurse asks the individual to look directly into the light source.

The Nose

Examination of the nose begins with inspection and palpation of the external structure. The nose is observed for symmetry and centrality. Any bulging, masses, or structural deformities are noted. Structural deformities should not be confused with expected variations in nose size and shape among various individuals. The nurse palpates bilaterally for structure and patency. Patency can be further assessed by asking the individual to occlude one nostril with a finger and to inhale through the open nostril while the mouth is closed. This is repeated on the other side. The nurse listens for sounds of obstruction and asks the individual for subjective feelings of patency.

The internal structure is then observed using a high-intensity penlight. The individual is asked to move the head backwards (hyperextend) while the nurse lifts the tip of the nose upward. The nurse next shines the light into one nostril and then the other, observing the mucous membrane for color, continuity, and drainage. The mucous membrane is expected to be deep pink in color and intact; it may have clear serous drainage. The septum is observed for deviation from the center. The septum should fall approximately midway between the two nasal canals. The lateral wall of the nasal canal is observed for the inferior and middle turbinates (the superior cannot be visualized by this method). The turbinates should not occlude the nasal canal or be inflamed. Throughout the examination, the entire nose canal is observed for signs of foreign bodies, masses, or any other type of obstruction. The individual is asked about the frequency, type, and amount of drainage, bleeding (epistaxis), history of trauma to the nose, feelings of obstruction, and pain.

The Ears

The external ear (auricle) is inspected for size, shape, and position. The presence of any masses, structural deformities, or drainage is noted. Like the nose, ears vary widely in size and shape. However, the end of the earlobe is expected to be in a plane slightly below the tip of the nose. The mastoid and tragus are firmly but gently palpated for tenderness and masses, which are not expected findings.

The nurse then inspects the ear canal and eardrum with the otoscope. The individual is asked to tip the head in a direction away from the ear being examined. When examining an adult, the nurse firmly grasps the middle of the auricle, pulls it upward and backward. With the infant and child, the auricle is only pulled backward. The speculum of the otoscope is then gently inserted into the ear canal. Care is taken not to damage or put pressure on the very sensitive epithelial lining. The canal is observed for color, drainage, continuity, masses, and foreign bodies. The canal is expected to be pale pink, without drainage, intact, and free of masses and foreign objects. The eardrum and attendant structures (Fig. 13-1) are identified and observed for signs of inflammation and structural deformity. The eardrum is expected to be shiny, translucent, and grayish in color. Any pain on examination or history of drainage or pain is recorded.

Nursing assessment related to physical assessment of the neurologic system and special senses includes descriptions of:

- cranial nerve testing
    presenting findings
    relationship between presenting and expected findings
- reflexes
    absence or presence of reflexes
    intensity of reflex
    appropriateness of reflex to level of growth and development
    relationship between presenting and expected findings
- sensations
    equality of sensations
    symmetry of sensations
    intensity of sensations
    continuity of intensity on specific body parts
    relationship between presenting and expected findings
- muscle strength
    presenting findings (weight bearing, posture, coordination and symmetry of movement, agility)
    degree of muscle strength in each muscle group
        presence of paralysis and/or paresis
    subjective statements concerning muscle strength
    presence of involuntary movements (during purposeful movements, during rest)
    history of involuntary movements
- coordination and balance
    presenting findings
    relationship between presenting and expected findings
    presence of tremors or ataxia
- special senses
    eye
        presenting findings of external eye and surrounding structures and retinal structures
        relationship between presenting and expected findings
        subjective statements related to vision
    nose
        presenting findings of external nose, internal nose
        relationship between presenting and expected findings
        subjective statements related to patency and smell, including history
    ear
        presenting findings of external ear, middle ear, and eardrum
        relationship between presenting and expected findings
        subjective statements related to hearing and ear inflammation, including history

Diagnostic Tests

The neurologic assessment is the major diagnostic testing method used to identify interferences with neurologic functioning. However, several other tests are often used to differentiate and specify the exact location and type of interference present. These include the skull x-ray, vertebral x-rays, angiography, lumbar puncture, myelogram, brain scan, and computerized axial tomography (CAT scan).

SKULL AND VERTEBRAL X-RAYS

The skull and its contents can be visualized at a variety of angles (lateral, posteroanterior, and axial) by x-ray. An x-ray of the skull can detect breaks in its continuity; shifting of contents; and changes in size, bone formation and calcification, or vascularity. No special pretest preparation or posttest care is required for this procedure. Vertebral x-rays give similar information about the vertebrae and spinal cord. However, the individual may be required to assume and maintain several positions for accurate visualization of different views of spinal structures.

CEREBRAL ANGIOGRAPHY

Cerebral angiography is performed to visualize the cerebral blood vessels and the presence of any obstructive interferences. As with any type of angiography, a radiopaque dye is injected. In this instance the dye is injected into the cerebral circulation via the carotid and/or vertebral arteries, depending on the specific visualization desired.

LUMBAR PUNCTURE

The pressure of the cerebrospinal fluid (CSF) can be measured and specimens of CSF obtained through lumbar puncture. In addition, radiopaque substances or gases may be injected for other diagnostic tests. This procedure can be very frightening and anxiety-producing; thus careful step-by-step explanations of the procedure and the individual's part in it are necessary. Special emphasis is placed on the fact that the needle is not inserted into any area of vital function. Posttest care is also explained at this time. Many

health care facilities require a signed consent prior to this procedure.

Since the lumbar puncture is most commonly performed at the bedside, familiarity with the equipment and procedure is important.

Equipment

The equipment needed includes a lumbar puncture needle, a regular needle and syringe, a manometer, a local anesthetic, gloves, test tubes and/or culture tubes, skin disinfectant, sterile drapes, and a small sterile dressing. This equipment is frequently available in sterile disposable packs.

Procedure

Lumbar puncture is performed with the individual in a side-lying position with the knees brought up to the chest and the head and shoulders hunched forward so that the spine is maximally curved. The individual is assisted in assuming this position and made as comfortable as possible by the use of pillows and other supports under the head, knees, and any other location the individual desires (except along the spinal column). Weak and debilitated persons may have to be held in this position if they are unable to maintain it themselves. Infants and children must be held at all times during the procedure to prevent unexpected movements and to provide support and comfort. (Fig. 13.6).

The insertion site, usually the space between the third and fourth lumbar vertebrae, is cleansed with a disinfectant solution and the area around it draped with sterile towels. Any persons involved with the actual procedure put on sterile gloves at this time. A local anesthetic is injected intradermally at the insertion site. The lumbar puncture needle is then inserted between the vertebrae. Since the lumbar puncture needle consists of a cannula and a stylet (a solid probe which blocks the lumen of the cannula), once the needle reaches the subarchnoid space the stylet is removed and a small amount of CSF is allowed to drip.

Once proper placement of the cannula is attained, as evidenced by dripping of CSF, the manometer is attached and measurement of the opening CSF pressure is obtained (expected 60–180 mm H_2O). Accurate CSF pressure readings require that the individual be relaxed. The individual may be helped to relax through distraction, straightening the legs, touch or stroking, and deep breathing. The first (opening) pressure is validated by having the indi-

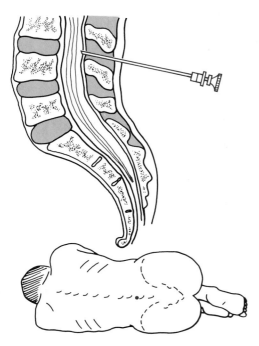

Figure 13.6
For a lumbar puncture, the individual is placed in a lateral position with head and knees flexed, allowing for maximal flexion of the lumbar vertebrae to facilitate insertion of the needle. The lumbar puncture needle is inserted into the subarachnoid space, usually between the third and fourth lumbar vertebrae. Injury to the spinal cord is avoided because, at this point of insertion, the cord has divided into a sheaf of nerves. (The cord ends between the first and second lumbar vertebrae.)

vidual bear down as if defecating (Valsalva maneuver) or by coughing. If the puncture system is patent, a temporary rise in pressure will occur.

The stopcock on the manometer is then turned to outflow and specimens of CSF are collected. Care is taken to prevent contamination of these specimens. A closing pressure reading is then obtained, the system removed, and a small dressing applied. The expected laboratory findings for CSF are listed below.

- color: none
- clarity: clear and translucent
- RBC: none
- WBC: 0–5 cu/mm^3
- protein: 15–45 mg/100 ml
- glucose: 60–80% blood level
- microorganisms: none

Different policies govern postprocedure care. They range from ambulation immediately after the procedure to strict, flat-lying position for several hours afterwards. Review of specific physician's orders and facility policies will clarify postprocedure care. Frequently, fluid intake is increased after this procedure to replace any fluid lost during the test.

MYELOGRAM

A myelogram is a test performed to visualize the spinal subarachnoid space for patency or obstruction. Pretest preparation includes careful explanation of the procedure and posttest care. Food and fluid are withheld 4 hours prior to the test. Sedatives may also be ordered to relieve anxiety and produce muscle relaxation.

The procedure is carried out in the radiology department, where a lumbar puncture is performed. After opening pressure is ascertained and any necessary specimens collected, a radiopaque dye is injected into the subarachnoid space and rapid serial pictures are taken. During the filming procedure the individual is expected to assume a variety of positions for complete visualization. After visualization is completed, the dye is removed. Its removal may cause pain for the individual as the needle must be manipulated to do this.

After the procedure is completed, the person is returned to his or her room to remain flat in bed for up to 24 hours. (As with the lumbar puncture, the time period may vary.) The individual may, however, turn from side to side and is assisted in doing so. Fluid intake may, again, be increased.

BRAIN SCAN

The brain scan, like other scans, detects the presence of tumors and lesions.

Computerized Axial Tomography
A newer, more versatile method is the CAT scan. In a CAT scan, an x-ray source emits rays which are picked up by a scanning device and transmitted to a computer where they are translated into a viewable picture. No special pre- or posttreatment care is required. However, the individual is required to lie mo-

tionless with a helmetlike device on the head for at least 30 min. During this time the head device rotates a full 360°. This allows for a three-dimensional view of brain tissue. Since this test involves x-ray emission, the individual may fear the possibility of radiation overdose. To help allay this fear the nurse can explain to the individual that this procedure involves no more radiation than a routine x-ray and should not be confused with other forms of radiation therapy.

Nursing assessment related to diagnostic tests includes descriptions of:

- level of understanding of tests (individual, family and/or significant others)
- preparations needed
- posttest care
- special equipment needed
- presenting test values
- the relationship between presenting values and expected values
- attitudes toward test (individual, family and/or significant others)
- reactions to tests
- nursing implications of the test results

NURSING DIAGNOSES

A 42-year-old divorced woman, Ms. Bosley, was hospitalized 2 days ago for multiple fractures of the femur as the result of an automobile accident. The fracture was surgically repaired on the day of admission and the affected leg was placed in balanced suspension traction (Chapter 14 discusses traction). For the past 2 days the fractured bone has been healing as expected (as evidenced by x-ray); she has experienced mild pain, which has been relieved by nursing measures; and nursing and medical assessments up to this point have revealed no unusual or unexpected behaviors. While the nurse is assisting Ms. Bosley with morning care, she states, "I didn't sleep well last night. I kept having these awful nightmares about big monsters coming to get me." The nurse observes that Ms. Bosley is distracted and keeps jumping from subject to subject in her conversation. Based on previous and present assessments, the nurse judges that Ms. Bosley may be showing some signs of impending sensory deprivation.

The nurse reviews previous assessments and reassesses the present situation to update the nursing diagnoses and plan. Following is that assessment of Ms. Bosley's expected and actual behaviors in relation to various levels of the sensory process.

ASSESSMENT FACTOR	EXPECTED BEHAVIOR	ACTUAL BEHAVIOR
Receptor sites		
Eyes, ears, nose, skin, deep tissues	Has full range of ability of accept stimuli from the environment—no structural or functional deficiencies.	Responds as expected, but ability to focus on stimuli has lessened.

Level of growth and development	Sight
	  acuity and accommodation begin to decline
	  color discrimination decreases, especially blues
	  greater occurrence of farsightedness
	Hearing
	  acuity begins to decline
		Recently started wearing glasses for reading and close work.

Perception and interpretation		
Cognitive processes	Can carry out cognitive processes such as memory, abstract reasoning, attention span, and orientation at previous level.	Attention span decreased. Moves quickly from subject to subject. Oriented × 3.

(continued)

ASSESSMENT FACTOR	EXPECTED BEHAVIOR	ACTUAL BEHAVIOR
Characteristics of Stimuli		
Past experience	—	Hospitalized 6 days for birth of son 19 years ago. "That was the last time I got a good rest." Hospitalized 5 years ago for 10 days for removal of gall bladder. "Not a pleasant experience but had to be done." States this is the first time in a private room.
Relevancy	—	"I'm bored to tears—each day is just like the one before it."
General state of mind	—	"Busiest time of year at work . . . used to being on the go."
Level of wellness	—	See previous assessment. Bone healing—see x-ray. Bone alignment being maintained. Scratches received during accident healing. No signs of infections. Lab values as expected.
Behavioral responses		
Neuromuscular responses	Appropriate in kind and strength to stimuli.	Same within limitations of traction.
Appropriateness of of behavior	—	Behavior appropriate to stimuli. States experienced nightmares previous night. Slept most of yesterday.
Level of consciousness	Alert and aware	Same
Affect	—	Irritable. Today complaining about breakfast, room, traction, people— this has not been her previous pattern.
Quality of stimuli	—	In a private room with radio and TV. Room is located at far end of hall away from activity center. Window faces another building. Receives several phone calls during day from co-workers, but none in evening. Has had one visitor since admission— close friend. Hospital 25 miles from home and work. Has left room only once to go to x-ray. Physician visits once each day. Does not use call bell except to request medication and bedpan.

(continued)

ASSESSMENT FACTOR	EXPECTED BEHAVIOR	ACTUAL BEHAVIOR
		Is used to: working in busy office 5 days per week traveling frequently for business and pleasure going out to dinner twice per week being active in business organization—attends meetings, is secretary of local buyers' union dating approximately one evening per week. States, "I date a lot, but there is no special person right now." Son presently away at college 1,000 miles away. States she is looking forward to his coming home for semester break. Jogs 3 times per week. Enjoys needlepoint.
Physical assessment		
Cranial nerve	See Chart 13.3.	No unexpected findings.
Reflexes	See Charts 13.4 and 13.5.	Reflexes as expected.
Sensation	Symmetrical, bilateral, superficial, and deep sensation	As expected. Mild pain in affected leg.
Muscle strength	Symmetrical, bilateral, equal	As expected. Decrease in quadriceps strength in affected leg.
Coordination and balance	Symmetrical, bilateral coordination with no ataxia	Ambulation cannot be evaluated. Other movements coordinated.
Special senses	No structural or functional deficiencies	Expected findings all present—see admission assessment.
Diagnostic tests		
Skull x-ray	No pathology	Same
Vertebral x-rays	No pathology	Same
X-ray of left femur	No pathology	Transverse, comminuted fracture of left femur.
Medical diagnoses	—	Fracture left femur.
Medical orders		Continuous balance suspension traction with 15-lb weight. Percodan tabs 1 Q3-4H PO p.r.n. for leg pain Chloral hydrate 500 mg PO h.s. p.r.n. Regular diet Strict bed rest

The resulting nursing diagnoses in the situation of Ms. Bosley might include:

- impending sensory deprivation related to a decrease in intensity and type of environmental stimuli
- possible social deprivation related to decrease in usual and familiar social interactions
- confinement deprivation related to decrease in muscle activity

PLANNING

Meeting sensory needs requires a plan which includes quality stimulation of all senses, safety measures, modifying the environment to compensate for sensory deficits, case finding, and teaching. Since most situations in which sensory deprivation occurs can be anticipated, the plan must include measures to prevent it. Many of the nursing interventions aimed toward reducing or preventing sensory deficits can be easily integrated into the plan for meeting other health care needs. It is the awareness of these actual and potential deficits which helps to make the nurse's actions more therapeutic and meaningful.

The plan for one of the nursing diagnoses in the situation of Ms. Bosley might look as follows:

NURSING DIAGNOSIS	GOAL	PLAN
Impending sensory deprivation related to a decrease in intensity and type of environmental stimuli.	1. Increased interaction with meaningful environmental stimuli within 24 hours as evidenced by increased ability to focus on stimuli and increased feelings of well-being.	1. Explore with individual ways to increase the amount and quality of stimuli within the hospital setting. 2. Devise with staff a plan for increasing interaction time with individual. 3. Move bed to various activity centers, e.g., day room, for meals and afternoon activity period. 4. Alternate routine of care. Devise TV and radio schedule with individual. 5. Arrange for recreational therapist to meet with individual to discuss leisure activities. 6. Devise exercise schedule with individual and staff. Suggest friend bring in needlepoint on next visit.
	2. Increased reports of restful sleep within 24 hours.	1. As above. 2. Provide activities to prevent sleeping during day. 3. Devise sleep-activity plan with individual. 4. Consult with physician about changing type and/or dose of sleeping medication.

INTERVENTION

Proper functioning of the sensory system requires continuous input with changes in quality and quantity of stimuli. Therefore, nursing intervention measures are directed toward recognition, prevention, and treatment of actual or potential interferences with the reception and utilization of stimuli. In addition, the nurse assists with maintaining a safe environment and teaches the individual to compensate for any sensory deficits.

Recognition of Sensory Deficits

Recognition of actual or potential sensory interferences can take place in any setting in which the nurse practices.

IN THE COMMUNITY

In the community, screening programs for detecting such things as glaucoma (pathology involving increased intraocular pressure), decreased visual and hearing acuity, environmental poisoning (e.g., lead poisoning), sound pollution, high-risk pregnant women, and persons at risk for cerebral vascular accidents (strokes) can be established. The clinic, school, and industrial settings provide opportunities for the nurse to observe behaviors which may be indicative of sensory deficits. The slow learner in school, the accident-prone worker, or the forgetful or "absent-minded" person who attends clinics may be manifesting behaviors which are representative of sensory deficits. In these situations, the nurse often acts as a referral person, using her knowledge of appropriate community resources.

IN HEALTH CARE FACILITIES

In health care facilities such as rehabilitation centers, nursing homes, and hospitals, the nurse can recognize interferences which may arise from, be related to, or occur coincidentally with other negative health behaviors. An example of a sensory deficit related to another condition is seen in the person who is placed in isolation. This person is much more prone to develop all types of sensory deprivation than the person who is not restricted in this way. An example of sensory interferences arising from pathology is the individual who is eye-patched after cataract surgery

and thus has an actual reduction in sensory input. A deficit which may occur coincidentally is the person who enters the hospital because of an acute myocardial infarction (heart attack) who is also deaf.

Prevention of Sensory Deficits

Preventive measures for neurologic and sensory deficits can be instituted at the same levels as recognition.

IN THE COMMUNITY

In the community the nurse can establish and support programs aimed at accident prevention, safety, and use of environmental supports. Sporting accidents in swimming, football, skateboarding, and skiing can frequently result in neurologic or sensory damage. Teaching the sportsperson to use proper safety equipment, safety measures, proper body conditioning, and emergency first aid is a nursing intervention which will increase the individual's level of knowledge in the prevention of sensory deficits. Since vehicular accidents are a major cause of neurologic injury, especially among adolescents and young adults, educational programs, driver-safety programs, and first-aid programs are interventions in which the nurse can participate.

Public education programs on environmental hazards and wellness promotion are other areas in which the nurse can take an active role. Environmental hazards which can lead to neurologic and sensory disturbances include poisoning, noise pollution, and unsafe industrial conditions. Nutrition, prenatal care, accident prevention, immunization programs, and screening programs for learning disabilities, hypertension, or glaucoma—all of which can result from or contribute to neurologic and sensory damage—are just a few of the wellness promotion aspects of nursing intervention.

The nurse in the community also has the opportunity to identify those persons who may be prone to various kinds of sensory deprivation and intervene directly or refer the individuals to such resources as community centers or clinics. These at-risk persons include the elderly living alone or in single-room occupancies, people newly discharged from psychiatric facilities, bedridden individuals with chronic illnesses, or people with perceptual disabilities such as blindness. Individuals in these circumstances are particularly susceptible to social deprivation, since the quantity and quality of their social interactions are significantly reduced. In addition, their limited physical activity may impose some type of confinement isolation. Furthermore, sensory and perceptual deprivations are not uncommon with these groups, since all types of meaningful stimuli may be reduced by concurrent perceptual difficulties.

IN THE HEALTH CARE FACILITY

Within the health care agency, the nurse can not only continue those activities carried out in the community, but can also work to prevent sensory and/or neurologic deficits on an individual basis. The nurse in the health care facility may be intervening with individuals with primary neurologic and/or sensory interferences to prevent further deficits or working with individuals whose health status makes them prone to neurologic or sensory impairments. The individual with intracranial pressure or perceptual disabilities or the unconscious person is an example of the former; persons who are immobilized, isolated, in an intensive-care unit, or, as a result of institutionalization, have an alteration in the quality and quantity of stimuli are examples of the latter.

Providing Safe Environments

A major nursing intervention for these individuals is the provision of a safe environment. The modifications that are necessary will be determined by the type and extent of sensory or neurologic interferences. The individual with a receptor or perceptual disturbance requires an environment which helps compensate for the sensory loss.

FOR INDIVIDUALS WITH VISUAL IMPAIRMENT

The visually impaired individual requires physically stable surroundings. That individual is oriented to the arrangement of furniture and objects and is consulted before any changes are made in their placement. Objects that are inadvertently placed in different locations or left in walk areas are particularly hazardous. Eyeglasses or contact lenses are kept clean and available for the individual's use. Eyeglasses are stored in a case and placed in an area where they are least likely to be broken. Contact lenses are stored according to manufacturer's directions.

This person also needs to be taught how to compensate for a change in vision. Teaching the individual to listen for sounds within the environment and to ask for assistance whenever new situations are encountered are examples of ways to make the individual safer. Referrals to such services as occupational therapy and associations for the visually impaired can assist the individual to learn skills necessary for long-term compensation. This is particularly true for the newly blind.

FOR INDIVIDUALS WITH HEARING DEFICITS

For the person who is hard of hearing or deaf, the nurse must directly face him or her when speaking and clearly enunciate words without screaming. Messages and instructions should be written if there is any question as to the individual's level of perception. The individual is taught to compensate for hearing loss by visually surveying the total surroundings. Turning the head or body in a wide arc is one way of achieving this. If the individual has a hearing aid, its function and the strength of its batteries should be tested frequently to allow for maximum hearing. If the individual is unable to place the hearing aid alone, the nurse does so. As with any other impairment, referral to the proper agency can assist the individual with a hearing deficit to learn skills to cope with the condition. Individuals who appear to be disoriented or who respond inappropriately to verbalizations are evaluated for hearing loss and not automatically assumed to be confused.

FOR INDIVIDUALS WITH LOSS OF SENSATION

People with loss of sensation require safeguards within the environment which protect them from extremes of temperature and pressure. Devices such as radiators should have covers, and heating pads should have maximum temperature control. The individual is taught to measure the temperature of bath water and hot-water bottles, to dress carefully for environmental extremes, and to visually check the environment for hazards the individual may not be able to perceive. For example, the paraplegic individual (paralysis of lower extremities) should look for objects which jut out, since the individual may bump into them and be seriously injured without realizing that any contact has been made. Unimpaired individuals shift their weight every few minutes without realizing it, maintaining a dynamic balance between circulation and pressure. Thus a schedule is devised with the individual who has a loss of pressure sensation to shift weight frequently when sitting or lying down.

Devices such as walkers, crutches, and canes can assist individuals with difficulty in coordination, equilibrium, and muscle strength. Teaching the individual to use handrails, walls, and stable pieces of furniture, aids that individual to walk about safely. Stray pieces of furniture, small area rugs, and sharp-edged or easily tipped furniture are particularly hazardous for persons with these impairments.

Individuals who have a decreased level of consciousness and/or disorientation have special requirements to make their environments safe. The nurse is responsible for structuring and modifying the environment for these individuals until they are oriented and able to act in their own behalf. Protective devices such as bed siderails and restraints may be needed to protect the individual. Illustration 13.3 shows commonly used restraints. State laws, agency policies, and common sense guide the nurse in the use of restraints. Regardless of these restrictions, certain guidelines are followed in the use of restraints. Restraints must be loose enough to provide adequate circulation and movement. They are completely removed as often as possible, but at least once a shift. The skin underneath the restraint is examined for any signs of circulatory impairment (Chap. 18), chafing, or bruising, and the extremity put through range of motion. Restraints can be removed when another person is with the individual, but the individual is never left unattended when the restraints are removed. Restraints are used only for the purposes for which they were made, and one type should not be substituted for another. Restraints are not used to punish or discipline the individual, or to replace nursing care and supervision. Often restraints, instead of protecting the individual, only increase the person's anxiety and acting-out behavior. It is necessary to explain the reason for the restraints to the individual and the family and/or significant others, to release the restraints whenever possible, and to use techniques of touch. Touching and talking with the individual may decrease anxiety. (Illustration 13.4)

Illustration 13.3

Devices that restrain an individual in bed must allow that person adequate movement and not interfere with circulation. *(Courtesy of J. T. Posey Co.)*

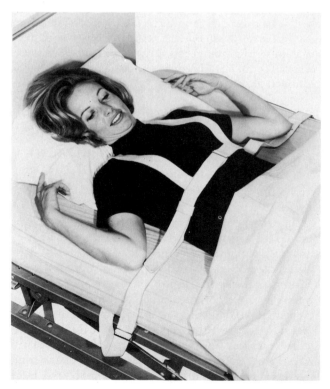
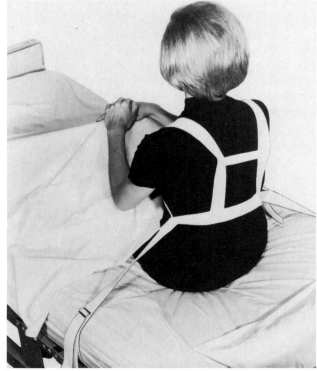

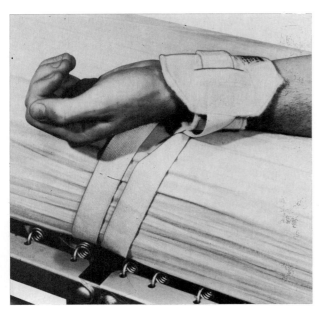

Illustration 13.4
Extremities that are restrained to protect an individual are checked by the nurse for chafing and bruising. Circulation is maintained by frequently putting the limb through range of motion. *(Courtesy of J. T. Posey Co.)*

FOR INDIVIDUALS WHO ARE DISORIENTED

The disoriented person requires continuous data about self, place, and time. This helps in reorienting the individual and decreasing confusion and the resulting anxiety. The nurse can orient individuals to self by calling them by name whenever speaking with them. The use of nicknames or the name that the individual is most accustomed to being called is more helpful in orienting the individual to self than the use of titles such as Ms. or Mr. Showing individuals envelopes addressed to them and having them practice writing their names may also be of assistance in orientation to self.

Orientation to place is accomplished by the nurse telling the individual his or her location. This is done specifically as well as generally. For example, the individual is told the name of the unit and the facility where he or she is located as well as the geographical location.

Identifying meal times, referring to the general time, as well as reference to specific clock time, helps orient the person to time. In addition, references to season of the year, forthcoming holidays, and days of the week are other ways of helping achieve time orientation. Calendars, daily newspapers, holiday decorations, and radios are some of the methods the nurse can use to help in orienting to time. When orienting the individual, the nurse intervenes in a way that is appropriate to the individual's level of growth and not in a condescending or inappropriately childish manner.

GENERAL SAFETY MEASURES

Certain safety measures are necessary regardless of the neurologic or sensory status of the individual. Such precautions as maintaining proper lighting, keeping beds at their lowest level, wiping up spills, being familiar with equipment, keeping work areas free of extraneous equipment, placing objects and possessions within the individual's reach, and suggesting proper-fitting nonskid shoes and slippers are some of the daily safety measures the nurse utilizes. The judicious use of central nervous system depressants and muscle relaxants is another area in which the nurse can protect the individual. Individuals receiving any of these medications are assessed for signs of drowsiness, decreased coordination, cognitive changes, decreased judgment, perceptual changes, and other similar reactions. These alterations may become exaggerated at night when there are fewer environmental cues for the individual to use for orientation. If any of these signs are noted, special safety precautions are instituted and consultation made with the physician for possible changes in medication or dosage. In addition, the nurse can be an active force in promoting the installation of such safety features as handrails in walkways and bathrooms; ramps; wide, easily accessible doorways; manually operated elevators; the use of nonskid floor wax; and equipment with brakes.

Prevention of Increased Intracranial Pressure

Head injury as well as any space-occupying mass in the brain frequently leads to neurologic and sensory dysfunctions. The nurse indirectly and directly helps to prevent these dysfunctions by early observation for ▶ signs and symptoms of intracranial pressure. **Intracranial pressure** (ICP) is the rise in pressure which occurs whenever the volume of contents of the cranium increases. Beyond the age of 18 months, when the fontanels close, the skull is a fixed bony structure which cannot expand to accommodate an increase in its content. Head trauma can result in swelling of the brain tissue (cerebral edema) and/or hemorrhage of blood into brain tissue. These, in turn, increase the volume of cranial contents, resulting in an increase in intracranial pressure. Increased intracranial pressure can subsequently result in damage to brain tissue.

The nurse indirectly intervenes to prevent the sequelae of intracranial pressure by teaching all individuals who receive head injuries and their families and/or significant others to observe for signs of ICP. Change in levels of consciousness, whether sudden or slow in onset; vomiting, with or without nausea; changes in pupil size; headache; neck stiffness (nuchal rigidity); and hemorrhage or leakage of cerebrospinal fluid are the signs that are taught. Leakage of cerebral spinal fluid can be observed as a clear drain-

age from the eye, ear or nose, or as a postnasal drip. Whenever a head injury occurs, the leakage of fluid should be suspected as having a relationship to ICP and not assumed to be a cold symptom. Any of these symptoms are immediately reported.

When directly intervening with individuals who have sustained a head injury, the nurse observes for all the signs and symptoms mentioned above. In addition, the nurse checks for PERLA and cranial nerve function, pulse, respiration, blood pressure, temperature, twitching and convulsions, bowel and bladder retention or incontinence, and changes in muscle strength or tone. In infants and young toddlers the nurse also observes for a bulging of the fontanels. Chart 13.7 outlines the signs and symptoms of intra-

---

Chart 13.7
Signs and Symptoms of Intracranial Pressure

FACTOR	RESPONSE WITH ICP	FACTOR	RESPONSE WITH ICP
Pupil equality	Dilation of one pupil frequently occurs on the same side as the area of pressure.	Twitching and convulsion	Can occur if pressure is on motor centers.
Reaction of pupils to light	May be constricted or dilated, depending on area of pressure.	Bowel and bladder function	Incontinence or retention, depending on area of pressure.
Accommodation of pupils	Commonly there is a decrease in ability to accommodate.	Level of consciousness	Diminishes.
Cranial nerve function	Diminished response in those nerves on which there is increased pressure.	Headache	Common occurrence.
		Vomiting	Usually projectile. May not be accompanied by nausea.
Pulse	Rate and quality decrease.	Nuchal rigidity	Stiff neck is present if there is pressure of hemorrhage or leakage of CSF into subarachnoid space.
Respiration	Rate and quality decrease.		
Blood pressure	Increases with a concurrent increase in pulse pressure.	Hemorrhage/leaking of CSF	Variable. May be seen as cough, runny nose, eyes.
Temperature	Can increase if there is pressure on hypothalamus.	Bulging fontanels	Present in infants to accommodate increase in volume.

cranial pressure. The exact findings will vary according to where the pressure occurs. Early recognition of these symptoms and prompt intervention can prevent subsequent brain damage.

Prevention of Sensory Deprivation

Since any individual who has a decrease in meaningful stimuli is susceptible to sensory deprivation, a major nursing intervention is the recognition and prevention of sensory deprivation. This intervention can take place in the home, community, or health care facility. Sensory deprivation can be prevented by providing a variety in the quantity and quality of stimuli. Stimuli that is meaningful to the individual are provided to all the senses. Chart 13.8 presents examples of ways the senses can be stimulated. Consideration of the individual's level of growth and development guides the nurse's choice of stimuli.

RECEPTIVE AND INTERPRETIVE DEPRIVATION

As previously mentioned, receptive and interpretive deprivation can be prevented by increasing the degree of the stimuli, supplying aids and devices which enhance the ability of individuals to pick up stimuli from the environment, assisting persons to compensate and seek out stimuli in other ways, orienting them, and providing some consistency and predictability of stimuli without producing white noise. The nurse can help prevent social deprivation by increasing the number of familiar objects in the individual's environment, increasing the individual's contact with significant others, and assisting the individual to seek out new and different social contacts and interactions. Familiar objects—furniture, clothing, pictures, and personal treasures—help the individual to feel a sense of security and orientation, especially in a new or unfamiliar environment. Contacts with or news about pets and other not usually recognized significant others, can help decrease feelings of social isolation.

CONFINEMENT DEPRIVATION

Since confinement deprivation is primarily the physical component of sensory deprivation, any activity which increases physical movement and stress will reduce its occurrence. Active and passive range of

---

Chart 13.8
Sensory Stimuli

SENSE	METHOD OF STIMULATION
Vision	Color, mobiles, changing pictures, changing room arrangement. Changing path of vision. Television,* visitors, colored uniforms, multicolored linen, changing light patterns.
Hearing	Radio, television, conversation, with a variety of voices. Movement to and from areas of high and low sound.
Smell	Foods, flowers, perfumes.
Taste	A wide variation in presentation of foods.
Tactile	Stroking, exercise, massage, change of position, changes in temperature and texture of room, linens, clothing, objects, cuddling, hugging, meaningful touch.

*Continuous playing of a radio or TV, as with any repetitive stimulation, results in its becoming meaningless white noise.

---

motion exercises, postural and position changes, massage, and occupational–recreational therapy can be utilized.

SENSORY OVERLOAD

Sensory overload can be decreased by restricting the amounts of white noise to which the individual is exposed. If the nurse becomes aware of those repetitive patterns in the environment, the nurse can intervene to reduce or vary them. Things such as constantly beeping monitors, unchanging light patterns, consistent machine gurgling, repetitive routines, continuous playing of radios, televisions, or record players can produce sensory overload, particularly when these factors are found in combination. Since sensory deprivation can be a potential or actual occurrence, the nurse intervenes both to prevent and to treat its sequelae.

EVALUATION

Evaluation for meeting sensory needs centers on the direction of change in the person's ability to receive, interpret, transmit, and respond to stimuli and the effectiveness of intervention in meeting these needs.

Specific criteria used in evaluating how sensory needs have been met include:

- How do physiologic changes relate to changes in the individual's ability to meet sensory needs? Psychologic changes? Environmental changes?
- Has the presenting level of reception moved closer to the expected? Interpretation and analysis? Transmission? Response? Cranial nerve function? Reflexes? Sensations? Muscle strength? Coordination and balance? Special senses? Diagnostic tests?
- Have the quantity and quality of stimuli changed?
- What is the relationship between change in the quality of stimuli and the behavioral responses?
- What are the changes in the ability to meet sensory needs?
- What are the changes in the individual's level of safety?
- What are the changes in compensatory mechanisms?
- What are the changes in knowledge about factors which precipitate sensory deficits?
- What are the changes in level of understanding about sensory needs?
- What are the changes in level of anxiety concerning meeting sensory needs?
- What are the changes in orientation? Level of consciousness?
- What skills have been acquired in utilizing methods to meet sensory needs?

RECORDING AND TEACHING–LEARNING ACTIVITIES

Teaching–Learning Topics

- rationale for therapeutic regimens
- methods to match capabilities with limitations

- ways to structure the environment to facilitate meeting sensory needs
- safety measures
- ways to assess ICP
- ways to assess sensory responses
- prevention of sensory deprivation
- appropriate use of central nervous system depressants and muscle relaxants
- factors which may precipitate sensory and neurologic deficits
- available resources and how to use them.

Charting

Using appropriate sensory need terminology, objectively describe such factors as:

- objective base-line data on reception, interpretation and analysis, transmission responses, stimuli, cranial nerve function, reflexes, sensations, muscle strength, coordination and balance, special senses.
- objective and subjective changes that occur in the person's ability to meet sensory needs
- subjective assessment data in the individual's ability to meet sensory needs
- attitudes toward sensory and neurologic deficits and treatment
- subjective and objective reactions and responses to treatment
- schedule and methods of care
- teaching carried out
- discharge planning done
- family's and/or significant others' interactions and responses

Update Kardex on changes in goals and plans for meeting sensory needs.

Medications to Review

- central nervous system depressants
   analgesics, e.g., meperidine (Demerol)
   hynoptics, e.g., flurazepam (Dalmane)
   sedatives, e.g., phenobarbital
   alcohol
   tranquilizers, e.g., chlorpromazine (Thorazine)

- central nervous system stimulants
    amphetamines, e.g., methylphenidate (Ritalin)
    antidepressants, e.g., amitriptyline (Elavil)
- muscle relaxants, e.g., carisoprodol (Soma)

CLINICAL APPLICATION

Nursing Care of the Unconscious Individual

Nursing care of the unconscious individual centers around meeting safety needs and providing for sensory input.

UNCONSCIOUSNESS

The unconscious person is one who is characterized as being in coma and thus incapable of performing any voluntary activities for meeting basic needs. The person in coma does not respond to environmental stimuli, including deep pain stimulation. Usually absent are superficial reflexes as well as some deep reflexes. The pupils may or may not respond to light, depending upon the depth of coma and the area of the brain affected. Bowel and bladder control is lost, and the swallow reflex is absent. The individual may have involuntary muscle twitches or even convulsions but does not carry out any purposeful movement. In addition, the individual has no way of communicating his or her needs to other persons around him and is thought to have reduced cognitive function as evidenced by irregularity in the electroencephalogram (monitoring of electrical impulses of the brain).

Unconsciousness is directly related to damage to some part of the brain tissue. This damage may result from a wide variety of factors, including head trauma, cerebral edema, infection of the brain or surrounding tissues, space-occupying lesions or masses, poisoning (including drug overdoses), waste-product buildup as a result of metabolic or other systemic pathophysiologies, or hypoxia.

INTERVENTION

Nursing intervention is, therefore, concerned with removing and treating the underlying pathology, meeting the individual's basic needs, providing a safe

---

Chart 13.9
First Aid for Epilepsy

1. Keep calm when a major seizure occurs. You cannot stop a seizure once it has started. Do not restrain the patient or try to revive him.

2. Clear the area around him of hard, sharp or hot objects which could injure him. Place a pillow or rolled-up coat under his head.

3. Do not force anything between the teeth. If his mouth is open, you might place a soft object like a handkerchief between his side teeth.

4. Turn the patient's head to the side, and make sure his breathing is not obstructed. Loosen necktie and tight clothing but do not interfere with his movements.

5. Do not be concerned if he seems to stop breathing. Do be concerned if the patient seems to pass from one seizure into another without gaining consciousness. This is rare but requires a doctor's help.

6. Carefully observe the patient's actions during the seizure for a full medical report later. When the seizure is over let the patient rest if he wishes.

Source: "Recognition and First Aid for Those With Epilepsy," pamphlet of the Epilepsy Foundation of America.

---

environment, maintaining vital functioning, and supplying sensory stimulation. The care of the unconscious individual is one example of nursing intervention which is done "for" the individual until the individual can intercede for him or herself. See Chart 13.9. The care for meeting the individual's basic needs and preventing the hazards of immobility are discussed in succeeding chapters.

Individual Safety

Modification of the environment to make it safe for the individual is a priority for care. Side rails are in up position when the individual is unattended and the bed in low position. This helps to prevent or minimize falls during involuntary movement of the individual. If the individual is prone to seizures or severe muscle twitching, side rails are padded with cotton batting, flannel blankets, pillows, or foam rubber. An airway or tongue blade that has been wrapped in gauze and covered with tape is kept in readiness, for instance, taped to the head of the bed. An airway or tongue blade is used to maintain a patent airway by preventing the tongue from falling back and occluding the pharynx and to prevent the individual from biting the tongue or cheek during the tonic-clonic (contraction and relaxation) movements of seizures. The tongue or airway blade is not forced into the individual's mouth, and fingers or hard objects are never used in place of either. Hard objects can break the individual's teeth, while the fingers can be severely hurt during the strong clench of a tonic phase of a seizure.

A suction machine with catheters is also set up and available to remove secretions or regurgitated food (Chap. 17). The individual is never restrained or held down during seizures as this can cause injury to soft tissues and bones.

Temperature Regulation

If pyrexia (fever) is present as a result of damage to the hypothalamus or infection, regulation of temperature by external means is necessary. Hypothermic devices which cool the body surfaces (see Chap. 15 for one type of mechanism for external temperature control). Tepid water baths are another external control. Avoiding exposure to extreme temperature is also necessary to protect the individual from burning or frostbite. Extreme temperatures can damage the individual because the individual cannot avoid them nor can the diminished circulation accommodate the changes.

Coma Evaluation

The level of consciousness, cranial nerve function, and reflexes are frequently assessed to determine if there are any changes in the depth of coma and to evaluate the effectiveness of interventions. Findings are precisely recorded, as minute differences may indicate changes in the individual's health status. Flow sheets can be of particular value here.

Sensory Stimulation

Stimulation of all senses helps prevent further deterioration of the individual. The sense of hearing is thought to remain in the unconscious individual. Thus conversation is directed toward the person and care is taken to avoid conversations which discuss the individual. Procedures are explained to the unconscious person as they are to any other person. Touching and stroking the individual helps to communicate a sense of safety, security, and caring, as well as giving tactile stimulation. Family and/or significant others are encouraged to talk with, touch, and provide care for the individual. Family and/or significant others are frequently frightened and anxious about the individual's condition and, therefore, need explanations of what is happening and the rationale for interacting with the individual.

Orienting the Individual

Orientation of the individual to self, place, and time is another aspect of care. Approximating the individual's daily routine by such things as dimming the lights at night and bathing at a usual time may also assist in raising the individual's level of consciousness. In other words, the nurse attempts to give the same individualized and competent care to the unconscious individual as would be given to any other individual.

SELECTED REFERENCES

Adams, Nancy. "Prolonged Coma." *Nursing 1977,* 7:20, August, 1977.

Bellam, Gwendoline. "The Nursing Challenge of the Child with Neurological Problems." *Nursing Forum,* 11(4):396, 1972.

Bolin, Karen. "Assessing the Status of Neurological Patients." *American Journal of Nursing,* 77:1478, September, 1977.

Bolin, Rose. "Sensory Deprivation: An Overview." *Nursing Forum,* 13(3):240, March, 1974.

Conway, Barbara Lang. *Neurological and Neurosurgical Nursing,* 7th ed. St. Louis, Mosby, 1978.

Downs, Florence. "Bed Rest and Sensory Disturbances." *American Journal of Nursing,* 74:434, March, 1974.

"Essentials of the Neurological Examination," Smith, Kline and French Pharmaceutical Company Booklet.

Hogan, Leola and Beland, Irene. "Cervical Spine Syndrome." *American Journal of Nursing,* 76:1104, July, 1976.

Huston, Janet. "Overcoming the Learning Disabilities of Stroke." *Nursing 75,* 5:66, September, 1975.

Mitchell, Pamela and Mauss, Nancy. "Intracranial Pressure." *Nursing 76,* 6:53, June, 1976.

Ohns, Mary. "The Eye-Patched Patient." *American Journal of Nursing,* 71:271, February, 1971.

"Patient Assessment: Neurological Examination." *Ameri-*

can Journal of Nursing, 75:supplement, September, 1975 (Part 1); 76:supplement, November, 1975 (Part 2); April, 1976 (Part 3).

Perron, Denise. "Deprived of Sound." *American Journal of Nursing,* 74:1057, June, 1974.

Pohutsky, Lorraine and Puhutsky, Karen. "Computerized Axial Tomography of the Brain." *American Journal of Nursing,* 75:1341, August, 1975.

Rudy, Ellen. "Early Omens of Cerebral Disaster." *Nursing 77,* 7:58, February, 1977.

Slater, Marianne Costopoulos. "Nursing Assessment and Intervention for the Patient with Central Nervous System Dysfunction." In *Advanced Concepts in Clinical Nursing,* 2nd ed., Kay Corman Kintzel, ed., Philadelphia, Lippincott, 1977, p. 639–700.

Strub, Richard and Black, F. William. *The Mental Status Examination in Neurology.* Philadelphia, Davis, 1977.

"Symposium: Neurological and Neurosurgical Nursing." *Nursing Clinics of North America,* 9(4), December, 1974.

"Symposium: Sensory Defects." *Nursing Clinics of North America,* 6(3):402, September, 1970.

"The Person with a Spinal Cord Injury." *American Journal of Nursing,* 77:1319, August, 1977.

"Working with the Confused or Delirious Patient." *American Journal of Nursing (Suppl.),* 78:1491, September, 1978.

Worrell, Judith Deignan. "Nursing Implications in the Care of the Patient Experiencing Sensory Deprivation." In *Advanced Concepts in Clinical Nursing,* 2nd ed., Kay Corman Kintzel, ed. Philadelphia, Lippincott, 1977, pp. 618–638.

UNIT IV
Safety Needs

Movement is a fundamental dimension of human behavior . . . . human behavior appears to be upon a continuum from functions which seem largely "motion" to those which involve no observable movements.

—E. L. Thorndike

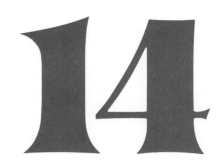

BODY KINETICS

PRINCIPLES RELATED TO BODY KINETICS

The stress of weight bearing and muscle contraction is necessary for the maintenance and growth of bones.

The stress of weight bearing and muscle contraction maintains the balance between osteoblasts (bone building and osteoclasts (bone resorption).

The maintenance and growth of bones are influenced by nutrients (minerals, vitamins, oxygen).

Circulation, nutrition, alignment, immobilization of the part, bone size, and protection from infection and further damage are related to bone healing.

Different bone articulations have different functions.

Normal range of motion of a joint prevents limitation of movement and loss of joint function.

Bones are moved by contraction of the skeletal muscles which perform mechanical work.

Muscles are always in a mild state of contraction *(tonus).*

Muscle contraction is under central nervous system control.

Muscle contraction is influenced by the transport of nutrients and oxygen and by the removal of waste byproducts.

Muscle fatigue is caused by the buildup of waste products.

Muscles need alternate periods of rest and work.

Almost every muscle has an antagonist that works in the opposite direction.

Muscles act in groups to perform work.

▶ The strongest of any muscle group will dominate when there is insufficient stress placed on the group (**contracture**).

▶ If muscles are not used, they degenerate in size, shape, and strength (**atrophy**).

If muscles are overused, they increase in size and shape (hypertrophy).

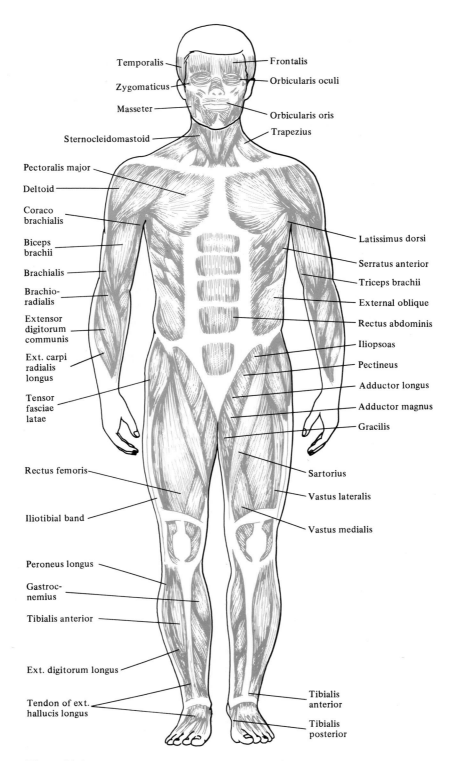

Figure 14.1

A. Muscles (anterior view).

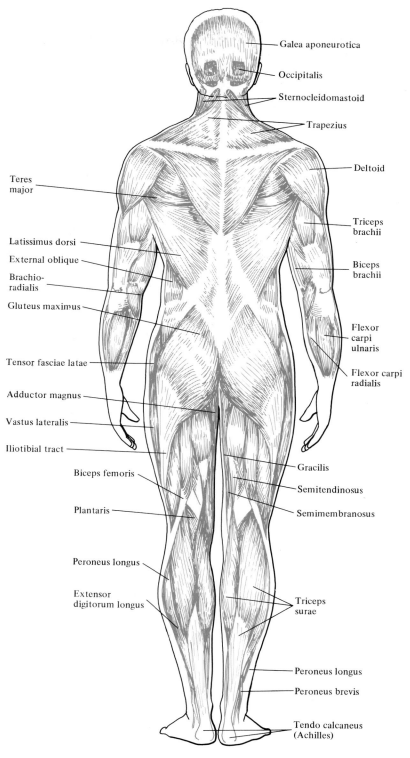

Figure 14.1
B. Muscles (posterior view).

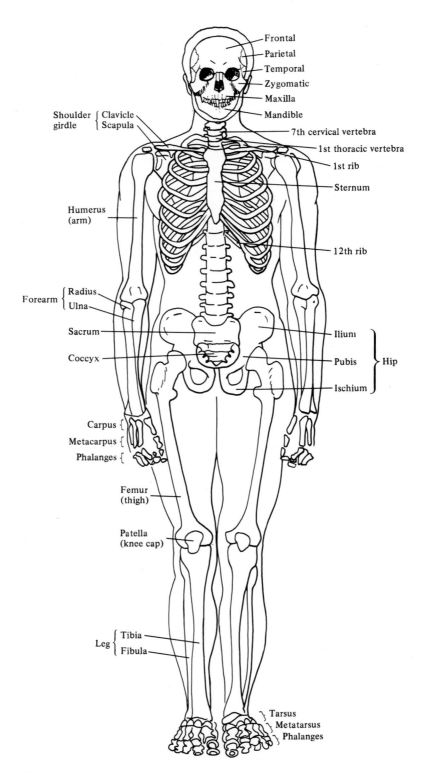

Figure 14.1.
C. Skeletal system.

Muscle weakness and atrophy result in limited range of motion for the related joint.

Passive exercises provide only for joint mobility, not muscle tone.

Active exercises provide for joint mobility and muscle tone.

Moving a muscle beyond its elastic limits will result in tearing or damage.

Decreased activity affects all body systems.

Decreased activity leads to increased work load of the heart, resulting in increased pulse rate.

Decreased activity leads to a decrease in peripheral vascular resistance, resulting in orthostatic hypotension.

▶ The use of **Valsalva maneuver** increases with immobility.

Circulatory stasis results in dependent edema.

Immobility leads to decreased stimulus for deep breathing.

Decreased stimulus for deep breathing contributes to carbon dioxide buildup, leading to respiratory acidosis.

Immobilization in the supine position increases the work of respiration.

Immobilization leads to stasis of respiratory secretions, resulting in a drying of the upper respiratory tract and helps to create hypostatic pneumonia.

Immobilization causes an increased decalcification of the long bones and leads to osteoporosis.

Lack of activity causes loss of protein from muscle and leads to a negative nitrogen balance.

Lack of activity decreases metabolic activity and oxygen consumption.

Immobility leads to anorexia, resulting in poor nutritional status.

Urinary stasis and increased calcium excretion lead to an increased urinary pH, resulting in the formation of renal calculi.

Immobilization in the supine position leads to urinary stasis, increasing the possibility of urinary retention and infection.

Immobility leads to a loss of tonus of bowel and bladder sphincters.

Decreased muscle activity and suppression of the defecation reflex lead to constipation.

Immobility creates pressure over bony prominences, leading to decreased blood supply to the area and causing local *ischemia* and *necrosis* (decubitus ulcer).

Inactivity contributes to feelings of boredom and apathy.

Immobility contributes to loss of role activity, leading to feelings of inadequacy, dependency, anxiety, and helplessness (loss of self-esteem).

Immobility contributes to distortion of body image.

Immobility contributes to sensory disturbances.

Immobility contributes to alterations in pain threshold.

▶ The point at which the body's mass is concentrated is the **center of gravity** (second sacral vertebra), which remains in the same vertical line whether in a standing or sitting position.

▶ A stable **base of support** occurs when a vertical line drawn from the center of gravity falls within the base of support (Fig. 14.2).

A wide base of support lowers the center of gravity and increases balance and stability.

Since gravity exerts a downward force, it is easier to push or pull an object than to lift it.

The closer a force is applied to the center of gravity, the more effective and stable that force is.

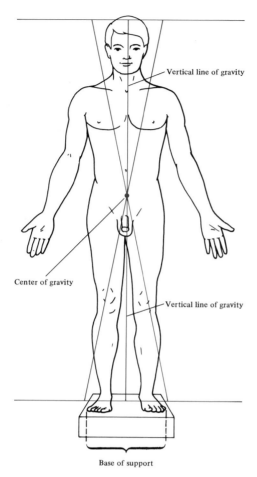

Vertical line of gravity

Center of gravity

Vertical line of gravity

Base of support

Figure 14.2
The center of gravity in human beings, usually located in the pelvis just anterior to the upper edge of the sacrum, must fall within the individual's base of support for him or her to be balanced, or stable. A wide base of support will promote good body mechanics.

Friction is resistive force between two objects. Rough and sticky surfaces increase the amount of friction.

The amount of work required to move an object is directly related to the amount of resistance and gravitational pull.

The use of the larger muscles is less fatiguing than the use of the smaller muscles in performing work.

The basic movements of the body are bending, twisting, and stretching: all activities are combinations of these three motions.

Movement is a basic process of the living organism. It underlies all human activity from the barely observable transport of the blood through the vascular system to the gross motor activity of the football player making a touchdown. The study of the movement of ► the human body is termed **body kinetics.** Body kinetics is the dynamic interaction of all systems and parts of the body in movement and the potential of the body for movement.

Many studies have investigated the phenomenon of body kinetics. As early as 1909 Thorndike hypothesized that the sensation of movement (**kinesthesis**) was relative to and subjective for the individual.[1] Modern research has validated this theory, and thus no firm laws can be made about kinesthesis.

Cratty[2] has theorized that there are four major variables which influence the actual movement an individual performs. They are (1) "basic behavioral supports," which deal with such physiologic factors as muscle tension and such cognitive skills as the ability to analyze a movement situation; (2) personal preferences as to speed and type of activity; (3) ability of the person to perform a movement task; and (4) "the unique performance factors" such as time and space, characteristics of the task, instructions given, and feedback about the task performance.[3]

The relationship between motivation and movement has also been explored. The specific motivation must be individualized, considering such factors as the importance of the activity to the individual. Fatigue plays an important role in motivation. The actual presence of fatigue or the anticipation of fatigue will discourage the individual from participating in activities. Interestingly, it is not always the level of activity that is tiring, but rather the degree of boredom it creates. Inactivity and movement restriction can lead to boredom and also to a greater need for movement. This produces a viscious cycle of frustration and fatigue.

The most recent studies of movement have centered around the relationship between time and movement. These studies have demonstrated the indivisibility of time and movement by showing how the individual views the passing of time by the quality and quantity of movement.

Much research is still needed to provide a unified theory of human movement and its implications for nursing practice.

ASSESSMENT

Nursing assessment of body kinetics is necessary not only for individuals with potential or actual movement interferences, but also of the body kinetic principles utilized by the nurse in carrying out nursing actions.

Body Alignment

▶ The nursing assessment begins by focusing on **body alignment.** Body alignment is the anatomical relationship between body parts regardless of the position assumed. The body is divided into interdependent segments. (Fig. 14.3.) Proper alignment occurs when the body segments are positioned one with another in such a way that muscle stress, strain, and fatigue are minimized, while function is maximized.

▶ When erect or **recumbent,** the body should be in an anatomical position to maintain proper alignment. In other positions, such as sitting and side lying, the *center of gravity, base of support,* and *physiologic function* must be taken into consideration along with proper alignment.

Structural deformities which interfere with body alignment and the functioning of body subsystems
▶ are also assessed. Such deformities as **kyphosis** (increased convexity of the posterior curve of the spine),
▶ **scoliosis** (side or lateral deviation of the spine), and
▶ **lordosis** (increased concavity of the lumbar spine) are commonly observed. These alterations in alignment (Fig. 17.4) can be frequently assessed in young children and treatment instituted to prevent lifelong disability and interference with other functions such as respiration.

Nursing assessment of an individual's body alignment includes descriptions of:

- the type of alignment naturally assumed (Is it proper? What is the relationship to the level of growth and development?)
- the ability to assume proper alignment (Are there obstacles preventing this, e.g., pain, deformities, traction, casts, paralysis?)
- degree of help needed in assuming proper alignment (type)
- devices needed to assume proper alignment (*hoyerlift, trapeze,* stool)

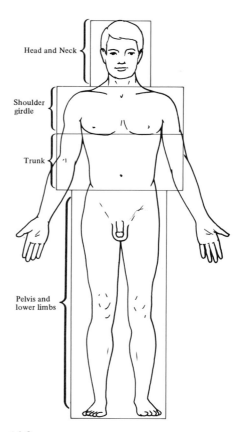

Figure 14.3
Body Segments. Good alignment of the interdependent body segments will promote efficiency in muscle function.

- ability to maintain proper alignment (obstacles)
- devices needed to maintain proper alignment (*trochanter rolls, sand bags,* pillows, *bed boards, foot blocks*)
- effects of position assumed on other body subsystems
- attitude toward body alignment
- knowledge of proper alignment

Joint Mobility

Joint mobility, along with body alignment, plays a major role in the physiologic functioning of the musculoskeletal subsystem. Each joint of the body is of a
▶ specific type and has a corresponding **range of motion**

Chart 14.1
Joint Mobility

BODY PART	TYPE OF JOINT	ACTION	MOVEMENT*	ROM (DEG)
Neck	Pivot (uniaxial)	Rotation along one plane	Flexion	90
			(extension)	90
			Hyperextension	90
			Lateral bending to the right and left	90
			Rotation to the right and left	90
Shoulders	Ball and socket (triaxial joint)	Side to side, back and forth and rotation along three planes	Flexion and extension	180
			Hyperextension	50
			Abduction and adduction	180
			Internal rotation	90
			External rotation	90
			Circumduction	360
Elbow	Hinge (uniaxial)	Back and forth along one plane	Flexion and extension	180
Forearm	Pivot		Supination	90
			Pronation	90
Wrist	Condyloid (ovoid, biaxial)	Side to side and back and forth along two planes	Flexion	90
			Extension	90
			Abduction (radial flexion)	45
			Adduction (ulnar flexion)	45
Fingers Metacarpophalangeal joint	Pivot		Flexion	90
			Extension	90
			Hyperextension	45
			Abduction (adduction)	30
Interphalangeal joint	Hinge		Flexion and extension	180

(continued)

(Chart 14.1 and Figure 14.4). Range of motion (ROM) constitutes the movement capabilities of a joint and is commonly measured by degrees along an axis. If a joint is not put through its ROM several times a day, atrophy and contractions of the surrounding muscles and ligaments will result. Range of motion can be accomplished through activities of daily living, as well as through a formal exercise routine.

Nursing assessment of the joint mobility of an individual includes descriptions of:

- degree of ROM
- obstacles to full ROM
- activities of daily living performed (ties shoelaces, brushes teeth, combs hair)
- restrictions on ROM (physician's orders, physical condition)

Chart 14.1 (Cont.)
Joint Mobility

BODY PART	TYPE OF JOINT	ACTION	MOVEMENT*	ROM (DEG)
Thumb				
Carpometacarpal joint	Saddle (biaxial)		Abduction	90
			Adduction	90
			Opposition (thumb to fifth finger)	
metacarpophalangeal and interphalangeal joints	Hinge		Flexion (extension)	90
Trunk	Gliding (biaxial, arthrodial)		Flexion	90
			Extension	30
			Lateral flexion	90
			Rotation	360
Hip	Ball and socket		Flexion (extension)	180
			Hyperextension	50
			Abduction (adduction)	45
			Internal and external rotation	90
			Circumduction	90
Knee	Hinge		Flexion and extension	90
Ankle	Hinge		Dorsiflexion	90
			Plantar flexion	90
Foot	Gliding		Inversion	
			Eversion	
Toes				
metatarsophalangeal joint	Condyloid (modified ball and socket)		Flexion (extension)	90
			Abduction	30
			Adduction	30

*Parentheses denote return to resting position.

- frequency of ROM
- reaction to ROM (endurance, pain, facial expression)
- attitudes toward motion

Mobility

Mobility is the next factor considered in the nursing assessment of body kinetics. Mobility is the capability to move from one location to another. It involves not only physical factors such as gait and endurance, but also such psychosocial factors such as feelings of independence and self-control. Mobility is related to the whole person—how he or she sees himself or herself and feels physically. Individuals will often evaluate their health status by their mobility. "I was so sick I could hardly move" is a frequently heard comment. Independence is often a function of the person's feelings of self-worth, and a limitation of

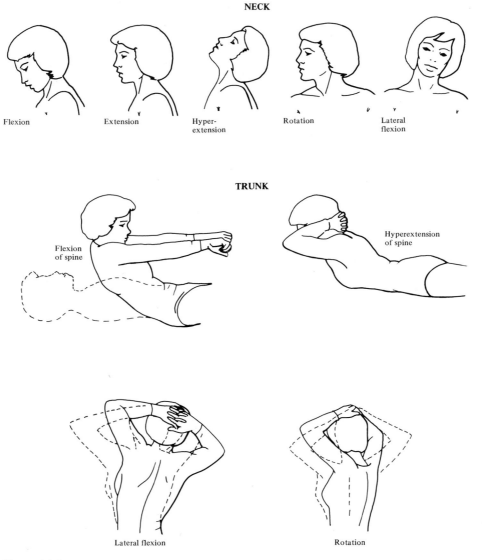

NECK

Flexion   Extension   Hyper-extension   Rotation   Lateral flexion

TRUNK

Flexion of spine   Hyperextension of spine

Lateral flexion   Rotation

Figure 14.4
Range of motion exercises.

movement affects these feelings. The hospital environment, therefore, can automatically interfere with these feelings by restricting the individual's mobility.

The way that a person moves when ambulating gives the nurse many clues as to the musculoskeletal status of the individual.

GAIT

▶ **Gait,** one area that should be observed, is the way that the person walks. Expected gait for an adult begins with both feet flat and parallel; weight is then shifted to one foot while the other foot swings forward. The body moves toward the standing foot, and the arm opposite the swinging foot moves at the same time to maintain balance. The foot hits the ground with the heel first, and then weight is borne along the outer edge of the foot to the ball of the foot and toes. The weight is now shifted to the forward foot and the process is repeated. The condition of the individual's shoes is often a reliable index of how the weight is distributed while walking.

Gait is described in terms of smoothness, ba-

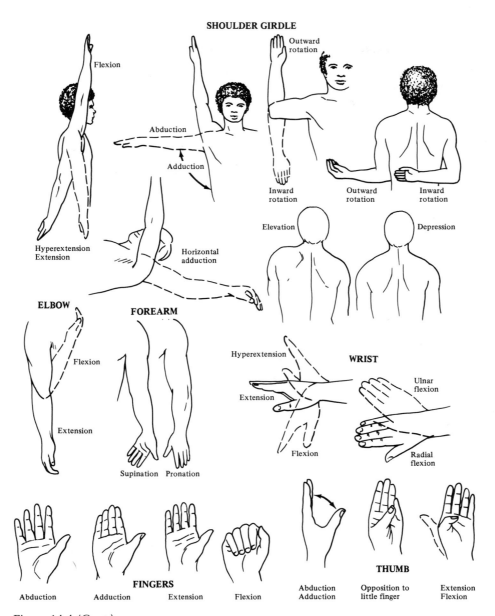

Figure 14.4 (Cont.)
Range of motion exercises

lance, arm movement, effectiveness, number of steps taken (pace) per minute (expected: 70–100/minute), and the length and width of the step.

ENDURANCE

Endurance, another major factor in mobility, is the ability to withstand movement in terms of duration and absence of fatigue. Reactions such as pain, fear, changes in mood, and changes in respiratory and circulatory status are important in mobility. Oxygen consumption increases during muscle activity. Therefore, the individual's need for more oxygen and its transport is reflected in his or her pulse and respiration. While increases in these rates and rhythms are the usual patterns of response, the degree of occurrence and time required to return to the resting rates are significant factors to include in the nursing assessment of mobility (Chap. 17).

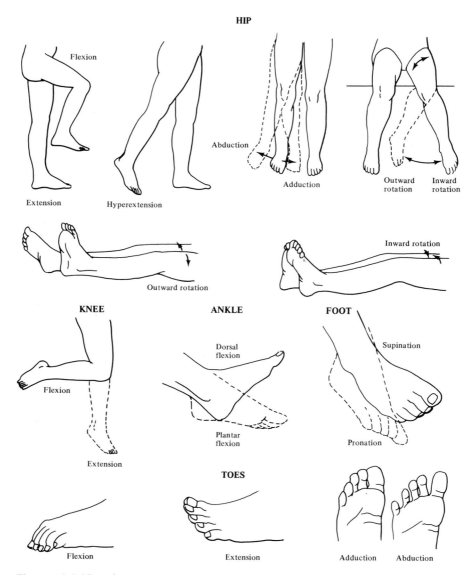

Figure 14.4 (Cont.)
Range of motion exercises.

SAFETY

Safety is a vital concern in mobility. The environment must be checked for slippery floors, inappropriately placed objects, handrails, and bed and chair heights. Equipment and assistive devices must be kept in good working order and used according to instructions. The individual's clothing and shoes should be appropriate to the activity. For example, paper slippers are often used in place of properly fit-ting shoes; however, slippers could present a hazard to the individual when walking. The individual's physical condition and awareness of the environment are also important factors in safety. Weak, disoriented individuals must be assisted in many movement activities to prevent accidents.

Devices are frequently used to assist the individual in moving. Trapezes, wheelchairs, walkers, canes, braces, and crutches are some of the more common ones. Both the nurse and the individual must be aware of the proper use and purpose of equipment.

Nursing assessment of the mobility of an individual includes descriptions of:

- the individual's mobility status (bedridden, ambulates with devices, ambulates alone)
- usual activity pattern (sedentary, active)
- activities ordered (bedrest, out of bed with assistance, out of bed without restrictions)
- obstacles to mobility (pain, fear, deformities):
  duration of limitation
  what increases/decreases limitation
  circumstances of occurrence (time of day, specific movement)
- gait
- posture
- endurance (pulse, respiration)
- safety factors
- reactions to ambulation
- devices used in mobility (and knowledge of devices)
- assistance required
- attitudes toward mobility

Fatigue

Since fatigue plays a large role in determining the amount of musculoskeletal activity undertaken, consideration of those factors which influence fatigue is necessary in any nursing assessment of body kinetic needs.

The degree to which the individual participates in activity is significant in determining the fatigue experienced. Activities that the individual enjoys are less likely to produce fatigue than are those activities which hold no interest for the person. Preferences, therefore, must be matched with capabilities. The physical condition of the person, his or her psychomotor skills, emotional state, and level of growth and development all influence the individual's capabilities.

The level of debilitation, the ability to meet oxygen and nutrient needs and to remove waste buildup are some of the physical determinations which must be made in assessing fatigue.

The individual's environment can contribute to fatigue as well. The degree of stimulation offered by the environment greatly influences the amount of fatigue present. Sensory under- or overload (Chap. 13) can produce monotony, which leads to boredom. Boredom or its anticipation has been directly related to fatigue.

Nursing assessment of fatigue includes descriptions of:

- activities which produce fatigue
- activities which do not produce fatigue
- sensory stimulation within the environment
- physical capabilities
- evidences of fatigue (through verbalization, posture, attention span)
- beliefs about fatigue (positive and negative)
- expressions of boredom

Growth and Development

In the nursing assessment of body kinetic needs, the individual's level of growth and development must be considered. The usual posture seen in a toddler would not be expected in an adolescent, just as the joint mobility of an adolescent would not be that of an older adult. Each level must be considered in terms of expected patterns of behavior and variations from them. Chart 14.2 outlines the patterns relevant to body kinetics at each level of growth and development.

Nursing assessment of growth and development in body kinetics involves comparing the presenting patterns with the expected patterns of behavior. The patterns are assessed in relation to:

- need for movement
- body alignment
- joint capability
- type of mobility
- degree of mobility
- gait
- endurance
- physical responses to movement
- psychologic responses to movement
- safety factors
- assistive devices needed

Chart 14.2
Development Patterns in Body Kinetics

LEVEL OF DEVELOPMENT	RELATIONSHIP TO BODY KINETICS
Infancy	
1–3 months	Limbs function as a unit but not separately; plays with own fingers and hands; in prone position turns head laterally; reaches for bright objects; at end of this time holds head erect and raises chest off bed, sits when supported by someone.
3–6 months	Supports head when sitting; rolls over; relative symmetry of movement; attempts to bear weight when held in standing position; hand-to-hand transfer of objects; begins to sit alone; moves along surfaces by rolling or shifting weight.
6–9 months	Holds own bottle; accurate hand-to-mouth movement; begins to feed self; crawls; walks along by holding on to objects.
9–12 months	Pulls up body; stands alone; walks; feeds self; legs bow; helps in dressing self.
Toddler (15 months–3 years)	Stair climbing; running; jumping; feeds self; carries out many basic ADL skills; becomes toilet trained: bowel first, then bladder.
Preschool (3–5 years)	Skips; hops; uses ride-on toys; dances; has increased hand coordination; dresses self; muscle growth.
School age (6–12 years)	Refines gross and minute motor skills; engages in athletics; long bones growing.
Adolescence (13–18 years)	Ossification of bones; poor posture; clumsiness; decreased coordination; daredevil activities.
Young adulthood (18–45 years)	Reaches full growth; posture erect.
Middle adulthood (45–65 years)	Osteoporotic changes; kyphosis; muscle disuse; decreases sustained endurance.
Later adulthood (65+ years)	Osteoporotic changes; ligament calcification; decreased muscle size; decreased muscle strength; decreased endurance.

- types of activities engaged in
- capabilities
- types of environmental stimulation needed
- special activity needs

Physical Assessment

Physical assessment for body kinetic needs is approached in two ways. First, the nurse observes the individual as he or she performs the usual activities of daily living, such as bathing, dressing, eating, combing hair, or turning on a faucet. Second, the nurse physically examines the individual for musculoskeletal functioning and alteration. Examination of the musculoskeletal system is interdependent with the neurologic examination, particularly in relationship to muscular strength and function. Chapter 13 provides a discussion of the neurologic examination.

The nurse looks at seven general aspects of musculoskeletal functioning: joint mobility, alignment, symmetry, deformity, tenderness, **crepitation** (the grating sound of two bone surfaces rubbing together), and unusual movement. The joints are put through their full range of motion, and the nurse observes for limitation of movement, pain, tenderness, and crepitation. The spine is checked for alignment, symmetry, and deformities by observing posture and palpating with the fingers along the vertebrae from the base of the neck (seventh cervical vertebrae) to the gluteal cleft. The spine is also percussed lightly to determine if there is any tenderness or discomfort. Muscle strength and tone are also assessed at this time. Throughout the exam the nurse notes the usual pattern of response and variations from it in terms of such factors as tenderness, deformity, unusual movements, pain, and resistance. In performing the examination the individual is in a sitting position for assessment of the upper extremities (head, neck, shoulders, arms, and hands), in lying position for assessment of the lower extremities (hips, legs, ankles, and feet), and in a standing position for assessment of the spine.

Diagnostic Tests

The diagnostic test specific to body kinetic needs is the x-ray. Bones, joints, and connective tissue are visualized to assess their integrity and alignment. X-rays help the physician in making a medical diagnosis and assist the health team in planning care. Although special preparations for these x-rays are rare, the nurse has the responsibility to explain the procedure to the individual and to position him or her as comfortably and safely as the circumstances permit for transport to the x-ray department. When the individual returns from the x-ray department, the nurse again positions him or her for comfort and safety and checks for any changes in care regimen.

Serum calcium and phosphorus levels may be drawn to assess changes in body kinetic status. Serum calcium levels can indicate the degree of decalcification of the bone and changes in muscle contractibility (expected serum calcium value, 4.8–5.2 mEq/liter). Serum phosphorus levels vary inversely with calcium and can indicate changes in bone formation (expected serum phosphorus value, 1.7–2.6 mEq/liter).

Nursing assessment related to diagnostic testing describes:

- special preparation for x-rays
- positioning of individual
- x-ray results

- the expected serum phosphorus and calcium range compared with the individual's values
- change in care regimen
- correlation of diagnostic tests with the individual's condition

Self-Assessment

There must be concern for the body kinetic needs of the nurse as well as those of the individual for whom the nurse is caring. When providing care, the nurse must assess his or her own movement needs and capabilities. This insures the nurse's safety and the safety of the individual in the care activities and prevents damage or trauma to both nurse and patient. It also enhances the nurse's function as a role model in that the same principles are used to assess the individual's body kinetic needs as are used to assess the nurse's kinetic needs.

NURSING DIAGNOSIS

A 20-year-old male college student, Mr. Jay, comes to the university health service complaining of pain and limited movement of his right arm after a fall.

The nursing assessment which follows on pages 264 and 265 is a comparison of the young man's presenting (actual) kinetic behaviors and those that the nurse would expect to find in a man of the same level of growth and development who has no interference with mobility.

Related nursing diagnoses might be:

- pain related to tissue trauma
- limited ROM related to tissue trauma
- improper body alignment related to tissue trauma
- interference with activities of daily living related to tissue trauma
- anxiety related to interference with activities of daily living

Variations on the above nursing diagnoses are possible, depending on the grouping and interpretation of data. For example, interference with the respiratory

ASSESSMENT FACTOR	EXPECTED BEHAVIOR	ACTUAL BEHAVIOR
Alignment	Shoulders abducted with spine midline.	Right shoulder adducted and internally rotated.
Effect on body systems	Erect position enhances respiration.	Lungs unable to expand fully as a result of body posture.
Attitude	Correct posture enhances feelings of well-being.	Same
Range of motion (ROM)	Shoulder and arm can be rotated 360°.	Shoulder and arm rotate 30°.
	Shoulder and arm can be abducted and adducted.	Can abduct shoulder, abduction is painful (stabbing pain when he moves shoulder).
	Shoulder can internally and externally rotate.	Shoulder can internally rotate, can't rotate externally.
	Shoulder and arm can flex and extend.	Can flex and extend lower arm.
Activities of daily living	Full activities.	Can brush teeth, cannot comb hair, cannot place clothes on right side.
Reaction to ROM	No pain, discomfort.	Screams with anguish when attempt is made by personnel to move joint, can move by self but grimaces and winces.
Gait	Arms swing when ambulating.	Holds right arm immobile when walking, swings left arm.
Oxygen consumption	No distress.	Respiratory rate increases to 28/minute, shallow; pulse 92, regular, full when ambulating, returns to usual rate when sitting for 3 minutes.
Duration		Fell yesterday AM while jogging, pain in shoulder since then (26 hours).
Growth and development	Age 20, male student uses right arm to write and to do most activities of daily living (ADL).	Cannot use right arm to write at present, upset at missing school work.
Physical assessment	Full ROM, no swelling or pain, posture erect.	Limited ROM (see above); shoulder painful to touch and movement; ecchymotic (black and blue) around entire shoulder; shoulder measurements: right, circumference 57 cm (22½ in.), upper arm distal to shoulder 42 cm (16½ in.); left, circumference 52 cm (20½ in.), upper arm distal to shoulder 37 cm (14½ in.); posture, see above.

(continued)

ASSESSMENT FACTOR	EXPECTED BEHAVIOR	ACTUAL BEHAVIOR
X-ray (right shoulder)	No pathology	Same
Physician's orders		Right arm in sling (ASA) Aspirin 10 g PO q4h. p.r.n. for pain Warm water soaks to right shoulder for 20 minutes t.i.d.

subsystem is not dealt with separately here because alleviating the pain and poor alignment through nursing and medical management will most probably relieve the respiratory symptoms. In addition, Mr. Jay's overall health status does not warrant specific consideration of the respiratory subsystem at this time.

PLANNING

Planning for meeting body kinetic needs centers on maintaining neuromuscular capabilities and prevent-

ing deformities in the individual. Factors such as endurance, fatigue, capabilities, and limitations are important determinants. Recognition of the potential for the hazards of immobility also guides the nurse in the plan of care. Individuals who have interferences with mobility are particularly prone to threats to safety. Thus consideration of both environmental and physical safety are additional components of planning for meeting body kinetic needs.

Using the situation of Mr. Jay, a plan for one nursing diagnosis listed above follows:

NURSING DIAGNOSIS	SHORT-TERM GOAL	PLAN
Limited mobility related to tissue trauma	180° ROM of right shoulder within 4 days	1. Teach rationale for use of sling. 2. Teach how to apply. 3. Give opportunity for return demonstration. 4. Teach rationale for warm water soaks. 5. Teach how to apply warm water soaks, including safety factors, e.g., maintain water temperature below 110° F. 6. Teach rationale for active assistive ROM of shoulder. 7. Teach how to do active assistive ROM until first point of pain. 8. Give opportunity for return demonstration. 9. Explain need for maintaining proper alignment to prevent "freezing" of shoulder muscles. 10. Explain relationship between taking ASA one half-hour before exercise and increased mobility as a result of reduced pain. 11. Demonstrate how to support arm and shoulder during sleep.

INTERVENTION

Maintaining Proper Alignment

Much of the nurse's activity in meeting body kinetic needs focuses on maintaining a person in proper alignment. Proper body alignment is necessary to prevent deformities, fatigue, and undue stress and injury, to promote physiologic function of body systems, and to maintain the functional relationships between body parts.

MEASURES TO PREVENT DEFORMITIES

Each muscle has an antagonist that works in the opposite direction, and when proper body alignment is not maintained the stronger muscle will predominate, causing contracture deformities. Hyperflexion of the neck (sternocleidomastoid muscle group), *claudication* of the wrist (hyperflexion of the flexor carpi ulnaris and radialis muscle group), clawing of the hand (palmar flexion of the lumbricales 1—4 muscle group), external rotation of the hips (obturator internus muscle group), and foot drop (plantar flexion of the gastrocnemius and soleus muscle groups) are all examples of contracture deformities caused by improper body alignment. These conditions may permanently interfere with the individual's ability to function in daily life.

The nurse is accountable for deformities that result from improper alignment. It is the nurse who is responsible for the proper body alignment of the individual regardless of the person's ability to tolerate activity and certain position changes or regardless of the medical orders written limiting movement for that individual.

MEASURES TO PREVENT FATIGUE

Improper alignment creates fatigue because of the increases in the stress and strain placed on the muscles. The stress and strain are a result of the body's attempt to compensate for the imbalance created by the shifting center of gravity. For example, if the body's base of support is narrowed, the body tends to wobble, which shifts the vertical line of gravity outside the base of support. The body tries to maintain its balance by contracting the muscles on the side opposite its weight concentration. This causes fatigue in the contracted muscle groups. If the stress and strain is great enough, injury occurs.

MEASURES TO PROMOTE PHYSIOLOGIC FUNCTIONING

Proper alignment promotes physiologic functioning of the body subsystems by allowing full expansion of the thorax and relaxation of the diaphragm to facilitate respiration; circulation is not restricted by external pressures and the abdominal organs are not compressed.

RELATIONSHIPS OF BODY SEGMENTS

To properly align the individual in any position, attention is paid to the relationships of the body segments to each other, the normal curvatures of the spine (dorsal convexity, lumbar concavity, and sacral convexity) and the correct angles of the joints. Therefore, the head should be in usual extension, the shoulders slightly abducted with the chest brought forward, the wrists extended with the fingers slightly flexed as if to grasp an object, the trunk straight with the elongated S-shape of the spine maintained, the shoulders and hips parallel to each other, the pelvis tipped slightly downward and at a right angle to the axis of the spine, the feet at right angles to the calves in dorsiflexion and no two body parts should lie directly on each other. Figure 14.5 illustrates these relationships.

To maintain proper alignment as described, weak muscle groups are supported by devices such as trochanter rolls, pillows, sandbags, braces, splints, casts, and traction. Chart 14.3 describes correct body positions and how devices are used to maintain and support those positions.

Considerations in Selecting Position

The actual position in which the individual is placed depends on several factors. (Fig. 14.6)

PERSON'S STATE OF HEALTH

One major consideration is the restriction placed on movement because of the individual's health state.

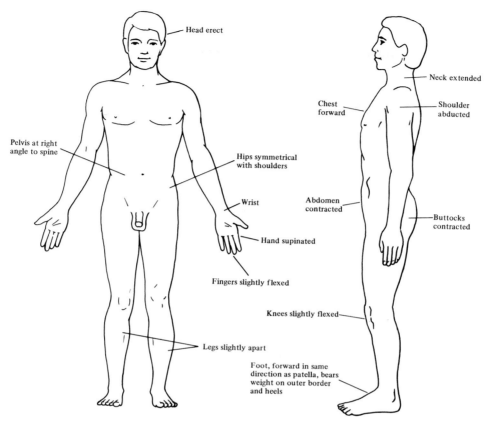

Figure 14.5
Correct anatomical body alignment in standing position (lateral and frontal views).

For example, if the person has a sacral decubitus ulcer, then the supine position will be avoided. Most individuals find the supine position comfortable. This is both a positive and negative aspect of the position, since many individuals are reluctant to assume other positions and thus are prone to pressure problems. (See Chart 14.6 concerning the hazards of immobility.) The prone position may be uncomfortable for long periods of time, as the individual may feel restricted or smothered. Because the individual may feel that way and because of the nurse's lack of familiarity with the proper procedure, nurses often overlook the benefits of the prone position. However, as a change, individuals find it gives a welcome relief to the entire body as it shifts all pressure points and utilizes different muscle groups. The majority of people sleep on their side and thus find the lateral position most conducive to sleep. This position also relieves pressure

from the posterior side of the body but can create ischial pressure if maintained for too long. No matter how the person is positioned the nurse checks for comfort. Often by observation alone the nurse can assess if the individual is comfortable and make changes accordingly.

FREQUENCY OF REPOSITIONING

A second consideration is the frequency of repositioning necessitated by the individual's health state. If the person is able to voluntarily move and shift position, then he or she may not have to be repositioned as often as the person who has limited voluntary movement. It has been shown that well tissue can **necrose** within 2 hours of no movement and unrelieved pressure. Thus the debilitated, unconscious, para-

(continued on page 273)

Chart 14.3
Body Alignment

POSITION	DEVICES	POINTS TO NOTE
SUPINE (Back lying, or dorsal recumbent—Fig. 14.6)		Bed is flat and mattress firm to maintain alignment.
Head is in extension.	A small pillow is placed under the head and shoulders (pillow extends from the 6th cervical to 1st thoracic vertebra).	A pillow should not cause neck flexion or hyperextension.
Shoulder slightly abducted.		Avoid inward rotation and adduction of the shoulder girdle.
Elbows are slightly flexed with forearms.	Place a pillow under forearm.	Position helps to maintain the physiologic function of the arm and shoulder and helps to prevent **claudication** of the wrist by virtue of gravitational pull. Special note: If forearms are kept supinated, the use of a pillow will cause unwanted adduction of the shoulders.
Fingers are slightly flexed with the thumbs adducted in extension.	Place large handroll in palm of the hand with fingers encircling it.	A small handroll encourages clawing of the fingers. Properly sized handrolls prevent palmar flexion of the hands. Loss of opposition of thumb to fingers results in inability to grasp objects.
The trunk is straight and the concave lumbar curve is maintained.	A small pillow or pad is placed under the lumbar curve.	Pad maintains the lumbar curve and helps to bring the chest forward with shoulders abducted.
Hips are parallel with the shoulders and symmetrical to each other.		Maintaining the trunk in alignment promotes proper hip placement.
Legs are in neutral position, neither externally nor internally rotated.	A trochanter roll is placed along each thigh to prevent external rotation. A small pillow between the knees prevents internal rotation.	Position of the feet indicates direction of the rotation.

External rotation

Internal rotation

(continued)

Chart 14.3 (Cont.)
Body Alignment

POSITION	DEVICES	POINTS TO NOTE
Knees are slightly flexed (not more than 5°–10°)	A small roll is placed behind the knees.	A roll maintains slight flexion but does not cause pressure on popliteal nerves and vessels.
Feet are at a 90° angle to the calves.	Footboard or footstraps.	The whole foot must rest against the footboard and not just the balls of the feet, because this causes automatic plantar reflex.
PRONE (Front lying) Head turned to one side in extension.	A folded towel is placed under the head.	Bed is flat and mattress firm to maintain alignment. Use of a pillow may cause lateral hyperextension of the neck and lumbar spine. No support causes cervical flexion of the neck and internal rotation of the shoulder, as well as restriction of chest movement.
Arms are pronated and sharply flexed at the elbows with hands at the level of the head.		Position supports adduction of the shoulders, facilitates expansion of the thorax, and helps prevent claudication of the wrist.
Fingers are slightly flexed with thumbs adducted in extension.	Handroll.	As above.
The trunk is straight and the lumbar curve is maintained.	A pillow is placed under the abdomen.	A pillow minimizes pressure on the thorax, prevents hyperextension of the cervical spine, and protects the breasts of women.
Legs are in a straight line with the trunk.	Pillows can be placed between the knees.	A pillow prevents the internal rotation of the femur.
Feet are at a 90° angle to the calves.	The feet can hang between the mattress and footboard or a pillow may be placed under the anterior calf.	Maintains the 90° angle and prevents plantar flexion.
LATERAL POSITION (Side lying) Head is on the side and in extension.	A pillow is placed under the head.	The bed is flat and the mattress firm to maintain alignment. Pillow maintains alignment of the neck.
The lower arm is supinated and flexed at the elbow with hand level with the head.		The arm does not rest under the body.

(continued)

Chart 14.3 (Cont.)
Body Alignment

POSITION	DEVICES	POINTS TO NOTE
LATERAL POSITION (cont.)		
The upper arm is pronated and flexed at the elbow.	A pillow supports the upper arm.	A pillow prevents pull on the shoulder girdle caused by internal rotation of the shoulder. Breathing is facilitated.
The fingers are slightly flexed with the thumbs adducted in extension.	Large handroll.	Same as above.
The trunk is straight and the lumbar curve is maintained.	Pillow is placed at the small of the back. Note: If individual is obese or has had abdominal surgery, a pillow is placed in front of the abdomen.	Maintains lumbar curve and helps to prevent the individual from rolling onto his back. Pillow by abdomen provides support by preventing gravitational pull on the abdomen.
The hips and shoulders are parallel and symmetrical.		Follows if trunk is straight.
Lower leg is slightly flexed.		
Upper leg is flexed at 90° angle.	A pillow is placed under the upper leg so that the knee is in a straight line with the corresponding hip.	Knee is flexed to provide a wide base of support, thereby promoting stability. Pillow prevents knee from pulling on hip joint, pelvis, or low back caused by internal rotation of the femur. Also helps to keep abdominal and pelvic viscera in a functional position.
Feet are at a 90° angle at calves.	Sandbags, footboard, or splint is placed for each foot.	Prevents plantar flexion.
FOWLER'S POSITION (Semisitting)		
Head of bed elevated at 45°.		At this angle the individual tends to slide down in bed, creating pull on the hamstring muscles, especially if the knees remain extended. Can cause friction burns and problems with **shearing force.**
Head is in extension.	A small pillow under head.	Maintains alignment. However, be careful to avoid flexion of neck.

(continued)

Chart 14.3 (Cont.)
Body Alignment

POSITION	DEVICES	POINTS TO NOTE
FOWLER'S POSITION (cont.)		
Shoulders are abducted, and forearms are flexed at the elbows with the forearms pronated.	Pillow under forearm	Prevents pull on shoulder girdle caused by internal rotation of shoulder.
Wrists are in extension, and fingers are slightly flexed with the thumbs adducted in extension.	Handroll	As above.
Trunk is straight. Hips and buttocks are deep into the angle of the bed with the weight resting on the buttocks and thighs so that the hips and shoulders are in a straight line and symmetrical.		Position prevents sliding and maintains lumbar curvature.
Knees are extended.		The individual in this position tends to slide down in bed, creating pull on the hamstring muscles especially when the knees are in extension.
Calves and feet are at 90° to each other.	Footboard	Prevents plantar flexion.
CHAIR SITTING		
Head is erect, shoulders are symmetrical and in a straight line with the hips.		Maintains alignment. Keeps hips and shoulders symmetrical.
Arms are supported. Hands and wrists as above.	Arms are supported by the chair at elbow.	Chair arms should not be so high that they cause elevation of the shoulder girdle.
Buttocks are deep into the angle of the chair.		Maintains alignment.
Hips, knees, and ankles are fixed at right angles. Feet are flat on floor or support.	Chair height should be such that a 90° angle is maintained. If chair is too short, place cushion in seat; if too tall, place some support under feet so that feet are flat and 90° angle of lower joints is maintained.	If chair height is too low, the angle of hip flexion increases, causing poor alignment. If the chair is too high, the thigh slants downward and pressure is created on the posterior thigh and popliteal area. Feet will dangle, encouraging the development of planter flexion.

Note: In **semi-Fowler's position,** the alignment is the same as in Fowler's but the hips and knees are flexed to prevent sliding and pull on the hamstring muscles. The flexion should not be so great that it causes pressure on the ischial and popliteal areas.

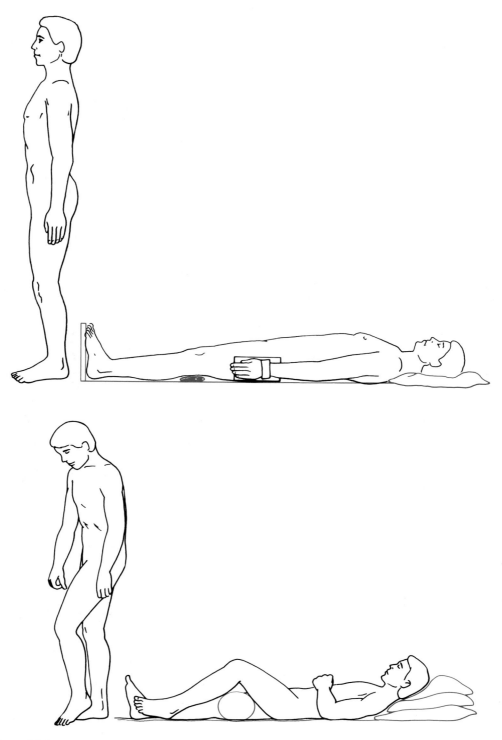

Figure 14.6

(Top) Proper supine positioning is shown along with a similar erect stance. Incorrect alignments are also demonstrated (bottom). The nurse is responsible for helping to maintain the individual in proper alignment while he is confined to bed, so that when the individual is erect, improper positioning does not result.

lyzed, or anesthetized individual whose tissue state may not be good and who cannot move voluntarily will certainly require position changes at least every 2 hours. This does not mean that the person on a 2-hour repositioning schedule does not require slight shifts of weight and position in between the 2-hour intervals. Slight repositioning helps to redistribute body weight and prevents unrelieved pressure while promoting passive muscle contraction. Any time movement takes place, the metabolic rate increases, circulation is promoted, and respiration is enhanced. In addition, the time periods between position changes are often perceived as being longer than the actual clock time.

Body Kinetics for the Nurse While Providing Care

A knowledge of lifting and moving is basic to any position change in order to protect both the individual and the nurse. The nurse's body weight and arm, hip, and knee muscles, as well as gravitational pull, are utilized in moving individuals and objects. Whenever the nurse moves anything, a good base of support must be maintained by assuming a broad stance. (Illustration 14.1)

In moving objects or people, the nurse's center of gravity is lowered by flexing the knees, and the vertical line of gravity is kept within the nurse's base of support by having the trunk straight and within the support base. The nurse also contracts the lower abdominal and gluteal muscles to serve as a sort of internal girdle. This contraction may be referred to as "putting on the internal girdle." These actions are done to increase the nurse's stability and prevent injury to the nurse and the individual. Bending at the waist and not at the knees, shifts the vertical line of gravity out of the base of support, thus decreasing stability, and places strain on the smaller, weaker sacrospinal muscles and joints, rather than on the longer, stronger gluteal and quadriceps muscles.

The nurse always works with the force of gravity rather than against it by pushing, pulling, and lowering instead of lifting. When moving an object the nurse holds it close to his or her body at the center of gravity in order to increase stability, maintain the vertical line of gravity within the base of support, and have better control of the object being moved. In this way the nurse's weight acts as a counterbalance for the weight of the object. The nurse turns his or her

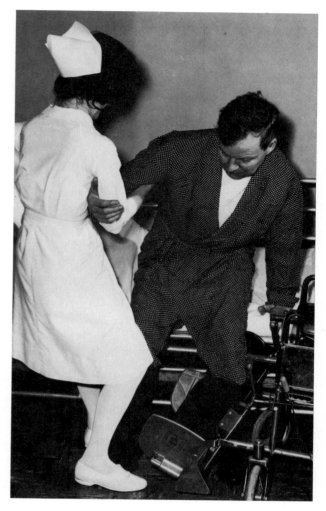

Illustration 14.1
Many principles of body kinetics come into play when a nurse assists an individual to move. In addition to maneuvering so that one's own safety is protected, proper movement by the nurse and individual will also help each person to avoid injuring the other. *(Photo © Lester V. Bergman & Assoc.)*

entire body to face the object being moved. Facing the object prevents rotation of the spine, which causes injury to the spinal muscles and joints.

The principles described above for nursing action are utilized in reaching, stooping, carrying, pushing, and pulling. For example, when reaching for an object on a high shelf, the nurse utilizes a steady stool placed as close as possible to the object in order to decrease the distance and to be able to reach above with both hands, maintaining the vertical line of gravity within the base of support and promoting good body alignment (Figure 14.7 and 14.8).

Friction acts as a major resistive force to movement; therefore, when pushing or pulling an object the adjacent surfaces should be as level and smooth as possible. For example, when moving an individual up in bed, the bed is kept flat (assuming there is no physical contraindication), the sheets wrinkle free, and the skin surface lubricated. A flat bed also aids in working with the force of gravity.

Devices that aid movement such as a mechanical lift or turn sheet can save the nurse and the individual energy and prevents strain and injury.

Moving An Individual

Movement is associated with well-being and independence; therefore, whenever the individual's degree of movement is maintained or increased, feelings of self-esteem are enhanced. For example, the individual who has experienced a restriction of voluntary movement may feel helpless, frustrated, and anxious if left

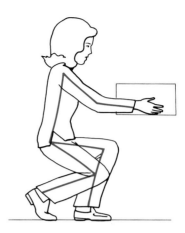

Figure 14.8
Body alignment for stooping. To maintain balance when stooping, the nurse must maintain a wide base of support, keep the trunk straight so that the vertical line of gravity remains within that base, and contract the gluteal and abdominal muscles.

lying in one position for long periods of time. These feelings are a result of an internal sensory deprivation.

When preparing to move an individual the nurse always informs him or her as to what will occur and explains his or her role in the move. This tends to lessen anxiety because it meets the need for security and predictability and allows the individual to participate more fully.

Chart 14.4 outlines various methods for moving an individual and the particular points to note in each technique. The procedures include moving an individual up in bed; moving to the side of the bed; turning to a lateral position; assisting the individual to sit on the side of the bed (dangle); moving to a chair; assisting with ambulation; transferring an individual to a stretcher; and using a mechanical lifter. (Illustration 14.2)

Assisting with Crutch Walking

Whenever crutch walking is anticipated (see Chart 14.5), the individual is first taught exercises to increase the strength of the shoulder, arm, and chest muscles (triceps, biceps, deltoid, trapezius, and pectoral muscles). Exercises such as pushups, pullups on the trapeze, weight lifting and hip lifts are used to strengthen these muscle groups. (Different exercises are discussed on pp. 283–284.) Muscles of the lower

(continued on page 282)

Figure 14.7
Proper body position for reaching. The nurse helps to prevent injury to self by using proper body mechanics when reaching. Being as close as possible to the object that is reached for and keeping one's center of gravity within the base of support are two important principles.

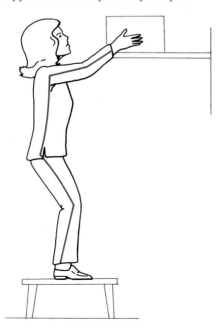

Chart 14.4
Methods of Moving an Individual

TECHNIQUE

POINTS TO NOTE

MOVING UP IN BED
Explain procedure to individual.

Helps decrease anxiety from fear of unknown and increases cooperation.

Adjust bed to flat position and correct working height. Lower the side rail on the side you are working on.

Bed is flat to decrease gravitational pull and resistance. The height of the bed is at the nurse's center of gravity to increase stability and prevent injury from stooping or reaching.

Place individual in a supine position and remove all pillows and appropriate devices.

Having individual flat promotes safety through increased control during movement; reduces friction.

Flex both knees of the individual. If individual can assist, ask him to dig in at the heels, lift buttocks off bed, and push upward during movement. Instruct individual to blow out through mouth while pushing upward.

Knee flexion reduces resistence. Individual pushing upward reduces the amount of work required by nurse.
Prevents use of *Valsalva maneuver.*

If individual can assist, have him place his chin on his chest and place one hand on bed and the other on the raised side rail
or
grasp head of bed during movement
or
place both hands on trapeze and lifts buttocks up.

Having individual assist with moving decreases the nurse's energy expenditure, decreases friction, and helps the individual to exercise and feel more independent.

If the individual cannot assist, place his arms crosswise across chest.

Arms folded across chest reduces the resistance (drag).

Assume a broad stance facing the head of the bed by putting one foot a step in front of the other with the rear foot closer to the bed.

Facing in correct direction prevents injury to spine. Broad stance increases the base of support.

Stand at the side of the bed with rear thigh braced against the bed.

Thigh serves as the pivotal point for movement.

Put on internal girdle.

Prevents injury to the nurse and increases stability and control.

Place hand closest to head of bed under individual's shoulders and the other hand under his thighs.

Hands in this position help distribute individual's weight evenly and support his heaviest part.

Rock back and forth, then shift weight toward the head of the bed while individual lifts buttocks, pushes upward with his heels, pulls with his arms, and blows out through his mouth.

Rocking overcomes inertia. Actions of the nurse and the individual must be coordinated for smooth movement.

(continued)

Chart 14.4 (Cont.)
Methods of Moving an Individual

TECHNIQUE	POINTS TO NOTE
MOVING UP IN BED (cont.) If the weight or condition of the individual requires two people to move him up in bed, the above procedure is followed except: one nurse stands on each side of the bed and, when ready to move, interlock hands under the individual's shoulders and thighs.	
A turn sheet may be used by two people to move an individual up in bed. Place a sheet folded in half across the width of the bed, extending the sheet from under the shoulders of the individual to under the thighs.	A turn sheet decreases friction, distributes body weight more evenly, supports heaviest part of the body, and decreases the energy expended by the nurses.
When using a turn sheet the same procedure is followed as above except: the nurse rolls the sheet close to the individual's body and then grasps it next to the individual's shoulder and thigh and then proceeds.	The turn sheet is grasped close to the individual's body to increase control, stability, and ease of movement.
MOVING INDIVIDUAL TO SIDE OF BED Explain procedure to individual.	Helps decrease anxiety from fear of unknown, helps increase cooperation.
Lock wheels of bed.	Prevents bed from rolling during movement.
Bed is flat, adjust bed height, and remove all appropriate obstacles to movement.	Decreases resistance, helps overcome gravitational pull, and helps bring object closer to center of gravity.
Stand facing bed and assume a broad stance with one foot in front of the other with body in proper alignment.	Prevents rotation of the spine, provides stability, prevents injury, and allows you to view the individual's reactions.
Fold individual's arms across his chest.	Decreases resistance.
Flex knees with front thigh against the bed.	Knee flexion lowers center of gravity, increasing stability; thigh acts as a pivotal point for movement.
Place arm nearest head of bed under individual's neck so your hand grasps his distal shoulder and his head is cradled in the crook of your elbow. Place other arm under the thoracic curvature.	Position of hands gives better support and control of individual's head and helps to distribute and balance weight of the individual.
Put on internal girdle. Rock back and forth, then shift weight toward the rear foot, bringing the individual's head and shoulders to edge of the bed with a pulling motion.	Rocking overcomes inertia and helps to counterbalance individual's weight with the nurse's weight. Avoid lifting, which attempts to work against gravity (pulling counterbalances weight of individual).

(continued)

Chart 14.4 (Cont.)
Methods of Moving an Individual

TECHNIQUE	POINTS TO NOTE

MOVING INDIVIDUAL TO SIDE OF BED (cont.)

Proceed in same manner to move trunk and hips (one hand under the small of back, other hand under the thighs). Then move legs and feet (one hand under knees, other hand under ankle).

Moving the individual in segments makes it possible for one nurse to move person of any size with ease. **Note:** Segmental moving is not used for individuals with spinal injuries.

Check for and position in proper alignment.

See supine alignment.

TURNING INDIVIDUAL TO A LATERAL POSITION

First individual is moved to the side of the bed, then:

Explain procedure to individual.

Helps decrease anxiety from fear of unkown, helps increase cooperation.

Put up side rails on side closest to individual.

Prevents falling.

Move to opposite side of bed and lower side rail on this side.

Side rails are lowered to increase control and stability when moving individual and prevents stretching movements and injury.

Face bed and assume broad stance with one foot only slightly ahead of the other and brace forward thigh against bed. Body is in proper alignment.

Prevents rotation of the spine, provides stability, and prevents injury; thigh acts as a pivotal point for movement.

Fold individual's arms across chest and place the distal ankle across the proximal ankle.

Decreases resistance and base of support while increasing the potential for movement. Folded arms also prevents lower arm from getting caught under the body.

Grasp distal shoulder with hand nearest the head of the bed and grasp hip with other hand.

Positioning hands in this manner reduces resistance and distributes the individual's body weight.

Put on internal girdle. Rock back and forth, then shift weight to rear foot, rolling the individual toward you.

Prevents injury. Rocking overcomes inertia and moves individual. Rolling toward you allows you to view the individual's reaction to movement.

Position individual in proper alignment for lateral position.

See lateral alignment.

MOVING INDIVIDUAL TO PRONE POSITION

For turning an individual to the prone position proceed as in turning to the lateral position *except:*

Place individual's arms straight at his side and roll individual onto his stomach.

Prevents pulling on joints and pinning arms under body.

Position individual in proper body alignment for prone position.

See prone alignment.

(continued)

Chart 14.4 (Cont.)
Methods of Moving an Individual

TECHNIQUE	POINTS TO NOTE
ASSISTING INDIVIDUAL TO SIT ON SIDE OF BED (DANGLE)	
Explain procedure to individual.	Helps decrease anxiety from fear of unknown and helps to increase cooperation.
Lower bed and lock wheels.	Prevents bed from rolling during movement.
Place individual in Fowler's position (Chart 14.3).	Decreases individual's energy output by decreasing the distance he has to sit up.
Facing the head of the bed, assume broad stance with the leg distal to the bed forward.	Stance prevents rotation of the spine and provides stability.
Place your distal hand on the individual's proximal shoulder. Place your proximal hand under individual's axilla.	Position of hands increases support and control of the individual.
Flex knees with proximal thigh against bed, put on internal girdle.	Lowers center of gravity and prevents injury; thigh acts as fulcrum for movement.
Rock back and forth, then shift weight back, bringing individual to a full sitting position.	Overcomes inertia and counterbalances individual's weight with nurse's weight.
Place your distal hand behind individual's neck to support sitting position. Reach with proximal hand behind individual's distal knee.	Position of hands prevents individual from falling back in bed.
Put on internal girdle. Brace your proximal thigh against the bed and pivot on proximal foot to swing individual's legs over the side of the bed and to pivot his trunk on his buttocks.	Proximal thigh acts as a brace, distal foot acts as a counterbalance during pivoting.
Note: If individual has one weak or paralyzed leg, cross that ankle over the other one while pivoting.	Decreases resistance.
If individual is to dangle, check that weight is equally distributed on both buttocks.	Maintains balance.
Remain with individual, providing support as necessary; check pulse, respiration, skin color, and moisture.	Individual may experience orthostatic hypotension.
MOVING INDIVIDUAL TO CHAIR	
Place chair of proper height and with arms at a 45° angle to bed (if wheelchair is used lock wheels).	Decreases distance individual has to move, especially if he is in a weakened state. Chair is readily accessible if individual starts to fall.
Evaluate if feet will be at a 90° angle to the calf and parallel to the floor; if not, place a footstool at bedside.	Footstool decreases the distance between bed and floor, thus decreasing the chance of falling.
Lower bed as low as it will go.	Decreases distance between bed and floor, decreasing the chance of falling.
Proceed as for dangling.	

(continued)

Chart 14.4 (Cont.)
Methods of Moving an Individual

TECHNIQUE	POINTS TO NOTE
MOVING INDIVITUAL TO CHAIR (cont.)	
Place robe and properly fitting slippers with nonskid soles on individual.	Prevents chilling and exposure. Slippers provide support and prevent slipping.
Facing the individual, assume a broad stance with the foot closest to the chair forward.	Prevents rotation of the spine, provides stability, and prevents injury.
Flex knees and place your hands under the individual's axillas or around his waist. Instruct individual to place his hands on your shoulders.	Knee flexion lowers center of gravity. Place your hands in the position that is most comfortable to you and that provides the most support and stability to the individual. Do not grasp upper arms of the individual to avoid dislocating his shoulder joint.
Instruct individual to inch off the bed until his feet are flat on the floor or stool.	Feet should be flat to give more support and to keep vertical line of gravity within the base of support.
Flex knees so forward knee is against the individual's knee.	Your knee serves as a brace in case the individual starts to fall. If a fall is inevitable, go with the fall by lowering yourself with the individual to ease him down.
Put on internal girdle and pivot with the individual so that his back is to the chair. Keep forward knee braced against the individual's knee.	Pivot uses the minimum amount of movement necessary to carry out the task. Bracing the individual's knee helps to support and lock his knee to prevent falling.
Instruct individual to place his hands on the arms of the chair.	Provides support to the individual as he lowers himself into the chair. Also serves to take full weight of individual off the nurse.
Continue to flex knees as you help lower the individual into the chair.	Prevents pull on back muscles.
Position individual in proper body alignment for chair sitting (Chart 14.3).	
ASSISTING WITH AMBULATION	
Proceed as for moving an individual to a chair, and on assumption of the standing position: Check individual's body alignment and instruct for any adjustments.	Individuals, when beginning to ambulate, tend to look at feet rather than straight ahead. Remind individual to hold head erect and to look forward.
If one nurse is assisting individual: stand alongside individual and place the hand nearest to him around his waist and grasp his forearm on the side opposite you; your other hand grasps the individual's upper arm nearest you.	Hands in this position give maximum support to the individual and help to brace him if he should fall.

(continued)

Chart 14.4 (Cont.)
Methods of Moving an Individual

TECHNIQUE	POINTS TO NOTE
ASSISTING WITH AMBULATION (cont.)	
Proceed with ambulation at a pace which the individual sets.	Too fast a pace can tire the individual as well as causing him to lose his balance. Too slow a pace can be frustrating to the individual.
If two nurses are assisting with ambulation: each nurse stands on one side of the individual and follows the above technique.	Walk in unison at individual's pace.
TRANSFERRING INDIVIDUAL TO STRETCHER (UTILIZING THREE PEOPLE)	
Adjust bed to height of stretcher. Bed is flat with side rails lowered.	Bed and stretcher at same height increases ease of movement (both should be at your center of gravity to increase stability and control). Lowered side rails prevent stretching movements and injury.
Place turn sheet under the individual and move him to the side of the bed nearest to where the stretcher will be placed.	Turn sheet distributes body weight, increases ease of movement, and decreases friction.
Position stretcher alongside bed and lock wheels of bed and stretcher.	Prevents bed and stretcher from rolling during movement.
Person 1 stands by the middle of the bed facing the bed. Person 2 stands opposite alongside the stretcher. Person 3 stands at the foot of the bed.	Individual's weight will be distributed by stance of the three nurses.
Remove top linen and place individual's arms across his chest.	Removing linen prevents tangling. Position of arms decreases resistance.
Persons 1 and 2 roll turn sheet close to the individual's body. (Person 2 is reaching across stretcher—internal girdle is in place.)	The turnsheet is grasped close to individual's body to increase control, stability, and ease of movement.
Assume broad stance and put on internal girdle.	Provides stability and prevents injury.
Persons 1 and 2 grasp rolled turn sheet at individual's shoulder and hip. Person 3 grasps ankles and feet.	Distributes body weight.
On the count of three, all persons move the individual onto the stretcher using smooth movements and acting in unison: person 1 using a rocking motion shifts weight forward and kneels on the bed while reaching across the bed; person 2 using a rocking motion shifts weight backward to move the individual on to the stretcher; person 3 moves along the bottom of the bed and stretcher supporting the individual's legs and feet.	Moving in unison supports the individual and provides for safe and effective transfer of individual.

(continued)

Chart 14.4 (Cont.)
Methods of Moving an Individual

TECHNIQUE	POINTS TO NOTE
TRANSFERING INDIVIDUAL TO STRETCHER (cont.) Place individual in proper supine alignment (Chart 14.3).	
Cover him with sheet and place necessary supportive devices. Buckle in individual and raise side rails.	Prevents chilling and exposure. Increases comfort and safety.
TRANSFERRING INDIVIDUAL FROM BED TO CHAIR WITH A MECHANICAL LIFTER (e.g., Hoyer lifter—two people are necessary to carry out this procedure safely.)	
Explain procedure to individual.	Helps decrease anxiety from fear of unknown, helps increase cooperation.
Obtain and check equipment.	Check that S hooks, chains, and canvas seat are intact and in place.
Place chair parallel to the bed (if wheelchair is used, lock wheels).	Leave enough room for lifter and individual to clear the bed and chair.
Position canvas seat under individual: top part goes under mid-third of back (in line with the axilla); bottom part goes under thighs.	Distributes body weight.
Put lifter in place: place footbars under the bed (at right angles to the side of the bed); place overhead bar over the midline of the individual.	Maintains stability and control of the individual and effectiveness of equipment.
Fasten hooks to corresponding openings on canvas seat.	Make sure that all hooks are in place and the chain is of equal length in all sections.
Put on internal girdle. Person 1: release pressure valve and slowly pump up the lifter until the individual's body is suspended above the bed.	Motion is smooth and is not frightening to the individual, thus increasing control and safety.
Person 2: manually guide the individual as he moves.	Gives security to individual and increases control.
Person 1: close valve and slowly roll lifter to the chair. Person 2: guide individual directly over chair.	Decreases fear and ensures smooth transfer.
Person 1: release pressure valve. Person 2: guide individual down into chair.	Decreases fear and ensures smooth transfer.
Remove hooks from canvas seat leaving seat in place.	Individual will be ready for return transfer.
Check for position in proper alignment.	See chair alignment in Chart 14.3.

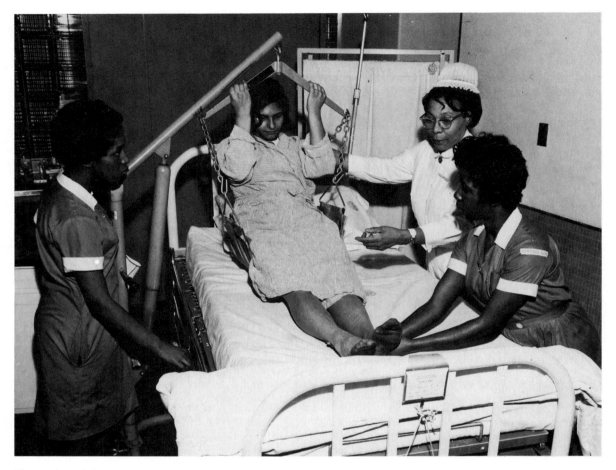

Illustration 14.2
The mechanical lift is one device used to assure an individual's mobility. *(Courtesy of Taurus Photos)*

extremities (quadriceps, gluteal, and gastrocnemius) may also be exercised to aid in balance and weight bearing. Such exercises as quadriceps and gluteal setting and dorsiflexion of the ankle help strengthen these muscle groups.

CRUTCH GAITS

Four-point gait is the most stable gait but requires partial weight bearing on both legs and the ability to move each leg separately. With four-point gait the four points are the individual's two feet and the tips of the two crutches; three of the points are always resting on the floor while the fourth point is being moved. Normal walking is most like this gait.

(Fig. 14.9.A.) In the diagrams below, shaded areas indicate where weight is placed. Normal walking is most like this gait.

Three-point gait is used when full weight bearing is possible on one leg while the other leg can bear no or only partial weight. The three points are the full weight bearing leg and the two crutches. (Fig. 14.9.B.)

Two-point gait requires partial weight bearing on both legs. The two points are the right leg—left crutch and the left leg—right crutch. (Fig. 14.9.C.)

Swing through gait is used when the individual is able to bear weight on either or both legs (with or without braces) and is utilized most commonly for rapid ambulation. (Fig. 14.9.D.)

Chart 14.5
Assisting Individual with Crutch Walking

TECHNIQUE	POINTS TO NOTE
Measure individual for proper crutch length.	Crutches should reach from about 2 in. below the axilla to a point 6–8 in. out from the foot.
	Measurements are taken with the individual wearing shoes.
	Handbars are positioned to prevent weight resting on axilla.
	Tips of crutches are nonskid.
Check for good standing alignment.	Make sure individual avoids adduction of shoulder and hip flexion to prevent backache and muscle strain.
	Keeps vertical line of gravity in place and aids stability.
Instruct individual to bear weight of body on arms and hands by stiffening and slightly flexing his elbows and hyperextending wrists.	▶ If weight rests on axilla, **crutch palsy** (damage to and paresis of radial nerve) occurs—sometimes within 4 hours.
Instruct individual to walk with usual gait.	Maintains balance and prevents muscle strain and plantar flexion.
Instruct individual to place crutches 4 in. ahead and 4 in. to the side.	Proper placement of crutches prevent tripping.
Instruct individual to walk rhythmically with short, equal steps.	Prevent stress and maintains balance.

Promoting Exercise

Another activity of the nurse in meeting body kinetic needs focused on maintaining the individual's muscle tone and joint mobility through exercise. The general purposes of exercise are (1) to maintain tone, strength, and elasticity of the muscles, joints, and surrounding tissues (e.g., ligaments), (2) to provide stress for the maintenance and growth of bones, and (3) to help promote the functioning of all other body subsystems (e.g., respiratory, circulatory, and digestive). Feelings of well-being are thus enhanced by exercise.

RANGE OF MOTION

Range of motion exercises are basic exercises which the nurse provides for the individual. They can be either passive, active, or active assistive.

Passive exercises are those in which the nurse supplies the energy for movement by putting an individual's joint through its full range of motion. The individual expends little energy of his or her own. Although muscles contract, tension is not sufficient to maintain the size and tone of muscle tissue. (Muscles need at least 75% maximal tension for muscle fibers to develop.[4]) Passive exercises do serve to maintain the mobility of joints by keeping the connective tissue surrounding the joints pliable and by preventing ▶ **fibrosis** (increased density and loss of elasticity of connective tissue).

Active exercises are those in which the individual supplies the energy in performing ROM exercise. Muscle size, shape, and strength are maintained and atrophy and contractures are prevented because the muscle tension is sufficient. The nurse has the responsibility to teach the individual how to perform active

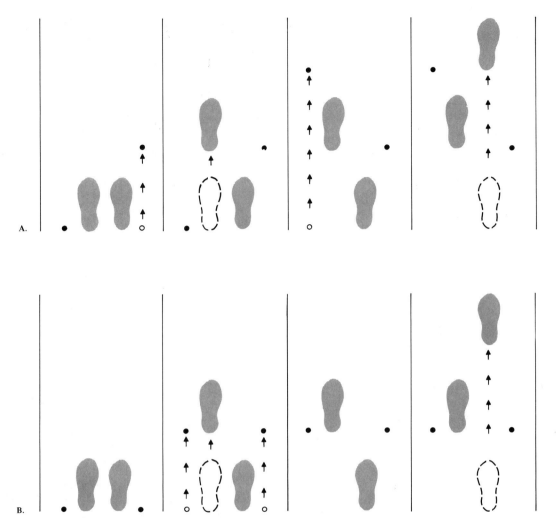

Figure 14.9
A. Four-point gait used in crutch walking. **B.** Three-point gait. *(continued)*

ROM and to encourage him or her to carry out the exercise program throughout the day.

Active assistive exercises are those in which the individual and the nurse both supply the energy to perform ROM. The individual performs the exercise as far as he or she is able and then the nurse aids in completing the full range.

Nursing Action

In performing any of the ROM exercises the nurse must know the expected range of motion for the joint (Chart 14.1), the individual's presenting ROM and the factors that create the difference. Limitations in movement can result from the actual physi-

cal state of the individual (e.g., fracture, fibrosis) or the externally imposed restrictions on movement (e.g., written orders, casts, traction, IVs). The assessment of endurance plays an important part in planning the frequency, duration, and type of exercise program. For example, a very debilitated person may become fatigued if all the joints of the body are put through ROM at one time. Thus the scheduling would be interspersed over a period of time.

The individual's presenting ROM for each joint is recorded to provide a base for evaluating progress.

In the actual performance of ROM, the nurse supports, with one hand, the joint distal to the one being exercised and with the other holds the joint to

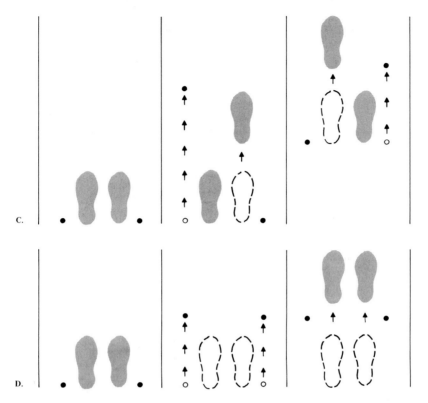

Figure 14.9 (Cont.)
C. Two-point gait. D. Swing through gait.

be exercised while putting it through its ROM. The grasp is firm but not constricting. The movement should be smooth, slow, and rhythmical. In carrying out the exercise, the nurse feels the joint and adjacent muscles for tightness, resistance, and spasm. The individual is informed that a slight sensation of stretching may be experienced, and the nurse observes for any signs of pain or discomfort. To prevent injury, a joint is never moved beyond the point of resistance. If an individual has pain during exercise of a joint, the nurse stops exercising that joint. This is important not only to prevent injury, but also to prevent the individual from associating exercise with pain.

MUSCLE CONDITIONING

Other types of exercise the nurse may help the individual perform are muscle conditioning exercises. They include resistive, isotonic, and isometric (muscle-setting) exercises.

Resistive exercises are those in which the individual contracts the muscle while pushing against a stationary object or resisting the movement of an object. They build the strength, size, and shape of the muscle and provide the necessary stress for bone maintenance and growth. Sufficient stress against the bone is needed to maintain a balance between osteoblasts (bone-forming cells) and osteoclasts (cells responsible for bone tissue absorption). Without sufficient stress the balance of power shifts in favor of the osteoclasts and demineralization of the bone takes place (osteoporosis), leading to bone fragility.

Examples of resistive exercises are pushups, pushing against a footboard to move up in bed, and hip lifting. In hip lifting the individual, while sitting, pushes with his or her hands against the sitting surface (e.g., chair, bed) to raise the hips.

Isometric exercises are those in which the individual contracts a muscle group without increasing the length of the muscle fibers. The individual usually holds the contractions for 10 seconds and then relaxes. Isometric exercises can be likened to a sponge being squeezed. They help to maintain muscle tone and strength.

Examples of isometric exercises are quadricep setting (contraction of the quadricep muscle group), gluteal setting, and tricep setting. The exercises can be performed while carrying out other activities. For example, as you read this you might try contracting your gluteal muscles.

Individuals performing isometric exercises should be instructed to exhale during the muscle contraction to avoid Valsalva maneuver.

Isotonic exercises, in contrast, cause not only muscle contraction but also a change in muscle length. This occurs when a person lifts an object such as a weight and continues to hold it for a brief period of time. While he or she is holding it, the contraction may stop, but the lengthening of the muscle fibers continues for a while. Guyton points out that isotonic exercise "entails the performance of external work. . . [thus] a greater amount of energy is used by the muscle" as compared with isometric exercise.[5] Isotonic exercises help to maintain and increase muscle tone, strength, and shape. Examples of isotonic exercises are weight lifting and working with pulleys.

Nursing Action

In an exercise program the principles of body alignment are utilized for the nurse and the individual. The nurse also recognizes that exercise requires increased energy output, and therefore, the individual's physiologic response to exercise must be assessed. The nurse does this by evaluating the individual's pulse, respiration, and sometimes blood pressure. Studies have indicated that blood pressure rises during isometric exercise.[6]

Creating an Environment Conducive to Meeting Kinetic Needs

Part of nursing intervention for meeting body kinetic needs is creating for the individual a conducive internal and external environment.

THE INTERNAL ENVIRONMENT

In considering the individual's internal environment, the nurse intervenes by utilizing those factors which the nurse has assessed as interfering with or aiding the individual's ability to deal positively with changes in his or her motor status. These factors include levels of anxiety and frustration, the impact the condition has on his or her lifestyle and family and/or significant others, understanding of the situation, and attitudes and values concerning movement. The nurse tailors the intervention accordingly, to both support and reinforce the individual's positive coping behaviors and help supplement and repattern those behaviors that interfere with progress. For example, the individual who wants to begin ambulation as soon as possible, yet refuses to do so because of a fear of falling is taught muscle-setting exercises to increase strength, instructed in the proper use of the walker to increase the safety level, ambulated progressively to increase confidence, and accompanied by the nurse during the first walks out of bed. This individualization of the care "routine" not only meets the person's physical needs and assists his or her progress, but also fulfills psychologic needs.

THE EXTERNAL ENVIRONMENT

The external environment can either support the individual's progress or impede it. The nurse has the capacity to directly control much of this environment by designing it so that it fosters independence, self-esteem, confidence, security, and achievement of developmental tasks. Independence can be encouraged by providing self-help devices such as a trapeze and by collaborating with the individual to set up his or her own care goals. Self-esteem can be enhanced by providing privacy, accepting the individual as he or she is, and willingly spending time with the person. The nurse who safely and effectively utilizes principles in intervention does much to increase the individual's confidence in those caring for him or her. Having familiar objects with which the individual can structure the environment greatly increases feelings of security. If allowed to participate in the individual's care, significant people such as family members or friends also help to increase feelings of security. The person can be assisted to achieve developmental tasks by the nurse's providing age-appropriate activities and help in maintaining and building on tasks already achieved.

INTEGRATING ACTION

The nurse accomplishes environmental intervention through his or her interaction style by providing activities and competent care, and by being aware of the uniqueness of the individual. This all serves to provide a stimulating environment for the individual, in which he or she can successfully move to a pattern of functioning which is more compatible with internal and external environmental demands. (Illustration 14.3)

EVALUATION

Evaluation of whether body kinetic needs are being met focuses on the direction of change that has occurred in the individual's movement abilities. Other major evaluation factors are activity modifications that are required; the influences of mobility alterations on other body systems (and vice versa); and changes in activity capabilities. Modifications in the environment which either enhance or threaten safety for the individual are also important evaluation considerations.

Specific criteria for evaluating an individual's kinetic needs include:

- How do the physiologic changes relate to changes in the body kinetic status? Psychosocial changes? Environmental changes?
- Has the presenting body alignment moved closer to the expected? Range of motion? Mobility? Endurance? Physical exam? Diagnostic test results? Level of growth and development?
- What is the direction of change towards independence in assuming proper alignment? Carrying out ROM and other exercises? Mobility?
- What skills have been acquired in utilizing devices? Carrying out exercises? Communicating body kinetic needs?
- What are the changes in attitude toward body alignment? Exercise? Mobility? Limitations? Body image?
- What are the changes in knowledge about alignment? Exercise? Mobility? Restrictions?
- What are the changes in the degree of ROM? Other exercises? Mobility? ADL? Activity pattern? Endurance? Limitations?
- How long after movement does it take for vital functions (i.e., pulse, respiration, blood pressure) to return to resting state?
- What are the changes in coping with increased activity? Limitations?
- Can the person function safely in the existing environment?
- Have sensory stimulation needs changed?

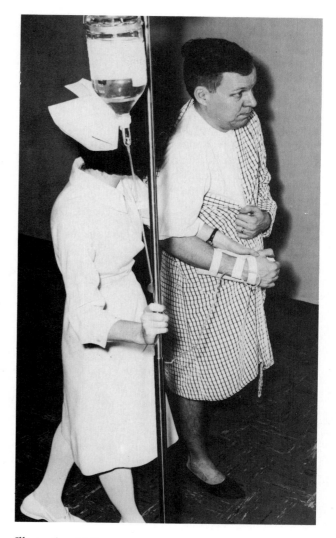

Illustration 14.3
Safe, effective intervention by the nurse will support the individual's progress toward independence. *(Photo © Lester V. Bergman & Assoc.)*

RECORDING AND TEACHING– LEARNING ACTIVITIES

Teaching–Learning Topics

- The rationale for restriction/limitations of body movement.
- The rationale for treatments used in meeting body kinetic needs.
- The importance of maintaining proper alignment while sitting, lying, or standing.

- How to use assistive devices in walking, turning, moving in bed, positioning in bed, etc.
- How the individual can assist in positioning, turning, and moving.
- Positions the individual can assume unassisted.
- How to shift and distribute body weight between position changes.
- The importance of exercises in maintaining muscle tone, strength, size, and joint mobility.
- How to perform exercises unassisted.
- How to make modifications in ADL.
- Safety factors related to exercise (e.g., fatigue, resistance, pain).
- Safety factors related to mobility (e.g., proper shoes, removal of obstacles, lighting, handrails, pace).
- Safety factors related to crutch walking.
- Types of activities available to the individual.
- How to structure a stimulating environment appropriate to his or her level of growth and development.
- How to improvise assistive devices in the home setting.
- What the available resources are and how to use them.

Charting and Recording

Using appropriate body kinetic terms, objectively describe such factors as:

- Objective base-line data on alignment, joint mobility, mobility, devices, help needed, environmental stimuli, level of growth and development, physical examination, physiologic responses, previous pattern of activity
- Subjective assessment data on responses to movement, preferences, and attitudes
- Objective and subjective changes that occur in the person's ability to meet body kinetic needs
- Objective and subjective changes in the frequency needed for movement and positioning
- Objective and subjective interferences with mobility and responses to these interferences
- Schedule and methods of care

Update Kardex concerning changes in goals and plans for meeting body kinetic needs.

Medications to Review

Muscle relaxants

- carisoprodol (Soma)
- chlordiazepoxide (Librium)
- chlorphensin carbamate (Maolate)
- diazepam (Valium)
- methocarbamol (Robaxin)

Analgesics

- acetylsalicylic acid (aspirin)
- aceteminophen (Tylenol)
- ethoheptazene citrate (Zactane)
- meperidine hydrochloride (Demerol)
- pentazocaine (Talwin)
- phenylbutazone (Butazolodin)
- propoxyphene (Darvon)

Diets to Review (see Appendix)

- high protein
- acid ash diets
- high residue/high fiber

CLINICAL APPLICATION A: IMMOBILITY

Immobilization is any actual or perceived restriction of movement. Movement, as a basic life process, influences the total being of the individual. Therefore, any immobilization will involve not only the part directly affected, but the whole person. Actual immobility can be therapeutically desirable as part of the individual's health care or it may be the result of a nontherapeutic care environment. (Fig. 14.10)

It is often therapeutic to immobilize the individual in order to repair or heal a body part (e.g., casting a fracture); decrease energy output by decreasing metabolic activity (e.g., debilitation); or increase venous return by altering the body's position in relation to gravity (e.g., elevating the legs when there is edema—swelling).

Actual immobilization also occurs when the individual is unconscious, paralyzed, and debilitated. It is within these latter situations that one most often

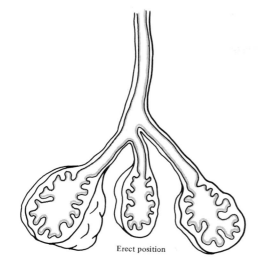

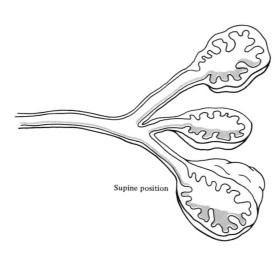

Figure 14.10
The pooling of respiratory secretions in the tracheobronchial tree (shaded areas pictured at bottom) is a negative health behavior that occurs when an individual is immobilized and supine. Gravity encourages this pooling. It requires nursing intervention to insure that the individual obtains an adequate supply of oxygen. When a person is erect, cilia more easily move mucus evenly along the tracheobronchial tree (see at top) and facilitate expectoration of secretions.

sees instances of nontherapeutic immobility. Examples of this are infrequent turning of the unconscious person, restraining the paralyzed individual in a chair for long periods of time, or doing everything for the weakened individual and not allowing him or her any independence.

Perceived immobility occurs when there is no physical restriction on movement, but the person feels immobilized by time, space, and/or situation. An example of this is the parent of a child with a handicap and because of anxiety does not allow the child to move along the growth and development continuum of which he or she is capable.

Immobility is a relative concept because the degree of its impact on the total person will depend on the person's own reactions to stress, coping abilities, age, and health state, as well as the characteristics of the immobility. Immobility can be characterized according to extent, e.g., the entire body versus a single part; type, e.g., physical versus social and voluntary versus forced; and duration, e.g., permanent versus short term.

One of the most common types of immobility the nurse encounters is actual immobility which can create many negative health behaviors. Chart 14.6 outlines these behaviors, their causes, and appropriate nursing interventions.

CLINICAL APPLICATION B: CASTS AND TRACTION

The treatment of a fracture by means of a cast or traction is a direct example of an intervention that results in immobility. Fractures are any discontinuity in the bone tissue. Chart 14.7 outlines the types and general causes of the major categories of fractures.

One method of treating fractures is by the application of a plaster cast. (See Fig. 14.11 for types of casts.) Casts serve three purposes. The first is to immobilize the affected limb and hold bone fragments in proper alignment (**reduction**). Second, they apply uniform pressure to the soft tissue surrounding the fractured bone. This prevents swelling and deformity by maintaining the functional position of the tissues. Third, casts often permit early weight bearing on the affected limb by providing external support to the bone and surrounding tissues.

After a cast is applied, nursing measures will include allowing sufficient time for the cast to dry before any pressure, however slight, is applied and allowing uniform drying of the cast. Usually drying takes 24–48 hours. Uniform drying of the cast is promoted by leaving the cast uncovered and not letting the cast rest directly on the bed. Pillows are used

Chart 14.6
Behaviors Presented in Actual Immobilization and Interventions

PRESENTING BEHAVIOR	MECHANISM OF OCCURRENCE	NURSING INTERVENTION	RATIONALE FOR INTERVENTION
Joint stiffness	Without usual patterns of movement, collagen tissues at joints become fixed and surrounding muscle tissue contracts and atrophies.	Full ROM to all joints	Normal ROM of a joint prevents limitation of movement and loss of joint function.
Atrophy	If muscles are not used they decrease in size, shape, and strength through protein loss. Decreased muscular contractions affect the transport of nutrients and oxygen and the removal of waste by-products necessary for healthy muscle tissue.	Active ROM Isometric and isotonic exercises	Active exercises provide for joint mobility and muscle tone (75 percent maximal tension is needed to maintain muscle size and tone).
Contractures	When there is insufficient stress placed on a muscle group, the stronger of that group will dominate because of shortening of the muscle.	Proper alignment Position changes Active exercises ROM Assistive devices which maintain function positions	Maintains balance of muscle groups. Prevents fatigue, encourages circulation, and shifts body weight. Provides joint mobility and muscle tone. Supplements weakened muscle groups.
Bone fragility	Stress of weight bearing and muscle contraction is necessary for maintenance and growth of bone. Without this stress calcium is lost from the bone, creating a negative calcium balance and increased serum calcium levels. Lack of exercise decreases the supply of nutrients and oxygen and removal of waste by-products necessary for healthy bone.	Resistive, isometric and weight-bearing exercises	Provides adequate stress for bone maintenance and growth.

Increased pulse rate	Cardiac muscles lose tone, as do all muscle groups with insufficient activity. In the supine position, gravity works to return more circulating blood to the heart, creating increased cardiac volume and increased cardiac output. The heart pumps faster to accommodate the increased load.	Change position in relation to gravity (e.g., tilt table, circoelectric bed, dangling) Stand and ambulate as soon as possible Active exercises	Helps maintain distribution of circulating blood. Prevents occurrence. Maintains tone of all muscles.
Increased fatigue	Decreased muscle tone creates loss of muscle strength. Lack of muscle tone creates a decrease in venous return, which decreases removal of muscle waste by-products and leads to fatigue. (May be evidenced by tachycardia on resumption of activity.)	Resistive, isometric, and isotonic exercises	Aids circulation and maintains muscle tone and strength.
Orthostatic (postural) hypotension (drop in blood pressure on rising from a supine position)—gives rise to feelings of syncope (faintness) and dizziness	Lack of movement creates a decreased vasoconstrictive reflex mechanism in the splanchnic and peripheral blood vessels, so when the individual stands peripheral vascular resistance is decreased and pooling of blood (*venous stasis*) occurs, causing a drop in blood pressure and decreased blood flow to the brain.	Change position in relation to gravity Resistive exercises, especially of the legs Elastic stockings Early standing and ambulation Change position slowly and gradually when resuming a standing position	Prevents loss of vasoconstrictive reflex mechanism. Maintains peripheral resistance by maintaining muscle tone. Supplements muscle tone and peripheral resistance. Prevents occurrence. Allows pooled blood to be circulated and reflex mechanism to respond.
Dependent edema (increase in interstitial fluid in an area that is lower than the heart) In supine individual occurs in the sacrum, scrotum, or labia In sitting or standing position occurs in ankles and feet	Loss of muscle tone results in poor venous return and therefore in venous stasis. Venous stasis changes the hydrostatic pressure gradient within the vessel and the plasma leaves the vessel and moves into the tissues (fluid moves from areas of higher pressure to areas of lower pressure).	Resistive and isometric exercises, especially of the lower legs Elastic stockings Change position in relation to gravity.	Helps maintain tone and allows muscle contraction to aid venous return ("muscle pump" effect). Supplements muscle tone and muscle pump action. Prevents venous stasis and resultant change in hydrostatic pressure.

(continued)

Chart 14.6 (Cont.)
Behaviors Presented in Actual Immobilization and Interventions

PRESENTING BEHAVIOR	MECHANISM OF OCCURRENCE	NURSING INTERVENTION	RATIONALE FOR INTERVENTION
Increased use of the Valsalva maneuver (attempted expiration with a closed glottis)	When the individual holds his breath while attempting activity the intrathoracic pressure rises significantly causing a decrease in venous return to heart and coronary arteries; when the breath is released, intrathoracic pressure falls sharply causing a rapid increase of blood to the heart; this can result in tachycardia and cardiac arrest.	Instruct individual to exhale while pulling up in bed, using a trapeze, defecating. Prevent constipation. Utilize the sitting position for elimination when possible.	Exhaling prevents closure of glottis. May result in straining at stool. Prevents straining and decreases work load on the heart.
Thrombus formation (blood clot attached to vein wall)	Controversy exists concerning the actual method of occurrence; however, increased viscosity of the blood (as a result of plasma loss from the circulating blood because of venous stasis and increased hydrostatic pressure) contributes to the formation of the thrombus. Increased serum calcium *may* lead to increased conversion of prothrombin into thrombin, producing more fibrinogen and resulting in hypercoagulability of the blood. Vein trauma resulting from excessive pressure damages the intima of the vessels causing platelets to catch on roughened traumatized surfaces.	Elastic stockings Exercise Change position in relation to gravity Proper position	Helps prevent venous stasis by supplementing muscle tone and muscle pump action. Helps maintain tone of muscle, aids circulation and venous return Prevents venous stasis and resultant change in hydrostatic pressure Decreases pressure on veins

292

Problem	Nursing Measures	Rationale
Shallow, slower respirations	Provide activity and position changes	Compensatory mechanism for decreased basal metabolic rate and decreased carbon dioxide production. Provides stimulus for deeper, more effective respirations
Decreased respiratory effectiveness	Position change to relieve constriction of respiratory effort; Exercise; Coughing and deep breathing exercises; Position change in relation to gravity; Avoid using constricting binders when possible; Avoid gas-forming foods	Poor muscle tone of muscles of respiration and impediment of full respiratory expansion by bed or chair helps to decrease vital capacity. Supine position raises diaphragm to highest level (any abdominal distention or constriction further decreases diaphragmatic excursion), increasing intrathoracic pressure and making the work of breathing more difficult. Decreases work of breathing. Provides stimulus for deeper, more effective respirations. Strengthens abdominal and respiratory muscles and allows better respiratory exchange. Decreases work of breathing by decreasing the pressure on the diaphragm and thorax. Decreases pressure and constriction on diaphragmatic excursion.
Pooling of respiratory secretions	Observe rate, character, and quality of respirations (See Chap. 17.); Coughing and deep breathing exercises; Give intermittent positive pressure breathing treatment (IPPB) as ordered.; Provide humidity.; Increase fluids if secretions are thick and tenacious.; Give percussion and vibration as ordered.; Give postural drainage as ordered (See Chap. 17.); Change position in relation to gravity.; Careful use of narcotics and sedatives	In the supine position, cilia are not as effective in moving mucus up the respiratory tract. Gravity pulls the mucus downward instead of equally distributing it along the tracheobronchial tree (see Fig. 14.9). Loss of muscle tone decreases effectiveness of cough and other mechanisms to rid tracheobronchial tree of mucus. Gives evidence of respiratory difficulty. Strengthens abdominal and respiratory muscles. Decreases intrathoracic pressure, mobilizes secretions and increases gas exchange. Loosens secretions. Moistens the tracheobronchial tree. Loosens secretions. Moves secretions, especially from the lower lobes of the lung. Helps mobilize secretions. Decreases respiratory stimulus even further.
Increased secretions	Same nursing measures as for pooling of secretions.	Compensatory mechanism to drying of the tracheobronchial tree. Same rationales.

293

(continued)

Chart 14.6 (Cont.)
Behaviors Presented in Actual Immobilization and Interventions

PRESENTING BEHAVIOR	MECHANISM OF OCCURRENCE	NURSING INTERVENTION	RATIONALE FOR INTERVENTION
Hypostatic pneumonia with rapid, shallow respirations	Dryness of the tracheobronchial tree decreases resistance to infection. Pooled secretions increase airway resistance, increasing respiratory effort and thereby increasing oxygen consumption and carbon dioxide production. Pooled secretions provide an excellent medium for bacterial growth.	Coughing and deep breathing exercises

Encourage fluids.

Exercise
Change position in relation to gravity.
Administer antibiotics as ordered.
Administer antipyretics as ordered.
Give IPPB as ordered.

Administer oxygen if ordered. | Strengthens abdominal and respiratory muscles and aids in improved respiratory gas exchange.
Moistens tracheobronchial tree, thins secretions.
Increases stimulus to breathing.
Mobilizes secretions.

Inhibits the growth of microorganisms.
Reduces fever.
Decreases intrathoracic pressure, mobilizes secretions, and increases gas exchange.
Provides necessary oxygen for energy need.
Decreases the respiratory effort. |
| Respiratory acidosis | As a result of increased respiratory effort and decreased respiratory effectiveness, there is increased oxygen consumption and carbon dioxide production. Along with the pooling of secretions, these factors prevent the blowing off of carbon dioxide and the uptake of oxygen so that carbon dioxide is retained and the pH balance decreases. | Same measures as above (See Chap. 17 & 21). | |
| Anorexia | Decreased basal metabolic rate, increased protein loss, and increased fatigability decreases appetite. | Small, frequent, desirable meals.
Increase protein intake.
Find out food preferences, pattern of eating (Chap. 19).
Exercise | More appealing to individual.
Offsets negative nitrogen balance.
To serve foods which individual will more likely eat.
Stimulates appetite. |

Constipation	Loss of muscle tone decreases peristaltic movement. Embarrassment in needing assistance in elimination causes individual to ignore defecation reflex.	Exercise Provide privacy for defecation. Increase bulk in diet and encourage fluids. Use proper physiologic position during elimination (Chap. 20). Prevent straining at stool. Selected use of stool softeners. Offer bedpan after meals, especially breakfast. Teach importance of not ignoring the defecation reflex.	Prevents loss of muscle tone. Decreases embarrassment. Increases peristalsis. Fluids prevent drying of feces and aid in elimination. Prevents use of Valsalva maneuver. Softens stool, prevents constipation and use of Valsalva maneuver. Utilizes gastrocolic reflex. Avoids constipation.
Urinary retention and/or incontinence	Loss of muscle tone causes the bladder to become dilated and thus inhibits urinary reflex, thereby leading to urinary retention. Loss of muscle tone may also cause loss of urinary sphincter control. Retention may lead to urinary tract infections and calculi.	Activity Offer bedpan. Use a sitting position to void.	Maintains muscle tone. Encourages voiding at regular intervals. In supine position, voiding must overcome the force of gravity. Sitting position aids flow by gravity.
Urinary calculi	Supine position aids in the pooling of urine and the increased serum calcium level raises the urine pH while the citric acid concentration does not change. Urinary stasis, along with decreased urinary volume, increased calcium, pH, and concentration of phosphorous, causes precipitation and coalescence of minerals.	Use sitting position to void. Exercise Increase fluids. Acid-ash diet If stones appear, strain urine.	Allows more complete emptying of bladder by gravity. Maintains muscle tone. Increases urinary volume. Maintains acidity of the urine so that minerals are not as likely to precipitate out. Helps diagnose the presence and type of stones and makes it possible to see when stone is passed.
Proteinuria	Increased protein loss from muscles is excreted in urine.	Exercise Test urine with TesTape. Look at color, consistancy, odor of urine (Chap. 20).	Maintains tone of muscle and prevents loss of protein. Shows degree of protein loss in urine.

(continued)

Chart 14.6 (Cont.)
Behaviors Presented in Actual Immobilization and Interventions

PRESENTING BEHAVIOR	MECHANISM OF OCCURRENCE	NURSING INTERVENTION	RATIONALE FOR INTERVENTION
Increased urine specific gravity	Increased mineral constituents of the urine and decreased urinary volume increase ratio of solute to solvent.	Encourage fluids. Check specific gravity of urine.	Increases urinary volume. A means of keeping a record of changes.
Altered blood chemistries Increased BUN Increased serum calcium Increased serum phosphate	Increased catabolism of protein, muscle, and bone causes a rise in blood levels of these constituents.	Observe for changes in these values (Chap. 21). Increase mobility and activities.	Indicates status of individual and need for intervention. Prevents changes.
Increased diaphoresis with increased loss of potassium, sodium, and chlorides (decreased serum potassium, sodium, and chloride levels)	In an attempt to maintain temperature, thermal regulatory mechanisms (e.g., anterior hypothalamus) of the body compensate by dilating peripheral blood vessels, leading to heat loss through evaporation; the fluid that is lost contains these electrolytes (Chap. 21).	Maintain comfortable room temperature. Avoid overuse of heavy bedclothes, covers. Check serum electrolyte levels.	Helps prevent overheating or chilling. Helps avoid overheating. Indicates status of the individual and need for intervention.
Decubitus ulcers	Increased pressure on bony prominences and uneven weight distribution reduces circulation to the tissues, resulting in necrosis.	Turn individual frequently. Shift body weight frequently. Avoid shearing force when moving individuals (overriding of tissue surfaces with blood vessel compressed in between). Use turn sheet. Massage skin around bony prominences. Careful use of antipressure devices. Keep skin clean and dry (Chap. 22). Encourage well-balanced diet. Encourage fluids.	Prevents prolonged pressure. Prevents uneven weight distribution. Decreases blood supply to body part. Turn sheet distributes body weight more evenly and helps to prevent shearing force. Increases circulation to the area. Antipressure devices create pressure. Helps prevent skin breakdown. Provides necessary nutrients for skin integrity and helps to maintain skin turgor and elasticity.

Peripheral nerve palsy (paresis or paralysis of peripheral nerves) manifested by tingling, numbness, weakness, paralysis	Relieve pressure areas. Turn frequently and reposition. Avoid use of devices and positions (e.g., knee gatch) which put prolonged pressure on nerves.	Prevents damage. Prevents pressure. Avoids pressure.
Pressure on nerves which cross over bony prominences damages the nerve (occurs particularly in popliteal and elbow regions).		
Perceptual changes manifested by: Time distortion Decreased sense of place in time and space Decreased discrimination of objects and people Decreased weight discrimination Decreased problem-solving ability Body-image distortions (see Chap. 22) Mood changes Increased use of coping mechanisms (e.g. anxiety, hostility, depression, dependency) Changes in sleep patterns	Change plane of individual's position. Exercise Increase use of touch in providing care. Provide time-orienting devices (e.g., clocks, calendars, radio, TV, newspaper). Provide interactions that direct individual as to time, place, and person. Provide meaningful activity appropriate to level of growth and development. Attempt to provide individual's usual habits of daily life. Provide familiar objects. Encourage visits from family and/or significant others.	These interventions provide increased proprioceptive stimuli for the individual.
Decreased proprioceptive stimulation, especially in the supine position, appears to alter the ability of the individual to interpret sensory input (see Chap. 13).		
Changes in interaction patterns with family and/or significant others (role changes) manifested by: Mood changes Increased use of coping mechanisms	Promote active participation in own care. Encourage individual to continue independence in any areas in which he is capable (e.g., decision making). Encourage family and/or significant others to include individual in plans and decision making. Allow individual to vent feelings concerning immobility, role changes, hospitalization, care, restrictions, etc.	These interventions serve to maintain the individual's interaction patterns and his self-esteem.
The individual has a loss in his ability to function in his usual role patterns; thus he cannot utilize his usual interaction patterns.		

Chart 14.7
Major Categories of Fractures and Their Causes

TYPE OF FRACTURE	CAUSE OF FRACTURE	DESCRIPTION
COMPLETE 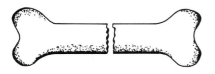	Fall, trauma	A clean break all the way through the bone shaft with no bone fragments (simple fracture).
INCOMPLETE 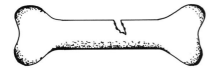	A soft fall, trauma	Bone shaft partially cracked, "cracked bone."
CLOSED COMPLETE 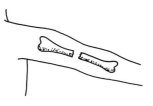	A fall, trauma	Overlying tissue remains intact, but there is a clean break all the way through the bone shaft.
OPEN COMPLETE 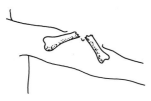	A severe trauma, usually with an impact	The bone ends pierce overlying tissue including the skin; Susceptible to infection.

(continued)

Chart 14.7 (Cont.)

Major Categories of Fractures and Their Causes

TYPE OF FRACTURE	CAUSE OF FRACTURE	DESCRIPTION
GREENSTICK	A fall, trauma	Usually found in children. One side of bone bends, while the opposite side cracks (incomplete fracture).

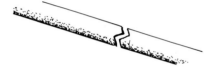

TRANSVERSE	Trauma, fall	The fracture is at a right angle to the shaft of the bone.

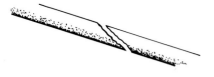

OBLIQUE (COMPLETE)	Fall, often on the limb	The break is at an angle greater than 90° to the shaft.

SPIRAL	Wrenching or twisting trauma	The bone fragments rotate around one another in any direction putting the bone out of alignment. Surrounding tissue can be extensively damaged.

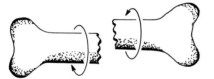

(continued)

Chart 14.7 (Cont.)
Major Categories of Fractures and Their Causes

TYPE OF FRACTURE	CAUSE OF FRACTURE	DESCRIPTION
COMMINUTED 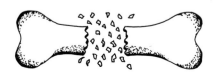	Severe trauma, hard blow	Bone fragments of varying sizes are scattered into surrounding tissue making realignment difficult. Often found in the elderly or people with osteoporosis.
DEPRESSED 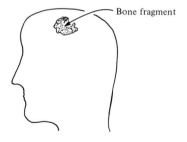	Localized sharp blow most often to the skull	Bone fragment falls downward, leaving an opening in bone.
IMPACTED 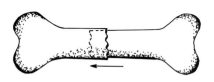	Severe pressure in the same plane as the shaft of the bone	One end of the bone is rammed into the other.
COMPRESSED 	Severe downward jolt to the spinal vertebrae	Two or more vertebrae are forced together, causing shattering or cracking of the vertebrae.

Bone fragment

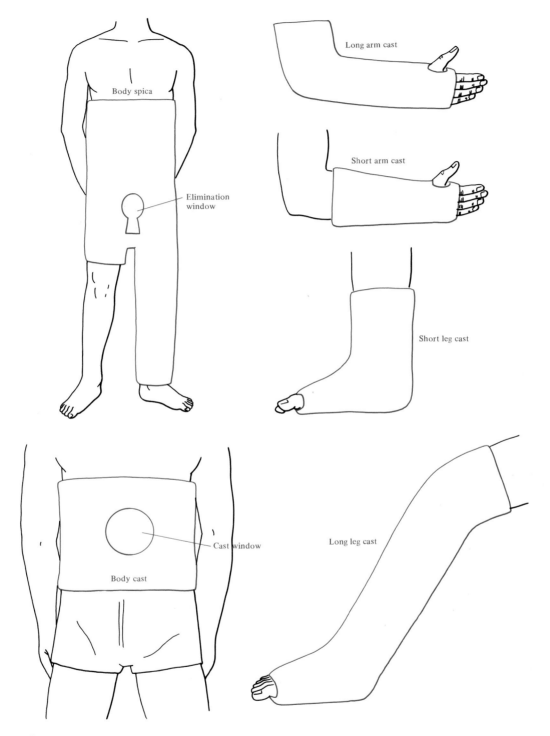

Figure 14.11
Types of casts.

Chart 14.8
Complications Caused by Casts and Nursing Interventions

PRESENTING BEHAVIOR	MECHANISM OF OCCURRENCE	NURSING INTERVENTION

Circulatory embarrassment* manifested by:
   Numbness
   Coldness
   Tingling
	Cast pressure on a vessel.
	
	 Maintanence of one position for extended periods.
		Proper positioning with the least amount of pressure points.
		 Change position as often as allowed.

Swelling Blanching Pain Cyanosis Decrease in pulses distal to the pressure Decrease in sensation distal to the pressure	Pressure against the cast wall created by swollen tissues. (Swelling can be a physiologic response to trauma and usually occurs soon after injury.) See Chapter 15.	Elevate limb to aid venous return. Observe carefully and frequently by comparing one extremity with the other as to color, size, and sensation. Notify physician immediately if any of these signs or symptoms occur—the cast may need to be removed.

Necrosis and decubitus ulcers manifested by:
   Odors from cast
   Hot areas on the surface of the cast
   Drainage on or from the cast
   Itching
   Pain
	Pressure on skin and blood vessels can cause skin breakdown and necrosis.
	 Irritation from jagged cast edges may also cause skin trauma.
		Circle all cast discolorations with a pen to provide a base for comparison.
		 Prevent pressure by use of methods described above.
		 Teach individuals not to use objects to scratch the skin under the cast, as objects can break off or become "lost" in the cast and cause skin trauma.
		 Observe for and pad any jagged or broken cast edges to prevent skin trauma.
		 Observe for signs of impending skin breakdown and report immediately to the physician.

Nerve damage manifested by:
   Numbness
   Tingling
   Loss of sensation distal to the point of pressure
	Pressure on the nerve supplying the area.
	 Pressure can come from the same factors that apply to circulatory embarrassment.
		Observe same care as for circulatory embarrassment.

Complications of immobility	See Chart 14.6.	

*Note: If circulatory embarrassment continues, the function of the limb can be permanently damaged and the limb itself may be lost.

to prop it. Chart 14.8 outlines the complications resulting from casts and preventive nursing measures for them.

Nursing Measures in Cast Care

General nursing measures for the care of the individual with a cast includes keeping the cast clean and dry to prevent deterioration of the cast, providing exercises to the affected limb (usually isometric) and providing for exercise and ROM to the joints not affected. If the cast is on the lower limbs, then care will include preparation of the individual for crutch walking.

Traction

Traction may also be used in the treatment of fractures by applying an external force (usually weights) to the affected limb. Traction is used to reduce fractures, maintain alignment, lessen muscle spasm, regain normal length of the limb shortened by muscle spasm and contractures, and prevent fracture deformities caused by spasm, contracture, and atrophy.

Traction may be applied by attaching the traction apparatus directly to the skin by means of adhesive tape or moleskin (skin traction) or by inserting special wires, pins, or tongs directly into the bone to which the traction apparatus is then attached (skeletal traction). Skeletal traction is a more effective method for accomplishing the purposes of traction.

The external force of traction can be applied in one of two ways—running traction or balanced suspension traction.

RUNNING TRACTION

Running traction is the application of a weight to a traction frame (Fig. 14.12). The frame may be applied by either the skeletal or skin method. With running traction the weight of the individual acts as a counterforce to the weight that is applied externally. Counterforce is a force that is applied in an opposite direction to maintain a system in balance, or equilibrium. These opposing forces can be likened to the child's game of tug of war. With this type of traction the individual must remain in the same position without turning, sitting up, or sliding down in bed in order to maintain the balance of the opposing forces.

BALANCED SUSPENSION TRACTION

In balanced suspension traction, the counterforce is provided, not by the individual's body weight, but by a series of weights placed along the traction setup (Fig. 14.13.) In this type of traction the affected limb is suspended on a canvas hammock so that it is only under the control of the weight system and not affected by the individual's own body weight. Therefore, the individual on balanced suspension traction may sit up in bed, turn slightly from side to side, and move up and down in bed since body weight has little influence on the weight system and force on the limb. It is important, however, to maintain the

Figure 14.12
Running traction.

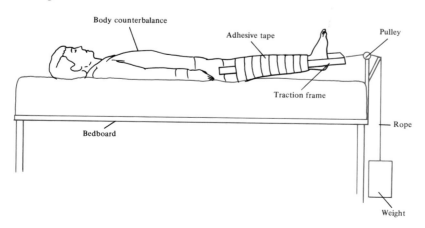

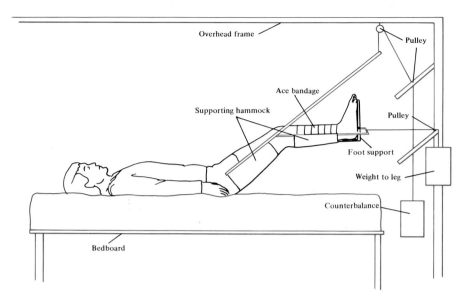

Figure 14.13
Balanced suspension traction.

exact relationship of the weights to each other. As in running traction, balanced suspension traction can be used with both skeletal and skin traction.

COMPLICATIONS OF IMMOBILITY

Complications of immobility are possible with both types of traction but occur more frequently in the individual with running traction because of the total restriction on movement. Complications that can occur as a result of traction immobilization are those already mentioned in Chart 14.8 as complications of casts. In addition, the individual with skeletal traction is prone to the development of an infection at the point where the wire, pin, or tong is inserted. Meticulous cleansing of the insertion site is a necessary part of nursing intervention to prevent infection.

NOTES

1. E. L. Thorndike. "A Note on the Accuracy of Discrimination of Weights and Lengths." *Psychological Review*, 16:340, 1909.
2. Bryant J. Cratty. *Movement, Behavior and Motor Learning*, 2nd ed. Philadelphia, Lea & Febiger, 1967, p. 3.
3. *Ibid.*, pp. 227–228.
4. Arthur C. Guyton. *Textbook of Medical Physiology*, 4th ed. Philadelphia, Saunders, 1971, p. 91.
5. *Ibid.* p. 86.
6. R. L. Bartels, E. L. Fox, R. W. Bowers, and E. P. Hiatt. "Effects of Isometric Work on Heart Rate, Blood Pressure, and Net Oxygen Cost." *The Research Quarterly*, 39:437, 1968.

SELECTED REFERENCES

Bartels, R. L., Fox, E. L., Bowers, R. W., and Hiatt, E. P. "Effects of Isometric Work on Heart Rate, Blood Pressure and Net Oxygen Cost." *The Research Quarterly*, 39:437, 1968.

Bilger, Anneta J. and Greene, Ellen H. *Winters' Protective Body Mechanics*. New York, Springer, 1973.

Carnevali, Doris and Brueckner, Susan. "Immobilization: Reassessment of a Concept." *American Journal of Nursing*, 70:1502, July, 1970.

Cratty, Bryant J. *Movement Behavior and Motor Learning*, 2nd ed. Philadelphia, Lea & Febiger, 1967.

Cuica, Rudy, Bradish, Jennie, and Trombley, Suzanne. "Passive Range of Motion Exercises: A Handbook." *Nursing 78*, 8:59, July, 1978.

———. "Active Range of Motion Exercises: A Handbook." *Nursing 78,* 8:45, August, 1978.

Dugas, Barbara W. "Movement and Exercise Needs," in *Introduction to Patient Care,* 3rd ed. Philadelphia, Saunders, 1977, p. 290–319.

Dison, Norma. *Clinical Nursing Techniques.* St. Louis, Mosby, 1975.

Farrell, Jane. "Casts, Your Patients, and You" (Part 1). *Nursing 78,* 8:65, October, 1978.

———. "Casts, Your Patients and You" (Part 2). *Nursing 78,* 8:57, November, 1978.

———. "Casts, Your Patients and You" (Part 3). *Nursing 78,* 8:53m, December, 1978.

Gordon, Margery. "Assessing Activity Tolerance." *American Journal of Nursing,* 76:72, January, 1976.

Guyton, Arthur C. *Textbook of Medical Physiology.* Philadelphia, Saunders, 1971.

Hirschberg, Gerald, Lewis, Leon, and Vaughn, Patricia. "Promoting Patient Mobility and Preventing Secondary Disabilities." *Nursing 77,* 7:42, May, 1977.

"How to Negotiate the Ups and Downs, Ins and Outs of Body Alignment." *Nursing 74,* 4:46, October, 1974.

Jungreis, Sidney. "Exercises for Expediting Mobility in Bedridden Patients." *Nursing 77,* 7:47, August, 1977.

Kerr, Avice. *Orthopedic Nursing Procedures,* 2nd ed. New York, Springer, 1969.

Kottke, Frederick J. "The Effects of Limitation of Activity Upon the Human Body." *Journal of the American Medical Association,* 196:117, June 6, 1966.

Latchau, Marjorie and Egstrom, Glen. *Human Movement.* Englewood Cliffs, N.J., Prentice-Hall, 1969.

Long, Barbara and Buergin, Patricia S. "The Pivot Transfer." *American Journal of Nursing,* 77:980, June, 1970.

Mitchell, Pamela H. "Motor Status," in *Concepts Basic to Nursing,* 2nd ed. New York, McGraw-Hill, 1977, p. 290–319.

Olsen, Edith. "Hazards of Immobility." *American Journal of Nursing,* 67:780, April, 1967.

Rantz, Marilyn J. and Courtial, Donald. *Lifting, Moving and Transferring Patients.* St. Louis, Mosby, 1977.

Snyder, Mariah, and Baum, Rebecca. "Assessing Station and Gait." *American Journal of Nursing,* 74:1256, July, 1974.

Spencer, W. A., Valbona, C., and Carter, R. E., Jr. "Physiologic Concepts of Immobilization." *Journal of Physical Medicine and Rehabilitation,* 46:89, 1965.

Wood, Lucille A. and Rambo, Beverly J., eds. *Nursing Skills for Allied Health Services.* Philadelphia, Saunders, 1977.

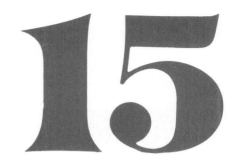

15

The Antiseptic Baby and the Prophylactic Pup
Were playing in the garden when the Bunny gamboled up.
They looked upon the Creature with a loathing undisguised;—
It wasn't Disinfected and it wasn't sterilized.
They said it was a Microbe and a Hotbed of Disease;
They steamed it in a vapor of a thousand-odd degrees;
And washed it in permanganate with carbolated soap.
　　　　Arthur Guiterman—*"Strictly Germ-Proof"*

BIOLOGIC SAFETY

PRINCIPLES RELATED TO BIOLOGIC SAFETY

Pathogenic and nonpathogenic organisms constantly exist in the internal and external environments.

Ability of microorganisms to cause disease is related to agent characteristic, host defense, and environmental support.

Any factor which increases agent viability, decreases host resistance, or reduces environmental supports increases the likelihood of infection.

Any factor which decreases agent viability, increases host resistance, or increases environmental supports decreases the likelihood of infection.

The skin is the major protective barrier against invasion of microorganisms.

The skin or body tissues cannot be sterilized.

The body's secretions of tears, digestive juices, and mucus have bacteriostatic and bacteriocidal properties which protect against invasion.

Inflammation is a naturally occurring defense of the body to invasion by any type of foreign agents.

An agent is any mechanical, chemical, biologic, physical, or psychosocial stressor.

An intact immune system is necessary for successful defense against invading microorganisms.

Antigen—antibody reactions are responsible for immunity.

Passive immunity is temporary and acquired.

Active immunity is permanent or long-term and produced through exposure to some form of antigen.

Healing is related to the amount of tissue damage and the level of wellness of the individual.

Healing cannot occur in the presence of infection.

Infants, children, and older adults are more susceptible to skin damage and infection than other age groups are.

Level of growth and development is directly related to healing ability.

Body cavities have naturally occurring resident flora.

Frequent handwashing significantly decreases the number of transient bacteria.

Hygiene habits are learned.

Dry, cool, well-ventilated areas are less conducive to microbial growth than moist, warm, unventilated areas.

Isolation techniques can set up a barrier to the transfer of microorganisms.

Portals of entry and exit of microorganisms determine the type of isolation precautions.

Isolation precautions increase susceptibility to sensory deprivation.

Maintenance of sterile technique requires that only sterile objects come in contact with sterile objects.

Maintenance of clean technique requires that only clean or sterile objects come in contact with clean objects.

Contamination in sterile technique occurs if unsterile objects come in contact with sterile objects.

Contamination in clean technique occurs if dirty objects come in contact with clean objects.

Cleansing of any object proceeds from clean to dirty areas.

Body temperature is a balance between heat produced and heat lost.

Heat is lost through the body by conduction, convection, evaporation, and radiation.

Heat is produced in the body by cellular metabolism.

Peripheral vasoconstriction results in conservation of body heat.

Peripheral vasodilation results in loss of body heat.

The hypothalamus is the thermoregulator center of the body.

The posterior hypothalamus regulates heat conservation.

The anterior hypothalamus regulates heat loss.

Brain cells are damaged by extremes of heat and cold.

Centigrade = 5/9 (Fahrenheit − 32)

Fahrenheit = 9/5 centigrade + 32

The internal and external environments of individuals are constantly exposed to a variety of microorganisms which have the potential for creating alterations in individuals' levels of wellness. The impact of these microorganisms at any given time will depend on agent−host−environmental interactions. Individuals (host) have many defenses which protect them from disease when changes occur in the agent or the environment. The skin, tears, digestive juices, and the immune system, including phagocytosis, are some of these defenses. In addition, the nutritional state, blood supply, and general health state contribute greatly to an individual's ability to resist the sequelae of invasion by microorganisms.

    ▶ The maintenance of the individual's defense system, the reduction of agents, and the support of a therapeutic environment are the focal points for the nurse in promoting biologic safety. **Biologic safety** is the protection of the individual against invasion from potentially harmful microorganisms and the possible sequelae of this invasion. Sequelae of invasion include inflammation, localized and systemic infection, and failure of body subsystems to function.

ASSESSMENT

Nursing assessment for biologic safety is directed toward assessing the agent, host, and environment and their dynamic interactions.

Agent Assessment

The ability of a microorganism to produce disease depends on having an environment where it can grow and multiply, a mode of transmission from that environment to a host, a method of entering the host, and the ability to grow, multiply, and produce symptoms within the host. Thus the nurse needs to assess these agent characteristics in order to prevent their spread, reduce their opportunities to enter people, and limit their disease-producing capabilities.

ENVIRONMENT (RESERVOIR)

Microorganisms require an environment which is conducive to their growth and multiplication. This environment is known as a **reservoir** and can be plants, animals, humans, insects, soil, or other nonliving organic matter. These reservoirs provide the elements necessary for the survival of the organism—nutrients, water, oxygen, and proper temperature.

MODE OF TRANSMISSION

Microorganisms are transmitted from these reservoirs to the host by means of direct or indirect contact, a vehicle, or vector or through the air. **Direct contact** involves the host actually coming in contact with the contaminated reservoir, while **indirect contact** occurs when the host touches an object which has been exposed to the reservoir. A **vehicle** is an inanimate object which carries the agent from the reservoir to the host. Milk, food, water, serum, or plasma can be vehicles. A **vector,** on the other hand, is any insect or other living thing which transmits the agent from the reservoir to the host. Agents can also be transmitted from the reservoir to the host through the air. Airborne agents may be directly inhaled by the host or may settle, as dust, on objects in the environment where the host comes in contact with them.

PORTAL OF ENTRY

Microorganisms can invade the body through the skin, mucous membranes, respiratory system, and gastrointestinal tract. Any interruption in the skin or mucous membrane can provide a portal of entry for microorganisms causing staphylococcal infections, venereal disease, and tetanus. Insect or animal bites can also be responsible for the entry of vector-transmitted diseases such as anthrax, malaria, Rocky Mountain spotted fever, typhoid, and rabies.

Airborne microorganisms can be conveyed through droplets or dust into the respiratory tract. People with airborne diseases can transmit these organisms through sneezing, coughing, spitting, or im-

properly disposing of contaminated tissues. Examples of airborne diseases are varicella (chicken pox), rubella (German measles), measles, tuberculosis, influenza, and the common cold.

Diseases contracted through the gastrointestinal tract include dysentery, salmonellosis, gastroenteritis, botulism, and infectious hepatitis. Food and water and feces may act as vehicles for transmission of these diseases.

CAPACITY TO PRODUCE DISEASE

One of the major factors determining the disease-producing capability of an organism is its ability to enter the body and find an environment suitable for growth. Some organisms are very specific to a particular type of body tissue. Such an organism is the influenza virus, which causes disease only when it contacts the columnar epithelium of the tracheobronchial tract. However, other organisms such as streptococci, staphylococci, and tubercle bacilli may have several different portals of entry and cause disease in a variety of body tissues.

Organisms differ in their abilities to produce disease and in the severity of illness they cause. Also, some diseases are more communicable than others. A **communicable disease,** as defined by the American Public Health Association, is "an illness due to a specific infectious agent or its toxic products, arising through transmission of that agent or its products from reservoir to susceptible host, either directly as from an infected person or animal, or indirectly through the agency of an intermediate plant or animal host, or the inanimate environment." The ability of the organism to enter the body, find an environment suitable for rapid growth, resist the host's defenses, and produce disease depends, in part, on the species of the organism, the strain within the species, and the susceptibility of the host. Chicken pox, measles, and the common cold, for instance, are more communicable than tuberculosis and leprosy.

SURVIVAL ABILITY

Each microorganism has its own requirements for survival and its own degree of resistance to destruction. The requirements for survival include proper environmental temperature range, sufficient amounts of oxygen and moisture, an appropriate chemical milieu and nutritional intake. When these requirements are interfered with, the organism may either cease to multiply or die. The ability of micro-organisms to withstand threats depends on their resistive properties. These properties include toxin and antigen production, ability to form spores, ability to mutate, and mobility.

Some microorganisms release toxins into the host which may act to protect the agent against the host's defense system. Microorganisms can also cause the host to develop antigens. These antigens may make the host immune to infection by the organism but may also create in the host a hyperresponse (allergic reaction) and a resulting sensitivity to subsequent invasions by the organism.

Under adverse conditions some organisms can form spores to survive, while other microorganisms may mutate when the environmental or chemical conditions change. Also, certain microorganisms can move more rapidly than others within the host, from host to host, and from reservoir to reservoir when environmental conditions are not suitable to their survival.

Nursing assessment of agent characteristics includes descriptions of:

- reservoir
- mode of transmission
- mode of entry
- communicability
- ability to cause disease
- organism requirements for survival
- resistive properties of the organism

Host Assessment

Since microorganisms are always present in both internal and external environments, individuals have certain defenses to protect themselves from invasion by microorganisms, to prevent their growth, and to limit their effects. These defenses include the inflammatory response, the immune response, the healing process, and the general physical and physiologic characteristics of the individual. The nurse therefore assesses the probability of the individual's coming in contact with injurious agents, as well as the individual's ability to mobilize and maintain defenses once contact with these agents has been made. This enables the nurse to promote, restore, and maintain the individual's defense system and to limit the effects of the agents.

INFLAMMATORY RESPONSE

Once agents have invaded the body, the body reacts by attempting to neutralize, destroy, and limit the effects of the invasion through the **inflammatory response**. This response is an expected one and is necessary for the survival of the host. The inflammatory response occurs in an orderly fashion. First, there is a brief period of localized vasoconstriction. Then the injured cells release histamine, kinin, and other substances; these responses result in localized vasodilation and increased capillary permeability. The increase in vasodilation helps bring more blood into the area. Neutrophils circulating in the blood and histiocytes in the surrounding tissues are attracted to the area, where they begin to engulf and digest bacteria and toxins by phagocytosis. The histiocytes become macrophages. These macrophages are highly phagocytic and also produce antibodies which counteract the agents and their toxins. The macrophages also play a later role in the collagen formation needed for healing.

Increased capillary permeability allows for the entry of fluids and protein, including fibrinogen, into the affected area. A clot forms as a result, and the injured area is walled off, limiting the spread of microorganisms and toxins to the rest of the body. Local edema occurs and the site is red, swollen, warm to the touch, and tender. There may be a resultant loss of function of the affected part.

Two other processes occur as a result of invasion: neutrophilia and leukocytosis. **Neutrophilia** is the increase in the number of circulating neutrophils, while **leukocytosis** is the increase in the total number of white blood cells. These increases occur as a result of depletion of neutrophil and leukocyte storage in the body and the subsequent increased production of these cells by the bone marrow.

Nursing assessment of the inflammatory response includes descriptions of:

- precipitating conditions
- signs and symptoms
- adequacy of response
- interferences

THE IMMUNE RESPONSE

The body also attempts to limit, destroy, and neutralize the effects of biologic invasion through the immune response. The immune response is the production of antibodies or sensitized lymphocytes which help counteract the effects of material that is foreign to the body (**antigens**). When a particular microorganism or toxin enters the individual's body for the first time, the plasma cells in the lymphoid tissue respond by producing globulins (**antibodies**). These globulins can act on the agent to neutralize, precipitate, or agglutinate it; destroy its cell membrane; or decrease its resistance to phagocytosis.

The initial production of a specific antibody requires time. Thus the first contact with a microorganism or toxin may result in a disease process. However, subsequent contacts with these agents usually produce an immediate immune response to counteract their effects.

Allergic Response

The body may overreact to an antigen or group of antigens, creating a hypersensitivity of the body to them. This hypersensitive reaction is called an allergic response. The body appears to continue to produce antibodies against the offending agent long after these antibodies are needed. Allergic responses may be either immediate (anaphylactic type) or delayed. **Anaphylactic** shock is a life-threatening emergency which results in complete circulatory and respiratory collapse and requires immediate intervention. Signs and symptoms of allergic reactions include localized tissue swelling, itching, runny eyes and nose, wheezing, and cardiovascular collapse and possibly death.

Natural Immunity

Human beings as a species have natural immunity to certain diseases found in other species. Individuals also have genetically acquired immunity, and it is often difficult to differentiate between this inborn natural immunity and immunity acquired through exposure to an antigen. Infants have acquired passive immunity for several months after birth because their mothers' antibodies cross the placental barrier or are transmitted through breast milk.

Passive Immunity

Passive immunity occurs whenever an individual receives antibodies from an external source for protection against specific antigens. Passive immunity is temporary, since these acquired antibodies break down and are not replaced by the body. Another example of passive immunity results from the administration of gamma globulin after exposure to rubella.

Active Immunity

Active immunity can be acquired by specific exposure to an antigen. Exposure may be accomplished either by the individual's actual infection by the microorganism or by the administration of small amounts of the organism to which the body responds by forming its own antibodies. Active immunity is long-term, or permanent, since the body is then "programmed" to replace these antibodies as necessary.

Several types of antibody-stimulating substances are used to actively immunize the individual. They include full-strength, live microorganisms (e.g., smallpox vaccination); attenuated, or dilute, microorganisms (e.g., Sabin polio vaccination); inactivated microorganisms (e.g., Salk polio vaccine); or purified forms of toxins produced by microorganisms (e.g., tetanus toxoid).

Reticuloendothelial System

The reticuloendothelial system also plays an important part in the immune response of the individual. This system, which includes the Kupffer cells of the liver, some cells of the spleen and bone marrow, reticular cells of the lymph nodes, and the histiocytes, acts to engulf and destroy microorganisms through phagocytosis and also produces antibodies. Thus the immune system is integrated to counteract the effects of the invading microorganisms and to promote healing.

Nursing assessment of the immune response includes descriptions of:

- precipitating conditions
- immunization record (where appropriate)
- previous allergic history
- history of diseases which produce immunity
- signs and symptoms of allergic response
- white blood cell count
- interferences with reticuloendothelial system

THE HEALING PROCESS

When a wound occurs, resulting cellular debris and blood from traumatized vessels begin to fill the space that has been created by the injury. As the blood coagulates, the fibrinogen that is released interconnects to bring the wound edges together. This wound covering is very fragile and easily disrupted.

Within a few hours this network dehydrates to form a harder surface, the scab, which provides protection for the wound. Soon after, leukocytes migrate to the area and, through the process of phagocytosis, surround and partially digest bacteria and cellular debris.

Within 3–5 days, fibroblasts from the dermis intertwine throughout the fibrin network. These fibroblasts secrete collagen and other proteins which constitute scar tissue. In addition, collateral circulation develops to bring an additional blood supply to provide the needed nutrition and to remove waste products. The resulting blood vessels and the collagen form granulation tissue, which is bright pink and easily damaged. Simultaneously, epithelial tissue grows on top of the wound. The collagen is knitted together to form fibrils, which, in turn, join with other proteins to form scar tissue. As the scar (cicatrix) tissue becomes denser, it loses its red color due to a decrease in blood supply. Scar tissue is less elastic than the original skin but binds the sides of the wounded area strongly.

Healing can occur through primary, secondary, or tertiary intention depending on the size of the wound, the presence or absence of bacteria in the wound, and the nutrition and blood supply to the area. (Figs. 15.1 and 15.2)

Primary Intention

Primary intention occurs when there is little gap between the edges of the wound, no infection is present, and a good local blood supply exists. A minimal amount of granulation tissue forms, and the resultant scar is small. Surgical incisions usually heal this way, as the wound edges are maintained in close approximation by sutures, clamps, staples or tape.

Secondary Intention

Wound healing by **secondary intention** occurs when the edges of the wound do not approximate, wound infection occurs, or the tissues surrounding the wound are not well supplied with blood. The granulation tissue formed—and thus the scar—is more extensive in order to fill the gap between the wound edges. Secondary intention healing occurs from the bottom of the wound upward.

Tertiary Intention

Tertiary intention healing takes place when primary or secondary healing has been interrupted, or when a wound has not been sutured initially but left open for drainage or treatment. Some granulation tissue does form; however, the healing process is not complete. These wounds do not heal by the expected processes and therefore must be closed before healing can occur.

Nursing assessment of tissue healing includes descriptions of:

- number of days since onset
- stage of healing
- degree of intention
- factors related to degree of intention
- interferences with healing

PHYSICAL AND PHYSIOLOGIC CHARACTERISTICS

Age, general health state, local tissue factors, health habits, and socioeconomic status play major roles in susceptibility of individuals to biologic invasion, as well as in their response to tissue damage after invasion.

Level of Growth and Development

The younger person is generally more resistant to infection and heals more rapidly than the older adult. As individuals age, changes in the elasticity of the skin, blood supply, pulmonary function, metabolism, and responses to stress alter their ability to resist biologic invasion and to heal as quickly as younger individuals. With age, the skin thins, the underlying, adipose and subcutaneous tissues decrease, and the connective tissue becomes inelastic. As a result the skin is more easily damaged, and any trauma is likely to be more extensive because of the decrease in underlying protective tissue. The skin of the infant and young child, however, is also more susceptible to infection and trauma because of an undeveloped, thin epidermis and minimal sebaceous secretions.

The aging process produces changes in the walls of the blood vessels, thus affecting the blood supply to body parts, especially the periphery. **Atherosclerosis** (fatty plaque buildup on vessel walls) and **arteriosclerosis** (loss of elasticity of vessel walls) are the main changes in blood vessels which can decrease the body's blood supply. In addition, decreased cardiac output and loss of muscle tone slow down the flow of blood throughout the body. Therefore when any wound occurs, the amount of blood which is readily available for localized defense and

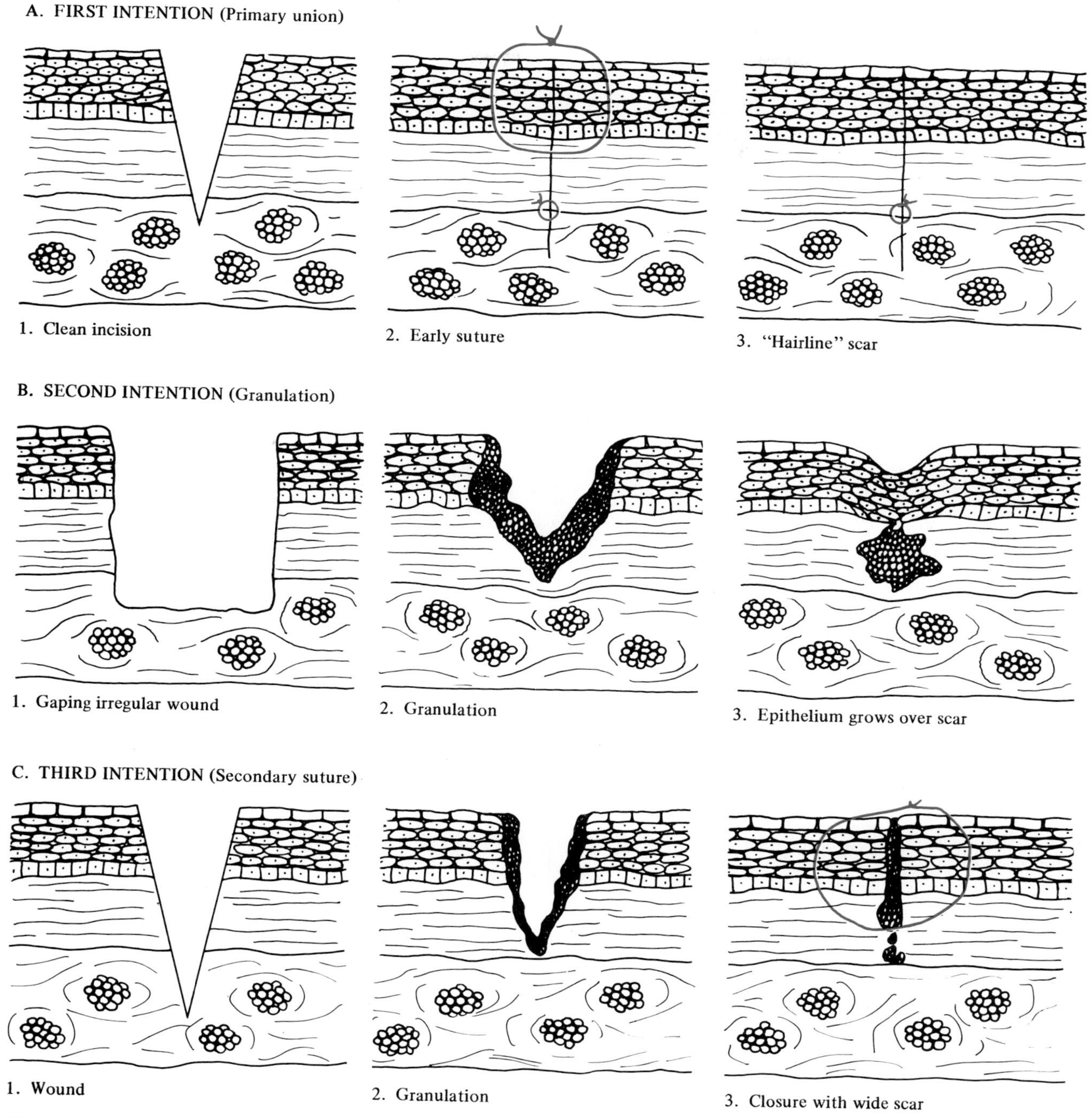

A. FIRST INTENTION (Primary union)

1. Clean incision
2. Early suture
3. "Hairline" scar

B. SECOND INTENTION (Granulation)

1. Gaping irregular wound
2. Granulation
3. Epithelium grows over scar

C. THIRD INTENTION (Secondary suture)

1. Wound
2. Granulation
3. Closure with wide scar

Figure 15.1
Types of wound healing.

tissue healing is decreased. Localized vasodilation, as a response to injury, may not occur as rapidly in the older person as in the younger person, causing a decrease in the effectiveness of the inflammatory response and a slower healing process.

Decreased lung expansion, tissue elasticity, and diffusion area as a result of the aging process reduce the amount of oxygen available for cell metabolism and maintenance. This, in turn, leads to a slower healing process since regenerating tissues require an adequate supply of oxygen for repair.

Starting around middle adulthood, metabolism

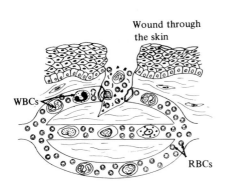

A wound through the skin results in bleeding

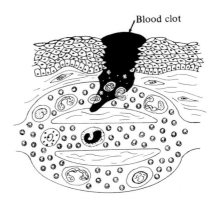

Inflammation of the capillary; formation of blood clot and growth of epithelial tissue

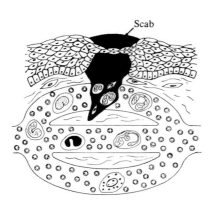

Production of new epithelial tissue and repair of capillary beneath scab

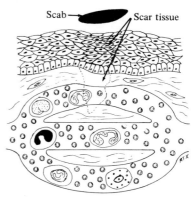

Sloughing off of scab; connection of blood capillaries; and formation of scar tissue

Figure 15.2

Stages of wound healing. *Reprinted with permission of Reston Publishing Company, Inc., a Prentice Hall Company, 11480 Sunset Hills Road, Reston, Va.*

decreases 5–10% every 10 years (Chart 19.2). There is also a decreased absorption of nutrients from the gastrointestinal tract as the individual ages. In addition, loss of teeth or poorly fitting dentures may change eating habits, thereby markedly influencing nutritional status. Individuals who are well nourished and in a positive nitrogen balance are less susceptible to disease and have a higher degree of reserve for tissue repair than those who are malnourished. The obese individual is particularly prone to poor healing, since adipose tissue has very few blood vessels running through it (**avascularity**) and therefore nutrients

and oxygen are not readily available. A good nutritional state provides for tissue growth and repair and supplies material for immunologic protection. In addition, adequate nutrition provides the needed fluids and electrolytes to maintain cell function and the raw materials for producing enzymes. Also, any change in metabolism or any dietary deficiency will alter the body's ability to heal rapidly and completely. Thus, any person of any age who has marginal nutrition or nutritional deficiencies will have a poor healing response. Proteins, vitamin C, and calcium as well as a positive nitrogen balance (Chap. 19) are particularly important for tissue repair. Since in the first few days of healing, protein catabolism outweighs protein anabolism, additional amounts of protein must be ingested to prevent a negative nitrogen balance and to promote healing.

The older person has a reduction in endocrine secretion, which may decrease the inflammatory and stress responses. This may make the older individual more prone to bacterial invasion and may therefore turn a seemingly minor wound into a complicated and dangerous threat.

Resistance to pathogens and healing in very young individuals may also be impeded by physical and physiologic immaturity in, for example, the renal, hematopoietic, and endocrine systems. In addition, their fluid and electrolyte and nutritional balances may be quickly compromised, thus affecting their ability to mobilize their defenses in order to respond to stressors and heal quickly.

Structural immaturity in infants and young children increases the susceptibility of these age groups to infection. Their short trachea and bronchi make them more prone to upper respiratory infections. The eustachian tube of the infant is shorter, wider, and straighter than that of adults, thus carrying microorganisms more readily from the upper respiratory tract to the middle ear, causing ear infections. Urinary tract infections in female children are very common because of their short urethrae. Irritation by bubble baths, masturbation, constipation, and improper bowel and bladder habits are factors which contribute to the occurrence of these infections.

Generally, therefore, younger but physiologically mature individuals have physiologic reserves and functional abilities which enable them, if no other interferences are present, to resist infection and heal more rapidly and completely. However, the individual's general health state, no matter what the age, is another consideration in assessing the individual's ability to withstand microbial attack and heal effectively.

Nursing assessment of an individual's level of growth and development related to resistance and healing includes descriptions of:

- the relationship of the level of growth and development to resistance and healing
- skin integrity
- blood supply
- respiratory function

- nutritional status
- endocrine function
- physical and physiologic maturity

General Health State

The presence of any disease process and the degree of accompanying debilitation influence the individual's ability to resist infection and heal. Contributing to an increased susceptibility to infection and a poor state of healing are such disease processes as metabolic disorders, which interfere with the ability of tissues to regenerate and thus alter the uptake and usage of cellular nutrients; anemias (changes in the oxygen-carrying potential of red blood cells); respiratory pathology and cardiovascular disorders, which decrease the amount of oxygen available to the cells for function and repair; renal dysfunction, which reduces the body's ability to remove waste products; endocrine malfunctions, which alter the inflammatory and stress responses of the body; and infections, either local or systemic.

Medications. Medications can either support or impede the healing process. Medications which promote metabolism (e.g., insulin) and the circulation of blood (e.g., digoxin) assist the body's defenses and the healing process. Antibiotics, both local and systemic, aid in destroying and controlling microorganisms, but they may also reduce the expected flora of the body. The expected flora of the body act to destroy other microorganisms (some potentially disease causing). Thus the destruction of the expected flora may give these invading organisms the opportunity to produce disease. Pharmacologic agents, such as steroids, depress the inflammatory response. While depression of the inflammatory response may be therapeutically desirable, as in cases where there is severe inflammation (e.g., arthritis), at other times these pharmacologic agents may reduce the ability of the body to respond to invading organisms. Other drugs, such as sedatives and tranquilizers, reduce metabolism and blood flow, alter the general health state, and impede the healing process.

Nursing assessment related to an individual's general health state, resistance to infection, and ability to heal includes descriptions of:

- presence of other infections
- presence of other diseases
- degree of debilitation

● medication
● relationship of medications to resistance and healing

Local Tissue Environment

The continuous nature of the skin and mucous membranes contributes to the body's defense system by providing a protective barrier against microorganisms. Secretions of the skin and mucous membranes are **bacteriostatic,** thus inhibiting the growth of microorganisms which are in constant contact with them (such as staphylococci). In addition the skin and underlying connective tissue act as a cushion against trauma. The brain is protected, in part, from invasion by microorganisms by the blood–brain barrier. The low permeability of the capillaries usually allows only movement of carbon dioxide, oxygen, and vital nutrients from the blood into the brain tissue.

The conjunctivae of the eyes are protected by the blink reflex and by the production of tears. Tears are **bactericidal** (destructive of microorganisms) and also help to wash out foreign bodies. The nose and mouth contain many potentially pathogenic microorganisms (e.g., streptococci and staphylococci), but the mucus and saliva of these organs help to prevent the pathogens' growth. The hairs in the nose act to filter out microorganisms. The respiratory tree is protected by cilia which help to move bacteria upward so they can be expelled. Here, too, the mucous secretions serve to limit bacterial growth. In addition, the reflexes of coughing and sneezing help to clear the airway of microorganisms.

The lymphatic system not only helps to produce antibodies and provides histiocytes for phagocytosis, but also helps to filter microorganisms from the lymph. The gastrointestinal tract has several types of secretions, such as digestive juices, hydrochloric acid, and digestive enzymes, which help to destroy microorganisms. In addition, the intestines contain a variety of microorganisms such as *Escherichia coli* and *Clostridium,* which, in part, help to prevent the overgrowth of other organisms. If these or other naturally occurring flora enter an area where they are not usually found, they will often produce disease.

The external genitalia also have natural flora such as *Mycobacterium* and *Trichomonas* and bacteriostatic secretions to protect the tissue from microbial invasion. The urinary tract is an enclosed system, helping to protect it from bacterial entry. The urine, which is usually sterile, continuously washes the ureters, bladder, and urethra to keep them free from microorganisms. Any interference with any of these natural protective barriers alters the body's ability to resist infection.

The local vascularity plays a great part in preventing the entry of microorganisms and in aiding the rapidity and degree with which healing occurs. Because an adequate blood supply is necessary to provide adequate amounts of oxygen and nutrients to the damaged area and to remove waste products, the greater the vascularity of an area, the less prone it is to infection and the more rapid and complete the healing process. Such areas as the head and neck region are highly vascular, while those in the lower extremities are less vascular. The obese individual will have slower healing because of the avascularity of adipose tissue.

A wound that is large and deep will take more time to heal than one that is small and superficial. The healing of a large wound requires a greater general bodily effort, while a deep wound involves several different layers of tissue which may have different healing rates. Deeper wounds are also more likely to have drainage tubes inserted in them, slowing the healing process and making the wounds more prone to infection. Extensive wounds are frequently second- and third-intention healers, which require more granulation and a larger scar tissue network.

The type of tissue that is injured determines, in part, the rate, type, and degree of healing. Skin and mucous membranes rapidly regenerate, while nerves, muscles, and connective tissues have a limited ability to regenerate and often heal by scar formation. Generally, the more highly specialized the cells, the less able they are to regenerate in a useful fashion.

Movement can both retard and enhance the healing process. General body movement increases the blood flow, thus aiding healing. However, displacement of the wound and the immediately surrounding tissues disrupts and slows the healing process.

Nursing assessment related to local tissue environment and an individual's resistance to infection and ability to heal includes descriptions of:

● presence of local defense systems (e.g., skin integrity, tears, mucus secretions)
● interferences with local defense systems
● local vascularity
● type of tissue injured

- depth and severity of wound
- degree of stress on wound caused by movement
- effects of stress on wounds caused by movement

Infection

Infection occurs when microorganisms invade the body and are not effectively counteracted by the body's defense system. These microorganisms multiply and produce cellular death. Infection can occur locally, as in a wound, or systemically. Localized infection is characterized by swelling, redness, warmth, tenderness, tissue death, wound drainage, and, possibly, by loss of function of that area. Systemic infection is manifested by fever, leukocytosis, malaise, and headache. Specific systemic infections will produce additional symptoms which are characteristic of that particular disease process. Localized infections can spread throughout the body by means of the vascular or lymphatic system or through extension of the infected area.

The presence of a wound infection retards healing. A wound may become infected because of its location, an inadequate inflammatory response, contamination at the time the wound occurred, poor wound dressing technique, local tissue factors, and/or debilitation. Wounds that are in or near the bowel or respiratory tree are more likely to become contaminated than other wounds, since the intestinal and respiratory tracts contain potentially disease-producing flora. These pathogens, when introduced into areas where they are not usually found, may produce infections. For example, if an individual coughs or sneezes over an open wound, a wound infection can result. Wounds that occur in a microorganism-free (**sterile**) area such as the bladder are also more likely to develop infections because the local defense system is incapable of handling the invasion of microorganisms.

If the individual's defense system is incapable of responding to invasion or becomes overwhelmed by the invasion, infection results. Individuals who are in a debilitated state prior to the onset of a wound are more likely to develop wound infection than those who are not debilitated, because their defense system may be so compromised that it cannot respond effectively.

Wounds that have occurred under nonsterile conditions are more likely to become infected than wounds produced in a sterile environment. Wounds that have accidentally occurred are most often more prone to infection that those that are surgically in-

duced. Local tissue condition and the depth and severity of the wound also contribute to infection, whether the wound is surgically or traumatically induced. Breaks in sterile procedure during surgery (Chap. 26) may also increase the likelihood of wound infections.

Conditions under which wounds are cared for also affect the individual's predisposition to infection. Wounds which are cared for using aseptic techniques are more likely to heal without infection than those which are not. Infected wounds, regardless of their mechanism of occurrence, will not heal until dead tissue is removed and the infection resolved.

Nursing assessment related to infection includes descriptions of:

- presence of infection
- local signs and symptoms of infection
- systemic signs and symptoms of infection
- factors which predispose to infection
- effects of infection on healing
- effectiveness of body defenses on severity of infection
- degree of debilitation from infection
- therapeutic measures used to prevent and treat infection
- effectiveness of therapeutic measures
- subjective reactions to infection

Health Habits

The individual's health habits and attitudes about health influence susceptibility to infection and physiologic reserve in combating infection when it occurs. Personal daily habits of bathing, teethbrushing, handwashing, hair and nail care, and cleaning procedures after urination and defecation are factors which affect the number and types of microorganisms present on the body at any given time. Inadequate personal hygiene increases the number of microorganisms on the body surfaces. When an injury occurs, or when any condition causes an increased susceptibility to microbial invasion, these microorganisms are readily available to infect the individual. In addition, poor hygiene habits increase the possibility that these microorganisms will be transmitted to others in such ways as food handling or child care.

People's knowledge, attitudes, and practices in relation to the prevention and spread of infection are major assessment areas for the nurse who is to help promote and maintain well-being. The individual's level of knowledge concerning how infection occurs and what measures help to reduce it can either increase or decrease the potential for infection. Persons of different educational, cultural, socioeconomic, and experiential backgrounds and levels of growth and development vary in their nutritional patterns, food-handling practices, household cleaning habits, and attainment of preventive health care. These habits and practices are determined not only by the individual's level of knowledge, but also by the resources that are available for carrying out activities that promote wellness. An individual may know the need for nutritionally well-balanced meals in preventing infection but may not have the money to purchase the foods or the facilities to store them properly.

Health practices which include immunization and screening for potential infections such as venereal disease and tuberculosis are important both in protecting the individual and in promoting community health. Health habits such as covering the mouth when coughing or sneezing, proper handling and disposal of used tissues, not spitting, handwashing, and cleaning clothes after they have been in contact with secretions and excreta are other important assessment factors. The extent of alcohol intake and cigarette smoking are also important assessment factors, since these habits increase the individual's susceptibility to infection.

Nursing assessment or an individual's health habits and susceptibility to spread of infection includes descriptions of:

- personal daily habits
  - frequency
  - how carried out
- knowledge about prevention and spread of infection
- attitudes toward infection and its spread
- relationship of educational background to health habits
- relationship of culture to health habits
- relationship of socioeconomic status to health habits
- relationship of previous experiences to health habits
- relationship of level of growth and development to health habits
- relationship of habits to susceptibility and spread of infection
- resources available for practicing positive health habits

- immunization history
- knowledge and use of infection screening resources
- respiratory hygiene habits
- relationship of alcohol ingestion and/or smoking to susceptibility to infection
- relationship of individual's personal habits to community health

Environment Assessment

Assessment of the internal and external environments of the individual completes the triad of agent—host—environment interaction for biologic safety. As discussed in previous sections, the individual's internal environment plays a major role in increasing either that person's susceptibility to infection and its spread or his or her resistance to these processes. Two aspects of the external environment need to be considered: those which influence the host's attempts to resist and limit infection, and those which affect the growth and spread of microbial agents.

THE HOST'S ENVIRONMENT

The individual's immediate personal environment directly influences the type and number of microorganisms the individual comes in contact with on a daily basis. The work and living areas of the individual can increase or decrease the likelihood of infection through their degree of cleanliness or contamination, state of crowding, sanitary facilities, food storage facilities, pollution levels, ventilation, humidity, and presence of infected persons. The community, state, national, and international environments of which the individual is a part also affect the individual's state of health. Public health laws covering such areas as sanitation, reporting of infectious disease, immunization, and public food handling protect the individual. Sewage control, water purification, mass immunization, and screening and educational programs are other community resources which help to decrease the chance of infection and its spread.

THE MICROORGANISMS' ENVIRONMENT

The immediate environment surrounding microorganisms can either support or deter their growth.

Generally, moist, warm, dark, dirty areas promote microbial growth, while dry, cool, well-ventilated, light (especially sunlit), frequently cleaned areas decrease the number of microbes present, as well as present an unsuitable environment for their growth. The geographic location and climate of an area also influence the presence and growth of microorganisms. Warm, wet climates enhance the growth of microorganisms more than cool, dry climates. The soil content, types of vegetation, and source of water supply influence the number of suitable reservoirs for agent growth.

The general economics of an area influences the quality and quantity of resources available to combat microorganisms and influences the type and number of agent reservoirs in that area. The degree of industrialization in an area will affect the number of pollutants and the number of people living within a given space.

Nursing assessment related to environment includes descriptions of:

- characteristics of internal environment which influence microbial growth and/or host resistance
- characteristics of immediate environment which influence host resistance and/or agent growth
- characteristics of community, national, and international environments which influence host resistance and/or agent growth

Physical Assessment

Each body subsystem, in one way or another, contributes to the protection of the individual against invasion and spread of microorganisms in an attempt to maintain biologic safety. Thus it is necessary to assess each subsystem as it relates to the promotion and maintenance of biologic safety. Physical assessment of the body subsystems is found in the related chapters. However, the skin and lymph nodes, which are major parts of the body's defense system, are discussed here.

SKIN

The skin provides an external barrier to microorganisms as well as helping to protect the internal environment from trauma and chemical damage. The skin is continuous with the mucous membranes of the nasal, oral, respiratory, gastrointestinal, and urogenital tracts. These mucous membranes are coated with mucous secretions which further reduce the chance of microorganisms entering the body, while inhibiting the growth of bacteria. When breaks in the skin occur through either thermal, chemical, mechanical, or physical means, microorganisms enter the body. Such breaks must be compensated for by the body's internal defense mechanisms.

Observation and Palpation

The integrity of the skin is assessed and compared bilaterally for turgor, texture, temperature, color, and disruption.

Turgor. The degree of elasticity and tone of the skin is called **turgor.** It reflects the degree of hydration, the condition of the underlying connective tissue, and the distribution of adipose tissue in the individual. Well-hydrated skin is firm, resilient, and cushiony. The nurse can assess turgor by pinching the individual's skin together, releasing it and observing the amount of time it takes for the skin to return to its original state. Usually the skin will bounce back immediately after release. However, if tissue turgor is poor, it remains in a pinched position, "tented," for several seconds after release. Elderly persons commonly have reduced tissue turgor because of redistribution of adipose tissue and a loss of underlying connective tissue. Skin with poor turgor is more subject to trauma and heals less rapidly.

Texture. The texture of an individual's skin consists of the degree of smoothness, the amount of lubrication, and the presence of furrows. The expected texture of the skin is smooth, lubricated, and slightly furrowed. The nurse assesses for texture by lightly running the backs of her fingers over the individual's skin surface. All parts of the body, not only those that are ordinarily exposed, are assessed. This is necessary since both environmental conditions and internal conditions may create differences in different parts of the body's surface. Dry, cracked, or chapped skin reduces the protective covering, making the body more prone to the invasion of microorganisms, as well as creating discomfort for the individual. Dry skin may be **pruritic** (itchy), thus causing the individual to scratch, which produces trauma. Overlubricated skin can result in clogged pores, which entrap bacteria and can cause localized infection.

Temperature. The temperature of the skin is assessed for signs of localized inflammation or infection. The skin is usually warm to the touch and any areas of increased warmth are further assessed for accompanying signs of inflammation or infection. The backs of the fingers are used in temperature assessment.

Color. Skin color is assessed for pigmentation, redness, cyanosis (Chap. 17 and 18), discoloration, and vascularity. Since each individual has a unique skin hue, there will be wide presenting variations ranging from pale, fair skin to dark skin; only changes from the individual's usual skin hue are significant. Difficulty arises when the nurse has no knowledge of the individual's normal skin hue. Thus it is necessary for the nurse to correlate the presenting skin color with other signs of inadequate gaseous exchange.

Discolorations from bruises result in ecchymotic areas which may be deep blue or purple immediately after injury, and yellow, green, and brown as blood absorption takes place. In dark-skinned individuals, these changes may not be as evident and may appear as darker areas. Accurate assessment may require asking the individual about recent traumas or bruises.

▶ **Vascularity** refers to the observable distribution of capillaries on body surfaces. Figure 15.3 shows and briefly describes common type s of vascular lesions.

Disruptions. The skin is observed for breaks in its surface. Wounds, eruptions, blisters, cracks, and ulcerations are examples of disruptions in skin integrity. Chart 15.1 describes some of these common skin disruptions.

Any skin disruption is described in terms of size, color, odor, location, configuration (shape), degree of elevation, amount and type of drainage, tenderness, temperature, duration, known precipitating causes, stage of healing, and the individual's subjective reactions to it. The size of the lesion is measured in centimeters and should not be approximated.

Drainage. Wound drainages fall into four
▶ general categories. **Serous drainage** is clear and straw-colored and consists of serum without fibrin-
▶ ogen. **Sanguineous drainage** is bloody and may be dark or bright red, depending on whether it is fresh or arterial (bright red) or old or venous (darker red).
▶ **Serosanguineous drainage** is a mixture of blood and serum and may be pink or flecked with blood, depending upon the proportions of blood and serum.
▶ **Purulent drainage** is the pus-containing debris from dead tissues and cells and indicates infection rather
▶ than the tissue trauma of other **exudates** (drainages).

LYMPH NODES

Observation and Palpation

Lymph nodes are found throughout the body, and are not usually observable or palpable. However, superficial lymph nodes may become enlarged when there are infecious processes or neoplasms present. Figure 15.4 shows the location of the superficial lymph nodes.

Superficial nodes are observed for enlargement and palpated for size, consistency, tenderness, and mobility (Chart 7.4). Palpation of lymph nodes is carried out in a cephalocaudal fashion. The nurse uses the pads of the first two or three fingers to lightly palpate each chain of nodes in a circular motion. For pal-

Figure 15.3

Examples of vascular lesions.

VASCULAR LESIONS

Cherry Angioma	Spider Angioma	Venous Star

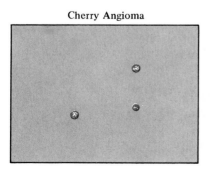
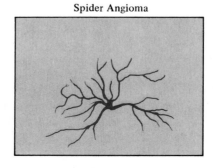
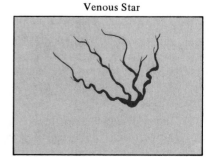

Chart 15.1
Common Skin Disruptions

TYPE	DESCRIPTION	EXAMPLE
Wound	A trauma-induced discontinuity in the skin or soft tissues of the body	
Abrasion	Superficial skin or mucous membranes rubbed away through friction with another surface	Chafing, scraped knee
Contusion	Damage to the soft tissues underlying the skin without a break in the skin surface; often characterized by the rupture of capillaries, leading to skin discoloration, swelling, and pain	Ecchymosis, hematoma, bruise
Incision	A smooth separation of skin and tissue surfaces made by a sharp instrument	
Clean	An incision made under aseptic or sterile conditions	Any surgical cut made under sterile conditions
Contaminated	A surgically induced incision: 1. made on an area which has not been surgically prepared 2. made with a break in sterile technique 3. made on a body part which cannot be surgically cleaned 4. made where there has been exposure to microorganisms after surgery	1. Emergency tracheostomy 2. Incision made with a contaminated scalpel 3. Bowel surgery 4. Postoperative wound infection
Laceration	Jagged-edged wound produced by trauma	Any cut made by a rough or blunt surface
Penetrating	Wound that passes through superficial body surfaces to enter deep body tissues, organs, or cavities	Any wound into deeper body structures
Puncture	Penetrating wound made by a sharp, narrow instrument	Stab wound
Septic	Any wound which is infected	
Lesion	A defined area of tissue alteration	
Primary lesions	Lesions that directly result from a pathologic process	Chicken pox, measles, blisters
Cyst	A firm, fixed fluid or semisolid sac below the surface of the skin	Sebaceous cyst

(continued)

Chart 15.1 (Cont.)
Common Skin Disruptions

TYPE	DESCRIPTION	EXAMPLE
Erythema	Skin redness as a result of vasodilation	Any kind of a blow, rash
Macule	A flat spot of skin color change	Nevi, roseola
Nodule	A solid elevation of the skin which extends into the dermis or subcutaneous tissue; larger than 0.5 cm in diameter	Swollen glands
Papule	A spot on the skin which can be felt; less than 0.5 cm in diameter	Measles, eczema
Plaque	A raised, flat series or cluster of nodules or papules	
Pustule	A small elevation filled with pus, or lymph	Acne, chicken pox
Vesicle	A small (up to 0.5 cm in diameter) sac within the layers of the skin filled with fluid; if larger than 0.5 cm in diameter, called a bulla	Chicken pox, poison ivy Blister, second-degree burn
Wheal	Elevations of the skin caused by edema in the dermis; can be red and warm to touch; may be characterized by itching	Hives, mosquito bites
Secondary lesions	Lesions resulting from changes in primary lesions	
Atrophy	Thinning of epidermis or dermis with resultant shining and translucency of skin	Arterial insuffiiency
Crust	Dried drainage from a wound or lesion	Seborrhea, impetigo
Erosion	Moist area of superficial tissue loss	Cervical erosion
Excoriation	Abrasion of a primary lesion with removal of the epidermis	Scratches of an itchy (pruritic) lesion
Fissure	Linear crack or break in the skin surface	Athelete's foot; anal fissure
Scales	A thin, dry flake shed from the epidermis	Dandruff, psoriasis, dry skin
Scar	Replacement of skin tissue by fibrous or connective tissue	
Keloid	Excessive or hypertrophied scar production	
Ulcer	Open lesion with loss of epidermis and upper dermis	Decubitus ulcer, stasis ulcer

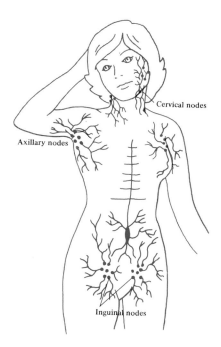

Figure 15.4
Location of superficial lymph nodes.

relationship of turgor to connective and adipose tissue
texture (exposed surfaces, nonexposed surfaces)
lubrication
temperature
color (exposed surfaces, nonexposed surfaces)
disruptions
   location
   size
   color
      redness
      cyanosis
      discolorations
      vascularity
   configuration
   degree of elevation
   drainage (amount, type)
   tenderness
   temperature
   duration
   stage of healing
   precipitating causes
   individual's subjective reactions
- Lymph nodes
   location of enlargement
   characteristics of nodes
      size
      shape
      consistency
      mobility
      tenderness
      symmetry
      color
      temperature
   factors which may contribute to changes in lymph node.

pation of the nodes in the head and neck region, the individual is placed in a sitting position. The nurse may use either the anterior or posterior approach. In the anterior approach, the nurse is in front of the individual and uses one hand to palpate while positioning the individual's head with the other hand. The individual's head is turned in the direction of the palpation to relax muscles. In the posterior approach, the nurse is behind the individual and uses both hands to feel the lymph nodes on each side.

The individual remains seated for examination of the axillary lymph nodes. The nurse palpates these nodes with the individual's upper arm at right angles to the body (abduction) and again with the upper arms parallel to the body (adduction). Examination of the breast is described in Chapter 17.

To examine the inguinal nodes, the nurse places the individual in a back-lying position, drapes the genitalia, and stands at the side being palpated. Using both hands, the nurse palpates for both the inferior and superior inguinal nodes.

Nursing assessment related to physical assessment includes descriptions of:

- Skin integrity
   relationship of turgor to nutritional state

Diagnostic Tests

Many tests used to diagnose inflammation and infection are specific to particular body subsystems and are discussed in the appropriate chapters. These include hematocrit, hemoglobin, reticulocyte count, chest x-ray, and urinalysis.

CULTURE AND SENSITIVITY

Wound drainage, sputum, mucous secretions, blood, urine, feces, and cerebrospinal fluid are fre-

▶ quently collected for **culture** and **sensitivity** (c/s). The specimens are placed in appropriate sterile containers and transported to the laboratory immediately. Caution is taken not to contaminate the specimens to avoid false readings, as well as to prevent contamination of the environment by the specimens. The specimens are placed on appropriate media and allowed to incubate (culture) for varying lengths of time, depending on the suspected organism. The resulting growths are microscopically identified as to type and number. At this time the organisms are placed on chemically heated disks. These disks may be treated with antibiotic, disinfectant, and other bacteriostatic and bacteriocidal agents. The disks are observed for the amount of growth which takes place. The organism is considered sensitive to any agent which limits or destroys it growth.

SPECIMEN COLLECTION

Wound, nose, throat, vaginal, cervical, and stool cultures are collected by placing a sterile cotton swab into the area from which a specimen is desired. Frequently these swabs are immediately placed in a transport medium, such as broth. However, each agency may have a different protocol for collecting these specimens so the nurse should be familiar with the procedure prior to collecting the specimen. This will avoid the necessity of repeating the collection process and slowing down the entire diagnostic procedure. Each specimen collected is carefully marked as to type of specimen and medications—especially antibiotics—the individual is receiving, along with other pertinent identifying data.

Blood cultures may be obtained in several ways, depending on specific agency protocol. However, use of a skin disinfectant and good skin cleansing prior to venipuncture are necessary to prevent contamination of the specimen. Sterile procedure is used in drawing the blood. If the blood has to be transferred from the syringe to the culture tube, the needle is changed before injecting the blood into the tube. Blood for culture is always immediately placed in a transport medium. This medium, like all others used for specimens, should be specific for the culture and should not be substituted with another. Cerebrospinal fluid is collected through a lumbar puncture (Chap. 13) using strict sterile technique. Chart 15.2 outlines the expected bacteriologic findings from these cultures.

Chart 15.2
Expected Bacteriologic Findings for Various Cultures

SPECIMEN	VALUE
Urine	Below 10,000 colonies
Blood	None
CSF	None
Wound	All wounds are contaminated. Significance of finding depends on type and amount.
Sputum	Same as wounds
Nose and throat	Same as wounds
Stool	All stool is contaminated. Significance of findings is dependent on types not usually found.
Vaginal	Same as wounds. Of significance are the venereal, yeast, and fungal organisms.

WHITE BLOOD CELL COUNT

Diagnostic studies of the white blood cells (WBCs) can be significant in determining the presence of an infection. During both inflammation and infection there is an increase in the total WBC count, as well as in counts of specific types of white blood cells such as leukocytes, monocytes, and neutrophils. No special pre- or posttest care is necessary. The expected range for a total WBC count is 4,000–11,000 cu mm. Chart 15.3 gives the expected values for WBC differential count.

TUBERCULIN TESTING

Intradermal skin testing is commonly done to indicate tuberculosis. Two types of tuberculin testing

Chart 15.3
WBC Differential Count

WHITE BLOOD CELLS	EXPECTED VALUE (%)
Neutrophils	54–62
Eosinophils	1–3
Basophils	0–1
Lymphocytes	25–33
Monocytes	0–9

From: Solomon Garb. *Laboratory Tests in Common Use,* 5th ed. New York, Springer, 1971, p. 49.

are the multiple puncture procedure (e.g., Tine test) and the Mantoux test.

Multiple Puncture

In the multiple puncture procedure the skin is punctured with prongs that have been coated with protein derived from the tubercle bacillus. The test is considered positive if an inflamed area larger than 2 mm is present 48–72 hours after puncture.

Mantoux Test

The second and preferred test is the Mantoux test. A small amount of protein derived from the tubercle bacillus is injected intradermally (usually into the underside of the forearm). This test initially produces a small inflamed area. However, if it is larger than 5 mm after 48–72 hours the test is considered positive.

Preparation of Individual

No pre- or posttest preparation is necessary but individuals receiving the multiple puncture test should be informed not to wash or scratch the test area. Positive test results indicate exposure to tuberculosis but do not necessarily mean the individual actually has the disease.

NURSING DIAGNOSIS

An 8-year-old girl, Kay, is brought by her father to the neighborhood health station. Kay's father states that his daughter has been running a fever and complains of a "stinging sensation when passing water."

Following on pages 326–327 is a nursing assessment of the actual (presenting) behaviors of 8-year-old Kay that reflect her ability to mobilize and maintain the defenses that promote her biologic safety, along with those behaviors that the nurse would expect to find in a person of a similar level of growth and development who has no interference in biologic safety. A physical assessment, diagnostic test results, and a medical diagnosis are included.

Nursing diagnoses based on the above assessment might include:

- Actual
  dyspuria (difficult urination) related to infectious process
  elevated temperature related to infectious process
  hazardous hygiene habits related to lack of knowledge and understanding
- Possible
  possibility of recurring urinary tract infections related to hazardous hygiene habits

PLANNING

Planning for biologic safety focuses on nursing actions which help to decrease the growth and spread of microorganisms while increasing the resistance of the individual. Interventions may be aimed at the agent, the environment, the individual, or a combination of all components of this dynamic interaction. Once the agent has infected the host, planning centers around prevention of further infection, debilitation, and spread. Planning for health teaching is an important component to assist individuals in changing personal habits that make them more susceptible to invasion and spread of microorganisms. Since the individual does not live in isolation but is part of a community,

ASSESSMENT FACTOR	EXPECTED BEHAVIOR	ACTUAL BEHAVIOR
Signs of Inflammation		
Temperature	98.6 F	100 F (oral)
Pain or tenderness	—	"Stinging" sensation when urinating. No back pain or frequency.
Duration of symptoms	—	One week
Previous history of illness		See record of previous illness and immunization. No recent history of illness.
Age	—	8 years, 3 months
General health state		No recent history of illness. No developmental or functional problems noted during last clinic visit 2 months earlier for complete school physical.
Health habits		
Hygiene		Uses bubble bath daily; frequently wipes perineum from back to front after urination or defecation. No history of constipation. Father states child doesn't wash hands unless reminded.
Nutrition		
Height	50 in.	47 in.
Weight	58 lb	50 lb
		Father states she eats three good meals a day and isn't much of a "snacker."
Level of knowledge	—	Father unaware of irritating effects of bubble baths.
	Wiping perineum from front to back after urination and defecation	Child states, "Mommy and Daddy keep telling me about wiping myself but I forget."
Environment	—	Shares room with 10-year-old sister. Four family members use same bathroom.
Physical assessment		Negative for all systems
Diagnostic tests		
Urinalysis		
Color	Yellow-amber	Yellow
Specific gravity	1.0003–1.030	1.025
pH	4.5–8.0	9
Clarity	Clear, transparent	Cloudy
Casts	None	—
Bacteria	None except by contamination	Many
WBCs	None	Many
Sugar/a	None	Same as expected
Acetone	None	Same as expected
Protein	None	Same as expected
		Clean-catch urine taken for c/s

(continued)

ASSESSMENT FACTOR	EXPECTED BEHAVIOR	ACTUAL BEHAVIOR
WBC	4,000–11,000/cu mm Average for 8-year-old 8,000 cu/mm	12,000 cu/mm Urinary tract infection Ampicillin 500 mg, p.o. Q6H × 2 weeks Repeat urine culture in 2 and 18 days Bed rest until fever subsides
Medical Diagnosis	—	
Physician's Orders		

the plan must also include the broader aspects of community or public health. In planning the individual's care, the nurse must consider himself or herself a possible source of contamination and thus must continuously plan interventions that will help break the chain of the agent–host–environment interaction.

The care plan for one of the nursing diagnoses listed above in the situation of 8-year-old Kay might look as follows:

INTERVENTION

Limitation of Reservoirs

Many actions which are aimed at reducing the strength and infectivity of the agent are carried out through modifying the environment. By creating and maintaining environments which do not support microbial growth, the nurse decreases the probability of microorganisms coming in contact with the individual.

NURSING DIAGNOSIS	GOAL	PLAN
Hazardous hygiene habits related to lack of understanding and knowledge	*Short term* Bubble baths within 1 day 1. No bubble baths within 1 day	1. a. Explain irritating effects of bubble bath on urethra and bladder to father and child. b. Explain relationship between symptoms and bubble baths through use of color diagrams and anatomic doll. c. Explore alternate ways of making bath time fun (e.g., soap crayons, squirt guns, bath toys).
	2. Wipes perineum from front to back after urinating or defecating, within 1 day.	2. a. Explain to child relationship between symptoms and wiping perineum by use of color diagrams and anatomic doll. b. Demonstrate proper wiping techniques. c. Allow child time for return demonstration on doll.

(continued)

NURSING DIAGNOSIS	GOAL	PLAN
		d. Discuss with father need for reinforcement of positive hygiene behavior in a nonpunitive manner.
	3. Washes hands after urinating or defecating within 1 day.	3. a. Explain relationship between handwashing and symptoms and general health.
		b. Demonstrate handwashing technique.
		c. Allow time for return demonstration.
	4. Increases understanding of factors contributing to urinary tract infection, as evidenced by follow-through on goals 1–3.	
	Long term 1. Stops using bubble bath.	*Long term* 1. As above
	2. Continues to wipe perineum from front to back.	2. Return demonstration of perineal wiping and handwashing at next clinic visit.
	3. Continues to wash hands after urinating or defecating.	3. Supplement knowledge where needed.

STERILE AND CLEAN

Such measures as sterilization, disinfection, maintenance of clean- and dirty-equipment areas, and general maintenance of a clean health care environment are important in decreasing microbial reservoirs. **Sterilization** is the removal of all microorganisms, including their spores. It can be accomplished through chemicals, heat, heat and steam, steam under pressure, irradiation, and gas. The type of organism to be destroyed and the characteristics of the object to be sterilized will determine the specific technique used. For example, rubber tubing cannot be submitted to high temperatures without deterioration; therefore, it is necessary to use gas sterilization. The use of disposable equipment has brought great changes in sterilization practices, since equipment is sterilized by the manufacturer and disposed of after a single use.

Disinfection is the process of killing microorganisms but not their spores. Most commonly disinfection is done through chemical means, but moist heat, radiation, and filtration can be used. Disinfectants are used on such objects as examining tables, counters, and thermometers. Since skin cannot be sterilized, disinfection is used to clean the skin, particularly prior to any surgical or sterile procedure.

Antisepsis is used to retard the growth of organisms rather than to kill them.

Areas where sterile or clean supplies are stored or utilized are separated from areas where contaminated supplies are kept. For example, places where specimens are tested, bedpans stored and emptied, and dirty linen collected should not be the same as those where sterile supplies are kept. In health care agencies two different rooms are usually maintained on each unit to separate these kinds of activities. In general an environment that is kept dry, dust-free, and clean from dirt, drainage, and other contaminants decreases the number of reservoirs for microbial growth. While in health care agencies the housekeeping department is responsible for maintaining the overall clean environment, the nurse is responsible for the proper disposal of equipment and supplies and for the maintenance of a clean immediate work environment. In addition, the nurse reports any special cleaning needs and gaps in cleaning procedures to the housekeeping department.

Principles of sterilization, disinfection, and cleanliness can be applied in the home environment. The nurse teaches individuals to identify possible reservoirs within the home, in bathroom, garbage cans, and improperly stored food and suggests methods to eliminate them through sterilization, disinfection, and antisepsis. As in the hospital situation the best way to prevent the formation of reservoirs is frequent cleaning with soap and water and exposure of surfaces to sunlight.

Reduction of Microbial Transmission

Since microorganisms can be transmitted in a variety of ways, methods which are specific to reducing or eliminating each mode of transmission are utilized.

HANDWASHING

Handwashing is the single most important deterrent to the spread of microorganisms through direct transmission. Handwashing helps to remove any transient bacteria that the individual may have come in contact with while handling contaminated surfaces, food, clothing, or other objects. The nurse needs to use handwashing before and after every direct contact with individuals in the direct care situation, after handling possibly contaminated equipment, and after urinating or defecating. Chart 15.4 outlines the procedure for handwashing. The individual and family and/or significant others are taught handwashing technique to help prevent the spread of microorganisms within the home.

BARRIER TECHNIQUES

When the individual has an infectious process which may be transmitted by contact or inhalation, certain precautions may be necessary to prevent its spread to other people. **Isolation** (barrier technique) is the term used to describe the process of protection used to prevent contamination by microorganisms. Chart 15.5 outlines the types of precautions neces-

sary for various microorganisms and pathologic states.

Strict Isolation

The use of protective precautions to prevent the spread of highly communicable microorganisms through contact or the airborne route is strict isolation. All equipment or other objects must be disinfected or destroyed at the end of the isolation term. Used linen is placed into two linen bags (double-bagged) and tagged. This allows for appropriate cleaning and disposal of contaminated items. The used linen is placed into one bag inside the isolation unit and then, using aseptic technique, placed into another bag outside the unit. The same procedure is used for soiled dressings and tissues.

Respiratory Isolation

To prevent the spread of airborne microorganisms, respiratory isolation is used. People entering the isolation unit wear masks and frequently wash their hands. Respiratory secretions are handled with gloves and are double-bagged.

Enteric Precautions

The use of enteric precautions avoids contamination with feces or feces-soiled articles containing pathogenic organisms. All persons giving direct care or handling feces-soiled articles wear gloves. Excreta are immediately disposed of into the sewer system. At the termination of isolation, dishes, bedpans, urinals, and related articles are bagged and tagged as contaminated.

Wound and Skin Precautions

Similar to strict isolation are wound and skin precautions, but gowns, gloves, and masks are worn only when direct contact is made. These precautions are used in cases of infected and/or profusely draining wounds. All objects soiled with the secretions are either disinfected or double-bagged.

Excretion and Secretion Precautions

With excretion and secretion precautions the potential for comtamination is decreased, and thus only articles directly contaminated need to be double-bagged or disinfected.

Blood Precautions

When microorganisms are actively borne in the blood, blood precautions are used. Therefore, any contact is avoided with the blood or objects such as needles which have been contaminated by blood. Contaminated objects are double-bagged, destroyed, or

Chart 15.4
Handwashing

TECHNIQUE	POINTS TO NOTE
Collect equipment: soap or antiseptic cleanser, towels.	Soap lowers surface tension to facilitate cleaning; antiseptic solutions act as bacteriostatics.
Remove jewelry.	Allows for cleaning of total skin surface.
Thoroughly wet hands and wrists with comfortably warm water.	Increases lathering potential; warm water is less drying to skin than hot or cold water.
Lather hands with soap or antiseptic.	Lather helps free bacteria and other organisms on skin surface.
Work up lather by rubbing hands in a circular motion; work lather between fingers; clean palms and backs of hands thoroughly.	First handwashing before giving care should last approximately 2 min. to remove bacteria and other organisms which have collected; succeeding washings last 30–60 sec, depending on degree of contamination. All skin surfaces are washed equally to prevent collection of bacteria and other organisms.
Clean nails by rubbing nails of one hand in the palm of the other hand to work lather under them (this is a "scratching" type of motion).	Nails are also be cleaned frequently with orange stick to prevent buildup of bacteria, other organisms, and dirt. Scratching motion forces lather under nails.
Rinse hands and wrists under running water, moving from fingertips to wrist.	Moving from clean to dirty area prevents backflow of contaminated water. Thorough rinsing removes dirt, bacteria, and other organisms.
Thoroughly dry hands with clean towel.	Thorough drying prevents chapping.
Use fresh towel to turn off faucet.	Prevents contaimination of hands by contact with "dirty" faucets. Use of clean towel prevents movement of organisms by capillary action.
Apply lotion as necessary.	Prevents chapping and drying of skin.

disinfected. If a used needle sticks the nurse, the nurse reports it to health services so that appropriate preventive measures (e.g., gamma globulin injections) can be taken.

Protective Isolation

The technique that protects the susceptible individual from being contaminated by persons or objects in his environment is called protective isolation (reverse isolation). This method is used with persons who, as a result of pathology or treatment, have a decreased resistance to infection. All objects are disinfected or sterilized before they are placed in the unit, and all persons entering the unit wear sterile gowns, gloves, and masks to prevent their spreading organisms to the ill individual. Chart 15.6 describes the procedure for masking, gowning, and gloving. (Illustrations 15.1, 15.2, and 15.3)

NURSING IMPLICATIONS

Sensory Deprivation

Individuals placed on isolation precautions of any type are prone to sensory deprivation (Chap. 13). The number of visitors is often limited either because of restrictions on numbers or others' reluctance to come in contact with the individual. Staff contact may be decreased because of the time involved in gowning and gloving and the possible negative attitudes of the staff. While limiting the number of people exposed to the individual or to whom the individual is exposed may be therapeutically desirable or necessary, the individual may still experience a sense of removal from meaningful interactions and social contacts. Isolated individuals may come to feel as if they were "dirty" or "contaminated." In addition, an individual may be limited in physical movement or restricted within a confined physical area which will result in confinement deprivation. The use of gowns, gloves, and masks limits direct physical contact and thus further deprives the individual of stimulation. Since many personal articles cannot be sterilized or disinfected, the individual is often denied access to significant familiar objects.

In addition to the nursing interventions discussed in Chapter 13, the nurse teaches the individual and the family and/or significant others proper isolation techniques so that contact can be safely increased. The nurse suggests other interaction techniques, such as telephoning and letter writing, and attempts to create ways for personal items to be introduced into the isolation environment.

In order to decrease the staff's reluctance and fear in interacting with the individual in isolation, it is necessary that they be carefully oriented to proper isolation techniques, the need for interaction with the individual, and ways to increase interaction without donning isolation equipment, such as standing at the doorway.

To help increase the individual's feeling of self-worth, avoid use of words with negative connotations such as dirty, contaminated, and isolation.

TEACHING IMPROVED HEALTH HABITS

Other measures specific to the host which help to reduce microbial transmission are respiratory and perineal hygiene. The nurse teaches the individual to sneeze, cough, expectorate, and blow the nose into disposable tissues. These used tissues are in turn placed in a receptable specifically designated for this purpose, such as a paper or plastic bag. The receptacle is emptied or changed as often as necessary to eliminate a reservoir for growth of microorganisms. Explanations are given of the need for frequent handwashing after handling respiratory secretions, particularly before handling food or coming in direct contact with other people. The nurse explains to the individual and family and/or significant others the relationship between the spread of droplet infection and respiratory secretions.

Since fecal material contains pathogenic, as well as nonpathogenic, organisms, special care is taken to prevent the spread of fecal material to the vagina, the urethra and, via the mouth, to the gastrointestinal tract. The individual and family and/or significant others are therefore taught to wipe the perineal area from front to back after urinating and defecating and to wash their hands immediately afterwards. Proper handwashing prevents transfer of organisms from the feces to the gastrointestinal tract through ingestion. This is particularly important for food handlers, who can transmit organisms to a wide number of people.

Increasing Host Resistance

The nurse can help increase the individual's resistance to infection in several ways. By assisting the individual to maintain adequate nutrition and fluid balance, the nurse not only helps promote biologic safety but also fosters tissue repair when microbial invasion has occurred. Maintenance of skin integrity and circulation also increases resistance. Therefore, teaching the individual and the family and/or significant others ways of promoting nutrition (Chap. 19), maintaining skin integrity (Chap. 22), and supporting oxygenation to cells (Chaps. 17 and 18) is an important intervention for biologic safety.

SUPPORTING OR CHANGING HEALTH HABITS

The nurse supports and reinforces those health habits the individual has which promote biologic safety and aids the individual in modifying those habits that interfere with wellness and decrease resistance. Interventions focused on health habits must take into consideration the individual's level of growth and development, cultural, societal, and family attitudes and values, living conditions, economic status, and actual and potential threats to biologic safety. The nurse can carry out biologic safety teaching with the individual and group in the home, community, school, work setting, clinic, or hospital.

Chart 15.5
Infectious Diseases Grouped According to Degree of Recommended Isolation

	PRIVATE ROOM	MASK	GOWN	GLOVES	EXCRETA AND EXCRETA-SOILED ARTICLES	BLOOD	SECRETA AND SECRETA-SOILED ARTICLES
STRICT ISOLATION							
Anthrax, inhalation; Eczema vaccinatum; Melioidosis, pulmonary, or extrapulmonary with draining sinus(es); Plague, pulmonary or bubonic; Smallpox; Vaccinia, generalized and progressive	X	X	X	X			X
Burns, extensive—infected with *Staphylococcus aureus* or Group A streptococcus	X	DC	DC	DC			X
Staphylococcal enterocolitis; Staphylococcal or streptococcal pneumonia	X	X	DC	DC			X
Diphtheria	X	X	DC				X
Neonatal vesicular disease (herpes simplex); Rubella; Congenital syndrome	X	DC	DC		X	X	X
Rabies	X			DC			X
RESPIRATORY ISOLATION							
Tuberculosis, pulmonary—sputum-positive (or suspect); Venezuelan equine encephalomyelitis	X	X					X
Meningitis, meningococcal; Meningococcemia	X	X					
Chickenpox; Herpes zoster; Measles (rubeola); Mumps; Rubella (German measles); Pertussis (whooping cough)	X	S					X
ENTERIC PRECAUTIONS							
Cholera; *Escherichia coli* gastroenteritis; Salmonellosis, including typhoid fever; Shigellosis	O		DC	DC	X		
Hepatitis, infectious or serum	O				X	X	
WOUND AND SKIN PRECAUTIONS							
Gas gangrene	O						X

Staphylococcal skin or wound disease

Impetigo; Streptococcal skin infection; Wound infections, extensive—other than staphylococcal; Burns, extensive—infected other than with *Staphylococcus aureus* or Group A streptococcus

DISCHARGE PRECAUTIONS

EXCRETION PRECAUTIONS

Herpangina; Leptospirosis; Meningitis, aspetic; Pleurodynia; Poliomyelitis; Taeniasis, pork; Viral diseases, enteric—if not covered elsewhere

SECRETION PRECAUTIONS

Actinomycosis with draining lesions; Anthrax, cutaneous; Brucellosis with draining lesions; Burns and wounds, minor-infected; *Clostridium perfringens* food poisoning; Coccidioidomycosis with draining wounds; Conjunctivitis, acute bacterial (including gonococcal); Cryptococcosis; Gonococcal ophthalmia neonatorum; Gonorrhea; Granuloma inguinale; Herpes simplex; Keratoconjunctivitis, infectious; Listeriosis; Lymphogranuloma venereum; Pneumonia, bacterial—if not covered elsewhere; Psittacosis; Q fever; Scarlet fever; Staphylococcal food poisoning; Streptococcal pharyngitis; Syphilis, mucocutaneous; Trachoma, acute; Tuberculosis, extrapulmonary with open lesions; Tularemia, cutaneous; Viral diseases, respiratory—if not covered elsewhere; Wound infections, not extensive—other than staphylococcal

BLOOD PRECAUTIONS

Arthropod-borne viral fever (dengue, etc.); Arthropod-borne viral hemorrhagic fever; Hepatitis, infectious or serum; Malaria

Marks by row:

- Staphylococcal skin or wound disease — O; DC; DC
- Impetigo; Streptococcal skin infection; ... — O; DC; DC; DC
- EXCRETION PRECAUTIONS (Herpangina...) — X
- SECRETION PRECAUTIONS (Actinomycosis...) — X
- BLOOD PRECAUTIONS (Arthropod-borne viral fever...) — X

X, Recommended; DC, With direct contact; S, For susceptibles; O, Desirable, but optional.
From: Department of Health, Education and Welfare, Isolation Techniques for Use in Hospitals., *Washington, D.C., U.S. Government Printing Office, 1970, pp. 66–67.*

Chart 15.6
Masking, Gowning, and Gloving

TECHNIQUE	POINTS TO NOTE
Masking	
Collect all equipment needed in isolation unit.	Increased organization. Prevents need to regown, reglove, and remask to get needed articles.
Wash hands.	Removes transient microorganisms.
Unfold mask and place securely over nose and mouth.	Makes tight seal to prevent escape of microorganisms.
Firmly tie upper ties, then lower ties.	Prevents mask from slipping. Masks are changed whenever they become wet or soiled; they are never removed and put on again.
Gowning	
Grasp neck and allow it to unfold without touching uniform, with wrong side of gown facing uniform.	Gown should reach below knees to prevent contamination of uniform. Any time outside of gown is touched it becomes contaminated and must be discarded, and procedure repeated with fresh gown.
Put one arm then the other through the armholes of gown without touching the outside of gown.	Work arms all the way into gown arms so gown does not have to be adjusted any more than necessary. Avoid touching outside of gown with hands.
Adjust shoulders and neck of gown.	Insures complete coverage of uniform.
Tie securely.	Prevents gown from slipping.
Arrange back of gown so it covers all of uniform.	Gown is changed when it becomes wet or contaminated. Gown is removed by reversing procedure, taking care to avoid touching outside. Discard gown after each use. (When paper disposal gowns are used, care is taken to avoid tearing when gowning.)

(continued)

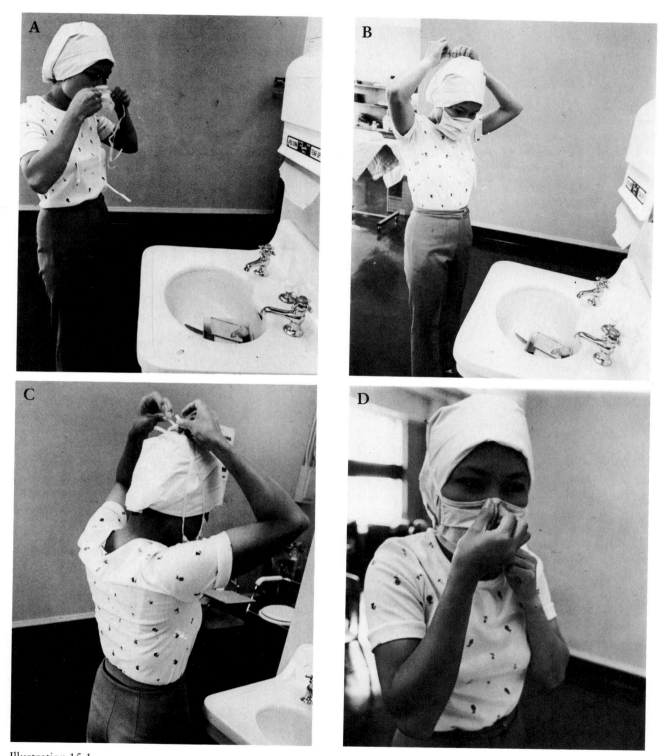

Illustration 15.1

Masking. To prevent the transmission of airborne pathogens, masks are worn in barrier technique. **A.** After hands have been washed, the mask is placed over nose and mouth; **B.** The upper ties are tied; and **C.** The lower ties crossed over the upper and fastened above them. **D.** Finally, the nurse fits the mask snuggly about her face, securing it by pressing thin wire that is in the fabric closely over the bridge of the nose. *(Photo © Leonard Speier, 1979)*

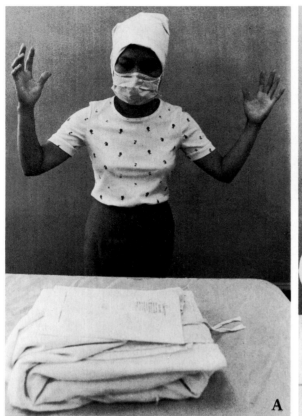
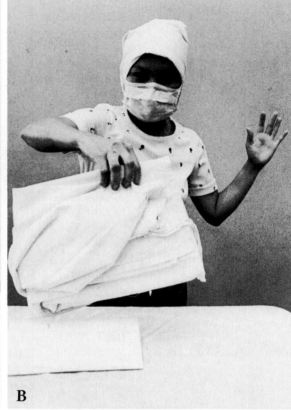
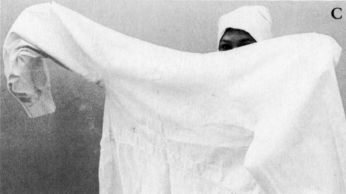
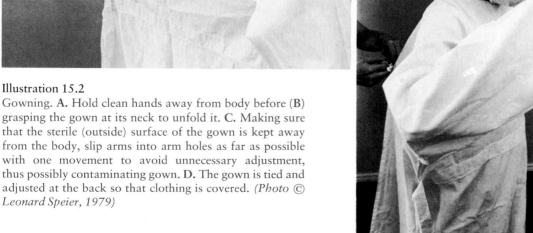

Illustration 15.2

Gowning. **A.** Hold clean hands away from body before (**B**) grasping the gown at its neck to unfold it. **C.** Making sure that the sterile (outside) surface of the gown is kept away from the body, slip arms into arm holes as far as possible with one movement to avoid unnecessary adjustment, thus possibly contaminating gown. **D.** The gown is tied and adjusted at the back so that clothing is covered. *(Photo © Leonard Speier, 1979)*

Chart 15.6 (Cont.)
Masking, Gowning, and Gloving

TECHNIQUE	POINTS TO NOTE
Gloving	
Remove inner packet containing gloves from outer wrapper.	Gloves are double wrapped to insure sterility.
Place inner packet on a clean, dry, flat surface.	Prevents contamination through capillary action or direct contact. Provides working space.
Open packet as if opening a book.	Touch only edges of wrapper. If inner aspect is touched or wrapper folds back, it is contaminated.
Arrange packet so cuff ends of gloves are closest to body.	Facilitates gloving and maintaining sterile field.
If necessary open wrapper to reveal gloves—do not touch gloves or inner surface of wrapper.	Glove packages vary in wrapping technique; determine type before opening.
Use one hand to glove the other.	Pick up gloves with hand not being gloved.
Grasp fold of glove cuff with one hand. Slip other hand into glove taking care not to touch outside of glove.	Inner aspects of gloves are considered clean whether folded or not and should not touch sterile outer surface of gloves. Do not adjust gloves at this point.
Using gloved hand, slide gloved fingers under other cuff edge.	As above.
Adjust gloves as necessary without touching skin, inner surface of glove, or any other nonsterile surface.	As above.
Remove gloves by peeling gloves inside out.	Outer glove is now considered contaminated and should not come into contact with skin or other clean surfaces.
Wash hands.	Reduces transient microorganisms. If only parts of masking, gowning, or gloving techniques are necessary, wash hands after each procedure used.

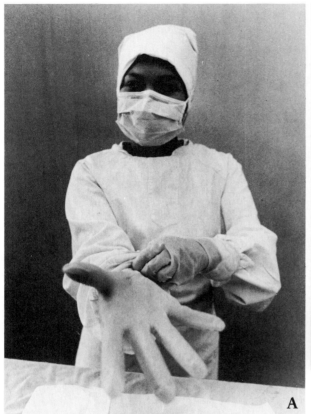

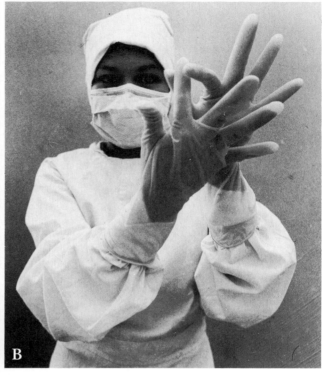

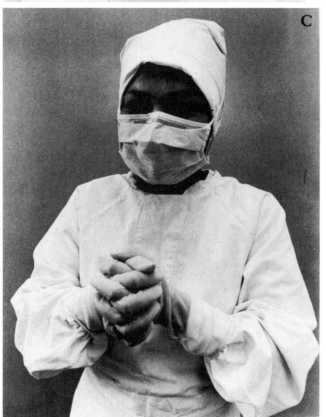

Illustration 15.3

Gloving. Glove first hand as the procedure is outlined in Chart 15.6. **A.** With gloved fingers under cuff edge of second sterile glove (pictured above as the right glove), slide hand into it, being careful not to touch contaminated areas in the environment. **B.** If necessary, adjust gloves after both gloves are on. In adjustment, do not touch skin or inner surface of glove, and make sure that fingers are comfortable and sufficiently flexible to perform procedure. **C.** Hands are kept folded at chest level to prevent contamination until procedure begins. *(Photo © Leonard Speier, 1979)*

IMMUNIZATION

By explaining the need for and scheduling and availability of immunizations, the nurse helps the individual to gain immunity to many contagious diseases. In addition, mass immunization helps protect the general public and prevents epidemics. Since the frequencies of some of these diseases have decreased markedly, many people believe the diseases have been eradicated and that immunizations against them are therefore no longer necessary. This is a misconception, since continued immunization of susceptible populations is necessary to maintain a low incidence. By explaining the relationship between decreased incidence and immunization, the nurse can help dispel these myths. Chart 15.7 gives the recommended immunization schedule for infants and children. This schedule does not imply that unimmunized adults cannot receive this protection at any age.

Support of Host Defenses

Once the individual has been invaded by microorganisms through any portal of entry, the nurse intervenes to limit the sequelae of invasion, to promote healing, and to restore high-level wellness. A major method of assessing responses and evaluating the effectiveness of treatment is the measurement of body temperature. One sign of inflammation or infection is fever, ► or **pyrexia** (increased body temperature).

FEVER

► Microorganisms often act as **pyrogens** to raise the basal metabolism with a resultant increase in production of heat. The heat produced is a further defense of the body in an attempt to create an unsuitable environment for the microorganism. However, this rise in temperature may reach a point where it becomes injurious to the host. Temperatures above 106 F result in damage to the cells and unless some type of intervention takes place and the temperature is lowered, the individual will die. Young children commonly respond to temperatures above 103 F (39.4 C) with convulsions. Once the temperature is lowered, the convulsions cease. Convulsions related to pyrexia should not be confused with convulsions resulting from underlying pathophysiologies.

There are three phases of fever.

Onset

The first phase, *onset,* occurs when the body temperature begins to rise as the body attempts to conserve and produce heat. The individual appears pale as a result of peripheral vasoconstriction, shivers to produce extra body heat through muscle activity, and feels cold.

The Fastigium, or Course

During the second stage, the *fastigium,* or *course,* the individual shows signs of fever as the body recognizes the rise in body temperature and attempts to give off heat to reduce the fever. The individual feels warm to the touch and is flushed as a result of peripheral vasodilation. The individual sweats in an attempt to lose body heat through evaporation and feels lethargic, headachy, and just plain sick.

Chart 15.7
Active Immunization Schedule
for Infants and Children

AGE	IMMUNIZATION
2 months	DTP†, TOPV‡
4 months	DTP, TOPV
6 months	DTP, TOPV
12 months	Tuberculin test, measles, mumps, rubella
18 months	DTP, TOPV
4–6 years	DTP, TOPV
14–16 years	Td§ and every 10 years thereafter

From 1974 Report of the Committee of Infectious Diseases of the American Academy of Pediatrics.
†DTP—Diphtheria and tetanus toxoids, and pertussis vaccine combined.
‡TOPV—Trivalent oral polio vaccine.
§Td—Adult type combined tetanus and diphtheria toxoids, containing less diphtheria component than TD.
From: Lillian S. Brunner and Doris S. Suddarth, *The Lippincott Manual of Nursing Practice,* ed. 2. Philadelphia: J. B. Lippincott Company, 1978, p. 1319.

Resolution

The final phase of the fever process is the *resolution* phase. If the temperature drops suddenly, it is called *crisis;* if it drops slowly, it is called *lysis.* During the period of falling temperature, the person may continue diaphoresis and other heat loss responses. However, once the temperature has returned to the expected level, the individual no longer has any signs or symptoms. Chart 15.8 outlines the procedures for measuring body temperature. (Figs. 15.5 and 15.6)

BODY TEMPERATURE MEASUREMENT

The rectal measurement of body temperature is the most accurate measure of internal body heat and is usually 1 degree F higher than measurements from other body sites. The rectal area is not affected as directly by the external environmental conditions as are the other measurement sites in the mouth and axilla. However, the rectal site is not always used because of pathology existing in the area and because exact temperture readings are not always needed. Having the rectal temperature measured can be embarrassing and uncomfortable for the individual. Thus this method is not used indiscriminately.

CARE OF THE FEBRILE INDIVIDUAL

The nursing care of the individual with fever focuses on removing the underlying pathology, maintaining fluid and electrolyte balance, promoting adequate nutrition, reducing the fever, and providing comfort.

Treating Pathology

Antibiotics are frequently utilized to treat the infectious process. Since a continuous supply of these medications must be maintained in the bloodstream for them to be fully effective, the nurse administers them at regular intervals. Often antibiotics are given for a period of time after the acute symptoms have disappeared, to insure that the disease is completely gone. Many individuals receive antibiotic therapy in the home setting. Thus, the nurse teaches people the rationale for taking their medications on schedule and for completing the full course of therapy even though they feel better.

Another way the nurse helps to treat underlying pathology is to assist in preventing reinfection. By teaching the individual handwashing, carrying out handwashing oneself, using appropriate isolation techniques, and improving the individual's level of health, the nurse decreases the chances for reinfection. If the infection has been caused by an infected wound, the wound may be *incised* (surgically opened) and drained. The drainage may be facilitated by the insertion of a drain into the wound (Fig. 15.7 shows some common wound drains) or the wound may be allowed to drain freely. When caring for draining wounds, precautions are taken not to dislodge any drains and to prevent contamination by the drainage. The amount, color, consistency, and odor of any drainage is recorded.

Maintaining Fluid and Electrolyte Balance

The febrile individual is losing water and electrolytes through diaphoresis and respiratory evaporation. Sodium is the major electrolyte lost in sweating. Thus the individual requires extra amounts of both water and electrolytes to compensate for losses. Intake and output are recorded to evaluate the relative balance between the two and to provide information on the individual's specific needs. Individualization is necessary to prevent overload or dehydration. Intravenous therapy is commonly used in more severe cases of fever to replace lost fluids and electrolytes and supplement oral intake. (Chapter 21 is a discussion of fluids and electrolytes.)

Promoting Nutrition

The individual with fever frequently has accompanying nausea and anorexia; thus nutritional intake is decreased. In addition, as a result of an increased basal metabolic rate, the person's energy needs are increased. Therefore, small, frequent feedings of foods desired by the individual (which are within the therapeutic regimen) are offered to the individual. Often explanations of the exact need for increased intake, plus a positive eating environment, will convince the person to increase food and fluid intake. (Chapter 19 discusses nutritional needs.)

Reducing Fever

Measures to reduce fever include administering antipyretics such as aspirin, giving tepid water or alcohol baths to lower the individual's body temperature by increasing evaporation and lowering skin temperature, and using other hypothermic techniques. Tepid water baths are carried out by covering large areas of the individual's body with towels soaked in tepid water. These towels are wrung so that they are not dripping. Drafts and chills are avoided

Chart 15.8
Measuring Temperature

TECHNIQUE	POINTS TO NOTE
For all methods of measuring temperature: Wash hands.	Removes transient bacteria.
Explain procedure.	Reduces anxiety and increases cooperation.
Determine method to be used.	Thermometers are not interchanged for different methods.
Collect equipment.	Allows working in orderly and organized manner.
Rinse the thermometer in cool water and dry from bulb to stem.	Removes transient particles and disinfectant. Prior to procedure, bulb end of thermometer is considered clean; stem end, dirty.
Shake down mercury in thermometer to below 94° F (34.4° C) by firmly holding end of stem and snapping wrist in a downward motion.	Shaking down prevents misreading. Snapping motion is required to move mercury into bulb. Stand clear of all objects to prevent hitting and breaking thermometer.
Check reading of mercury.	Ensures mercury is shaken down.
After temperature is measured: Wipe thermometer with tissue from stem to bulb.	Cleans stem for reading. After use, stem end is considered clean; bulb end, dirty.
Hold thermometer at eye level.	Best point for visualization of mercury.
Rotate until silver line of mercury can be clearly seen.	Brings line of mercury into full view.
Read temperature to nearest indicator line.	Gives most accurate reading.
Wash thermometer with soap and cool water; dry, place into appropriate container.	Removes surface organisms, aids in disinfection.
Record temperature, indicating method used, e.g., 98.6° F (R) or 99.0° F (O).	Maintains continuous updated record.
Measuring Oral Temperature Check to ascertain if individual has smoked, taken food or fluids orally, or chewed gum within last half-hour.	These can alter reading.
Place thermometer under tongue or ask individual to do so and to seal lips around stem.	If individual wets lips prior to insertion, thermometer won't stick to lips. Placement insures most accurate reading. Sealed lips prevent thermometer from slipping and maintains steady temperature of oral cavity.
Keep thermometer in place 5–7 min.	Allows time for accurate measurement.
Remove thermometer.	

Oral method of measurement of temperature is not used for infants and small children, confused, disoriented, or unconscious individuals, or when oral route is contraindicated.

(continued)

Chart 15.8 (Cont.)
Measuring Temperature

TECHNIQUE	POINTS TO NOTE
Measuring Rectal Temperature	
Close bed curtains or place screens around individual.	Maintains privacy.
Position individual in comfortable side-lying position or supine, with one leg flexed.	Exposes rectal opening.
Remove clothing and bed linen from around rectal opening.	Facilitates seeing rectal opening and inserting of thermometer.
Uncover smallest area possible.	Maintains privacy.
Lubricate bulb and lower portion of stem of thermometer.	Lubrication reduces friction and increases ease of insertion.
Lift upper buttock.	Increases view of area.
Insert thermometer approximately $1\frac{1}{2}$ in. for adults.	Allows for most accurate measurement with least chance of trauma.
Keep thermometer in place for 3−5 min.	Allows time for accurate measurement.
If individual is conscious and oriented, remind him or her not to roll onto thermometer.	Prevents injury to intestine through breakage or pressure.
If individual is infant, child, confused, disoriented, or unconscious, stand with individual, holding thermometer in place and prevent individual from rolling on it.	

Rectal method of measurement is not used for individuals who have had rectal or perineal surgery or when vagal stimulation is contraindicated.

Measuring Axillary Temperature	
Dry axilla using gentle patting.	Rubbing increases local circulation and alters readings.
Place bulb of thermometer in middle of axilla and adduct arm against side of chest.	Allows for most accurate measurement.
Keep axilla tightly closed.	Holds thermometer in place and maintains steady axillary temperature.
Hold in place 10 min.	Allows time for accurate measurement.

The axillary method of temperature taking is used for newborns and when other methods cannot be used.

ready... aim... fire...

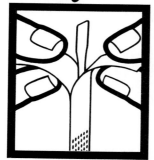

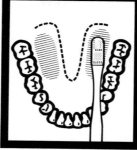

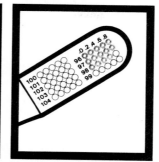

Remove thermometer from wrapper
Peel back paper wrapper to expose handle end of thermometer. Remove thermometer, taking care not to touch sterile indicator dots or shaft as these will go in patient's mouth.

Place thermometer under tongue
Insert thermometer under tongue as far back as possible into either heat pocket. Have patient press tongue down on thermometer, keeping mouth closed.
Remove thermometer after a minimum of 45 seconds.

Read temperature
Wait a few seconds to permit precise indicator color to develop. The last blue dot gives you the patient's temperature.

Importance of proper placement
A patient's oral temperature may vary widely in different areas of the mouth. In one study,* a low of 96.8°F was measured immediately behind the incisors and a high of 98.4°F in the right "heat pocket" at the base of and under the tongue. (These figures represent the averages of ten readings taken in each area.)

*Beck WC (MD), St Cyr B (RN): Oral thermometry, *The Guthrie Bulletin*, 43:170, 1974.

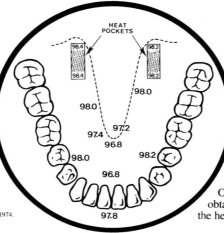

Therefore, to get the most accurate oral temperature, it is essential to insert the Tempa-DOT Ready Strip Thermometer deep into the heat pocket under the tongue on either side of the frenum. Otherwise, the temperature obtained may differ from that of the heat pocket by as much as 1.6°F.

Figure 15.5
Single-use oral thermometer. *(Used with permission of Organon Inc., West Orange, N.J.*

and the individual's temperature is measured frequently to prevent overcooling, which will produce shivering. Overcooling and shivering counteract the effects of the treatment. Alcohol baths are also used to lower body temperature and are done with a half-alcohol and half-water solution. The alcohol produces more rapid evaporation than water by itself. However, the fumes from alcohol may be toxic to the individual if inhaled in large doses and may produce disorientation and coma. For these reasons alcohol baths are used only when tepid water baths have been

ineffective. Family and/or significant others should be made aware of these effects to avoid indiscriminate use.

The most common hypothermic measure is the use of electric cooling blankets or pads. These blankets, filled with alcohol and distilled water and attached to a cooling unit, are placed under the individual. If body temperature is extremely high, a cooling blanket may also be placed over the individual. A sheet is placed between the individual and the blanket. The fluid continually circulates through the unit

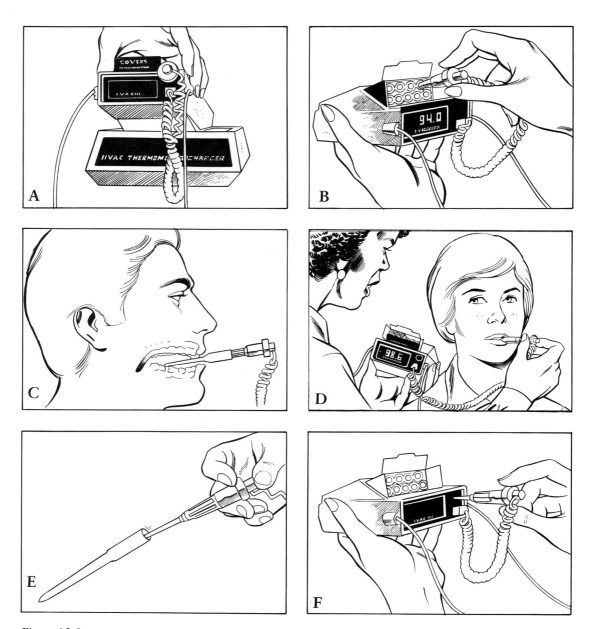

Figure 15.6

Using an electronic thermometer. **A.** Remove the thermometer from its charging base and place the carrying strap around the neck. **B.** Next, grasp the probe by the large ring *below* the attached wire and insert the probe firmly into a cover. *Do not* push the top of the probe as that is the ejection button. **C.** For oral temperatures, slowly slide probe under the individual's tongue, back to the sublingual pocket at the tongue's base. The individual's lips come to rest at the step on the probe cover. (Rectal temperatures may be determined with the electronic thermometer. A red probe is used. The technique for penetration is described in Chart 15.8.) **D.** Hold the probe while it is in the individual's mouth and watch the probe, not the digital display panel. An audible signal will notify the nurse when the individual's temperature is displayed. **E.** Remove probe from the individual's mouth. Discard probe cover by pushing ejection button with thumb. **F.** Read and record temperature. Then return probe to its storage well, which will automatically turn the thermometer off. After all temperatures have been taken, return thermometer to its charging base. *(Adapted with permission from IVAC® Corporation, San Diego, Calif.*

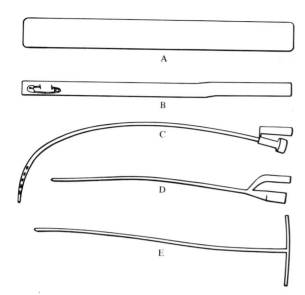

Figure 15.7
Wound drains. Wounds may be drained to relieve infection and remove drainage. Commonly used for wound drainage are: **A.** Penrose drain; **B.** cigarette drain; **C.** sump catheter; **D.** Foley catheter; and **E.** T-tube.

Chart 15.9	
Vocabulary Related to Body Temperature	
TERM	**MEANING**
Afebrile	Without fever
Constant fever	Continuous temperature elevation during a 24-hour period; shows little or no variation.
Febrile	Having fever
Hyperpyrexia	Excessively high temperature above 103 F.
Hyperthermia	Increased fever states; may be induced.
Hypothermia	Lowered body temperature; may be pathologic or induced.
Intermittent fever	Intervals of elevated temperatures which return to basal body temperature; interval may be days, hours, or weeks.
Pyrogen	Any agent which increases body temperature.
Remittent fever	Fluctuations of increased body temperature without returning to basal values.

and is kept at a constant preset temperature to cool the body. The same precautionary measures used with cooling baths are used with these devices. Care is also taken not to use pins or other sharp objects as they may puncture the blanket and cause leaks. These units can also be used for hyperthermic technique. When used for this purpose, care is taken not to burn or overheat the individual.

Providing Comfort

Comfort measures for the febrile individual include keeping the skin, clothing, and linen clean and dry, providing mouth care, and generally trying to increase the individual's feeling of well-being. Since the febrile person is diaphoretic, frequent sponge baths and changes of clothing and linens are necessary. Skin care measures (Chap. 22) are also used. The individual's mouth may become dry or foul-tasting. Thus frequent brushing of teeth, rinsing of mouth, and lubrication of lips are carried out to increase comfort and prevent breakdown of mucous membranes. Good mouth care may also work as an incentive to increased nutritional intake.

Chart 15.9 describes terms related to body temperature.

Other Interventions for Inflammation and Infection

Other accompanying signs of inflammation or infection are also focuses for nursing intervention. Rest and immobilization of the affected part, reduction of pain and swelling, promotion of circulation, care of any accompanying wounds, and promotion of healing are the areas of focus. If the inflammation is confined to one body part, that area may be splinted, casted, or bandaged to decrease movement. More generalized inflammation or infection may require completed bed rest or limitations on usual activities. Any accompanying pain and swelling may be treated with analgesics, anti-inflammatory drugs, immobilization, heat and cold, as well as treating the underlying cause. An attempt to limit swelling may be made by applying elastic bandages or stockings to the affected area (Chaps. 14 and 18). Whenever these techniques are used, the bandages or stockings are removed frequently to check the underlying skin. They are not applied so tightly that they interfere with circulation.

Measures to increase circulation in the affected part are instituted to increase the supply of nutrients and oxygen and to remove waste products and debris. Increased circulation promotes healing, reduces congestion in underlying tissues, and reduces swelling. In addition, heat may relax muscles and reduce spasm.

APPLICATION OF HEAT

A common method of increasing circulation is the use of heat, which causes peripheral vasodilation. Dry heat may be applied through heat lamps, hot-water bottles, and heating pads. Moist heat is more penetrating than dry heat, since water is a better conductor of heat than air. It is applied through soaks, compresses, and baths. Regardless of the method used, safety precautions are taken to prevent burning the skin. During treatment, the skin is observed for signs of redness or breakdown. The individual's statements concerning the temperature felt are carefully validated since the temperature experience is subjective and the individual may have sensory deficiencies that prevent accurate perception and reporting of temperature. Correlating subjective statements with known safety principles, observations of the skin, pathophysiologic processes present, and the individual's sensory abilities guides the nurse in determining appropriate actions. Any equipment used should be in good working order. The purposes and methods of heat application are explained to the individual, who is told to report any subjective signs of discomfort.

Heat Lamps

Heat lamp treatments are applied intermittently for periods of 15–20 minutes. The distance the lamp is kept from the skin surface depends on the size of the lamp and the condition of the skin. The closer the lamp is to the skin surface, the more intense the heat will be. Lamps are rarely placed less than 18 inches from the skin.

Hot-water Bottles

When hot-water bottles are used to apply heat, they are not filled completely—the air is removed after filling—and the cap is sealed tightly. Extremely hot water (above 125 F or 51.7 C) is not used, and cooler water is used for children and debilitated persons. The bottle is covered before being placed next to the skin. Hot water bottles may be applied continuously or intermittently. During continuous application, the water in the bottle is changed at least every 45 minutes to an hour to maintain a relatively comfortable temperature.

Heating Pads

Heating pads may also be applied either continuously or intermittently. These heating pads may be either the usual commercial pads or water-circulating hyperthermia pads. Whatever type is used, it must have a temperature control device to prevent it from overheating and burning the individual. The temperature of the heating pad is usually maintained at the low setting and the control device is checked frequently to assure that the setting has not been changed. Heating pads or hot-water bottles may be secured in place by wrapping them in a towel, placing the towel around the body part, and taping the ends of the towel.

Soaks

A soak is the immersion of a body part in heated water or the application of well-saturated towels or dressings to an affected part. If soaks are applied to an area where there is an open wound, sterile technique is maintained and sterile supplies used. When applying towels or dressings, bed linen and clothing are protected by plastic or underpads. To slow the cooling process, the soaks are often encased in plastic sheeting. If continuous warm soaks are required, a waterproof heating pad or hot-water bottle may be placed around the soaks. A thin layer of petroleum ointment may be patted on the skin surface prior to the application of soaks to prevent maceration and irritation of the skin.

Baths

Moist heat can be applied to large areas of the body by baths. In essence, these are large soaks. Because of vasodilation over a large portion of the body, the individual is observed for signs of fainting. These signs include dizziness, pallor, sweating, hypotension, and feelings of weakness. The safety guidelines for any bathing situation are followed (Chap. 22).

Nursing Implications

No matter what method of heat application is used, the individual's response to treatment is recorded. The treatment is discontinued whenever signs of tissue damage occur or the individual is unduly distressed by the accompanying sensations. Heat treatments are usually ordered by the physician. However, agency policy may allow the use of certain types of heat in specific situations. Thus the nurse needs to be familiar with the policies of a particular agency. Whether or not the use of heat requires a physician's order, the nurse is aware of the implications for the use of heat and its contraindications. Heat is not applied when prevention of swelling is desired, when it may increase the individual's discomfort, or if suppuration is not desired. Suppuration is the accumulation and drainage of pus.

APPLICATION OF COLD

Applications of cold produce vasoconstriction and lower tissue metabolism. Cold treatments are used to prevent swelling, reduce inflammation, decrease bleeding, and decrease sensitivity of nerve pain endings. Cold may be applied either dry or moist. Ice bags and hyperthermia pads are frequently used methods for applications of dry cold, while soaks and baths are common types of moist-cold applications. The same procedures and precautions are utilized with cold applications as with heat. Cold therapy is not used with individuals whose circulation is compromised, since the administration of cold may further deteriorate circulatory status. Signs of overcooling such as peripheral cyanosis, mottling, shivering, pain, decreased body temperature, total numbness (cold will produce some numbness), and tissue damage are indications that cold treatment should be discontinued.

ASEPTIC TECHNIQUES

Aseptic practices are used whenever the individual's defense systems have been lowered. **Aseptic practices** are those activities which prevent infection and are of two types—medical and surgical. **Medical asepsis** is the use of equipment and supplies which are free of pathogenic organisms in a clean environment while **surgical asepsis** is the use of strict sterile technique. In **sterile technique** all equipment and supplies are free from all organisms and their spores and are used in a clean environment.

The person utilizing sterile technique uses sterile protective barriers to prevent contamination of the individual and the environment. Masks, gloves, and gowns are the most common barriers used. Medical aseptic practices include frequent handwashing, respiratory and perineal measures, cleaning equipment after use, housekeeping activities such as damp dusting, personal care activities, and any other activity which helps to reduce or eliminate organisms in the environment or in direct contact with the individual.

In using aseptic techniques, sterility is maintained only when sterile objects touch sterile objects. If a sterile object touches a clean or dirty object, it is contaminated. Whenever contamination occurs, the contaminated equipment is replaced and the activity is restarted. There is no such thing as an object being slightly or a little contaminated (either it is or it isn't). If any doubt exists, the object is considered contaminated. An object is no longer considered clean if it touches a dirty object. However, if a clean object touches a sterile object, it is still clean. Any time a sterile object becomes wet, it is also considered contaminated because capillary action brings microorganisms up from the wet, nonsterile surface to the sterile object. Therefore, when following aseptic practices, the guidelines are: sterile to sterile maintains sterility; sterile to clean is contaminated, but clean to sterile is still clean; and clean to clean maintains cleanliness.

Medical asepsis is always used when caring for individuals. Surgical asepsis is used when caring for open wounds, during surgical procedures, in protective isolation, and in procedures which require entering sterile body cavities such as the bladder or body tissues such as muscle.

WOUND CARE

When the individual has a wound, the type of care given to that wound will depend on the physician's orders, the presence of drainage or infections, the degree of healing present, and the depth of the wound. Small, scabbed wounds may require no treatment or dressing or simply a dry, sterile dressing. Larger, more extensive wounds may require use of sterile dressing techniques, while large, draining, or infected wounds may require sterile technique and irrigation. Chart 15.10 outlines one technique used for

Chart 15.10
Sterile Wound Dressing and Irrigation

TECHNIQUE	POINTS TO NOTE
Collect equipment:	Allows procedure to be done in an organized, uninterrupted manner. All equipment coming in contact with wound is sterile.

Collect equipment:

1. Gloves (2 sets)	8. Bulb syringe and holder
2. Tape	9. Scissors
3. Gauze pads	10. Protective underpads
4. Sterile applicators	11. Kidney basin
5. Disinfectant	12. Pickup forceps
6. Bowl	13. Paper bag
7. Irrigating solution	14. Medication if ordered

Explain procedure.

Decreases anxiety, increases cooperation.

Wash hands.

Reduces surface microorganisms.

Position individual comfortably so that the maximum access to wound is possible.

Increases visualization of field, increases working area, and decreases opportunity for contamination.

Place protective pads under individual.

Prevents wetting and soiling of bed linen.

Set up sterile field on clean, dry, solid surface.

Provides sterile working area.

Open needed number of sterile gauze pads.

Total number will depend on size of wound to be covered and number needed for cleaning and drying.

Drop gauze from wrapper onto sterile field taking care not to touch sterile field with wrapper or hands (Fig. 15-7).

Prevents contamination of field and wound.

Open any other individually wrapped sterile equipment (e.g., applicators, basins) and place on sterile field.

Prevents contamination of field and wound by allowing procedure to continue without interruption

Cut needed tape strips and place over edge of solid surface away from sterile field.

Tape ready for use at end of dressing change.

Pour disinfecting solutions into basins on sterile field. Do not spill fluids on sterile field.

Solutions are poured from approximately 3–6 in. above basin. End pouring with a twisting motion to prevent drips on field. Do not touch bottle to basin or field.

If wound is to be irrigated, open disposable irrigating set. Pour irrigating solution into container.
Do not contaminate syringe or inside of container.

If syringe, inside of container, and solution are not contaminated, they may be reused.

Remove old dressing:
1. Pull tape off skin working from skin to dressing at all points.

Prevents tension on wound.

2. If outer dressing is clean and dry, gloves or forceps are not necessary if dressing is picked up by corners without touching center of dressing; otherwise use gloves or forceps to remove dressing.

Nurse does not touch contaminated areas.
Reduces chance of cross contamination.

3. Discard contaminated dressing, and gloves if they are used, in paper bag.

Prevents contamination of field and surrounding areas by soiled articles.

(continued)

Chart 15.10 (Cont.)
Sterile Wound Dressing and Irrigation

TECHNIQUE	POINTS TO NOTE
Glove using sterile technique.	Prevents contamination of field and wound.
Clean wound with solution as ordered or according to agency policy by:	Properly used, either gloves or forceps method prevents contamination. Prevents bringing microorganisms into wound from surrounding areas.
1. *Glove method*—Pick up gauze pad by its corners and wet center with solution. Cleanse wound using a circular motion, working from center of wound outward, if it is a circular or irregularly shaped wound.	
If it is a straight wound, clean from middle to wound edge, repeat with new pad on other side of wound.	
Use each gauze pad only once.	
2. *Forceps method*—Fold gauze and pick it up with forceps. Clean wound in above manner.	

Irrigating wound

Place kidney basin firmly against skin surface below wound.	This prevents solution from flowing on or contaminating surrounding skin or linen.
Flush wound with irrigating solution using bulb syringe.	Tip of syringe does not touch wound.
Pat wound dry with sterile gauze using hand with glove, which is still sterile, or sterile forceps. Do not let gloved hand touch skin surface.	Dry in same manner as cleansing.
Apply medication if ordered.	Use contaminated hand to hold medication container. Squeeze, pour, or shake medication on sterile pad.

Redressing

Using hand with glove or sterile forceps, which are still sterile, place sterile gauze pads on wound.	Prevents contamination of wound.
Once wound is completely covered with layer of gauze, gloves or forceps are not necessary.	First layer protects wound from contamination.
Cover wound with desired layers of gauze.	Number of layers will depend on orders, amount of drainage, and degree of protection desired.
Tape gauze securely in place.	Prevents displacement of dressing.
Place tape in direction that is in opposition to underlying tissue movement.	Prevents tension on skin and loosening of tape.
Remove underpads.	Promotes comfort.
Reposition individual comfortably.	
Assemble used supplies and dispose of appropriately.	Prevents contamination of environment.
Chart observations and procedure.	Updates records so information on the progress of wound healing is available.

▶ sterile dressing and **irrigation.** When using sterile technique or doing other procedures, the nurse avoids talking, sneezing, coughing, and reaching over the sterile field. Anything the nurse cannot keep within his or her line of vision is not considered sterile, since the nurse has no way of knowing if any contamination has occurred. Therefore, holding sterile gloved hands below the waist, above the head, or behind the back; reaching across a sterile field; and turning away from a sterile field are violations of the sterile technique.

PSYCHOSOCIAL CONSIDERATIONS

The nurse also intervenes with the individual in relation to that individual's psychosocial responses to infections and wounds. When the individual's body image is threatened as a result of disfigurement or deformity from the wound, measures to support self-esteem are initiated (Chap. 22). Increased anxiety levels as a result of the special procedures used and fears about the outcome of healing and interference with daily routines may be reduced by careful explanation of all procedures, listening to the individual's concerns, and following through with specific interventions for the individual's particular needs. Family and/or significant others may have similar reactions. They are included in all aspects of the care situation.

Overview

The nurse plays a major role in helping the individual meet his biologic safety needs. The nurse works to prevent disease, minimize sequelae of infection and inflammation, support host defenses, and maintain an environment which both facilitates the host's resistance and hinders the ability of the agent to cause disease.

EVALUATION

Evaluation of meeting biologic safety needs centers on the direction of change in the agent–host–environment interaction. The nurse also evaluates the effectiveness of intervention in reducing the agent's ability to invade and produce disease in the body, of measures to increase the host's resistance and defense system, and of intervention to maintain an environment which is supportive of the host and reduces the agent's viability at the same time.

Specific criteria for evaluating intervention to meet biologic safety needs include:

- What changes have occurred in the agent's characteristics?
- What changes have occurred in the host's defenses and resistance?
- What changes have occurred in the ability of the environment to support the host?
- Has the presenting agent–host–environment interaction moved closer to the expected?
- What are the changes in interferences with biologic safety?
- What are the changes in knowledge concerning agent–host–environment interactions?
- Are there modifications in personal habits?
- What skills have been acquired?
- What are the changes in attitude toward biologic safety? Body image? Treatments? Limitations?
- What are the changes in level of anxiety related to biologic safety (of the individual, of family and/or significant others)?

RECORDING AND TEACHING–LEARNING ACTIVITIES

Teaching–Learning Topics

- rationale for therapeutic regimen
- dressing changes
- ways to use aseptic technique
- ways to modify personal habits
- safety factors related to prevention of infections
- immunization rationale and schedules
- ways to take temperature
- care of the individual with fever
- ways to break the pathology-producing chain of agent–host–environment interaction
- available resources

Charting

Using appropriate biologic safety terms, objectively describe such factors as:

- objective base-line data for agent–host–environment interaction, inflammatory response, immune response, healing process, level of growth and development, health state, local tissue environment, infection, health habits, physical assessment, and diagnostic tests
- objective and subjective data on changes that occur in the individual's ability to meet biologic safety needs
- attitudes toward interference and treatment
- degree of healing
- responses to treatments which promote meeting the need
- schedule and methods of care
- teaching carried out
- discharge planning done
- interactions and responses of family and/or significant others

Update Kardex on changes in goals and plans for meeting biologic safety needs.

Medications to Review

- antibiotics, e.g., penicillin
- debriding agents, e.g., varidase
- disinfectants, e.g., povidone-iodine (Betadine)
- antiseptics, e.g., isopropyl alcohol
- anti-infectives, e.g., sulfonamide
- irrigating solution, e.g., normal saline
- oxydizing agents, e.g., hydrogen peroxide
- prophylactic agents, e.g., gamma globulin
- vaccines, e.g., DPT

Diets to Review

- high calorie
- high protein
- high vitamin and mineral

NOTES

1. The American Public Health Association. "Control of Communicable Diseases in Man." *Official Report,* 9th ed. New York, 1965, p. 117.

SELECTED REFERENCES

Aspinall, Mary Jo. "Scoring Against Nosocomial Infections." *American Journal of Nursing,* 78:1704, October, 1978.

Castle, Mary and Eatkins, Jane. "Fever: Understanding a Sinister Sign." *Nursing 79,* 9:26, February, 1979.

Castle, Mary. "Wound Care: Clear-Cut Ways to Speed Healing." *Nursing 75,* 5:40, August, 1975.

———. "Isolation: Precise Procedures for Better Protection." *Nursing 75,* 5:50, May, 1975.

Davis-Sharts, Jean. "Mechanisms and Manifestations of Fever," *American Journal of Nursing,* 79:1874, November, 1978.

"Hot and Cold Therapy." *Nursing 78,* 8:44, October, 1978.

Jenny, Jean. "What You Should Be Doing About Infection Control." *Nursing 76,* 6:78, November, 1976.

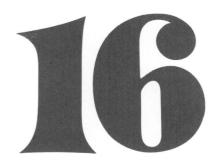

As crude a weapon as the caveman's club, the chemical barrage has been hurled against the fabric of life.

—Rachel Carson, Silent Spring

CHEMICAL SAFETY

PRINCIPLES RELATED TO CHEMICAL SAFETY

An individual's responses to medications are unique.

Medications given for therapeutic purposes may have effects other than those for which they are intended.

Medications interact with other chemicals in the body.

Placing medications toward the back of the tongue reduces unpleasant taste.

Accompanying oral medications with iced or cold water reduces the sensation of unpleasant taste.

Drug dosages are dependent on the size, weight, physiologic functioning, and maturity of the individual.

The liver is the major detoxifying organ of the body.

Medications must reach the bloodstream to produce systemic effects.

Degree and speed of absorption are related to the distance from point of administration to bloodstream, type of tissue between point of administration and bloodstream, and interferences with absorption.

Drug action takes place at the cellular levels.

Drug responses may be physical, physiologic, and/or psychosocial.

Attitudes toward chemical safety are learned.

Knowledge and attitudes about medications and the ability to purchase them influence medication patterns.

Drugs to increase appetite are given prior to meals.

Drugs to reduce gastric acidity are given after meals.

Administration of oral medications is carried out using clean technique.

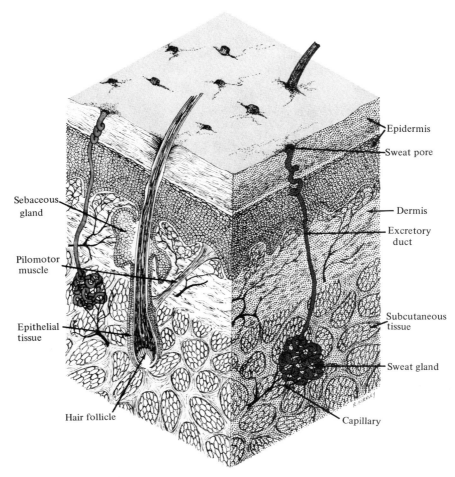

Figure 16.1
Layers of the skin, subcutaneous tissue, and structures within those areas. *(Reprinted with permission of Reston Publishing Company, Inc., a Prentice-Hall Company, 11480 Sunset Hills Road, Reston, Virginia)*

Administration of parenteral medications is carried out using sterile technique.

Any entry into the body may result in distortions of body image.

Chemical agent poisoning and accidents are preventable.

Chemical safety is a major concern for the nurse. Individuals frequently receive chemical agents or drugs to help in meeting their basic needs or to prevent or treat interferences in meeting these needs. Chemical agents can bring about both negative and positive changes in the individual's health state. Therefore,

the nurse needs to understand the uses of the drugs the individual is receiving and to be aware of the proper methods of preparation and administration of drugs, as well as to observe for the effects drugs have on the individual. In addition, the nurse has a role in teaching individuals about self-administration of drugs, whether they are prescribed or over-the-counter, and about prevention of household poisoning by other chemical agents. (Illustration 16.1)

Since nurses do not order the medications that individuals receive, many health care workers view the nurse's role in drug administration as a dependent one. However, in actuality, it is a collaborative role, since the nurse is responsible for ensuring that the individual receives the proper drug in the right dosage

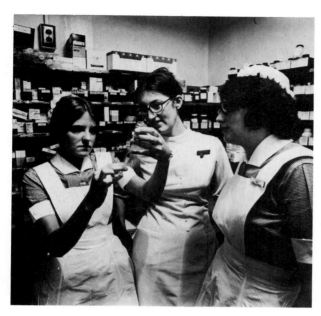

Illustration 16.1
In fulfilling her collaborative role in drug therapy, the nurse learns about many aspects of drug administration and evaluation to ensure individuals' safety and the optimum benefit of their therapy. *(Photo by Ellis Herwig, from Stock, Boston)*

at the appropriate time by the correct route. It is often the nurse's assessment of the individual which determines whether or not the individual receives a medication and which guides the physician's choice of prescribed drugs. The nurse's assessment also often provides the most consistent reports on the individual's responses to drugs.

ASSESSMENT

The individual's level of growth and development, state of health, body chemistry, size, and sex determine the need for a particular drug, its dosage, route of administration, and response.

Level of Growth and Development

The maturity of body subsystems at different levels of growth and development plays a role in the individu-

al's ability to metabolize, utilize, and excrete medications, and influences the response of body tissues to them. Those individuals at either end of the growth and development continuum are generally least able to detoxify, concentrate, dilute, metabolize, and excrete drugs.

Rapid tissue growth, subsystem immaturity, and increased metabolism account for these factors in the young child, while tissue loss, degeneration, and decreased metabolism are responsible in the older adult. Pregnancy is another developmental state which influences drug administration. Many drugs pass over the placental barrier and have a direct influence on the developing fetus. In addition, maternal hemodynamics and metabolism are altered during pregnancy, resulting in changes in drug concentration administered and its utilization. For example, the antibiotic tetracyline, when given to a young child or pregnant woman, can affect tooth development in the child or fetus and causes the teeth to be discolored. Frequently, dosages must therefore be adjusted, methods of administration modified, and certain drugs eliminated from use according to the individual's level of growth and development. The nurse makes sure, therefore, that any drug the nurse administers is appropriate in type, dosage, and method of administration for the individual and observes for any reactions which may be related to the level of growth and development.

Nursing assessment related to the effect of an individual's level of growth and development on chemical safety includes descriptions of:

- implications for drug choice
- implications for drug dosage
- implications for method of administration
- implications for drug utilization
- implications concerning response to drug
- relationship between drug restrictions (contraindications) and level of growth and development

State of Health

The individual's state of health influences not only how the body utilizes the medication, but also the type of drug given. Nutritional state, level of debilitation, pathophysiologic processes, activity level, and psychosocial status are all part of the person's state of health. Interferences with the individual's ability to meet basic needs often alters the form and function of the body, thus changing its physiologic response to a drug. Physiologic alterations may result in the drug having effects other than those for which it is intended. Such responses include accumulation, potentiation, synergism, antagonism, and idiosyncratic and allergic reactions. (Chart 16.2, in the section on drug side effects, explains these terms.)

Therefore, the nurse needs to know the intended action of a drug; how it is absorbed, metabolized, and excreted; and the expected response of the individual. This information provides a basis on which the nurse can correlate the person's response to the drug with the person's state of health. To do this, the nurse assesses how the individual's present state of health affects the above drug characteristics, what the individual's actual response to the drug is, and what potential alterations in response can occur as a result of the individual's state of health and any changes in it. For example, if an individual has been receiving fat-soluble vitamin supplements and the individual's diet is changed to one that is fat-free, the individual will not be able to absorb these vitamins from the gastrointestinal tract and thus their therapeutic action will be lost.

The type of medication ordered is a direct reflection of the individual's specific state of health. When the individual's body is not producing sufficient amounts of a vital substance such as hormones or cannot compensate for losses, the individual will need medications to replace these deficiencies. Pathophysiologic processes which alter body tissue, responses, and function are often treated with a medication that helps to reverse or counteract those changes. These drugs may produce such action as dilation or constriction of tissue, stimulation or depression of responses, concentration or dilution of body fluids, and inhibition or acceleration of reactions. Biologic or chemical agents which invade the body tissues can be destroyed, inhibited, precipitated, or counteracted by drugs. Drugs are also used to reduce (and occasionally support) inflammation, prevent disease states, and diagnose illness. (Chart 16.1 lists major drug categories.) Many of these drugs are multipurpose and may therefore be used in different circumstances to treat various pathophysiologies. For example, aspirin is commonly used as a nonnarcotic ► pain reliever (**analgesic**) but is also a very effective antipyretic agent and anti-inflammatory drug, depending on the circumstances in which it is used.

Nursing assessment of the effect of state of health on chemical safety includes descriptions of:

- individual's state of health
- intended action of drug
- drug absorption, metabolism, and excretion
- expected response of individual to drug
- relationship between present state of health and drug actions
- individual's actual response to drug
- potential alterations or response as a result of health state
- relationship between actual and expected responses

Physiologic Makeup

Other characteristics of the individual which influence drug selection, dosage, and administration include biorhythms, sex, biochemistry, body size, and weight.

BIORHYTHMS

The biorhythms influence the rate at which drugs are absorbed, metabolized, and excreted at various times of the individual's infradian, circadian, and ultradian cycles. (Chapter 23 further explains biorhythms.) The individual's cycle can potentiate or antagonize the effects of a drug. While conclusive research has not been done to determine the exact relationship between biorhythms and drug responses, the nurse, through observation, can often determine cyclic variations in the individual's response to drugs. Noting times when the action of the drug is more or less effective and when reactions and responses occur are some of the ways the nurse can establish profiles on the individual's biorhythms and drug-activity patterns.

SEX

The sex of the individual influences the biochemical interactions of the body, tissue distribution, and, to some degree, body weight and size. These factors in turn directly influence the types of drugs which can be used therapeutically, their dosages, and methods of administration. Individuals must function within a biologic range to survive; however, each individual is at different points within this range at various time. The differences in hormonal concentration in men and women affect these biochemical interactions and thus influence the pharmacologic interactions of chemical agents on body tissues.

SIZE

Since a heavier, larger-framed individual often requires a larger dose of a medication than a lighter, smaller-framed person, body surface area and weight are considered when selecting drugs and their dosages. Currently many drugs are being prescribed in terms of quantity of drug per kilogram of body weight to adjust for differences in body weight and size. Adipose tissue and muscle distribution also play a major role in the method of administration (see Intervention).

The distribution of drugs to body tissues is directly related to the blood supply of that tissue. Since adipose tissue is basically avascular, the more adipose tissue an individual has, the less evenly a medication will be distributed. This can result in drug effects other than those intended.

Nursing assessment related to the effect of physiologic makeup on chemical safety includes descriptions of:

- biorhythm profile of drug responses
- influence of sex on body chemistry
- influence of sex on tissue distribution
- body weight
- body size
- influence of body weight and size on drug actions

Drug Dependency

Many individuals become physiologically and/or psychosocially dependent on drugs. Such drugs range from caffeine to laxatives to narcotic analgesics. Drug dependency is often differentiated into the categories of habituation and addiction. **Habituation** is the process that results from prolonged use of a substance, in which continued use is an involuntary behavioral pattern. Attempts to break this habit create psychosocial and/or physical reactions. **Addiction,** on the other

hand, is the process that occurs when prolonged use of a substance creates a physiologic change of the body tissues. This change necessitates the continued use of the substance for body functioning. Withdrawal of the addictive substance causes severe and, sometimes, even life-threatening physiologic signs and symptoms. Closely related to habituation and addiction is drug tolerance. **Tolerance** is the process that results when increasing amounts of a drug are needed by an individual to produce previous drug responses.

Since some drugs have been identified as more addictive than others, laws have been established to restrict and control the use of these substances. The sale of alcohol and tobacco are controlled by (state) laws which prohibit their sale to "minors," with each state defining the term "minor." The federal government, however, sets the standards for the distribution and sale of controlled substances. **Controlled substances** are those which have potential for addiction. The Comprehensive Drug Abuse Prevention and Control Act of 1970 (also known as the Controlled Substances Act) is the law which currently regulates the production, dispensing, and sale of controlled substances. This act contains five schedules, or classifications, of drugs which rank these substances according to therapeutic applicability and potential for abuse. In addition to these federal standards, individual states may set more stringent regulations, as long as they do not violate federal laws.

Individuals who are drug dependent require special consideration in the selection and administration of medications. Certain drugs may need to be eliminated from use by these individuals and/or dosages adjusted. This is necessary because the drug on which the individual is dependent may interfere with or potentiate the actions of other drugs. In addition, if the dependent drug is to be used therapeutically, it is often necessary to increase doses to compensate for an acquired tolerance.

As a result of social attitudes and mores, many people are reluctant to freely discuss drug dependency within the health care system. Through careful observation and assessment, the nurse can often determine individual drug dependency and tolerance. Frequently, individuals who are maintaining their usual intake of the dependent substance may not exhibit any unexpected signs or symptoms. However, on withdrawal of the dependent substance, they will display increasing signs and symptoms of discomfort. The exact signs and symptoms will vary according to the specific substances and degree of dependency. By

Chart 16.1
Major Drug Categories

CATEGORY	GENERAL ACTION	EXAMPLES
Acidifiers	Decrease pH of body fluids; used especially in urinary tract diseases.	Ammonium chloride, hydrochloric acid
Alkalinizers	Increase pH of body fluids.	Sodium chloride
Antacids	Neutralize acid in gastrointestinal tract.	Aluminum hydroxide, milk of magnesia
Antiarrhythmics	Regulate cardiac impulses.	Lidocaine hydrochloride, procainamide hydrochloride, quinidine
Antibacterials	Inhibit or destroy the growth of bacterial organisms.	Antibiotics, e.g., penicillin; sulfanomides, e.g., sulfisoxazole
Anticoagulants	Increase clotting time of blood.	Warfarin, heparin.
Antidepressants	Reduce depression by acting on the central nervous system.	Monoamine oxidase inhibitors, e.g., isocarboxazide; tricyclics, e.g., imipramine hydrochloride
Antiemetic	Reduce nausea and vomiting.	Trimethobenzamide
Antihistamine	Reduce allergic response.	Diphenhydramine hydrochloride, promethazine hydrochloride
Antihypertensive	Reduce blood pressure primarily by acting on autonomic and/or central nervous system.	Sympathetic nervous system, e.g., reserpine; vascular smooth muscle, e.g., hydralazine hydrochloride
Anti-inflammatory	Reduce inflammatory response.	Corticosteroids, aspirin
Antineoplastics	Limit aberrant cellular growth through a variety of actions, depending on type of neoplasm.	Alkylating agents, e.g., chlorambucil; folic acid antagonizer, e.g., methotrexate
Antitussives	Decrease cough reflex and/or liquify respiratory secretions.	Terpin hydrate, glycerol guaiacolate
Cardiotonics	Strengthen cardiac contractions.	Digitalis
Cathartics/laxatives	Prevent or treat constipation through a variety of actions (Chap. 20).	Milk of magnesia, dioctyl sodium sulfosuccinate
Central nervous system depressants	Reduce activity of central nervous system; include many subcategories such as analgesics, anesthetics, antispasmodics, anticonvulsants, sedatives, and tranquilizers.	Analgesic, e.g., meperidine hydrochloride; anesthetic, e.g., sodium pentothal; anticonvulsant, e.g., phenobarbital; antispasmodic, e.g., methocarbamol; sedative, e.g., secobarbital; tranquilizers, e.g., diazepam
Central nervous system stimulants	Increase activity of central nervous system.	Amphetamine sulfate, caffeine
Diagnostic agents	Diagnose pathophysiologic processes.	Lopanoic acid, iodine 131; a wide variety of chemical agents, such as dyes and radioactive tracers

(continued)

Chart 16.1 (Cont.)
Major Drug Categories

CATEGORY	GENERAL ACTION	EXAMPLES
Diuretics	Increase excretion of fluid and electrolytes.	Thiazides, e.g., hydrochlorothiazide; mercurials, e.g., meralluride; miscellaneous, e.g., furosemide
Electrolytes	Supplement and replace electrolytes lost.	Potassium chloride, sodium chloride
Emetics	Promote vomiting to expel toxic substances from the stomach.	Ipecac, apomorphine hydrochloride
Enzymes	Supplement and replace enzymes which have been lost.	Pancreatin, pepsin, bile salts
Hormones	Supplement or replace hormones lost, or treat hormone-related pathophysiologies; may also be used to alter menstrual cycles for birth control.	Androgens, estrogen, insulin, thyroid hormone, adrenalin, cortisone
Local anesthetics	Act on peripheral nervous system to block innervation.	Lidocaine
Minerals	Supplement and replace minerals lost.	Iron, calcium, zinc
Nutrient supplements	Supplement and replace lost nutrients such as proteins, carbohydrates, and fats.	Sustagen, Vivonex, Meritine
Parasympatholytics (cholinergic blocking agents)	Depress the parasympathetic and stimulate the sympathetic nervous system.	Atropine sulfate, scopolamine, propantheline bromide
Parasympathomimetics (cholinergic agents)	Stimulate the parasympathetic and depress the sympathetic nervous system.	Bethanechol chloride, neostigmine bromide
Prophylactic agents	Any drug used to prevent a condition or pathophysiologic state.	Vaccines, antibiotics, oral contraceptives, Rhogam, gamma globulin
Sympatholytics	Depress the sympathetic and stimulate the parasympathetic nervous system.	Phentolamine, ergot extract, methyldopa
Sympathomimetics (adrenergic agents)	Stimulate the sympathetic and depress the parasympathetic nervous system.	Epinephrine, angiotensin amide, levarterenol bitartrate
Urinary antiseptics	Inhibit and destroy urinary tract bacteria.	Mandelic acid, methenamine-mandelate
Vitamins	Supplement and replace vitamins lost.	Vitamins B_{12}, C, and K

establishing a therapeutic relationship with the individual, the nurse frequently gains the individual's confidence and can thus obtain information about and insights into the dependency that assist the nurse in gathering a more complete and accurate assessment.

Nursing assessment related to the effects of drug dependency on chemical safety includes descriptions of:

- type of dependency
- degree of dependency
- signs and symptoms of dependency or withdrawal
- relationship of dependency to drug selection and dosage
- individual's attitude toward dependency
- individual's level of knowledge about dependency

Drug Characteristics and Individual Response

The second major area of nursing assessment in relation to chemical safety is assessing the drug itself and correlating the individual's actual response to it with the intended response.

CATEGORIES OF DRUG NAMES

Drugs are usually referred to by a variety of names. Each name category provides information about the drug. The **chemical name** of a drug identifies its chemical structure and composition. Once a drug has been developed, it is given a **generic name** which commonly reflects some aspect of its chemical composition. The generic name is within the public domain and can be utilized by anyone in referring to that drug.

When the drug has been recognized and approved by the Federal Food and Drug Administration and listed in the *United States Pharmacopeia* (U.S.P.) and/or the *National Formulary* (N.F.), it is assigned an **official name,** which is most frequently the same as the generic name. The U.S.P. and the N.F. are the official references which contain the standards for drugs in the United States.

In addition to the above-mentioned names, the company which develops the drug registers it under its **proprietary name** (trade or brand name). The use of this proprietary name is allowed under law only in reference to that specific company's product. Proprietary names are designated by the symbol ®, signifying brand name registration. The following example presents the various names of one drug:

- *chemical name:* 4 hydroxyacetanilide
- *generic name:* acetaminophen
- *official name:* acetaminophen
- *proprietary names:* Tylenol®, Tempra®, Liquiprin®, Datril®

CLINICAL USE OF DRUG

The first aspect of assessment is identifying the clinical use of the drug. As previously discussed, drugs have many uses, and identification of the intended use of the drug helps in determining its effectiveness with the individual. The *action* of the drug is the particular cellular activity produced by the drug to bring about the intended response. The action is often described in terms of whether it is local or systemic and the type of action produced in the target cells, such as depression or stimulation of cellular activity.

DOSAGE

Assessment of the dosage of the drug ordered is necessary to determine its appropriateness for the individual. The **therapeutic dosage** of a drug is one which will produce the desired action with the least amount of drug. Since there are variations among individuals, safe dosage ranges for most drugs have been ascertained. However, as each person is unique, a safe dose for one individual may be toxic or lethal for another even within these established ranges. A **toxic dose** is one which causes physical, physiologic, or psychosocial damage to the person; a **lethal dose** is one which will most likely result in the individual's death.

METHOD OF ABSORPTION

The nurse also looks at the method of absorption of the drug. *Absorption* is the process of drug movement from the point of administration until it reaches the bloodstream. This process is influenced by the route through which the drug is administered, the solubility of the drug, the ability of the drug to cross cell membranes, and the function of the tissue through which it must pass.

DISTRIBUTION

The *distribution,* of a drug, also assessed by the nurse, refers to the drug's transport from entry into the bloodstream until it arrives at the target cells. The degree of vascularity, pumping action of the heart, and the function of the tissue surrounding the target cells are all factors affecting drug distribution.

DRUG METABOLISM

The nurse assesses too the method of drug *metabolism,* which is the breakdown of a drug into its component parts for ease of excretion. The most common site of drug metabolism is the liver. The drug may be partially or completely broken down or it may be excreted unchanged. If the liver is damaged, it will not be able to adequately break down (detoxify) the drug. In addition, if drug degrading enzymes are decreased or absent, or if cardiovascular or renal disease is present, drug metabolism is hindered.

DRUG EXCRETION

Another factor for nursing assessment is drug excretion, i.e., the elimination of a drug from the body through one of the excretory systems. The renal system is the most common route of drug excretion. However, the lungs, gastrointestinal tract, salivary and sweat glands, and nursing mother's milk are other such routes. Any interference with these systems results in impaired excretion of drugs.

Assessment of the absorption, distribution, metabolism, and excretion of a drug helps the nurse determine the safety of the drug for the individual, potential interferences with the drug action, hazards to the individual's health, and possible rationales for the individual's responses to the medication.

SIDE EFFECTS

Beneficial effects may be derived from a drug other than those for which it is primarily given. Often

these side effects may make the drug the one of choice over a similar drug which does not have these similar actions. For example, an analgesic which not only relieves pain, but which also has a concurrent sedative effect, may be chosen over an analgesic without the additional relaxing effect. However, at times these same side effects may be undesirable. If, for instance, the individual needs to maintain alertness, the analgesic without a sedative would then be the drug of choice.

Drugs may also have side effects that are undesirable at any time. These are known as *untoward effects* or *reactions.* Untoward effects may range from temporary discomfort to long-term or permanent damage to tissues. The more severe untoward effects are often termed *toxic* effects. Common untoward effects are nausea, vomiting, skin rashes, diarrhea, constipation, and dizziness. Common toxic effects include respiratory depression, anaphalactic shock, hepatic and renal damage, and blood *dyscrasias* (an alteration in the type or amount of blood components).

Idiosyncratic reactions are also possible. These reactions are individual responses to medications which cannot be predicted in advance of the administration of the drug. A common idiosyncratic reaction is the production of a response opposite the intended one.

Frequently a drug is given in combination with other drugs, and often they interact with one another, producing responses different from the usual expected effect of each. These resultant responses may be desirable or untoward. Chart 16.2 lists some common terms used to describe interaction responses. In addition, certain drugs may interact with foods to produce undesirable responses (Chart 16.3).

The predictable effects of some drugs in certain conditions necessitate their elimination when these conditions are present. Whenever a specific circumstance or condition restricts or limits the use of a drug, it is said to be *contraindicated.* Pregnancy; periods of rapid tissue growth or regeneration; organ damage, particularly interferences with liver or kidney function; vascular insufficiencies; and immaturity of body subsystems are common causes for the contraindication of drugs.

NURSING IMPLICATIONS

The nurse assesses all these drug characteristics to determine the safety of the specific drug for the in-

Chart 16.2
Terminology for Common Drug Interactions

TERM	DESCRIPTION	TERM	DESCRIPTION
Additive effect	Use of two or more drugs to produce an effect greater than either drug by itself.	Inhibition (blocking effect)	When one drug interferes with another's action or its absorption, distribution, metabolism, or excretion.
Allergic response	Individual sensitivity to a drug or combination of drugs.	Potentiation	When one drug acts as a catalyst to increase the effect of another.
Antagonism	Use of one drug interferes with or counteracts the effect of another drug.	Synergism	A cooperative interaction between two or more drugs to produce the desired effects.
Cumulative effect	The buildup of a drug within the body; usually occurs when one dose of a drug is not metabolized or excreted before the next dose is given.		

Chart 16.3
Commonly Used Drugs with Nutritional Implications

DRUG	POTENTIAL NUTRIENT INTERFERENCE	SIDE EFFECTS WITH NUTRITIONAL IMPLICATIONS
Adrenal corticosteroids	Vitamins C, A, D; folic acid, pyridoxine, calcium, potassium, zinc	Gastric inflammation; may produce ulcers
Antibiotics		
Chloramphenicol	Folic acid, pyridoxine, riboflavin, vitamins B_{12}, A; iron	Aplastic and hypoplastic anemia, nausea, vomiting, diarrhea may occur; glossitis and stomatitis
Erythromycin		Inhibits protein synthesis; gastrointestinal discomfort, cramping. Nausea, vomiting, and diarrhea occur occasionally. May form salts with acids—avoid orange, lemon, cranberry juices and other acid drinks.
Neomycin	Vitamins B_{12}, A; iron, calcium, potassium	Glossitis, stomatitis, nausea, vomiting, diarrhea. May produce malabsorption with increased fecal fat.
Penicillin	Potassium	Nausea, vomiting, occasionally hemolytic anemia
Tetracycline	Vitamins C, K; folic acid, riboflavin, calcium, zinc, magnesium	If used during tooth development may cause permanent staining. May cause increased blood urea nitrogen, anorexia, nausea, vomiting, diarrhea, glossitis, dysphagia, hemolytic anemia. Should not be taken with milk, since calcium impairs absorption.
Anticoagulants (coumarin derivatives)	Vitamin K, alcohol	Gastrointestinal bleeding, nausea, vomiting, diarrhea
Anticonvulsants (phenobarbital)	Folic acid, pyridoxine, vitamins B_{12}, D, K; calcium	Nausea, megaloblastic anemia

(continued)

Chart 16.3 (Cont.)
Commonly Used Drugs with Nutritional Implications

DRUG	POTENTIAL NUTRIENT INTERFERENCE	SIDE EFFECTS WITH NUTRITIONAL IMPLICATIONS
Antidepressants (monoamine oxidase inhibitors) Phenelzine Tranylcypromine		Foods high in tyramine should be avoided as they may precipitate a hypertensive crisis. Foods to avoid: aged cheddar cheese, alcohol, yogurt, sour cream, yeast, bananas, broad beans, canned figs, raisins, chicken liver, chocolate, cola, coffee, tea, pickled herring, licorice
Antihypertensives, diuretics Chlorothiazide	Pyridoxine, riboflavin, zinc, potassium, sodium	Fluid and electrolyte imbalance
Furosemide Hydralazine		Fluid and electrolyte imbalance Anorexia, nausea, vomiting, diarrhea, constipation, reduction in hemoglobin
Antilipemic agents Cholestyramine	Vitamins A, B_{12}, D, K; calcium, iron	Binds bile acids; may interfere with normal fat absorption. Constipation, flatulence, nausea, diarrhea
Clofibrate	Vitamins A, B_{12}; iron	Nausea, diarrhea, vomiting, anemia
Cardiac glycosides (digitalis)	Calcium, magnesium	Nausea, vomiting
Levodopa	Vitamin C, pyridoxine, potassium	Drug effectiveness decreased by increased intakes of protein. Anorexia, nausea, vomiting, burning sensation of the tongue, bitter taste
Uricosuric agents Allopurinol	Riboflavin, calcium, magnesium, potassium	Increased fluid intake is desirable. Nausea, vomiting, diarrhea
Probenecid		Anorexia, nausea, vomiting, anemia

From: Rosanne B. Howard and Nancie H. Herbold. Nutrition and Clinical Care. New York, McGraw-Hill, 1978, p. 288.

dividual's use. Instances where the nurse notes possible chemical safety hazards require that the nurse be particularly alert to the implications of administering these drugs. It is necessary for the nurse to refer to resources such as current pharmacology textbooks, drug inserts, the *Physician's Desk Reference,* and the *Hospital Formulary* to be knowledgeable about the many drugs available.

Nursing assessment related to the effects of drug characteristics on chemical safety includes descriptions of:

- clinical use of drug
- drug action identified in individual
- method of drug action, absorption, distribution, metabolism, and excretion

- actual or potential interferences with drug action, absorption, distribution, metabolism, and excretion
- appropriateness of drug dosage ordered
- side effects of drug (beneficial, untoward, toxic)
- known idiosyncratic reactions of individual to drugs
- known sensitivity of individual to drug
- drug interaction
- drug–food interaction
- contraindications of drug
- relationship of contraindications to health state

Other Aspects of Chemical Safety

The nurse's assessment of the individual for chemical safety also includes the individual's level of knowledge and attitudes toward drug use, present and past history of drug use, exposure to other potentially dangerous chemical agents, and knowledge about the uses and abuses of these agents.

ATTITUDES TOWARD DRUG USE

The simple prescription of a drug does not imply that the individual will take the drug properly or even take it at all. The nurse therefore assesses the individual's attitudes toward the use of drugs, their social and cultural ramifications, the relevancy of the drug or the intended response of the individual, and the individual's level of knowledge concerning the drug, dosage, route, and time of administration. The assessment of these factors assists the nurse to intervene most effectively to insure safe self-administration of drugs. (Illustration 16.2)

HISTORY OF DRUG USE

By ascertaining the individual's past and present history of using both prescription and nonprescription drugs, the nurse can recognize potential safety hazards and anticipate possible untoward drug interactions. Many people today rely on frequent use of over-the-counter drugs for relief of daily discomforts and may become dependent on them over time. In addition, individuals may attempt to relieve symptoms of potentially serious pathologies with such drugs and may not seek appropriate health care. Therefore, identification of drug use patterns aids the

nurse in case finding, dependency prevention, and diagnosis of negative health behaviors.

CHEMICAL AGENTS IN THE ENVIRONMENT

A large variety of chemical agents surrounds us not only in the institutional setting but also in the home. The nurse needs to be aware of these agents and their potential effects on people. The nurse assesses the individual's use and storage of chemical agents. Drugs kept in the home, cleaning agents, paint, paint removers, bleach, and other common household substances are potentially lethal when improperly used. Young children are particularly prone to accidental poisoning when chemical agents are not properly stored. A more detailed discussion of this aspect of chemical safety is on pages 382–384.

Nursing assessment of general chemical safety includes descriptions of:

- level of knowledge about drug use
- attitudes toward drug use
- past and present drug history—prescription and nonprescription drugs
- exposure to chemical agents
- manner of using and storing chemical agents
- potential hazards posed by chemical agents in the environment
- knowledge about threats to health by chemical agents

PLANNING

In planning to meet chemical safety needs, the nurse correlates the assessment done of the individual's needs, the physician's orders, and the nurse's knowledge of the medication. Scheduling the administration of medication and the strategies for teaching the individual and family and/or significant others are also included in the planning phase. The plan for administering medications is influenced by the route by which the medication is to be given, its interactions with foods and other drugs, other therapies ordered,

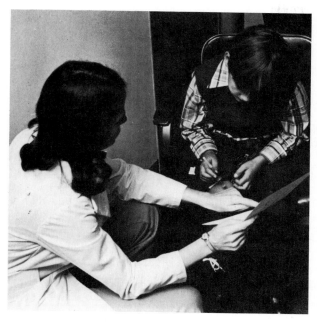

Illustration 16.2
When teaching an individual to administer his own medications at home, the nurse takes into account the person's level of growth and development and how much knowledge he has about drugs and their use. *(Photo © Bob Adelman)*

the individual's physical, physiologic, and psychosocial status, and activities that have to be carried out prior to and concurrently with drug administration.

Time Schedule for Administration

Some drugs are ordered with specific time intervals between administrations, while others are ordered to be given as needed (within a safe time span). When a drug is ordered as needed (p.r.n. order), the nurse needs to know the purpose of the drug (e.g., for abdominal pain, to induce sleep), its relationship to the other drugs the individual is receiving, how the individual communicates a need for the medication, and how this drug can best be utilized to maximize its benefits. For example, if the individual has an order for an antiemetic p.r.n., the nurse finds out the individual's pattern of nausea and vomiting, the relationship of activities such as eating to the nausea and vomiting, the person's previous responses to the antiemetic drug, and the individual's attitude toward both the nausea and vomiting and the medication. Once this information is collected, the nurse can best plan the times to give the medication.

Knowledge of Drug

A thorough knowledge of the drug itself is also necessary to plan for administration. Important information includes such factors as the relationship of the medication to a full or empty stomach, contraindications, the expected dose range, the expected response, and precautions needed before and after administration (e.g., if the drug makes individual drowsy, side rails may have to be raised after administration). Many medications require preadministration activities. Frequently, vital signs must be checked prior to giving a drug to assure they are within safe ranges. Lab values may need to be assessed to determine whether or not a drug is to be given.

Ascertaining Availability of Drugs and Other Supplies

The nurse ascertains the availability of the drug in its proper form and dose prior to time of administration, availability of supplies to give it with, and the presence of medications to be given concurrently. This prevents delay in administration of needed drugs. Delays not only waste the nurse's time, but also often result in the individual's discomfort and alter blood levels of medications. In addition, delays may alter the scheduling of subsequent drugs and treatments. For example, if an individual is to receive a tracer dye 2 hours before a diagnostic test and the drug is not available at this time, the test may have to be cancelled.

Checking Accuracy of Drug Order

Before administering any drug, the nurse checks the accuracy of the drug order. All drug orders must state clearly the name of the drug, the exact dosage, the route of administration, and time intervals for administration. In addition, some orders give specific instructions for situations when a drug should or should not be given. For example, the order may say do not give if apical pulse is below 60 beats per minute. Figure 16.2 shows an example of a properly written medication order. Incomplete or unclear drug orders are validated and rewritten prior to the drug's administration. Telephone orders are not acceptable. All medication orders are written except in situations of extreme emergency. Even in those situations the

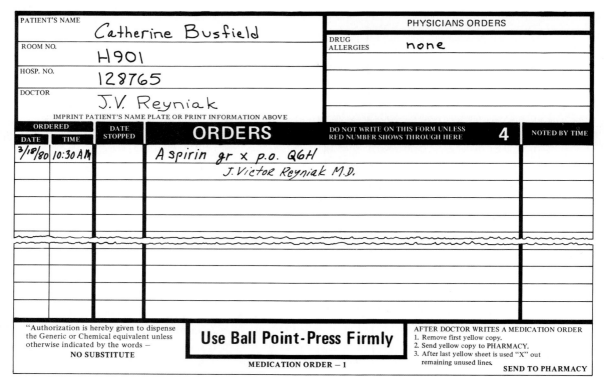

PATIENT'S NAME	Catherine Busfield	PHYSICIANS ORDERS	
ROOM NO.	H 901	DRUG ALLERGIES	none
HOSP. NO.	128765		
DOCTOR	J. V. Reyniak		

IMPRINT PATIENT'S NAME PLATE OR PRINT INFORMATION ABOVE

ORDERED		DATE STOPPED	ORDERS	DO NOT WRITE ON THIS FORM UNLESS RED NUMBER SHOWS THROUGH HERE	4	NOTED BY TIME
DATE	TIME					
3/18/80	10:30 AM		Aspirin gr x p.o. Q6H			
			J. Victor Reyniak M.D.			

"Authorization is hereby given to dispense the Generic or Chemical equivalent unless otherwise indicated by the words — **NO SUBSTITUTE**

Use Ball Point-Press Firmly

MEDICATION ORDER — 1

AFTER DOCTOR WRITES A MEDICATION ORDER
1. Remove first yellow copy.
2. Send yellow copy to PHARMACY.
3. After last yellow sheet is used "X" out remaining unused lines.
SEND TO PHARMACY

Figure 16.2

Medication order. Specific, accurate medication orders help to ensure chemical safety in an individual's care.

order must be written as soon as possible after the emergency situation is over.

In many agencies, physician's orders are transmitted to medication cards, medication Kardexes, or medication sheets. Figures 16.3–16.5 give examples of a medication sheet and a medication card. Regardless of the method used, the nurse administering medications is also responsible for comparing the medication sheet, card, or Kardex with the physician's orders for accuracy. This process helps eliminate errors that may have been made in transcribing the orders from the original source.

Preparing to Teach Safety

When it is necessary to teach the individual and family and/or significant others about the administration of medications or other facets of chemical safety, the nurse plans for the time and equipment necessary to do this teaching. Having all the needed supplies readily available and set up for teaching facilitates the process and prevents the loss of teaching opportunities. Teaching chemical safety is described on page 381.

INTERVENTION

Once the nurse is fully informed about a drug and its implications, and has ascertained the accuracy of the order and determined the individual's need, the nurse is ready to prepare and administer the medication. A variety of administration setups exist for preparing and giving medications. Medications may be prepared in a medication room and distributed via a tray or cart or prepared directly from a rolling cart which is taken to the bedside. Two major categories of preparation systems are used: stock medications and unit dose. In the stock medication systems, all medications are kept in multidose containers from which

BROOKLYN EYE & EAR HOSPITAL
BROOKLYN, N.Y. 11238
MEDICATION RECORD

1. Allow sufficient space between items to provide a blank line for each administration in the 24-hour-period.
2. Indicate "A.M." or "P.M." after the time.
3. At the end of 7 days draw a line under the last entry and redate on the next line.
4. Record pertinent reactions to medication on the "Nurses Note."

Case No. _123765_

Name _Catherine Busfield_   Admitted _3/17_ 19 _80_ Ward _H901_

Medication	DATE 3/18/80 Time—Init.	DATE Time—Init.	DATE Time—Init.	DATE Time—Init	DATE Time—Init.	DATE Time—Init.	DATE Time—Init.
Aspirin gr X̄ p.o. Q6H	12N DFK						
	6p E.L.B.						
	12m						
	6A						
DFK - Dawn F. Kilts							
E.L.B - Esther L. Brill							

MEDICATION RECORD (OVER)

Figure 16.3
The medication record provides a clear picture of drug dosages that have been administered to a particular individual.

all individuals medications are taken. Stock medications are usually kept in a locked cabinet. The unit dose system may be of two types. With the first type, each individual has his or her own containers of medication from which specific doses are taken, while with the second type, each individual has his or her own supply of individually wrapped single dose medications. Rolling carts are usually used for unit-dose administration. Each individual has a drawer in the cart. (Illustrations 16.3 and 16.4)

Routes of Administration

Medications may be administered by the oral route, intramuscularly, subcutaneously, intradermally, in-

10-15
NAME _John Smith_
ROOM _1032_
DRUG _Mandelamine_
DOSE _1 GM. P.O._
TIME _q6° 12-6, 12-6_

Figure 16.4
Medication card. *(Courtesy of The Brooklyn Hospital)*

N.S. 42							
DATE	MEDICATION	TIME	DISC.	DATE	MEDICATION	TIME	DISC.
10/15	Mandelamine 1 GM	12-6					
	p.o. Q6H	12-6					

NAME:	HOSP. #:	DOCTOR:	SERVICE:
Smith, John	48-19-27	J. McCarron	Urology

Figure 16.5
Medication Kardex. *(Courtesy of The Brooklyn Hospital)*

travenously, topically, and directly into a body cavity or organ either through inhalation, instillation, or application. The route of administration is determined by the way the drug is absorbed, the speed of action desired, the health state of the individual, and the ease of administration. Some drugs cannot be absorbed from the gastrointestinal tract or are destroyed by the digestive juices. Therefore, these drugs must be administered parenterally (any method other than through the gastrointestinal tract). On the other hand, some medications are more readily absorbed from the gastrointestinal tract or cannot be chemically prepared for administration through other routes.

Since systemic drugs must enter the bloodstream to reach target sites, direct entry into the bloodstream (**intravenous**) is the fastest route. The **intramuscular** route (injection of substances into muscular tissue) is the next most rapid route. Instillation, inhalation, or application of medications directly on vascular mucous membranes (e.g., the **sublingual** route—under the tongue) has a similarly rapid action. **Subcutaneous** administration (injection of substances into subcutaneous tissue) requires more absorption time than either intramuscular or intravenous administration, since the medication has to travel further to the bloodstream. **Intradermal** (administration of substances into the dermal layer of the skin) is the slowest route of parenteral administration and is most commonly used for diagnostic testing rather than for drug administration.

The oral route is a relatively slow route of administration, but absorption time depends on the amount of food in the stomach, the type of protective coating on the medication, the effectiveness of digestive juices, and the overall functioning of the digestive tract. The greater the amount of food in the stomach, the longer the absorption time. Liquid medications are more quickly absorbed than solid medications, while enterically coated medications are only slightly broken down in the stomach and must reach the intestines before absorption can take place. An alteration or decrease in digestive juices or gastrointestinal functioning will speed or slow the absorption of the medication, depending on the direction of the change.

While topical medications will eventually enter the bloodstream, they are usually applied for their actions on local tissues. Administration of medications directly into an organ or body cavity may take place through either instillation, application, or inhalation. ▶ **Instillation** is the administration of liquid medication through a tube, catheter, or syringe (Charts 16.4,

16.5, 16.6). This is commonly used for the bladder, ▶ ears and eyes, or the abdominal or pelvic cavity. **Inhalation** is the breathing in of a vapor containing a medication. The medication may be added as a liquid to a vaporizer and then converted into a vapor or may come prepared as a vapor. Medications may be applied directly onto body tissue in the form of suppositories, ointments, or creams. *Suppositories* are drugs mixed with a base which melts or dissolves at body temperature and are shaped for insertion into

---

Chart 16.4
Instillation of Eyedrops

PROCEDURE	POINTS TO NOTE
Check orders for drug, dosage, site, and time of administration.	Provides necessary information for preparing medication; prevents error.

Assemble equipment:
  medication card
  eyedrops
  gauze pads or absorbent tissues.
	Allows for orderly and organized procedure.

Identify individual.	Prevents medication error.
Ask individual to hyperextend neck and roll back eyes.	Places eye in proper position for instillation of drug and avoids damage to cornea of the eye.
With nondominant hand retract lower eyelid with gauze pad or tissue so that conjunctival sac is exposed.	Creates space for instillation of medication; gauze pad or tissue prevents damage to eyelid and eye and decreases chance for contamination by fingers.
Grasp eye dropper in dominant hand and position surface of hand across bridge of individual's nose so that dropper is directed toward designated eye.	Steadies hand for instillation and encourages upward gaze of individual; protects cornea and prevents corneal reflex.
Instruct individual to look up.	Prevents corneal reflex and damage.
Instill desired number of drops in designated eye into conjunctival sac without touching any eye surface with dropper.	Prevents contamination of eye and eyedropper for future use.
Instruct individual to close and rotate eye in a full circle.	Evenly distributes medication over eye surface.
Blot excess medication with clean gauze or tissue.	Prevents irritation of tissue and increases individual's level of comfort; blot from inner to outer canthus to prevent contamination of lacrimal duct.
Reposition individual comfortably.	Increases feelings of well-being.
Record.	Provides accurate record of procedure.

Chart 16.5
Instillation of Nose Drops

PROCEDURE	POINTS TO NOTE
Check orders for drug, dosage, site, and time of administration.	Provides necessary information for preparing medication; prevents error.

Assemble equipment:
    medication card
    nose drops
    gauze pads or absorbent tissue.
	Allows for orderly and organized procedure.

Identify individual.	Prevents medication error.
Ask individual to hyperextend neck.	Places nasal canal in proper position for instillation and distribution of medication.
Instruct individual to breathe through mouth.	Prevents direct inhalation of medication; decreases amount of medication swallowed.
Instill appropriate number of nose drops into designated nostril without touching dropper to nares.	Prevents contamination of dropper for future use.
Instruct individual to maintain position for approximately 5 minutes without blowing nose.	Provides for distribution and absorption of medication; supports such as pillows are provided to prevent fatigue and discomfort.
Blot any excess medication with gauze or tissue.	Prevents irritation of tissue and increases feelings of well-being.
Reposition individual comfortably.	Increases feelings of well-being.
Record.	Provides accurate record of procedure.

Chart 16.6
Instillation of Ear Drops

PROCEDURE	POINTS TO NOTE
Check orders for drug, dosage, site, and time of administration.	Provides necessary information for preparing medication; prevents error.

Assemble equipment:
    medication card
    ear drops
    gauze pads or absorbent tissues.
	Allows for orderly and organized procedure.

Identify individual.	Prevents medication error.
Position individual with designated ear in upward direction.	Places ear in proper position for instillation of drug.
Expose external ear canal by: for preschooler and older, firmly grasping middle of auricle of ear (pinna) and pulling it in an upward and backward direction; for toddler and younger, firmly grasping middle of auricle of ear and pulling in a backward direction.	Straightens ear canal and prevents damage to ear canal.

(continued)

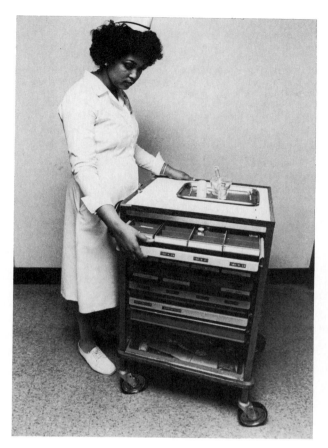

Illustration 16.3
There are many types of setups for administering
drugs in the institutional setting. In the cart shown
above, there is a labeled compartment for each individual, where unit doses can be stored. A unit
dose would then be prepared at bedside. *(Photo
© Leonard Speier)*

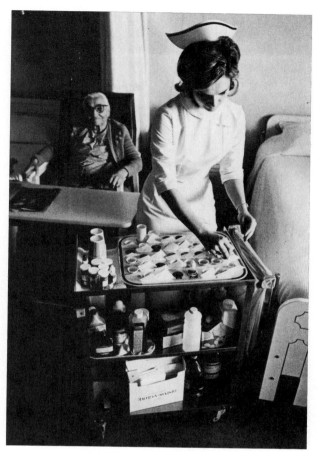

Illustration 16.4
The nurse is using a rolling cart to administer
medications at the bedside. *(Photo by Jean-Pierre
Ragot, from Stock, Boston)*

Chart 16.6 (Cont.)
Instillation of Ear Drops

PROCEDURE	POINTS TO NOTE
Insert dropper at opening of external canal.	Positions dropper for instillation of medication.
Instill appropriate number of drops into external canal without touching to ear surface.	Prevents contamination of ear and dropper and prevents damage to sensitive ear canal tissue.
Blot away excess medication with gauze or tissue.	Prevents irritation of canal tissue and increases individual's level of comfort.
Instruct individual to refrain from turning designated ear in downward direction for approximately 5 minutes.	Provides for distribution and absorption of medication.
Reposition individual comfortably.	Increases feelings of well-being.
Record.	Provides accurate record of procedure.

Chart 16.7
Major Medication Forms

FORM	DESCRIPTION
Capsule	Gelatinous shell containing powdered medications. Given orally
Liquid	A solution, emulsion, or suspension of medication in a fluid form. Used for all routes of administration, depending on type of substance and condition under which it is prepared
Ointment	Medication mixed with spreadable base for topical application
Powder	Crystallized or ground medication which dissolves in a liquid, usually sterile water or normal saline, for parenteral administration. May be directly applied topically
Tablet	Compressed or molded powders. Used orally or dissolved in liquid for instillation.

an orifice. Common suppository routes are rectal, vaginal, and urethral. Absorption by these routes is comparatively slow because of the surface conditions of these areas. Chart 16.7 describes various forms of medications.

Choice of Site

When administering drugs by parenteral routes, the site for administration and the size of the needle and syringe must be determined before preparing and administering the medications.

INTRAMUSCULAR INJECTIONS

The sites that are used for intramuscular injections are the mid-deltoid of the arm, the gluteus medius of the buttock, ventrogluteal of the hip, and the vastus lateralis of the thigh. These sites are used because of the presence of relatively large muscles, their ease of accessibility, and the relative distance of major blood vessels, nerves, and bones. The exact site chosen will depend on the amount of medication to be injected, the state of the muscle, and the condition of the skin and underlying tissues. No more than 5 cc of solution can be given at one time in one injection in one site. However, the mid-deltoid areas should not be used for amounts greater than 1 cc.

The age of the individual, muscle tone, and amount of muscle also determine the site. Children below the age of three do not have sufficient muscle development in the gluteal or deltoid muscle groups to withstand injections at these sites. Hence the vastus lateralis is the site of choice for this age group. The area with the greatest amount of intact muscle tissue is the site of choice for individuals with altered muscle size and tone. Muscle areas which have had repeated intramuscular injections or which have been damaged by trauma or pathology cannot be used for injection sites. To prevent trauma to muscle tissue and its breakdown, injection sites are rotated. Recording the exact site of injections provides the information necessary to choose site rotations. Areas where the skin or surrounding tissue is damaged from repeated injection or from other trauma are also avoided to prevent further breakdown or infection. Figure 16.6. A–E shows sites for intramuscular injection.

SUBCUTANEOUS INJECTIONS

Common sites for subcutaneous injections are the outer aspect of the upper arm, the abdominal region between the iliac crests, and the anterior aspect of the thigh. Other areas which can be used are the scapular areas and the inner aspects of the upper arm. Again, the condition of the skin and underlying tissue will determine the exact location for subcutaneous injections. Subcutaneous sites are also rotated. Since the subcutaneous route is used for long-term insulin therapy, it is particularly important not only for the nurse to rotate sites but also for the individuals to do so when administering their own insulin. This can be accomplished by preparing a diagram of all available sites and marking the location of each injection after it is given.

Choice of Needle and Syringe

The size of the syringe used is determined by the amount of medication to be injected. Except when using insulin syringes, syringes should be approximately 1 cc larger than the amount to be given. This

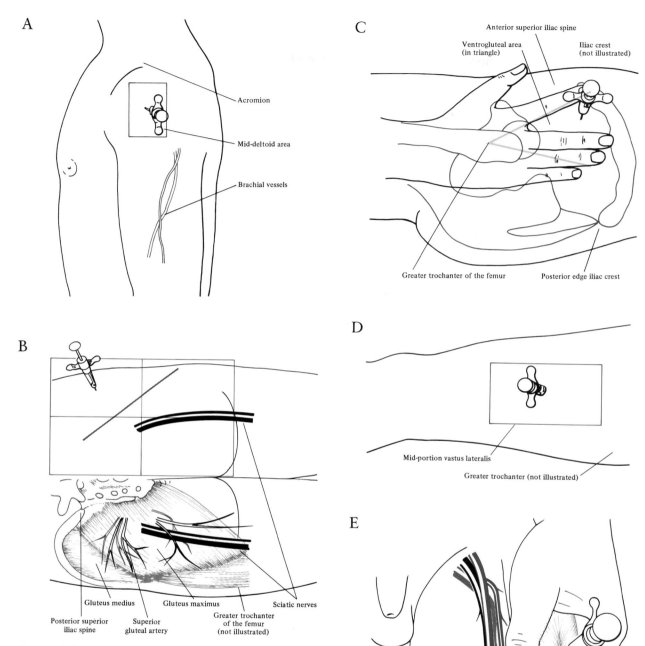

A

Acromion

Mid-deltoid area

Brachial vessels

C

Anterior superior iliac spine

Ventrogluteal area
(in triangle)

Iliac crest
(not illustrated)

Greater trochanter of the femur

Posterior edge iliac crest

B

Gluteus medius

Gluteus maximus

Sciatic nerves

Posterior superior
iliac spine

Superior
gluteal artery

Greater trochanter
of the femur
(not illustrated)

D

Mid-portion vastus lateralis

Greater trochanter (not illustrated)

E

Deep femoral artery

Sciatic nerve

Femoral artery and vein

Rectus femoris
muscle

Vastus lateralis
muscle

Figure 16.6

Sites for Intramuscular injections. **A.** Mid-deltoid site. **B.** Gluteus medius site. **C.** Ventrogluteal site. **D.** Vastus lateralis site (adult). **E.** Vastus lateralis site (infant). *(Courtesy of Wyeth Laboratories, Philadelphia, Pennsylvania)*

allows room for proper aspiration. This is not true for insulin syringes, since they come in only the 1-cc size. The length of the needle is determined by the degree of adipose tissue and the estimated distance between the skin and the interior of the muscle. Needle lengths range from ⅝ to 3 inches. Most commonly, however, needles 2–2½ inches long are used for intramuscular injections for well-nourished adults, and a needle ⅝ inch long for young infants. A ⅝-inch needle is almost always used for subcutaneous injections.

The diameter of the lumen of the needle is called the gauge. Needles range from 18 to 25 gauge. The largest diameter needle is 18 gauge, 25 gauge the smallest. The ideal choice is the smallest gauge which can be used, since the smaller gauges produce less trauma to the tissues. However, it is not always pos-

sible to use a small gauge when administering viscous medications such as penicillin. Therefore, the viscosity of the medication helps determine the gauge to be used. In addition, when a thick medication is forced through a small gauge needle, the pressure with which the medication is injected into the tissue is raised, and the likelihood of tissue damage is increased. Subcutaneous injections are most frequently given with a 25-gauge needle, as viscous medications are not usually given by this route.

Preparation and Administration of Medications

Regardless of the route of medication, certain rules are followed during the preparation and administra-

Chart 16.8
Medication Rules

RULE	RATIONALE
Wash hands before preparing medication.	Prevents contamination of medications, supplies.
Check medication card/sheet/Kardex with physician's orders.	Prevents continuing any errors made in transcribing.
Check and double check medication, dose, route, and time when preparing medication, by comparing medication order with medication container.	Prevents giving the wrong medication with the wrong dose, by the wrong route at the wrong time.
Use medical asepsis to prepare oral medications.	Prevents undue exposure to microorganisms.
Use sterile technique to prepare parenteral medications.	Prevents introduction of microorganisms into body tissue or cavity.
Do not prepare medications that are to be given at different times of the day at the same time.	Medication orders may be changed; person who prepares drugs may not be available to give them; drugs may become contaminated; and cups or syringes holding medications can become mixed up.
Do not prepare medication for someone else to give.	The individual giving medication has no way of validating the accuracy of the medication.
Do not give medications that someone else has prepared.	As above.
Identify individual receiving medication by checking identification or by asking the individual's name or its spelling.	Prevents giving wrong medication to wrong individual. Do not identify individual by asking "Are you Mr. Smith?" Individual may respond yes to voice or person but not to question itself.
Do not leave medications unattended.	Prevents contamination and individual's taking wrong medication.

(continued)

tion of drugs. Chart 16.8 lists these rules and the reasons for them. (Illustration 16.4)

CALCULATIONS

Frequently dose may have to be calculated because the dosage ordered by the physician is not the dosage available. The medication dosage may be known, but the volume to be given may have to be calculated. The general formula for these calculations is outlined in Chart 16.8.

Often medications are ordered in one system of measurement, while the available dose is in another measurement system or within the same system but not the same unit. In order to give the medications, it is necessary to convert to the same type of unit and system. The major systems used are the apothecary, the metric, and the household. Chart 16.9 gives common conversion factors.

PREPARING TABLETS

When preparing tablets from stock containers for oral use, the nurse pours the medication from the container into its cap. The exact number of tablets can be obtained by shifting the tablets back and forth between the container and the cap. The medication cup is not used to count out medication, since it may contain other tablets which may get mixed in with the medication being poured. This method also avoids

---

Chart 16.8 (Cont.)
Medication Rules

RULE	RATIONALE
Do not leave medication at bedside—watch individual actually take medication.	Prevents individual's forgetting, losing, or collecting medication.
Chart medications as soon as they are given.	Prevents repeating of doses, forgetting what has been given; and provides updated records.
Once medications have been poured, do not return them to the storage container; discard them appropriately.	Prevents contamination of medications. Disposing of narcotics should be witnessed.
Return any medication bottles with labels that are torn or illegible to the pharmacy.	Prevents errors in administering.

For determining the volume needed or the number of tablets, capsules, or ampules to use:

$$\frac{\text{Desired dose}}{\text{Available dose}} = \frac{\text{Amount of medication to be used}}{\text{Unit of available dose}}$$

Example:
Physician's order reads:
   Aspirin gr $\bar{x}$ P.O. Q6H
Available dose in stock:
   Aspirin gr V per tablet

Using the formula:
Desired dose   = 10 grains
Available dose   = 5 grains
Amount to be used = unknown
Unit of available dose = 1 tablet
$$\frac{10 \text{ gr}}{5 \text{ gr}} = \frac{x \text{ tablets}}{1 \text{ tablet}}$$
$$5x = 10$$
$$x = 2 \text{ tablets}$$

Example:
Physician's order:
   Demerol 75 mg I.M. Q3-4H p.r.n.
Available dose in stock:
   Demerol 50 mg/cc

Using the formula:
Desired dose   = 75 mg
Available dose   = 50 mg
Amount to be used = unknown
Unit of available dose = 1 cc
$$\frac{75 \text{ mg}}{50 \text{ mg}} = \frac{x \text{ cc}}{1 \text{ cc}}$$
$$50x = 75$$
$$x = 1.5 \text{ cc.}$$

touching the medication by hand. Once the correct number of tablets is in the cap the tablets are shifted from the cap into the medication cup. If a tablet is scored and needs to be divided, it is wrapped in a clean paper towel and briskly snapped apart. Tablets that are not scored can be divided by using tablet files.

PREPARING LIQUIDS

When pouring liquids, the medication cup is held at eye level with calibrations facing the nurse. The bottle is held with the label facing the palm so that the medication doesn't drip down the side and obscure the label. The bottle cap is placed top side

---

Chart 16.9
Most Commonly Used Equivalents

APOTHECARIES'		METRIC		HOUSEHOLD
Weight	Volume	Weight	Volume	
1 grain	1 minim	0.060 g	0.060 ml or cc	1 drop
15 grains	15 minims	1 g	1 ml or cc	15 drops
1 dram (60 grains)	1 fluidram	4 g	4 ml or cc	1 tsp (60 drops)
4 drams	4 fluidrams	15 g	15 ml or cc	1 tbsp
1 ounce	1 fluidounce	30 g	30 ml or cc	
1 pound	12 fluidounces	360 g	360 ml or cc	
	1 pint	500 g	500 ml or cc	
	1 quart	1 Kg	1 L	
	1 gallon	4 Kg	4 L	

APOTHECARIES'	METRIC		APOTHECARIES'	METRIC	
15 grains	=	1000 mg	$1/6$ grain	= 10	mg
10 grains	=	600 mg	$1/10$ grain	= 6	mg
5 grains	=	300 mg	$1/15$ grain	= 4	mg
$1\frac{1}{2}$ grains	=	100 mg	$1/20$ grain	= 3	mg
1 grain	=	60 mg *	$1/30$ grain	= 2	mg
$3/4$ grain	=	45 mg	$1/60$ grain	= 1	mg
$2/3$ grain	=	40 mg	$1/100$ grain	= 0.6	mg
$1/2$ grain	=	30 mg	$1/200$ grain	= 0.3	mg
$3/8$ grain	=	25 mg	$1/250$ grain	= 0.25	mg
$1/3$ grain	=	20 mg	$1/300$ grain	= 0.2	mg
$1/4$ grain	=	15 mg	$1/600$ grain	= 0.1	mg
$1/5$ grain	=	12 mg	$1/1000$ grain	= 0.06	mg

*These fractional apothecaries'–metric dose equivalents are approximate and represent quantities usually prescribed by physicians using one of these systems.

When a medication is prescribed in the metric system, the pharmacist and the nurse may dispense the corresponding equivalent in the apothecaries' system, and vice versa.

However, for prescriptions that require compounding or for converting a pharmaceutical formula from one system to the other, the following fractional equivalents are listed in the *United States Pharmacopeia*:

grains	milligrams	grains	milligrams
1	65	$1/10$	6.5
$3/4$	48.6	$1/20$	3.2
$1/2$	32.4	$1/30$	2.2
$1/4$	16.2	$1/64$	1.0
$1/8$	8.1	$1/100$	0.6

From: George I. Sackhein and Lewis Robins, Programed Mathematics for Nurses. *New York, Macmillan, 1974.*

down to prevent contamination of the inner surface. The liquid is poured until the meniscus reaches the desired calibration. To prevent errors during preparation, medication sheets, cards, and Kardexes are validated several times with the label on the medication container.

ADMINISTERING ORAL MEDICATION

When administering oral medications to the individual, the individual should be in an upright position to facilitate swallowing. The individual's identity is checked before drug administration. The nurse may have the individual take the medication, or if the individual is unable to do so, the nurse places the medication in the person's mouth. Water is given to facilitate swallowing. Since individuals differ in the number of tablets or capsules that they can take at one time, the nurse checks with them for their preferences. Some persons may not be able to take whole tablets or capsules. In such cases, the nurse can crush the tablet or open the capsule and mix it with a compatible fluid such as water or juice. Although it is not desirable to connect food with medicine taking, some persons prefer taking medications with their food. If medications are mixed with foods or fluids, small amounts of food or fluid are used and care is taken to ensure that the whole mixture is ingested.

ADMINISTERING PARENTERAL INJECTIONS

Chart 16.10 outlines the procedure for preparing intramuscular, subcutaneous, and intravenous medications. Figure 16.7 shows the special method of preparing Tubex® cartridges.

Intramuscular Injections

In administering intramuscular injections, the exact anatomic landmarks are ascertained to avoid injuring bone, nerves, or blood vessels. The area selected is fully visible so as to decrease the likelihood of injury.

The nurse can find the correct site for mid-deltoid injections by identifying the acromion process and then moving two finger widths directly below it. Since the width of fingers vary, palpating for the most muscular point immediately below the two fingers further ensures finding the correct site.

The upper outer aspect of the upper outer quad-

rant is used for gluteus medius injections and can be found by sectioning off a buttock into four equal quadrants. To find the exact spot within this quadrant, the nurse locates the iliac crest by palpation and injects the medication 2–3 inches below the iliac crest.

The ventrogluteal site of injection is ascertained

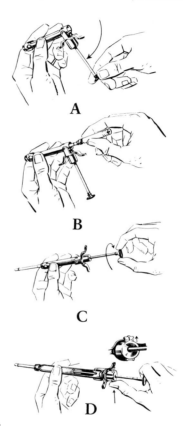

Figure 16.7

Preparing to give an injection. **A.** Grasp barrel of syringe in one hand. With the other hand, pull back firmly on plunger and swing the entire handle section downward so that it locks at a right angle to the barrel. **B.** Insert the needle end of the sterile cartridge-needle unit into the barrel. Rotate the cartridge clockwise until slight clicking sound indicates that the cartridge is threaded into front end of syringe. **C.** Swing plunger back into place and attach end to the threaded shaft of the piston. Hold the metal syringe barrel—not the glass cartridge—with one hand and rotate plunger until both ends of the cartridge-needle unit are fully, but lightly, engaged, and slight clicking is heard. To maintain sterility, leave the rubber sheath in place until ready to use. **D.** To adapt a 2 cc syringe to a 1 cc Tubex®, engage both ends of the Tubex® and push the slide through so that the number one (1) appears. After use, the syringe automatically resets itself for 2 cc. *Courtesy of Wyeth Laboratories, Philadelphia, Pennsylvania)*

by first palpating for the greater trochanter, the anterior superior iliac spine, and the iliac crest. The nurse places the palm of the dominant hand on the greater trochanter with the index finger at the anterior iliac spine. The middle finger is spread away from the index finger to form a wide V. The medication is injected in the middle or muscular point of the V.

In an adult, the vastus lateralis injection site can be found between the midpoint of the anterior aspect of the thigh and midpoint of the outer lateral aspect of the thigh. Once this area has been found, the nurse measures one hand width below the proximal end of the trochanter and one hand width above the distal end of the knee. The area between these landmarks can be used for injection purpose. The nurse can ascertain the thickest portion of muscle in this area by palpation.

In infants, the muscle site is determined by palpation. Once the muscle is identified, it is grasped and

---

Chart 16.10
Preparation of Parenteral Injections

TECHNIQUE	POINTS TO NOTE	TECHNIQUE	POINTS TO NOTE
Check medication order.	Provides necessary information for preparing medication; prevents error.	Remove needle cover (save it).	Exposes needle for use. (Cap is needed to protect needle from being contaminated after solution is drawn up.)
Calculate volume for administration if necessary.	Insures giving accurate amount of medication.	Without touching barrel of plunger or syringe or needle, pull out syringe plunger handle to the calibration on the syringe which correlates with the volume to be given.	Prevents contamination and fills syringe with air.
Gather equipment: Proper size syringe Proper size needle Alcohol swabs Medication tray Medication vial	Allows for orderly and organized procedure.		
Open syringe and needle packets by peeling back wrapper.	Prevents contamination.	Push needle into the center of the vial stopper.	Center of seal is less resistant to needle than other areas.
Do not touch open end of needle.		Inject air into vial.	Air displaces solution and assists withdrawal.
Remove cap of syringe.		Invert vial and needle and syringe (make sure the needle is fully covered by solution).	Hold vial in palm of one hand, securing with fingers.
Do not touch tip of syringe.			
Connect needle and syringe by twisting needle on tip of syringe.	Secures needle to syringe.	Slowly pull plunger out, until desired amount of solution fills syringe.	Hold handle of plunger securely with fingers of other hand. Slow withdrawal prevents accumulation of air.
Clean seal of vial with alcohol swab.	Reduces microorganisms on seal.		

secured. (Refer to Figure 16.6 for illustrations of the above-mentioned sites and landmarks.)

Whichever site is chosen, the individual is positioned so that the muscles are as relaxed as possible and no body part overrides another. The procedure is explained to the individual prior to injection. The nurse also explains that a certain amount of pain or discomfort may accompany the injection. Figure 16.8 outlines the procedure for administering an intramuscular injection.

Chart 16.10 (Cont.)
Preparation of Parenteral Injections

TECHNIQUE	POINTS TO NOTE
Do not touch the plunger of the syringe.	Prevents contamination.
Pull needle out of vial.	
Holding syringe with needle upward, remove any air bubbles from syringe by tapping the side of syringe until bubbles rise to hub of needle.	Position facilitates upward movement of air.
Force out all but 0.1 cc of air.	Excess air causes pain to individual. Air bubble retained to assure all medication is injected, seals medication in muscle, and prevents leakage of medication into tissues as needle is withdrawn.
Replace cap on needle.	Prevents contamination.
Recheck medication order with bottle label.	Prevents error.
Place syringe with needle, alcohol swabs, and identification card on tray.	Prepares for administration.

Z-Tract Method. A special technique for deep intramuscular injections is the Z-tract method of administration. Its purpose is to displace the layers of the tissue above the muscle. In so doing, the needle can be inserted more deeply into muscle tissue, damage to overlying tissue is prevented, and absorption of the medication is facilitated. Once the site has been determined, the nurse firmly places fingers on either side of the exact site and then "twists" or rotates the skin and underlying tissue. The needle is now inserted and the medication injected. The nurse waits approximately 10 sec before removing the needle. After the needle is removed, the skin and tissues are released. The site is not massaged.

Subcutaneous Injections
The procedure for subcutaneous injection is similar to that used for intramuscular injection, with the exception of the angle of needle insertion. In a subcutaneous injection the needle is inserted at a 45-degree angle, and the skin is always pinched prior to injection.

Intravenous Injection
Medications to be given intravenously are drawn up in the syringe in the same way as any other parenteral medication. There are several ways in which intravenous medications are administered: they may be added directly to an intravenous solution; added to a small bottle of intravenous solution and attached as a secondary bottle (Chap. 21); injected directly into the bloodstream; or added to a chamber which is attached to the intravenous tubing. (Figure 16.9 illustrates the chamber and its use.) Strict sterile technique is utilized for any type of intravenous drug administration. Any time a medication is added to an intravenous solution, a label is attached to the bottle which clearly states the type and amount of medication added, the time it was added, and who added it.

Recording of Medications

Once medications have been administered, the nurse observes the individual for responses to the medication, checking for expected responses, side effects, and untoward effects. Objective and subjective signs and symptoms are recorded and correlated with the nurse's observations and knowledge of expected outcomes. The specific activities and observations that the nurse carries out will depend on the exact drug given and the characteristics of the individual. For example, if an antihypertensive drug is given, the nurse checks the individual's blood pressure and

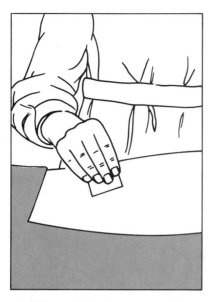

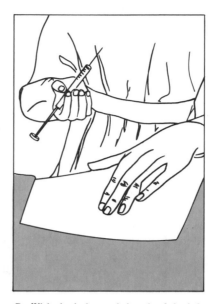

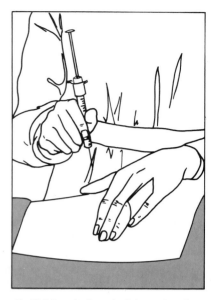

A. Using an alcohol sponge or swab, cleanse an area approximately two inches square around the proposed injection site.

B. With the index and thumb of the left hand spread or tense the skin in the injection area.

C. Holding the barrel of the syringe in the right hand* in a dart or pencil grip, introduce the needle into the skin with a quick thrust.

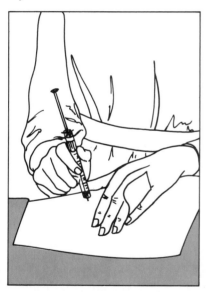

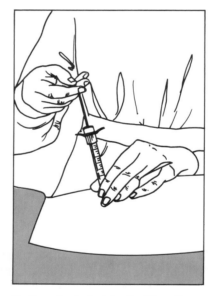

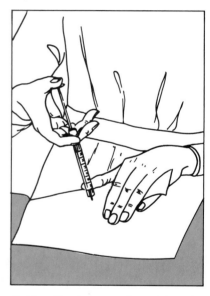

D. Once the surface of the skin has been punctured by the needle, the remainder of the penetration of the needle through the skin and into the muscle should be with a firm and steady pressure. In the case of average or heavy patients it is preferable to retain the pressure on the skin around the injection site with the thumb and index fingers of the left hand for the entire time the needle is being inserted. In thin patients, on the other hand, it is often preferable to release the pressure of the left hand once the puncture has been made, and change to a slight pinching grip in order to firm the injection site and avoid the possibility of going too deep and striking a bone, nerve or blood vessel.

Figure 16.8.   See legend opposite.

E. Once the desired depth of insertion has been reached, steady the syringe tip with the left hand and with the right hand pull back or out on the plunger approximately one-quarter inch for a few seconds, to see if any blood can be aspirated back into the syringe. Should blood appear in the syringe, the needle should be withdrawn and a new injection site selected.

*Dominant hand is intended when right hand is used, non-dominant hand when left hand is used.

F. If no blood appears, the position of the fingers on the right hand can be shifted so that the thumb covers the head of the plunger and the index and middle fingers are hooked under the side grips on the syringe barrel. With a firm pressure on the thumb move the plunger downward into the syringe as far as it will go. (The small air bubble that is last to disappear is an important part of the injection, since it helps to spread the medication, clear the medicine from the needle, seal the injection site and prevent tracking of the medication as the needle is withdrawn.)

pulse before and after administration and observes for possible signs and symptoms of hypotension.

Medications are recorded as soon as they are given. Records include the medication dosage, route, time, individual's response, and the name of the nurse administering the drug. Special sheets are often used to record such data (Figs. 16.3 to 16.5). If an individual refuses a medication, the refusal is indicated on the chart along with the reasons the individual states for refusal. If the medication is spit out or vomited, the nurse charts this and attempts to ascertain the amount that was lost. If the entire dosage was lost, the nurse checks with the physician to see if the drug should be given parenterally.

Narcotics and other controlled drugs are recorded both on the chart and on the narcotics count sheet. A *narcotics* and *controlled drug count sheet* is a federally required record of the administration of narcotics and controlled drugs, the ordering physician, and the administering person. This record is usually kept locked with the narcotics and controlled

drugs. A narcotic and controlled drug count of medications used and remaining is done at the beginning of each shift by one nurse from the ending shift and one nurse from the beginning shift.

Teaching Related to Chemical Safety

Many individuals take prescribed medications in the home environment. The nurse teaches the individual and his or her family and/or significant others the uses of these medications, their rationale for use, and ways to administer them. Related activities and safety precautions, expected responses, possible side and and untoward effects, and what to do if unexpected responses occur are also taught. Frequently, individuals are readmitted to hospitals or other health care agencies because medication schedules were not followed. Many studies, however, have shown that a major factor in the failure to take medications is a result of a lack of understanding of administration

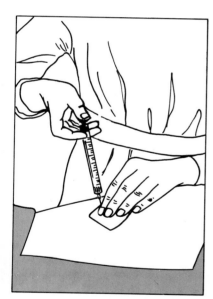

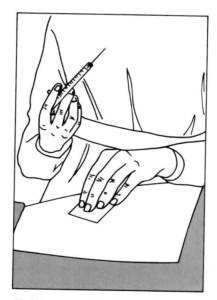

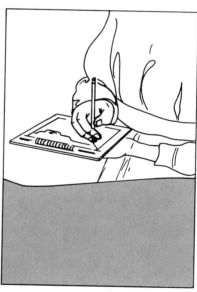

G. After the medication has been injected, apply pressure against the injection site with the alcohol sponge in the left hand as the needle is withdrawn by the right hand; this reduces the risk of medication leaking into the subcutaneous tissues and possibly forming abscesses.

H. Then proceed to cleanse the injection site, by massaging the area with the sponge to remove any blood or medication that might be present. If rapid absorption is desired, the massaging should be continued for about two minutes.

I. After the injection has been given, it is important that all the information be recorded on the patient's chart. This should include: the hour of injection, name of the medication, amount and strength, method of administration, specific site including which side of the body, any unusual reaction and your signature. No injection is complete until this has been done.

Figure 16.8
Administering intramuscular injections. (*Courtesy of Wyeth Laboratories, Philadelphia, Pennsylvania*)

Chart 16.11
Poison Treatment Chart

Acetone 2
Acids
Ingestion 5
Eye Contamination ...7
Topical 6
Inhalation if mixed with
bleach 9
Aerosols
Eye Contamination ...7
Inhalation 9
After Shave Lotions ...See
Cologne
Airplane Glue 10
Alcohol
Ingestion 2
Eye Contamination ...7
Ammonia
Ingestion 5
Eye Contamination ...7
Inhalation 9
Amphetamines 2, 8
Analgesics 10
Aniline Dyes
Ingestion 2, 8
Inhalation 8, 9
Topical 6, 8
Antacids 1
Antibiotics
Less than 2–3 times
total daily dose 1
More than 3 times total
daily dose 2
Antidepressants
Tricyclic 2, 8
Others 2
Antifreeze (Ethylene
Glycol)
Ingestion 2
Eye Contamination ...7
Antihistamines 2, 8
Antiseptics 2
Ant Trap
Kepone Type 1
Others 2
Aquarium Products 1
Arsenic 2, 8
Aspirin 2

Baby Oil 1
Ball Point Ink 1
Barbiturates
Short Acting 10
Long Acting 2

Bathroom Bowl Cleaner
Ingestion 5
Eye Contamination ...7
Inhalation if mixed with
bleach 9
Topical 6
Batteries
Dry Cell (Flash Light) .1
Mercury (Hearing Aid)
.................2
Wet Cell (Automobile)
.................5
Benzene
Ingestion 10
Inhalation 9
Topical 6
Birth Control Pills 1
Bleaches
Liquid Ingestion 1
Solid Ingestion 5
Eye Contamination ...7
Inhalation when mixed
with acids or alkalies ..9
Boric Acid.............2
Bromides 2
Bubble Bath 1

Camphor 2
Candles 1
Caps
Less than One Roll ...1
More than One Roll ..2
Carbon Monoxide 9
Carbon Tetrachloride
Ingestion 2
Inhalation 9
Topical 6
Chalk 1
Chlorine Bleach ......See
Bleaches
Cigarettes
Less than One 1
One or More 2
Clay 1
Cleaning Fluids 10
Cleanser (household) 1
Clinitest Tablets 5
Cold Remedies 10
Cologne
Less than 15cc 1
More than 15cc 2
Contraceptive Pills 1
Corn-Wart Removers ...5

Cosmetics ....See Specific
Type
Cough Medicines 10
Crayons
Children's 1
Others 2
Cyanide 8

Dandruff Shampoo 2
Dehumidfying Packets ..1
Denture Adhesives 1
Denture Cleansers 5
Deodorants
All types 1
Deodorizer Cakes 2
Deodorizers, Room 10
Desiccants 1
Detergents
Liquid-Powder
(General) 1
Electric Dishwasher &
Phosphate Free 5
Diaper Rash Ointment ..1
Dishwasher
Detergents ....See
Detergents
Disinfectants 3
Drain Cleaners ...See Lye
Dyes
Aniline .....See Aniline
Dyes
Others 2

**Electric Dishwasher
Detergent** See Detergents
Epoxy Glue
Catalyst 5
Resin or When
Mixed 10
Epsom Salts 2
Ethyl Alcohol See Alcohol
Ethylene Glycol .....See
Antifreeze
Eye Makeup 1

Fabric Softeners 2
Fertilizers 10
Fish Bowl Additives 1
Food Poisoning 4
Furniture Polish 10

Gas (Natural) 9
Gasoline 10
Glue 10
Gun Products 10

Hair Dyes
Ingestion 3
Eye Contamination ...7
Topical 6
Hallucinogens 5, 8
Hand Cream 1
Hand Lotions 1
Herbicides 10
Heroin 8, 11
Hormones 1
Hydrochloric Acid ....See
Acids

Inks
Ballpoint pen 1
Indelible 2
Laundry Marking ...2
Printer's 2
Insecticides
Ingestion 8
Topical 6, 8
Iodine 5, 8
Iron 10
Isopropyl Alcohol .....See
Alcohol

Kerosene 10

Laundry Marking Ink ...2
Laxatives 2
Lighter Fluid 10
Liniments 2
Lipstick 1
Lye
Ingestion 5
Eye Contamination ...7
Inhalation when mixed
with bleach 9
Topical 6

Magic Markers 1
Make-Up 1
Markers
Indelible 2
Water Soluble 1
Matches
Less than 12 wood or
20 paper 1
More than the above .2
Mercurochrome
Less than 15cc 1
More than 15cc 2
Mercury
Metallic
(Thermometer) 1

Chart 16.11 (Cont.)
Poison Treatment Chart

Mercury (cont.)
  Salts 2
Metal Cleaners 10
Methadone 8, 11
Merthiolate
  Less than 15 cc 1
  More than 15cc 2
Methyl Alcohol 2, 8
Methyl Salicylate 2
Model Cement 10
Modeling Clay 1
Morphine 8, 11
Moth Balls 2
Mushrooms 2, 8

Nail Polish 1
Nail Polish Remover
  Less than 15cc 1
  More 2
Narcotics 8, 11
Natural Gas 9
Nicotine ...See Cigarettes

Oil of Wintergreen 2
Opium 8, 11
Oven Cleaner ....See Lye

Paint
  Acrylic 10
  Latex 10
  Lead Base 10
  Oil Base 10
Paint Chips 10
Paint Thinner 10
Pencils 1
Perfume .....See Cologne
Permanent Wave Solution
  Ingestion 5
  Eye Contamination ...7
Pesticides
  Ingestion 8
  Topical 6, 8
Petroleum Distillates ...10
Polishes 10
Phosphate Free
  Detergents 5
Pine Oil 10
Plants 10
Polishes 10
Printer's Ink 2
Putty 1

Rodenticides 10
Rubbing Alcohol .....See
  Alcohol

Saccharin 1
Sachet 1
Sedatives 10
Shampoo
  Ingestion 1
  (See also Dandruff
  Shampoo)
Shaving Cream 1
Shaving Lotion ....See
  Cologne
Shoe Dyes 2
Shoe Polish 2
Sleep Aids 10
Soaps 1
Soldering Flux 5
Starch, Washing 1
Strychnine 10
Sulfuric Acid ...See Acids
Sun Tan Preparations ..10
Swimming Pool
  Chemicals 5

Talc
  Ingestion 1
  Inhalation 10
Teething Rings 1
Thermometers (All
  types) 1
Toilet Bowl Cleaner ...See
  Bathroom Bowl Cleaner
Toilet Water .See Cologne
Toothpaste 1
Toys, Fluid Filled 1
Tranquilizers 2, 10
Tricyclic
  Antidepressants 2, 8
Turpentine 10
Typewriter Cleaners ...10

Varnish 10
Vitamins
  Water Soluble 1
  Fat Soluble 2
  With Iron 10

Wart Removers 5
Weed Killers 10
Window Cleaner 10
Windshield Washer
  Fluid 2, 8
Wood Preservatives 5

SUGGESTED GENERAL TREATMENT FOR POISONING MANAGEMENT

1. There should be no problem in small amounts. No treatment necessary. Fluids may be given.

2. Induce vomiting. Give Syrup of Ipecac in the following dosages:
   Under one year of age: Two teaspoons followed by at least 2–3 glasses of fluid.
   One year and over: Give one tablespoon followed by at least 2–3 glasses of fluid.
   Do not induce vomiting if the patient is semicomatose, comatose, or convulsing. Call Poison Center for additional information.

3. Dilute or neutralize with water or milk. Do not induce vomiting. Gastric lavage is indicated. Call Poison Center for specific instructions.

4. Treat symptomatically unless botulism is suspected. Call Poison Center for specific information regarding botulism.

5. Dilute or neutralize with water or milk. Do not induce vomiting. Gastric lavage should be avoided. This substance may cause burns of the mucous membranes. Consult E.N.T. specialist following emergency treatment. Call Poison Center for specific information.

6. Immediately wash skin thoroughly with running water. Call Poison Center for further treatment.

7. Immediately wash eyes with a gentle stream of running water. Continue for 15 minutes. Call Poison Center for further treatment.

8. Specific antagonist may be indicated. Call Poison Center.

9. Remove to fresh air. Support respirations. Call Poison Center for further treatment.

10. Call Poison Center for specific instructions.

11. Symptomatic and supportive treatment. Do not induce vomiting for ingestions. I.V. Naloxone Hydrochloride (Narcan) to be given as indicated for respiratory depression.
    Dosage:
    Adult—0.4 mg I.V. May be repeated at 2–3 min. intervals.
    Child—0.01 mg/kg I.V. May be repeated at 5–10 min. intervals.

This chart is recommended for use by health professionals only.

National Poison Center Network, Children's Hospital of Pittsburgh, 125 DeSoto St. Pittsburgh, Pennsylvania 15213.

methods and the rationale for medication use. Therefore, the nurse plays an important role in creating positive change in the individual's ability to meet personal health care needs when the nurse carries out a comprehensive teaching plan with the individual and the family and/or significant others.

Another important aspect of teaching is the use and storage of all types of chemicals and related safety precautions. One of the major causes of death in toddlers and young children is poisoning by chemical agents found within the home. A few of the safety measures the nurse can teach are: keeping medications and other chemicals in locked, out-of-reach cabinets; discarding old or no longer needed chemicals; storing chemicals in their proper containers; and not mixing chemicals together. In addition, emergency treatment for poisoning and the telephone numbers of the nearest poison-control centers are taught to individuals and their family and/or significant others. (See Chart 16.11 for emergency poison interventions.) The nurse can carry out chemical safety teaching in a wide variety of settings: the home, school, community, industry, and health care agency.

EVALUATION

Evaluation for meeting chemical safety needs focuses on the direction of change in an individual's responses as a result of the administration of chemical

Via Venoset® Administration Set

1. Through air inlet

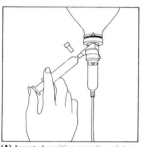

(A) Inverted position permits uninterrupted infusion: Remove air filter. Ball-check valve prevents leakage when container is inverted. Use syringe without needle. Observe aseptic technique. Swirl to mix thoroughly. Replace filter securely.

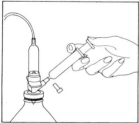

(B) Upright position (before attaching set to patient): Remove air filter. Use syringe without needle. Be sure to use aseptic technique. Replace filter securely. Mix thoroughly.

2. Through injection sites

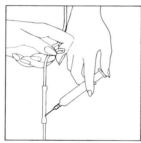

(A) Latex injection site: Cleanse resealing site with antiseptic. Syringe with 20- or 22-G needle is preferred. Pinch off or temporarily clamp tubing above site to prevent reverse flow and drip chamber flooding.

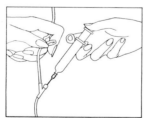

(B) "Y" injection site: Cleanse resealing site with antiseptic. Syringe with 20- or 22-G needle is preferred. One or more "Y" sites are provided depending on choice of Venoset.

Via Rubber Stopper of Abbo-Vac Bottle

1. From rubber stoppered vials

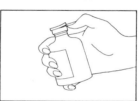

(A) Remove the protective top of Flip Top vial. Cleanse the rubber stopper with antiseptic.

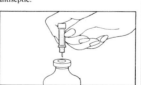

(B) Remove the plastic sheath from one end of double-ended transfer needle. Insert the needle into the stopper of the vial.

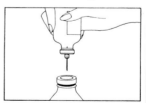

(C) Remove the overseal and metal disk from the Abbo-Vac container. Remove the sheath from the other end of the transfer needle and insert it into the Abbo-Vac "bull's eye." Vacuum in the Abbo-Vac container will automatically withdraw the contents from the vial.

2. From syringe with needle

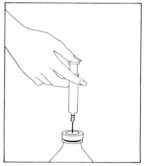

Medication may be added through the stopper of the Abbo-Vac bottle by sterile syringe and needle. Either conventional or pre-loaded syringe may be used. Vacuum helps withdraw the medication.

After additive procedure is completed, bottle should be properly relabeled, and either Additive Cap or Primary Venoset may be affixed. Use promptly.

Figure 16.9

Intravenous administration of medication. *(Courtesy of Abbott Laboratories, Chicago, Illinois)*

agents and focuses on the effectiveness of interventions in meeting chemical safety needs.

Specific criteria for evaluating how chemical safety needs have been met include:

- How do physiologic changes relate to the need for chemical agents? Psychologic changes? Environmental changes?
- Have the presenting behavioral responses for which medications are being given moved closer to the expected?
- What are the changes in degree of interferences?
- What are the changes in coping with interferences and related responses as a result of medication administration?
- What are the changes in knowledge related to chemical safety?
- What chemical safety skills have been acquired?
- What are the changes in attitude about chemical safety (in the individual, family and/or significant others)?

CHARTING AND TEACHING–LEARNING ACTIVITIES

Teaching–Learning Topics

- rationale for therapeutic regimen
- methods for matching capabilities with limitations
- ways to space medications for most beneficial effects
- drug and diet interactions
- administration of drugs
- expected responses
- untoward effects
- what to do in instances of untoward effects
- ways to potentiate effects of drugs, e.g., diet, relaxation techniques
- activities related to administration of drugs, e.g., how to take blood pressure, pulse
- ways to safely store chemical agents
- safety precautions related to chemical agents
- poison-control center numbers
- emergency poisoning treatment

Charting Related to Chemical Safety

Using appropriate chemical safety terms, objectively described such factors as:

- objective base-line data on individual's need for and response to chemical agents, the individual's size, level of growth and development, muscle tone, allergies, and previous history related to medications
- objective and subjective data on responses to chemical agents
- medication given
- dose given
- route used
- time given
- person administering
- preadministration and follow-through activities
- attitudes toward chemical safety
- teaching carried out
- discharge planning done
- interactions and responses of family and/or significant others

Update Kardex on changes in goals and plans for meeting chemical safety needs.

SELECTED REFERENCES

Boyles, Virginia. "Injection Aids for Blind Diabetic Patients." *American Journal of Nursing*, 77:1456, September, 1977.

Carr, Joseph, McElroy, Norman, and Carr, Bonita. "How to Solve Dosage Problems in One Easy Lesson." *American Journal of Nursing*, 76:1934, December, 1976.

Galton, Lawrence. "Drugs and the Elderly." *Nursing 76*, 6:38, August, 1976.

Geolot, Denise and McKinney, Nancy. "Administering Parenteral Drugs." *American Journal of Nursing*, 75:788, May, 1975.

Gotz, Bridget and Taylor, Ann Gill. "Drugs and the Elderly." *American Journal of Nursing*, 78:1347, August, 1978.

"Intravenous Therapy" (Special Feature). *American Journal of Nursing*, 79:1268, July, 1979.

Kelly, June, Stewart, Diane, and Dinel, Brian. "Unit-Dose Medication System: A Nursing Perspective." *American Journal of Nursing*, 76:1308, August, 1976.

Lambert, Martin. "Drug and Diet Interactions." *American Journal of Nursing,* 75:402, March, 1975.

Lanz, Susan, Zawacki, Ann, and Johnson, Jean. "Reducing Discomfort from IM Injections." *American Journal of Nursing,* 76:800, July, 1976.

Newton, David and Newton, Marian. "Route, Site and Technique: Three Key Decisions in Giving Parenteral Medications." *Nursing 79,* 9:18, July, 1979.

Newton, Marian. "Guidelines for Handling Drug Errors." *Nursing 77,* 7:62, September, 1977.

Parker, William. "Medication Histories." *American Journal of Nursing,* 76:1969, December, 1976.

Physician's Desk Reference. Medical Economics, Oradell, N.J. (latest edition).

Romankiewicz, John, et al. "To Improve Patient Adherence to Drug Regimens: An Interdisciplinary Approach." *American Journal of Nursing,* 78:1216, July, 1978.

"Topical Therapy: Choosing and Using the Proper Vehicle." *Nursing 77,* 7:8, November, 1977.

UNIT
V
Energy
Needs

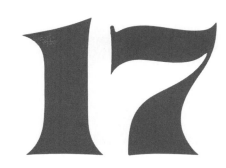

". . . As though to breath were life!"
—Tennyson

17

INTAKE OF OXYGEN

PRINCIPLES RELATED TO OXYGEN UPTAKE*

Respiratory centers in the medulla oblongata regulate inspiration and expiration.

The primary stimuli for respiration are the levels of CO_2 and H^+ (from the breakdown of carbonic acid) in the bloodstream.

The secondary stimulus for respiration is the decreased O_2 concentration in the bloodstream acting on the chemoreceptors in the aortic and carotid arteries (hypoxic drive).

The tertiary stimulus for respiration is the activation of stretch receptors in the bronchioles and lung tissues during inhalation and exhalation (Hering-Breuer reflexes).

An intact neurorespiratory system is necessary for efficient and effective respiration.

An intact, closed respiratory system is necessary for adequate ventilation.

Gases flow from areas of higher pressure to areas of lower pressure.

During the active process of inspiration the intra-alveolar pressure, in accordance with Boyle's law, falls below atmospheric pressure and air flows into the lungs.

Elastic recoil of the lung tissue is responsible for expiration, which is a passive process.

Maintenance of subatmospheric pressure within the thoracic cavities prevents lung collapse.

Effortless respiration is accomplished by low airway resistance and a high compliance.

Compliance is the elasticity of the lungs.

Gaseous exchange in the alveoli is dependent on diffusion and blood flow.

Adequate blood flow to the alveoli is maintained by subatmospheric hydrostatic pressure within the pulmonary arteries and veins.

---

*Figure 17.1 shows the anatomy of the respiratory subsystem and Figure 17.8 is a diagram of pulmonary volume relationships.

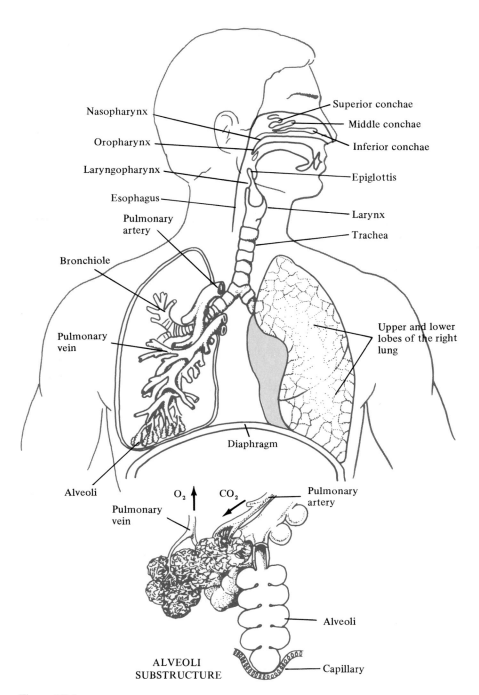

Figure 17.1
Anatomy of the respiratory subsystem illustrating the alveoli substructure.

Alveolar gaseous diffusion is inversely proportional to the thickness of the alveolar membrane.

Alveolar gaseous diffusion is directly proportional to the amount of alveolar surface area.

Airway resistance is the resistance produced by the respiratory tract to the flow of air.

Intrapleural pressure goes from 757.5 to 754 mm Hg during quiet inspiration.

CO_2 is diffused through the alveolar membrane 20 times more rapidly than O_2.

Alveolar gaseous exchange depends on the partial pressure of CO_2 and O_2 in the blood.
   a. In venous blood the partial pressure of CO_2 is higher than the partial pressure of O_2.
   b. In arterial blood the partial pressure of O_2 is higher than the partial pressure of CO_2.

Alveolar gaseous exchange is dependent on the partial pressure of the gases in the atmosphere.

Adequate hemoglobin is necessary for the transport of O_2 to the cells.

Patency of the respiratory tract is maintained by:
   a. cough reflex
   b. sneeze reflex
   c. cilia movement
   d. proper viscosity of mucus
   e. proper secretion of mucus
   f. swallowing
   g. anatomical structure
   h. sighing
   i. yawning

Activity acts as a stimulus to respiration.

Activity increases tissue demand for O_2.

Activity increases production of CO_2 by the tissues.

Activity maintains and improves respiratory muscle tone.

Respiratory rate is directly proportional to metabolic rate.

Emotional status affects the respiratory pattern.

A sitting or upright position facilitates the descent of the diaphragm, aiding lung expansion during inspiration.

Respiratory distress produces anxiety and apprehension.

Pain affects respiratory pattern.

Any sudden external environmental event can affect respiratory pattern.

Behavior is altered by O_2 deprivation.

O_2 supports combustion.

O_2 has a drying effect on mucous membrane.

A continuous supply of oxygen is necessary to sustain life. Oxygen deprivation for as little as three minutes can permanently affect vital functioning. Man instinctively and physiologically strives to satisfy this basic need above all others. Whenever there is a lack of oxygen we automatically seek out an open space or window where we can feel less confined. Our bodies reflexively increase our breathing rate in an attempt to supplement the existing supply of oxygen and to blow off carbon dioxide.

The implications of today's world on men and women's respiratory needs are numerous and complex. The advent of new treatment modalities and therapeutic agents has greatly reduced our chances of death from acute respiratory disorders (e.g., pneumonia) and makes it possible to maintain people with chronic respiratory problems (e.g., emphysema) for longer periods of time. Although modern technology has provided these benefits, it has also produced the stimuli for increased respiratory problems. These stimuli are the many pollutants resulting from industrialization such as sulfur dioxide, fluorocarbons, radioactivity, dust, and smoke.

These environmental hazards have increased the need for greater emphasis on the preventative aspects of respiratory care. Recognition of the roles that personal habits, environmental standards, and safety measures play is a major factor in the prevention of respiratory interferences. Thus behavioral modification teaching, legislation, case finding, and safety teaching become important nursing interventions in meeting the need for oxygen uptake. Therefore, the nurse requires a greater knowledge of the recognition and treatment of respiratory interferences and those factors related to their occurrence.

ASSESSMENT

Respiratory Pattern

Assessment of oxygen uptake begins with observation of the individual's respiratory pattern. The respiratory pattern is the rate, rhythm, depth, effort, and movement of the respiratory muscles as air is inhaled and exhaled. **Respiratory rate** is the number of respirations an individual takes in 1 minute. **Rhythm** refers to the pattern of recurrence of respirations, while **effort** is the degree of energy required to move air in and out of the lungs. **Depth** is the volume of air that is inhaled and exhaled with each respiration and is observed in relation to the amount of inspiratory effort and the distance the chest wall moves from frontal planes. Respiratory **movement** indicates whether the costal or abdominal muscles predominate in respiration.

Chart 17.1
Respiratory Patterns Related to Various Factors

FACTORS	RATE	MUSCLES USED	CHEST MOVEMENT	CHEST CONTOUR
Age				
Newborn	30–80/min	Diaphragm	Paradoxical movement of chest and abdomen	Perfectly round (1:1)
Young child	20–40/min	Diaphragm	Same	Roundish
Late childhood	15–25/min	Becomes adult pattern	Symmetrical	Oval
Adult	14–20/min	male: diaphragmatic female: costal	Symmetrical; females have more chest wall movement	Oval (becomes roundish with age)
Activity				
↑ Activity	Rate ↑ Depth ↑	Accessory muscles		
↓ Activity	Rate ↓ Depth ↓	As CO_2 builds up, accessory muscles may be used		
Metabolism				
↑ Metabolism (e.g., fever)	Rate ↑ Depth ↓	Dependent on O_2 supply and degree of metabolic change		
↓ Metabolism (e.g., hypothermia)	Rate ↓ Depth ↓	Same		
Tissue perfusion				
Decreased cardiac output	Rate ↑ (eventually will ↓)	Accessory muscles used		

The expected respiratory pattern *(eupnea)* is characterized as rhythmical (having equal intervals of time between respirations), effortless (no conscious awareness of the energy required for respiration), quiet (no overt *stertorous* or *adventitious* sounds) and symmetrical (the equal, coordinated movements of both sides of the chest and abdominal walls). The individual's respiratory pattern is related to his age, sex, activity, metabolic rate, size, tissue perfusion, drugs, pain, and level of wellness; these patterns are outlined in Chart 17.1.

Nursing assessment of the respiratory pat-

tern includes descriptions of:

- rate—Is it within the expected range? What is its relation to activity, metabolism, age, tissue perfusion?
- rhythm
- depth
- effort—Is it tiring? What is the person's awareness of the need to take a breath?
- what muscles the individual uses to breathe
- what sounds can be heard without instruments
- symmetry of chest movements
- what impairs/impedes lung expansion
- usual respiratory pattern
- presenting respiratory pattern in comparison with the expected
- factors influencing respiratory pattern (e.g., infection, pain, psychologic state)
- what the individual says about his or her respiratory pattern

---

Chart 17.1 (Cont.)
Respiratory Patterns Related to Various Factors

FACTORS	RATE	MUSCLES USED
Tissue Perfusion (cont.)		
Peripheral vasoconstriction	Rate ↑ (as a result of ↑ heart rate)	Accessory muscles used
Advanced shock	Rate ↑ with shallow respiration	Muscle tone decreased
Drugs		
CNS depressants	↓ Rate ↓ Depth *Biot's respirations* (alternate periods of apnea and normal breathing	Overdoses may cause failure of respiratory muscles
CNS stimulants	↑ Rate may alter depth	
Pain	Rate ↓ or ↑, rhythm and depth may be affected	

Observation of the respiratory pattern is a frequent nursing activity; however, in isolation, these observations provide little insight into the adequacy of oxygen uptake and carbon dioxide removal. These basic observations need to be supplemented with assessments of: circulatory transport and utilization of oxygen (Chap. 18), skin color changes, the relationship of position to respiratory function, adequacy of gaseous exchange in the alveoli, the behavior exhibited by the individual in response to oxygenation needs, environmental factors, and patency mechanisms. Physical examination of the respiratory tree provides added information as to the effectiveness of respiration and gaseous exchange.

Skin Color Changes

Changes in skin color represent a gross index of ventilation, alveolar gaseous exchange, and oxygen transport.

CENTRAL CYANOSIS

▶ **Central cyanosis** is the significant skin color change that results from inadequate oxygen uptake. Central cyanosis is the dusky or hazy bluish-gray color occurring, generally, all over the body. It differs
▶ from **peripheral cyanosis,** which is found mostly in the extremities and is a consequence of decreased

cardiac output or peripheral vascular changes. The physiologic mechanism of central cyanosis is the decrease in circulating oxyhemoglobin and the increase in reduced hemoglobin due to the inadequate gaseous exchange in the alveoli. Cyanosis is usually a relatively late-appearing sign of inadequate oxygen uptake, since it is not observable until oxygen saturation levels fall below 80% (expected: approximately 97%) with 5 g (per 100 ml of blood) of reduced hemoglobin present. The reduced hemoglobin is dark blue in color and when the levels rise above 5 g/100 ml of blood, the dark blue color predominates over the red of oxyhemoglobin, giving the skin a bluish hue. Therefore, by itself, the absence or presence of cyanosis is not a reliable indicator in assessing the adequacy of oxygen uptake.

In order to assess effectively for central cyanosis, the nurse looks at areas of the body which are not masked by pigmentation and where there is a high concentration of superficial blood vessels. These areas include the lips, nail beds, cheeks, ear lobes, lower eyelids (inferior **palpebral conjunctiva**), mucous membrane lining of the mouth *(buccal mucosa)*, soles of the feet, and palms of the hands.

Central cyanosis can be a difficult sign to assess since factors such as lowered environmental temperature, pigmentation patterns, and systemic disease (e.g., anemia) can mimic or obscure cyanosis. Close, frequent assessment of those body areas listed above will help the nurse to recognize the development and presence of central cyanosis.

Pallor is a skin color change which is frequently associated with respiratory inadequacy. However, it is actually a sign of cardiovascular function and is discussed in the next chapter.

Nursing assessment of skin color changes includes descriptions of:

- usual skin color (including ethnic characteristics and areas of pigmentation)
- presenting skin color (including location)
- color of the mucous membranes, lips, cheeks, earlobes, nail beds, etc.
- hemoglobin level
- presence of cyanosis (central? peripheral?)
- skin color changes related to environmental temperature
- any changes in skin color (including frequency of inspection)

Position

The individual with no impairment of respiratory function can assume upright, prone, supine, and lateral positions without thought to respiratory effort and with no respiratory difficulty. However, the individual with an interference in respiratory function may experience respiratory distress when taking any position which does not allow for full lung expansion and the maximum assistance of gravity. Lung expansion is altered by resistance from an object or surface, compression of the abdominal and thoracic organs, pain or discomfort, generalized debilitation, medications, and pathologic interferences (Chart 17.2). Gravity can increase the work of respiration in two ways: (1) by pooling secretions and preventing their distribution through the tracheobronchial tree and (2) by opposing the movement of the chest wall. For example, the person lying in a supine position must counter the resistance of the bed, as well as overcome the force of gravity on the diaphragm, the anterior chest wall, and the mucous secretions.

COMPENSATING FOR RESPIRATORY INTERFERENCE

Many people with respiratory difficulty automatically assume a position which compensates for these interferences. **Orthopnea** is the term used to describe the condition in which the individual must assume an upright position in order to breathe more effectively and comfortably. The upright position eases diaphragmatic excursion by working with gravity and downwardly displacing the abdominal organs. This position also allows for fuller diaphragmatic excursions, distribution of mucous secretions, and an increase in the efficiency of the cilia, and aids fuller chest expansion. The orthopneic person often further compensates by hunching forward with his shoulders and arms elevated in order to increase chest size and expansion. (Fig. 17.9)

Often difficulty in breathing in a flat, lying position may occur so subtly that the individual is unaware of any breathing change with the positions assumed. However, questioning the individual may reveal a tendency for him or her to use added pillows for comfort while lying down or an inability to rest in the usual sleep position. For example, persons who used to sleep on their stomach may find that they now sleep on their back. The nurse, in questioning the individual, may also find out that the bed has been recently moved so it is nearer a window. This furniture rearrangement is seemingly for decorative purposes, but in actuality it is to increase the individual's exposure to the air flow from the window.

Chart 17.2
Factors Which Impair/Impede
Lung Expansion

FACTOR	MECHANISM OF OCCURRENCE
Increased resistance	Bed surfaces Tight binders and dressings Pillows Casts
Crowding of organs	Gastric distention Ascites Pregnancy Obesity Position: supine, slumped, sitting Structural defects: kyphosis, scoliosis, lordosis, pigeon chest, funnel chest Restrictive clothing, e.g., girdles Casts
Pain/ discomfort	Pleurisy Respiratory infection Chest surgery High abdominal surgery Gas pains Hiatal hernia
General debilitation	Immobility Weakness Decreased energy
Pathology	Mechanical disruption, e.g., pneumothorax, fractured ribs Acute and chronic obstruction Neurologic impairment
Medications	CNS depressants: narcotics, anesthetics Respiratory muscle relaxants Cholinergics Analgesics, e.g., pentazocine

---

Nursing assessment of the relationship between position and respiratory function includes descriptions of:

- usual positions for sleeping and sitting
- presenting positions for sleeping and sitting
- relationship between presenting position and respiratory effort
- what may be impeding lung expansion
- conditions affecting the force of gravity which oppose movement of the chest wall
- conditions affecting the force of gravity which oppose movement of secretions
- number of pillows used
- modifications made in activities of daily living
- when changes in position and activity began
- progression, if any, of these changes

Ease of Respiratory Effort

Breathing is usually without effort, noise, or discomfort, but at times the individual may have a subjective awareness of difficulty in breathing. This is known as **dyspnea.** Dyspnea may or may not be related to a pathologic process, since anxiety, fear, and environmental gaseous changes may produce this symptom. The person may make such subjective statements as "I can't seem to catch my breath," "It hurts every time I try to take a breath," "I feel like I'm choking to death," or "I can't seem to move an inch without being short of breath."

NURSING OBSERVATIONS

The nurse cannot directly observe dyspnea, as it is a symptom the individual reports. However, she may observe for signs that indicate dyspnea such as gasping for breath, not being able to finish sentences without taking one or several deep breaths, changing respiratory pattern, **stertorous** (noisy) breathing, and using the accessory muscles of respiration.

Changes that occur in the respiratory pattern that denote changes in the ease of respiration are related to depth and rate. They include **hyperpnea,** increased depth; **bradypnea,** decreased respiratory rate; **tachypnea,** increased respiratory rate; and **hyperventilation,** increased rate and depth.

While noting respiratory pattern, the nurse also looks for signs that the accessory muscles are being

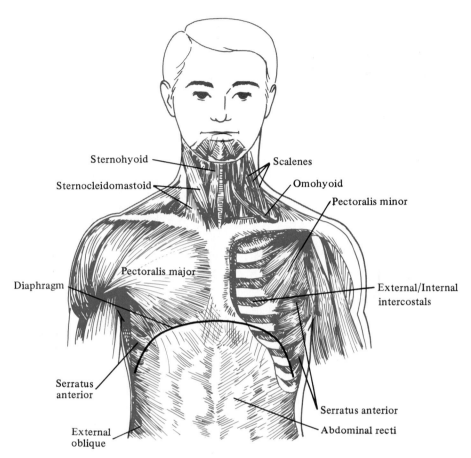

Figure 17.2
Muscles used in respiration.

used to augment respiratory effort. These muscles are the pectorals, the sternocleidomastoid and scalenes, and are found in the neck and shoulder girdle (Fig. 17.2). These muscles will bulge and enlarge with respirations, and if there is chronic difficulty in breathing, hypertrophy of these muscles will result. The nurse may also observe flaring of the nares accompanying use of the accessory muscles.

Nursing assessment related to an individual's ease of respiratory effort includes descriptions of:

- subjective awareness of breathing
- statements made to reflect awareness of breathing
- relationship of this awareness to respiratory pattern
- use of accessory muscles
- flaring of the nares during respiration
- factors interfering with ease of respiration (e.g., pathologic processes or anxiety)
- devices used to aid breathing (humidifier, oxygen, nebulizer)

Adequacy of Gaseous Exchange

Direct assessment of alveolar gaseous exchange is made by testing for blood gas levels (see Chart 17.8, Blood Gas Values). The nurse will include these values as part of the data base in assessing respiratory adequacy.

RESPONSE TO ACTIVITY

The nurse also indirectly assesses the adequacy of gaseous exchange by observing the individual's respiratory response to activity. Activity increases the oxygen demands of the tissues, while increasing the amount of carbon dioxide and heat produced. In response, the respiratory rate increases to meet the need for more oxygen, to blow off carbon dioxide, and to increase heat loss. This compensatory mechanism occurs in all individuals, and after strenuous exercise may take as long as 90 minutes to return to a resting rate.[1] For example, when a person runs up several flights of stairs, temporary shortness of breath and an increased respiratory rate and depth (hyperventilation) is experienced; but as the increased oxygen demands are met and the buildup of carbon dioxide is removed, the respiratory rate should return to the pre-exercise levels without exhaustion or prolonged respiratory difficulty. However, when there is an interference with alveolar gaseous exchange, even an activity of daily living such as eating can produce severe and prolonged tachypnea, dyspnea (conscious difficulty in breathing), fatigue, and an inability to proceed with further activity. In situations where distress is less pronounced, the person may appear to be functioning at a satisfactory level, while in reality the individual has actually changed his or her activities of daily living to compensate for inadequate gaseous exchange. The person who previously would walk the five blocks to the grocery now finds it is easier and less fatiguing to take the car. The person may not consciously identify the reason for this change in behavior or may choose to rationalize the change. Thus careful interviewing that includes a comparison of activities over a period of time will help to uncover any unrecognized behavioral changes.

Two other behaviors that influence alveolar gas exchange are hypo- and hyperventilation.

HYPOVENTILATION

▶ **Hypoventilation** is a decrease in the amount of oxygen-enriched air inspired, resulting in less oxygen being taken in and more carbon dioxide being retained. Therefore, carbon dioxide levels in the blood
▶ ($PaCO_2$) increase (**hypercapnea**) and oxygen levels in the blood decrease. Hypoventilation is usually the result of shallow, restricted breathing with or without a change in respiratory rate. If the hypoventilation is severe or prolonged, respiratory acidosis results.

Hypoventilation may be precipitated by pain or chest trauma, central nervous system drugs (e.g., barbiturates), tight chest dressing or binders, neurologic impairment, pathologic processes which decrease alveolar surfaces (e.g., emphysema or **atelectasis**—
▶ localized collapse of the alveoli) and respiratory obstructions.

HYPERVENTILATION

▶ Hyperventilation is an increase in the amount of air inspired, resulting in little or no change in the amount of oxygen taken in but with an increased amount of carbon dioxide being blown off. Therefore, PaO_2 levels in the arterial blood remain fairly
▶ constant, but $PaCO_2$ levels drop (**acapnea**). Hyperventilation usually results from deep, rapid breathing as seen in acute anxiety, acid–base imbalance (e.g., ketoacidosis), drug overdose (e.g., salicylate poisoning), hepatic coma, midbrain damage (e.g., cerebrovascular accident), and hypoxemia. Hyperventilation can lead to respiratory alkalosis.

Nursing assessment of the adequacy of gaseous exchange includes descriptions of:

- presenting blood gas levels in relation to expected levels
- effect of activity on respiratory pattern
- how long it takes for the respiratory pattern to return to the resting state
- any modifications in activity which have taken place (individual, family and/or significant others)
- presence of hyperventilation
- presence of hypoventilation
- factors influencing ventilation (e.g., pain, medication, pathologic processes, anxiety)
- whether the respiratory rate adequately compensates for increased activity

Behavioral Responses

There is a direct relationship between behavior and oxygen need. Mental functioning depends, in part, on an adequate oxygen supply to the brain. Whenever this supply is interfered with, there will be changes in the level of consciousness, orientation, cognitive functioning, mood, emotional state, and activity. These changes may be insidious and thus difficult to recognize if the oxygen deprivation is slow in onset. Rapidly occurring oxygen deprivation, however, often produces dramatic and sudden changes in behavior.

Whenever the individual is actually deprived of oxygen or perceives this to be so, anxiety and apprehension result. This anxiety may manifest itself as restlessness; a frightened, pinched, "scared" facial expression; hyperventilation; and the activation of the stress mechanisms. In turn, this makes for still greater oxygen demands on the body, resulting in a vicious cycle of increased oxygen need leading to anxiety leading to increased oxygen need.

Nursing assessment of an individual's behavior in response to oxygen uptake includes descriptions of:

- presenting level of consciousness
- usual level of consciousness
- changes in level of consciousness
- orientation to time, place, person (presenting, usual, changes)
- mood (presenting, usual, changes)
- cognitive functioning (presenting, usual, changes)
- activation of stress mechanism (e.g., hyperventilation, tachycardia, pallor, apprehension)
- onset of behavioral changes
- perceptions of oxygen insufficiency
- reaction to changes by family and/or significant others
- report of changes by family and/or significant others

Environmental Factors

The concentration of oxygen in the atmosphere must be approximately 21%, and the partial pressure of the gas at approximately 160 mm Hg—milligrams of mercury—(21% × 760 mm Hg at sea level), if an individual is to have an adequate supply of oxygen for uptake and a sufficient pressure for the oxygen to diffuse into the bloodstream. Thus the gaseous composition of the air in the environment greatly influences respiration. Such atmospheric pollutant hazards as temperature inversions, industrial wastes, automobile emissions, cigarette smoke, pollen, and dust reduce the ambient oxygen content and act as irritants to the respiratory tree. Crowded rooms with inadequate ventilation can also reduce the environmental oxygen concentration.

Whenever a person moves above sea level, the concentration of oxygen decreases, as does the barometric pressure, resulting in a lower partial pressure of oxygen and an impairing of the respiratory function.

The nurse looks at these factors to assess how they influence the individual's respiratory status. They are especially important for people with preexisting respiratory pathophysiologic changes. For example, the urban dweller with a respiratory impairment (e.g., emphysema) may have an exacerbation of symptoms and have to remain in an air-conditioned environment when the air quality index is reported as unacceptable. Since many of these factors are associated with the onset of respiratory pathology, a knowledge of them is necessary to provide preventive health teaching.

Nursing assessment of an individual's environment includes descriptions of:

- room ventilation
- living environment (e.g., industrial, rural, altitude)
- smoking habits
- pollen and pollutant levels
- preexisting respiratory pathology
- environmental modifications (e.g., air conditioning, humidifier, oxygen)
- circumstances necessitating use of modifications
- knowledge of the effects of pollution on respiratory systems
- attitudes toward environmental hazards (individual, family and/or significant others)
- how effects of respiratory hazards are communicated (individual, family and/or significant others)

Mechanisms Which Maintain A Patent Airway

In an attempt to keep the respiratory tree clear and open (patent), the body uses the mechanisms of coughing, sneezing, swallowing, and cilia movement, and maintains the proper viscosity and produces appropriate amounts of mucus.

COUGH

When secretions, foreign objects, or irritants interfere with the passage of air in the respiratory tree, the cough reflex is initiated. **Coughing** is the forceful expiration of air following an intake of air. During the cough the glottis is partially closed and the accessory muscles of respiration are used. While coughing is a protective mechanism, if prolonged or ineffective in clearing the airway, it can produce further irritation and markedly tire the individual. (See Chart 17.3 for types and characteristics of cough.)

Pain, CNS depressants (e.g., narcotics, sedatives, and anesthetics), lung pathology, and general debilitation can suppress or decrease the effectiveness of the cough reflex. When the cough reflex is interfered with, secretions build up, alveolar gaseous exchange decreases, and the airway becomes blocked. The secretions can become a focus of infection.

The nurse notes the type of cough, the effect of the cough on the individual, precipitating conditions, actions which relieve the cough reflex, and the type of sputum produced. **Sputum** is a mixture of the secretions of the respiratory tree, including mucus, saliva, bacteria, and cellular wastes.

Chart 17.3
Characteristics of Coughs

TYPE	DESCRIPTION
Asthmatic	Wheezing, labored dry cough
Dry	Cough that produces no sputum or mucus (synonym: nonproductive)
Explosive	Forceful, sudden, productive cough
Hacking	Frequent, dry, superficial cough
Harsh	Brassy, metallic sounding nonproductive cough
Paroxysmal	Episodes of forceful coughing
Productive	Cough that produces sputum or mucus
Reflex	Cough produced by any stimulation of the ear, pharynx, stomach, intestine, or uterus

---

CILIA MOVEMENT

The distribution and movement of mucus along the respiratory tree is necessary to maintain airway patency. The movement of the cilia helps with these actions. Several factors interfere with ciliary movement, such as smoking, alcohol ingestion, infection, unhumidified air, increased mucus viscosity, and pollutants. Although the nurse has no direct means of observing ciliary movement, she assesses those conditions which may indicate a loss of ciliary movement. Questioning the individual about smoking habits, history of colds and throat infections, and the humidity of the environment in which he or she lives or works gives clues about the ability of the cilia to distribute mucus.

ADEQUATE MUCOUS SECRETION AND VISCOSITY

When mucous secretions are altered through an increase or change in viscosity, the distribution and movement of mucus is affected. Viscosity of mucus increases any time the water content of the mucus is decreased. Water can be lost by inhaling dry, hot, or unhumidified air; anticholinergic drugs (e.g., atropine); and through dehydration. Mucous secretion is increased in infections, as a response to irritants, and with any pathology that causes *hyperplasia* of the goblet cells (e.g., chronic bronchitis).

Gravity may affect the distribution of mucus by preventing the even distribution of mucus along the respiratory tree. As a result, as secretions pool and alveolar gaseous exchange decreases, the airway becomes blocked and hypostatic pneumonia can develop. In addition, whenever mucus distribution along the respiratory tree is decreased, the mucous lining becomes dried out and more prone to trauma and infection. The nurse will look at the amount and quality of sputum **expectorated** (the expelling of sputum from the respiratory tree), as well as the factors that precipitate a change in mucus production and viscosity. Types of sputum are described in Chart 17.4.

Nursing assessment of mechanisms that help to maintain a patent airway includes descriptions of:

- Cough
    - frequency, quality, type, reaction to, precipitating factor, relief actions, type of sputum produced, amount of sputum produced
    - interferences with cough reflex (e.g., pain, medications, weakness)
    - effects of cough on gaseous exchange
    - attitude toward cough
    - knowledge about cough mechanism
    - aspectic practices related to cough
- Ciliary movement
    - factors which may interfere with movement of cilia (e.g., smoking, humidity)
    - indications of loss of ciliary movement (e.g., history of colds, throat infections)
    - related environmental conditions (humidity)
- Mucous secretions and viscosity
    - state of hydration (see Chap. 21)
    - conditions which increase water loss from the respiratory tract (e.g., drugs, dry air)

conditions which increase mucus production (e.g., infections, irritants, disease processes)
positions assumed which interfere with mucus distribution (e.g., supine)
effects of mucus production on gaseous exchange
type of sputum produced
amount of sputum produced
aseptic practices related to sputum production

Interferences with Oxygen Uptake (Chart 17.5)

In the nursing assessment of individuals' oxygen uptake, it is necessary to be familiar with the five major mechanisms which interfere with adequate gaseous exchange. In this way the nurse can effectively recognize signs and symptoms of interferences and thus be able to intervene appropriately in these life-threatening situations. The mechanisms are obstruction, mechanical damage and failure, circulatory impairment, inflammation, and reduction in available oxygen supply.

OBSTRUCTION

Airway obstruction is the occlusion of any part of the respiratory tree preventing the inhalation and exhalation of air and the diffusion of gases across the pulmonary membrane. Respiratory obstruction can be either acute or chronic.

Acute Respiratory Obstruction
In acute respiratory obstruction, onset is rapid and immediately life threatening. It usually results from a foreign object lodging in some part of the airway and is common in children who, while exploring the world, put objects into their noses and mouths. Airway obstruction in adults occurs most often when poorly masticated food is lodged in the airway. ▶ **Mucus plugs** (thick, sticky globules of mucus), although not a foreign object, can also cause airway obstruction. Frequently mucus plug obstructions are found in the alveoli and the bronchioles, but if the cough reflex is poor or the mucus secretions particularly ▶ **tenacious** (adhesive, sticky, and viscous), they may occur in the upper airway.

Chronic Obstruction
Chronic obstruction, on the other hand, is slower in onset and the result of a pathologic process.

Chart 17.4

Characteristics of Sputum

Bloody (hemoptysis)—Sputum that has flecks of blood in it. Characteristic of lung hemorrhage. Irritation of the tracheobronchial tree.

Currant jelly—beadlike clumps of sputum.

Mucoid—Thick, slimy, clear sputum having a high content of mucus. Characteristic of bronchitis.

Purulent—Thick sputum containing pus. Color dependent on offending organism. Characteristic of lung infection.

Serous—Watery clear sputum. Characteristic of allergies and upper respiratory infections.

Frothy—Soapsudsy type of sputum. Characteristic of pulmonary edema.

Muco-Purulent—Combination of mucus and pus.

Prune juice—Watery, brownish-red sputum. Characteristic of pneumonia and lung necrosis.

Rusty—Thick, reddish-orange sputum. Characteristic of pneumococcal pneumonia.

Chronic obstruction may occur when a lumen of the respiratory tree is slowly occluded, as with a tumor; when a buildup of fluid blocks the diffusion of gases as in *pulmonary edema;* or when the lung tissue loses elasticity and becomes fibrotic, blocking diffusion and increasing the distance the gases must diffuse, as in *chronic obstructive lung disease.*

MECHANICAL DAMAGE AND FAILURE

Mechanical failure is the partial or total loss of respiratory function. It occurs when the structures of ventilation—the lungs, respiratory muscles, and neuroregulatory centers and pathways—are damaged by trauma or chemical agents. These structures work through an integrated process that results in ventilation. Therefore, a change of function in one part will produce an impairment in the whole.

Developmental or cogenital deformities such as kyphosis (increased convexity of posterior curve of spine) and scoliosis (side or lateral deviation of the spine) also interfere with the mechanics of respiration.

INFLAMMATION

Inflammation is the major protective mechanism of the body against injurious agents such as bacteria, viruses, and irritants. Inflammation of the lungs results in localized vasodilation, tissue edema, and increased secretion. These responses act in a way similar to chronic obstruction by impairing diffusion of gases, thus increasing the alveolar–capillary distance, and by the buildup of secretions.

CIRCULATORY IMPAIRMENT

Systemic circulatory problems affect the uptake, transport, and utilization of oxygen and the removal of CO_2 and other byproducts of metabolism. (See Chap. 18 for transport, utilization, and removal.) The major pulmonary interference with uptake occurs when either an **embolus** (a blood clot floating in the bloodstream) or a clump of **sickled blood cells** (abnormal, crescent-shaped red blood cells) causes an **infarct** (localized damage or death of tissue resulting from the occlusion of the blood supply) in lung tissue, reducing the amount of usable alveolar diffusion area.

REDUCTION IN AVAILABLE ENVIRONMENTAL OXYGEN

Anything that decreases oxygen concentration in the environment, or the partial pressure of environmental oxygen, interferes with the amount of oxygen inspired and diffused. Changes in altitude or in the gaseous composition of the atmosphere, smoke inhalation, or any hazard mentioned under environmental factors (page 398) can result in respiratory difficulty because of a decrease in the arterial oxygen partial pressure (PaO_2).

By interfering with oxygen uptake and diffusion, these conditions result in a lowered oxygen saturation level in the blood (**hypoxemia**) and a decrease in the oxygenation of body tissue (**hypoxia**) and even respiratory acidosis (see Chap. 21).

Hypoxia is the insufficient oxygenation of the body that occurs when oxygen needs are greater than the oxygen available for uptake, delivery, or use. Hypoxia results in changes in mental functioning, as discussed in Behavioral Responses (pages 397–398), and in the ability to carry out activity as discussed in Adequacy of Gaseous Exchange (page 396). If hypoxia is prolonged and severe, it can lead to death.

Hypoxia can be categorized several ways, depending on whether the interference is with uptake, transport, or utilization. When oxygen uptake is impaired, the Pao_2 is decreased (often referred to as hypoxemia). Since other types of hypoxia are related to transport and utilization, they are discussed in Chapter 18.

Nursing assessment of interferences with oxygen uptake includes descriptions of:

- existing interference, i.e., acute obstruction, chronic obstruction, mechanical damage and failure, inflammation, circulatory impairment, reduction in available oxygen supply
- effects of interference on gaseous exchange
- relationship of growth and development to interference
- relationship of interference to any body image changes
- conditions precipitating interference
- blood gas levels
- signs and symptoms of hypoxia
- assessment by family and/or significant others of interferences
- effect of interference on interactions with family and/or significant others

Chart 17.5
Interferences with Oxygen Uptake

INTERFERENCES	CAUSE	EXAMPLES	ASSESSMENT FACTORS	SEQUELAE
Acute obstruction	Mucous plugs Food Fluid Beans Buttons Any foreign object	Acute airway obstruction	Color changes Choking sensation Voice loss Grasping the throat	Cessation of breathing Death if not immediately treated Hypoventilation
Chronic obstruction	Tumor Secretions Increased fluids and secretions Loss of lung elasticity Lung tissue fibrosis Increase in surface diffusion area Alveolar capillary distance increases	Lung or airway tumor Pulmonary edema Chronic obstructive pulmonary disease Pulmonary effusion Pulmonary edema	Blood gas levels Signs and symptoms of hypoxia Coughing Change in anterior–posterior diameter Use of accessory muscles Chest sounds Respiratory pattern Inability to assume all positions	Respiratory failure Alveolar–capillary diffusion block Hypoventilation Abnormal ventilation perfusion ratio
Mechanical damage/failure	Chest trauma	Gunshot Crushing blows	Change in respiration Change in symmetry Hypoventilation or hyperventilation Contour	Hypoventilation

Mechanism	Cause	Condition	Signs/Symptoms	Outcome
Neurologic damage	Cerebrovascular accident, Multiple sclerosis, Myasthenia gravis, Guillain-Barré syndrome			
Congenital deformity	Kyphosis, Scoliosis, Lordosis			
Drug reactions	Salicylate poisoning, Narcotics			
Inflammation	Infection, Tissue damage, Aspiration, Autoimmune reaction	Bronchitis, Pneumonia	Increased temperature, Increased respiration, Cough, Pain, Increased secretions	Alveolar–capillary diffusion block
Circulatory impairment	Sickled cells, Decreased clotting time, Immobility, Fat released from fracture of long bones, Vascular occlusion, Decreased Hgb blood levels	Sickle cell anemia, Pulmonary emboli, Fat emboli, Pulmonary infarct, Anemia	Pain, Changes in respiratory pattern, Blood gas changes	Hypoxemia
Reduction in available environmental oxygen	Pollution, High altitudes, Smoke inhalation	Same	Decrease in PaO_2	Hypoxemia

Physical Assessment

The physical assessment of the individual's lungs and thorax include inspection, palpation, percussion, and auscultation. The entire subsystem can be examined while the person is sitting; however, he or she may wish to lie down for certain parts.

INSPECTION

Inspection begins with an overall assessment of the individual's respiratory response to activity and position, the position he or she naturally assumes, ease of breathing, behavioral responses, and skin color.

After getting a general impression of the person's respiratory functioning, the nurse can then focus on more specific observations.

Breasts

Moving caudally, the breasts are inspected. With the woman sitting and her arms at her side, the shape, size, symmetry, and skin characteristics are observed. Typically, a degree of asymmetry can be expected. Questioning the woman can ascertain whether the assymmetry is simply a developmental variation or a change related to possible pathology. Shape is inspected for signs of masses, **dimpling** (skin puckering), or changes. The skin is observed for erythema, changes in texture, and increased vascularity. The areolas are observed for masses or changes in size, color, or skin texture. The nipples should be noted for **inversion** (turning inward), discharge, skin texture, and direction (usually both point in same direction). This inspection is repeated with the arms raised and with hands on the hips in order to observe for variations which are obscured by position.

The breasts of males are inspected in a similar

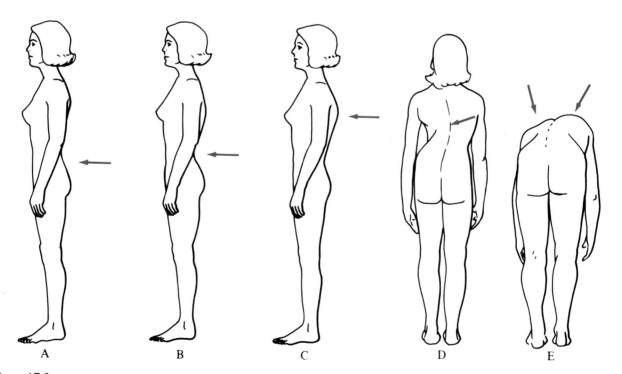

Figure 17.3

Structural interferences with respiration. Proper expansion of the chest wall does not occur if an individual exhibits any of the abnormal spinal curvatures pictures above (B - G). **A.** Expected posture. **B.** Lumbar lordosis, which is an accentuation of the noramal lumbar curve. **C.** Kyphosis, rounded thoracic convexity. **D.** Scoliosis, lateral curvature of the spine, this illustration with convexity to the right. **E.** Scoliosis demonstrated with body in forward flexion.

manner. The axilla are observed for any signs of masses and for rashes.

Posture

Posture both influences and is affected by respiratory functioning. Structural defects in posture, such as *kyphosis, scoliosis,* and *lordosis* (Fig. 17.3) interfere with proper expansion of the chest wall, while respiratory pathology often forces the individual to assume a particular posture such as that of orthopnea and the hunched foward, shoulders elevated position.

Contour

In adults the shape of the chest is slightly oval, while in young children it is barrel-shaped or nearly rounded. The relationship of the anterior–posterior (A–P) diameter of the chest wall (front to back) to the transverse-horizontal (side to side) diameter is expected to range from 1:2 to 5:7 in the adult. In other words, the A-P diameter is expected to be less than the transverse-horizontal diameter. Structural deformities, such as pigeon chest, funnel chest, and barrel chest (Fig. 17.4), prevent the adequate expansion of the chest wall and thus interfere with respiration.

Chest Wall Movement

Respiration is expected to be symmetrical with equal and synchronous movements of the chest wall during inspiration and expiration. Men are usually abdominal breathers, while women are usually costal breathers. Observation of the movement of one part of the chest wall in relationship to the other is also

▶ made. Conditions such as **paradoxical breathing** (one part of the lung moves in the opposite direction to the rest of the lung), or asymmetrical breathing, indicate respiratory impairment due to trauma, atelectasis, or pain. The nurse also observes for synchronous movements of the chest wall and the abdomen, as lack of synchrony may indicate lung pathology. In infants, however, this is an expected finding. Chest wall movement is assessed both during regular respiration and when the individual is taking deep breaths.

The intercostal interspaces are observed for retraction (sinking inward) during inspiration and bulging during expiration as they are indicative of increased respiration effort as in respiratory obstruction.

Respiratory Pattern

The respiratory rate, rhythm, depth, ease, and sound are also assessed. Charts 17.1 and 17.6 outline

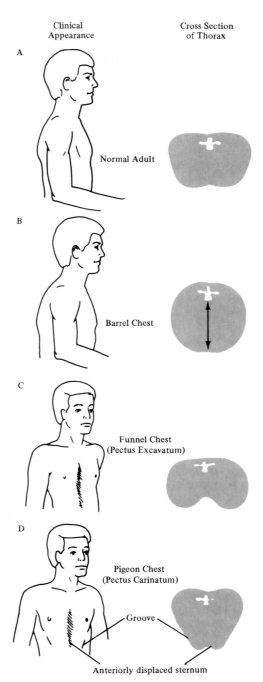

Figure 17.4
Deformities of the thorax.

the expected respiratory patterns and common variations.

Skin Color

See page 393 for nursing assessment of skin color changes.

PALPATION

Any area that the nurse observes to be different from the expected or where pain has been reported, is palpated for texture, tenderness, temperature, and masses. The nurse also palpates for respiratory excursion, tactile, or vocal fremitus, level of the diaphragm, and crepitations.

The axillary lymph nodes are palpated as discussed in Chapter 15. Masses or lesion should be noted and described.

Figure 17.5 shows the procedure for self-examination of the breast. The procedure for examining another person's breast is similar.

Respiratory Excursion

In palpating for respiratory excursion, the nurse places his or her palms, with thumbs facing the central axis (i.e., xiphoid process anteriorly, spine posteriorly) on the chest wall, allowing the hands to move freely with chest wall movement. As the person breathes, the nurse notes the distance his or her fingers move apart, as well as the symmetry of the two sides of the chest wall. The nurse does this for the upper, middle, and lower portions of the chest, both back and front, when the individual breathes in the usual respiratory pattern and when deep breaths are taken.

Tactile (Vocal) Fremitus

▶ **Tactile fremitus** is the palpable vibration of air passing through the vocal cords as they resound on the chest wall. To elicit tactile fremitus, the nurse asks the individual to repeat a resonant phrase (e.g., "99,

---

Chart 17.6
Common Variations in Respiratory Pattern

TERM	DESCRIPTION	MECHANISM OF OCCURRENCE
Apnea	Absence of respirations	Severe illness
Apneustic	Long, gasping inspirations following a short expiration	Brain damage
Bradypnea	Decreased respiratory rate	CNS depressants Brain tumors
Brachypnea	Shortness of breath	Respiratory pathology
Biot's	Cheyne-Stokes respirations but with inspirations having same depth	Neurologic damage Increased intracranial pressure
Cheyne-Stokes	Periods of increased rate and depth of respiration followed by periods of decreased rate and depth ending with periods of apnea	Unknown, but accompanies severe illness
Dyspnea	Conscious difficulty in breathing	Anxiety, respiratory distress
Eupnea	Normal respiratory pattern	
Hyperpnea	Increased respiratory depth	Increased activity Emotions Decreased environmental oxygen Various diseases
Hyperventilation	Increased respiratory rate and depth	Increased carbon dioxide blown off
Hypoventilation	Shallow, restricted breathing with or without a change in respiratory rate	Decreased inspiration of oxygen Retention of carbon dioxide
Kussmaul's	Labored respiration having an increased rate and depth	Metabolic acidosis
Tachypnea	Increased respiratory rate	Anxiety; Respiratory pathology

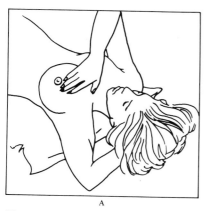
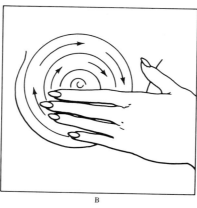
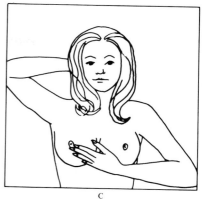

Figure 17.5

Self examination of the breast. **A.** Lie down. Put one hand behind head. With other hand, fingers flattened, gently feel your breast. Press ever so slightly. **B.** This illustration shows you how to check each breast. Begin where you see the A and follow the arrows, feeling gently for a lump or thickening. **C.** Now repeat the same procedure sitting up with the hand still behind the head. *(Courtesy of the American Cancer Society)*

1, 2, 3, Blue Moon") while the nurse systematically palpates the chest wall, moving from one side of the chest to the corresponding side in a downward zigzag course (Fig. 17.6).

Although several techniques can be effectively used, the simplest method is to use the open palm flat against the chest wall. The individual should attempt to maintain the same volume and pitch (low) throughout this examination for fremitus. The nurse notes the location of any area of increased or decreased fremitus.

Level of Diaphragm

With the person repeating a resonant sound, the nurse places the ulnar surface of his or her extended hand on the posterior chest wall. Moving the hand downward, the nurse notes where fremitus disappears. This is the approximate level of the diaphragm. It should be noted that it is difficult to elicit fremitus if the voice pitch is too high.

Crepitation

Crepitation is the crackling sound and feeling which may be elicited when the nurse palpates areas of the chest wall. It occurs when small pockets of air are trapped in the subcutaneous tissue because of a pathologic process *(subcutaneous emphysema)*. The crackling is often likened to the sound of wadding a piece of plastic wrap.

PERCUSSION

The nurse percusses in order to note areas of the chest that are air or fluid filled or solid. These differ-

ent densities will give sounds of differing pitch, intensity, duration, and quality. The nurse percusses at 5-cm intervals down the anterior and posterior chest wall in a zigzag pattern, noting the changing sounds. (Fig. 17.7.) The nurse notes the locations and the

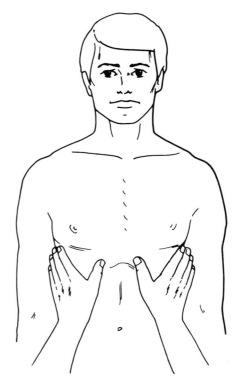

Figure 17.6

Placement of hands in palpating for tactile fremitus.

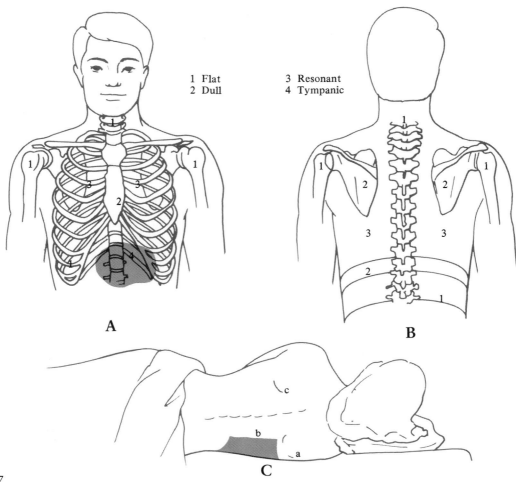

1 Flat   3 Resonant
2 Dull   4 Tympanic

A

B

C

Figure 17.7

Expected percussion findings in chest areas. **A.** Anterior view. **B.** Posterior view. **C.** Lateral recumbent position, which dulls the sounds usually detected while percussing the chest. (a=dull zone caused by the deadening effect of the mattress. b=area of dullness due to the weight of the body compressing the chest. c=dull zone due to crowding of the ribs.)

quality and type of any departures from the expected sounds. As the nurse percusses, he or she attempts to visualize the expected underlying tissue to give meaning to the findings.

AUSCULTATION

The nurse auscultates both the anterior and posterior aspects of the chest to listen for **breath sounds** (the usual movement of air through the respiratory tree) and **adventitious sounds** (unexpected sounds produced by trapped air or secretions). The stethoscope is placed in a zigzag fashion, similar to the placement used in percussion, and the person is asked to take deeper than usual breaths through the mouth. Again, knowledge of the underlying structures will help the nurse in identifying the differing breath sounds. Chart 17.7 identifies the types and locations of these sounds. (Illustration 17.1)

Adventitious Sounds

Some of the adventitious sounds the nurse might hear are rales, rhonchi, wheezes, gurgling, and friction rubs. **Rales** are the intermittent crackling sounds produced by air moving through excessive secretions in the bronchioles and alveoli. Their crackling sound can be simulated by rubbing a lock of hair between the fingers or listening to the fizz of a carbonated beverage being opened. Rales are most often heard on in-

Chart 17.7
Breath Sounds

SOUND	PITCH INTENSITY	LOCATION	CHARACTERISTIC
Vesicular	Low pitch, soft intensity	Most of chest surface	Inspiratory sound is three times longer than expiratory sound
Bronchovesicular	Medium pitch and intensity	Posterior: between scapula Anterior: between sternum and clavicle Where tracheobronchial tree is closest to surface	Inspiratory sound is equal to expiratory sound
Bronchial	High pitch, loud intensity	Over trachea	Inspiratory sound is slightly shorter than expiratory sound (2:3)

spiration. If the individual is too weak or too ill to clear the trachea, wet or gurgling rales (death rattle) may be heard. If this is pronounced enough, gurgling may be heard without a stethoscope.

Rhonchi are the continuous low-pitched, bubbling sounds heard as air passes through bronchi that are narrowed by secretions, obstructions, or inflammation. These sounds are heard more distinctly during expiration. Rhonchi produce sounds similar to snoring. Wheezes are high-pitched rhonchi.

Friction rubs are the rubbing sounds heard when inflamed pleural surfaces come in contact with each other. They can be heard either on inspiration or expiration and are not altered by coughing. These sounds can be simulated by rubbing the dry thumb and forefinger together.

The nurse notes the type, quality, and location of adventitious sounds and any situation that alters them.

Nursing assessment related to the physical assessment of the respiratory system includes descriptions of:

- Inspection
    general inspection factors
    posture used to assist respiration (e.g., orthopnea)
    posture which interferes with respiration
    relationship of chest contour to growth and development
    structural deformities which interfere with respiration

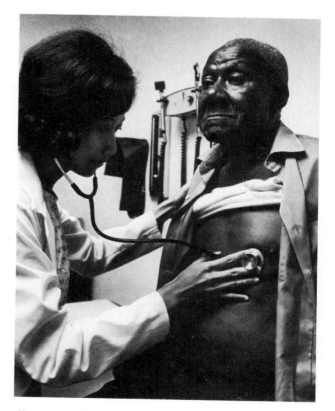

Illustration 17.1

To auscultate for breath sounds and adventitious sounds, the nurse zigzags the stethoscope across an individual's anterior and posterior chest, listening at points approximate to those used in percussing the chest. The individual takes deep breaths through his mouth and is asked to hold them. *(Photo © Stephen L. Feldman, from Rapho/Photo Researchers)*

symmetry of breathing
type of chest wall movement (costal, diaphragmatic, abdominal)
relationship of movement of chest wall parts to each other
retraction and bulging of interspaces during respiration
respiratory pattern
skin color
- Palpation
texture, temperature, tenderness, and masses in areas where unexpected responses such as pain were reported
areas of altered fremitus
level of diaphragm
area of crepitation
- Percussion
quality and location of sounds
- Auscultation
quality and location of sounds

Diagnostic Tests

There are many tests which can be used to assess for interferences with oxygen uptake.

CHEST X-RAYS

The most common diagnostic measure is the x-ray of the P-A and lateral (side view) chest. It is part of the routine physical examination in addition to being used specifically to diagnose a pathologic process. Chest x-rays outline the structures of the lungs and thorax to help identify any changes in their mechanical integrity. There is no special preparation of the individual for this examination. However, the individual will need to be informed that all neck jewelry will have to be removed, as will clothing from the waist up, and that he or she will have to take and hold deep breaths during the procedure. The person should also be told that he or she will be left alone while the x-ray is actually being taken. A description of the equipment used may also be helpful to decrease anxiety.

A specialized form of chest x-ray is the lung tomogram. It is used to visualize several planes of lung tissue in contrast to the single dimension chest x-ray to help identify growths, cavities, and changes in density.

EXAMINATION OF ARTERIAL BLOOD GASES

One of the most definitive tests of adequacy of gaseous exchange is examination of the arterial blood gases. Blood gases measure the arterial oxygen and carbon dioxide tensions of the blood, oxygen saturation of the blood, the pH of the blood, and the bicarbonate (HCO_3^-) levels. Oxygen and carbon dioxide tension levels are reported as partial pressures, abbreviated as PaO_2 and $PaCO_2$, respectively. Oxygen saturation (O_2 Sat) is reported as a percentage. (Chart 17.8 lists expected ranges.)

Arterial blood is used for the test because the adequacy of O_2 uptake is the focus point and not the ability to transport or utilize the oxygen. The major arteries from which blood is taken are the radial (at the wrist), brachial (at the antecubital fossa), and the femoral (at the groin) arteries. Since an artery is punctured, pressure will have to be applied to the site for at least 5 minutes after the needle has been removed to prevent hemorrhage.

Equipment necessary for this procedure are a heparinized syringe with needle, a container of ice, skin antiseptic, and sterile sponges. The person doing the procedure may wish to use sterile gloves to help maintain sterile technique. Heparin, an anticoagulant, is used to prevent coagulation of the drawn blood. After the procedure, the blood specimen is placed in ice to prevent diffusion of the oxygen from the blood into the air. The specimen must be sent to the laboratory immediately to prevent distortion of findings.

The individual needs to have the procedure explained and understood, in particular, the necessity for remaining still throughout the procedure to prevent increased discomfort and possible damage to the arterial wall. The individual should also be informed

---

Chart 17.8
Blood Gas Values

	NEWBORN	ADULT
PaO_2	60–70 mm/Hg	80–100 mm/Hg
PCO_2	35–45 mm/Hg	Same
ph	7.35–7.45	Same
O_2 Sat.		95% (approx.)
HCO_3^-		25 meq/liter

of the discomfort involved and the need for pressure to be applied after the procedure. It should be noted that any discomfort experienced by the individual during the procedure can lead to hyperventilation, thus distorting test results.

SPUTUM

▶ Sputum is frequently collected from the individual with respiratory interference. The sputum is obtained to test for gross observation, culture and sensitivity, and cytology. **Cytology** is the examination of cell structure and function done to identify any abnormal cells, as in lung cancer. The collection of the sputum specimen will be made when the individual first wakes up in the morning. It must be obtained before he has eaten, drunk, or brushed his teeth. First, the person is instructed to rinse out his mouth with water and then cough deeply to bring up secretions deep in the respiratory tree. Then the person is asked to expectorate in the appropriate container.

The first morning sputum specimen is used because secretions pool during sleep, and thus bacteria or cells are more highly concentrated. Food and mouthwash disturb and dilute the findings. Suctioning is used to obtain sputum specimens from infants, small children, and anyone who is unable to cough productively.

Sputum containers should be wide-mouthed and waterproof and kept closed after use. In addition, containers for culture and sensitivity must be sterile. Principles of good respiratory hygiene are followed throughout the collection procedure.

PULMONARY FUNCTION TESTS

Pulmonary function tests are used to evaluate the degree of lung pathology. These tests assess the lung's capacity to carry out ventilation by measuring lung volumes, degree of compliance, air flow rates, airway resistance, and the effects of exercise on ventilation. (Fig. 17.8 diagrams the pulmonary volume relationships.) Pulmonary function tests are usually done in the respiratory lab. These tests require exertion and cooperation on the part of the individual. The nurse's role is to inform individuals about the nature of these tests and how their assistance can aid the tests and their results.

LUNG SCAN AND BRONCHOSCOPY

Other diagnostic tests of the respiratory system include lung scan and bronchoscopy.

Nursing assessment related to diagnostic tests includes:

- the individual's level of understanding of the tests
- preparations needed
- posttest care
- special equipment needed
- the relationship between expected test results and the presenting results
- the relationship of interferences to test results
- the individual's attitude towards the tests
- the nursing implications of the test results

NURSING DIAGNOSIS

A 60-year-old black man, Mr. Em, enters the emergency room and states that he has shortness of breath and difficulty breathing.

The nursing assessment that follows compares Mr. Em's presenting (actual) behaviors that are related to his oxygen uptake with those behaviors that the nurse would expect to find when assessing a man of similar age and development who has no interference in oxygen uptake.

ASSESSMENT FACTOR	EXPECTED BEHAVIOR	ACTUAL BEHAVIOR
Respiratory pattern		
Rate	18/min	30/min
Rhythm	Regular, even	Uneven, gasps when speaking after every fifth word
Depth	Moderate—neither shallow nor deep	Hyperpnea

(continued)

ASSESSMENT FACTOR	EXPECTED BEHAVIOR	ACTUAL BEHAVIOR
Effort	No conscious awareness	States: "It takes so much energy to catch my breath." "I never felt like this before."
Muscles	Male—abdominal; no accessory muscles in use	Neck muscles bulging; flaring of nares; predominantly abdominal breathing
Sounds	No overt sounds	Stertorous
Skin color		
Character	Translucent, "healthy glow"	
Pigmentation	Highly pigmented	Café au lait coloration; grayish hue
Nail beds, mucous membranes, palpebral conjunctiva, etc.	Pink	Pink
Position	Assumes any position without respiratory distress or awareness	More comfortable breathing in a sitting position
Lung expansion	Full, unimpeded	Same
Response to activity	Respiratory rate increases but steadily returns to resting state with cessation of activity	States: "I get so short of breath if I try to move at all. I'm short of breath all the time."
Behavioral responses	Alert, oriented, responsive, calm	Excited; restless, quick movements; keeps tugging at his tie to loosen it.
Environmental		
Habits	—	Smokes two packs of cigarettes per day (for 40 years)
Modifications	—	
Cough	—	Coughs several times within 15 minutes; productive; states, "My chest hurts from coughing so much."
Mucus secretions and viscosity	Unaware of presence	Thick, tenacious, clear; uses three tissues in five minutes
Interferences with O_2 uptake	None	Inflammation: temp., 100.6 F; throat red
Physical examination		
Posture	For 60-year old: erect, with possible lordosis	Same
Contour	A-P/transverse 1:2 to 5:7	A-P less than transverse
Chest wall movement	Symmetrical, no retraction or bulging of interspaces	Same
Palpation	No tenderness, masses, pain	Same

(continued)

ASSESSMENT FACTOR	EXPECTED BEHAVIOR	ACTUAL BEHAVIOR
Tactile fremitus	Complementing areas have same intensity; decreases in intensity as you move away from neck region	*Tussive* fremitus (fremitus caused by coughing)
Auscultation	No adventitious sounds	Rales in upper bronchi region
Duration of symptoms	—	2 days
Chest x-ray	No pathology	Same
Attitudes toward respiratory changes	—	States: "This is probably just the beginning of my problems. I'll end up like my brother who died last month from lung cancer."
Physician's diagnosis		Upper respiratory infection
Doctor's Orders	—	Ampicillin 250 mg, p.o., B.I.D. × 10 days; elixir terpin hydrate, 15 cc, p.o., q4h prn; salt water gargles prn

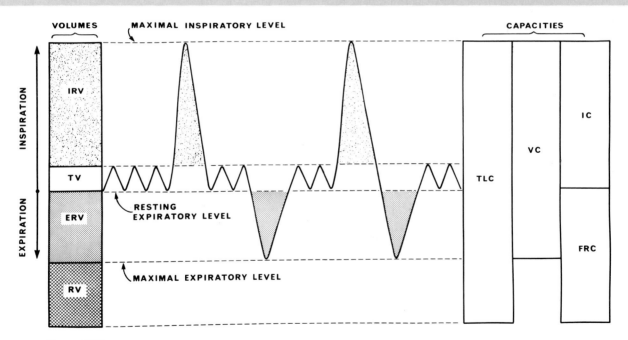

Figure 17.8

The principle lung volumes include: *residual volume* (RV), the volume of gas that remains in lungs following maximal expiration; *expiratory reserve volume* (ERV), the maximal volume of gas that can be expired following normal expiration; *tidal volume* (TV), the volume of gas inspired and expired during a normal respiratory cycle; and *inspiratory reserve volume* (IRV), the maximal volume of gas, besides tidal volume, that can be inspired. The lung capacities are: *total lung capacity* (TLC), the amount of gas in lung after maximal inspiration; *vital capacity* (VC), the amount of gas that can be forcefully expelled after maximal expiration; *inspiratory capacity* (IC), the maximal amount of gas that can be inspired following normal inspiration; and *functional residual capacity* (FRC), the amount of gas in lungs following normal expiration. *(Courtesy of David Jensen,* The Principles of Physiology, *Appleton, New York, 1976)*

Resulting nursing diagnoses, in order of priority, might include:

- anxiety related to reaction to family history and present symptoms
- chest discomfort related to inflammatory process
- dyspnea related to anxiety
- dyspnea related to inflammatory process
- increased respiratory hazard related to smoking habits

PLANNING

Interference with oxygen uptake is potentially life threatening. The degree of respiratory interference, degree of anxiety, level of growth and development, underlying respiratory pathology, and the individual's general health state determine the specific goal and immediacy of the course of intervention. For example, respiratory crisis (e.g., complete airway obstruction) takes precedence over any other need interference. However, regardless of the severity of the respiratory interference, planning priorities are based on maintaining a patent airway and ensuring respiratory adequacy. This is true because the survival of all other body systems depends on preservation of respiratory functioning. In addition, plans should include structuring the environment so it assists the individual in meeting his or her oxygen uptake needs.

In the situation of Mr. Em, the plan for one of the nursing diagnoses listed above might look like the one on page 415.

INTERVENTION

Observing Respiratory Pattern

Observing the individual's respiratory pattern is usually the first activity the nurse does in assessing oxygen uptake needs. To measure the respiratory rate, the nurse counts the number of respiratory cycles per minute. A respiratory cycle is one inspiration and one expiration. By counting the entire cycle, the nurse is able to obtain additional information about the quality, depth, rhythm, symmetry, effort, and overt sounds of the respiratory pattern. When first taking a respiratory rate, it is difficult to integrate all these factors into one observation. However, repeated practice with a variety of individuals will help to acquire this skill. Chart 17.9 outlines the techniques used for counting the respiratory rate. (Illustration 17.2)

Chart 17.9
Counting Respiratory Rate

TECHNIQUE	POINTS TO NOTE
Make sure individual is unaware of respiratory observation.	Individual should be unaware that respiration rate is being observed, since breathing is partially under voluntary control. A good time would be just before or after taking the pulse.
Count respiratory cycles for 1 minute (may be counted for 30 sec and the value multiplied by two, if no respiratory distress is suspected).	Counting respirations for less than 30 sec can result in a high deviation from actual.
Respirations that are difficult to observe can be measured by auscultation or when taking individual's pulse by placing his or her hand across the chest and counting the respiratory cycles by feeling the movement of the chest wall.	This method also aids in more accurately assessing depth.
Listen for overt breath sounds; observe for symmetry, effort, and rhythm.	Identification of timing of these factors in the respiratory cycle can be diagnostically significant.

Determining Skin Color Changes

In observing for skin color changes, the nurse may have to differentiate between cyanosis and other conditions which may mimic cyanosis. In addition, it is necessary to determine whether the presenting cyanosis is central or peripheral. Charts 17.10 and 17.11 describe methods for making these determinations.

Easing Respiratory Effort

POSITIONING

Positioning may be an effective technique in assisting the individual in easier, more efficient breathing. Any position in which the individual is placed should allow for maximum lung expansion (see

NURSING DIAGNOSIS	SHORT-TERM GOALS	NURSING PLAN

Chest discomfort related to inflammatory process	Decreased amount of coughing within 3 days
	
	Relief of chest discomfort within 1 week
	
	Temperature return to usual within 2 days
		1. Give first dose of cough medicine.
		
		2. Instruct in use of cough medicine:
		    How often to take
		    Benefits
		    Dosage limits
		    Wait 30 minutes before drinking liquids
		
		3. Instruct how to cough effectively
		    Procedure
		    Splinting
		    Disposal of tissues
		
		4. ASA for pain
		
		5. Increased humidification
		    Benefits
		    Procedure
		
		6. Increase fluids to 2500 cc/day
		    Benefits
		    Types
		    Frequency
		
		7. Rest
		    Benefits
		    Coordination with medications
		    Difference between rest and sleep
		
		8. Give first dose of antibiotic
		
		9. Instruct in:
		    Use of antibiotics
		    Frequency
		    Dosage limits
		    Need for full course of therapy
		    Reporting side effects
		
		10. Provide clinic number to report back if symptoms not relieved within stated time.
		
		11. Explain relationship between smoking and chest discomfort
		    Irritations
		    Decreased immunity

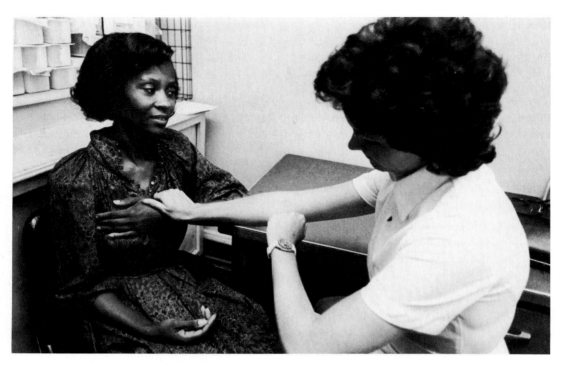

Illustration 17.2
So that an individual is not aware that his or her respiratory rate is being measured, respirations are often counted in conjunction with pulse taking. Here, the nurse feels the individual's expirations and inspirations with her hand, while it seems to the woman that her pulse is being measured. *(Photo © Leonard Speier)*

Chap. 14). For example, in the lateral position, the upper arm is supported away from the chest, and the individual is tipped so he or she faces the ceiling rather than the bed. If the sitting position feels more comfortable or if it is therapeutically desirable, the individual can be placed in a *high semi-Fowler's* position (head of bed elevated at 90° angle). To further maximize lung expansion of the individual, the over-bed table can be placed in front of the individual at chest level, helping him or her to hunch shoulders

---

Chart 17.10
Determination of True Cyanosis

TECHNIQUE	POINTS TO NOTE
Choose an area of skin where cyanosis can be easily detected (e.g., nail bed, earlobe).	Areas where superficial blood vessels are plentiful and not masked by pigmentation.
Press area lightly with finger until area becomes pale.	Pressure prevents capillary filling.
Release pressure and closely observe color changes.	Capillaries refill when pressure is released, spontaneously filling from both the sides and the area below the spot pressed.
	In true cyanosis refilling is slower and filling occurs from sides to middle of area.
	In other conditions, discoloration remains.

Chart 17.11
Differentiation between Central
And Peripheral Cyanosis

TECHNIQUE	POINTS TO NOTE
Massage cyanotic area.	Stimulates peripheral vasodilation.
Observe color changes.	In peripheral cyanosis, blood supply returns to area, causing cyanosis to disappear. In central cyanosis, discoloration remains.

and elevate arms (Fig. 17.0). Pillows should be placed for support and comfort. The orthopneic or dyspneic individual often finds that this position is the only one in which he or she can sleep. Therefore, the individual should be permitted to maintain this position whenever he or she feels it necessary.

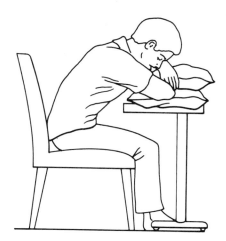

Figure 17.9
The individual with an interference in oxygen intake may rest and be helped to breathe more easily by sitting down at a table and leaning over it, resting arms and head on pillows that have been placed on the table. In this position, the hunched shoulders and elevated arms facilitate lung expansion.

FREE RESTRICTIVE COVERING

If the person is having difficulty breathing, the nurse checks for clothing, dressings, or binders which may be restricting lung expansion. Loosening or repositioning them can often be sufficient to ease breathing.

RELIEVING PAIN

Pain is carefully evaluated as a possible source of respiratory interference. Nursing actions such as administration of analgesics, repositioning, and modifying the environmental stimuli may be helpful in decreasing the pain and thus enhancing respiratory ease. It should be remembered that certain analgesics may further interfere with respiration by depressing the respiratory center.

PROVIDE OPEN ENVIRONMENT

The individual with respiratory difficulty may find it psychologically beneficial to be in an airy, uncluttered environment. Placing the bed near a window, keeping the bedside curtains open when possible, and minimizing the amount of equipment kept at the bedside may provide this open atmosphere. (Illustration 17.3)

LESSEN ANXIETY

Any interference with respiratory ease creates feelings of anxiety. The anxiety in turn can increase respiratory difficulty. Nursing intervention for anxiety will be based on the individual's specific needs. However, one major fear that is often felt by the individual is that no one will be available in the event of a respiratory crisis. If the individual knows that someone is available in case of need, anxiety about this concern is lessened. Such nursing actions as answering the call bell promptly and checking the individual frequently helps the individual to feel more secure.

ASSIST IN RECOGNIZING LIMITS

Individuals with respiratory difficulty must match their capabilities with their limitations. The nurse can help by assisting the individual to recognize activities which produce dyspnea and to modify his

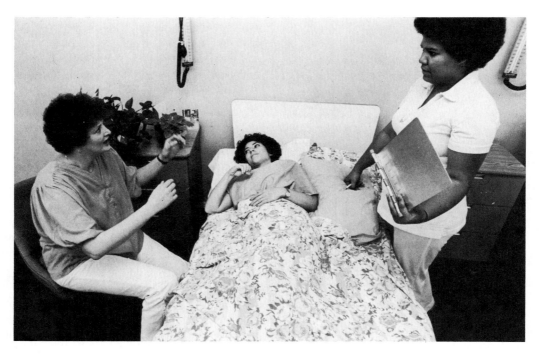

Illustration 17.3
An individual who is having respiratory difficulty finds psychological and physical comfort in being positioned properly, having friends visit, and being in an uncluttered, attractive environment. *(Photo © Leonard Speier)*

or her activities of daily living accordingly. Scheduling care to allow for periods of rest and to minimize exertion is also necessary.

Promoting Effective Cough

When the cough reflex is depressed or when secretions interfere with gaseous exchange, the nurse can intervene by teaching the individual to cough more effectively. Teaching the individual the proper technique conserves his or her energy while helping to keep the airway patent. (Chart 17.12 and Fig. 17.10)

Promoting Gaseous Exchange

BREATHING EXERCISES

Breathing exercises can be done in conjunction with coughing or as a separate intervention. These exercises help to inflate the lungs in order to promote gaseous exchange and strengthen respiratory and abdominal muscles. Before beginning breathing exer-

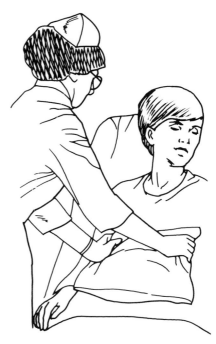

Figure 17.10
The individual who has had a recent abdominal incision is taught by the nurse how to splint the wound with a pillow to ease the discomfort of deep breathing and coughing.

Chart 17.12
Effective Cough Technique

TECHNIQUE	POINTS TO NOTE
Explain need for effective cough and procedure.	Anxiety is lessened when individual is aware of what is expected of him or her and why it its necessary. Information increases cooperation.
Administer appropriate medications (e.g., analgesics, expectorants).	Pain may prevent the individual from effectively coughing and may reduce cooperation because of fear of pain. Expectorants loosen secretions so that they can be brought up more easily.
Assist individual to a sitting position.	Upright position facilitates lung expansion and movement of secretions.
Teach and assist individual to splint abdominal area by one of the following methods: (Fig. 17.8)	If an incision or pain is present, splinting provides support to the area and also provides comfort and protection to area. External splinting prevents muscular contraction which inhibits lung expansion.

Pillow method
    Place small pillow over area of incision or pain.
    Apply steady pressure, sufficient to counter the resistance of the cough.
    Remind individual to splint during cough and deep breathing. (Fig. 17.8)
	Pillow provides support.
	Pressure prevents strain on muscles. Pressure varies with size of the individual and personal preference.
	Support is necessary during cough itself and for deep breathing.

Hand method Place hands, one on top of the other, over area of incision or pain (see Fig. 17.10) and proceed as with a pillow.	Pillow may not be available. Provides support and pressure of pillow. Nurse may provide splinting if individual is unable to do it unaided.
Instruct individual to take deep breaths: Ask individual to inhale slowly and deeply through nose.	Breathing through the nose warms, humidifies, and filters air. Deep breaths aerate lungs, especially portions not aerated during regular respirations.
No more than five times	More than five breaths can fatigue the individual and may result in hyperventilation. Watch relationship of number of breaths to fatigue.
After the fifth inhalation, instruct individual to exhale as fully as possible and then to cough.	Prolonged expiration helps move secretions up respiratory tree. May also stimulate natural coughing.
Instruct individual to expectorate any sputum raised.	Have container and tissues available. Expectorating sputum prevents it from flowing back into respiratory tree or being swallowed. Observe color and amount of sputum.
Repeat as necessary allowing for rest periods between each set of coughs.	Check for fatigue and hyperventilation. Match effort with capabilities.
Give oral hygiene.	Aesthetically pleasing, as well as preventing growth of microorganisms.

Note: Coughing may be stimulated by firmly stroking the throat near the cricoid cartilage of the trachea.

Marie E. Collart and Janice K. Brennerman, "Preventing Post Operative Atelectasis," *American Journal of Nursing,* 71:1982, October, 1971.

Chart 17.13
Pursed-Lip Breathing

TECHNIQUE	POINTS TO NOTE
Explain procedure.	As above.
Instruct individual to breathe in through the nose.	As above.
Instruct individual to purse (pucker) lips and to exhale for a count of seven:	Exhaling through pursed lips increases the intra-alveolar pressure and prolongs expiration and the increased removal of CO_2. Exhaling for a count of seven prolongs expiration and mimics normal respiratory pattern.
Instruct individual to lean slightly forward while exhaling or to press firmly on abdomen while exhaling.	Assists in exhalation.
Repeat procedure, allowing for periods of rest.	Matches effort with capabilities. Observe for fatigue, hyperventilation.

---

cises, the individual should attempt to clear nasal secretions from the upper respiratory tree in order to decrease resistance to air flow. A steady and rhythmical pattern should be maintained throughout the exercises. The nurse observes for signs of any anxiety, respiratory distress or discomfort, and intervenes appropriately. Two major types of breathing exercises —pursed-lip breathing and diaphragmatic breathing —are outlined in Charts 17.13 and 17.14. However, other breathing techniques are also used to inflate specific parts of the lung.

OTHER TECHNIQUES TO INFLATE LUNGS

Other techniques to help inflate the lungs and to promote gaseous exchange are the use of blow bottles, intermittent positive pressure breathing (IPPB), and incentive respiratory devices. Blow bottles (see Illustration 17.4) specifically aid expansion of the alveolar sac and strengthen the muscles of expiration. To prepare the bottles for use, one bottle is filled with colored water (to aid observation) and all connections are closed securely to prevent dispersion of air. The individual is instructed to blow the water from one bottle to the other. Each expiratory effort is aimed at displacing approximately 100 ml of water. Ensuring that individuals form a tight seal with their lips around the blowing tube prevents wasted effort. Individuals are reminded to release their lips from the ▶ tube during inspiration to prevent **aspiration** or swal-

lowing of the water. (Aspiration is the inhalation of fluids, food, or foreign objects into the lungs.) This procedure is repeated according to physician's orders and the individual's level of tolerance. The nurse notes how much water is displaced with each exhalation and the individual's reactions to the procedure, such as dizziness or a change in blood pressure. If this technique is ordered for children, blowing up baloons or blowing bubbles with a straw in a glass of water may make it more fun, thereby increasing cooperation.

Incentive Respiratory Devices
The object of incentive respiratory devices (e.g., spirometers) is also to inflate the alveoli and strengthen the muscles of respiration in order to prevent atelectasis. When using these devices, the individual first exhales as completely as possible to empty the lungs in preparation for deep inspiration. After placing the mouthpiece firmly between the teeth with lips forming a tight seal, the individual takes as deep an inspiration as possible. He or she holds the inspiration for at least 5 sec and then slowly exhales. Holding the inspiration allows for maximum aeration and expansion of the alveoli.

Intermittent Positive Pressure Breathing
IPPB is a technique which aids alveolar gaseous exchange through the application of positive pressure. The positive pressure that is delivered helps expand the alveoli, lessens the effort of inspiration, and

Chart 17.14
Diaphragmatic Breathing

TECHNIQUE	POINTS TO NOTE
Explain procedure.	As above.
Place individual in supine position.	Provides counterresistance, forcing use of abdominal muscles.
Instruct individual to place one hand on middle of chest and the other hand on the abdomen.	Helps individual become aware of breathing pattern.
Instruct individual to inhale slowly and deeply through nose while raising the abdomen.	As above. Raising the abdomen increases the descent of the diaphragm, allowing for fuller lung expansion. Strengthens abdominal muscles.
Instruct individual to exhale slowly and deeply through mouth (may be pursed lips) while lowering abdomen and pressing inward and upward with hands.	As above. Strengthens abdominal muscles. Aids exhalation of gases.
Repeat as tolerated, allowing for periods of rest.	As above.
Provide oral hygiene as necessary.	As above.

Note: After individual has become proficient in use of technique in supine position, progress to sitting, then standing positions, until individual can use diaphragmatic breathing without conscious awareness.

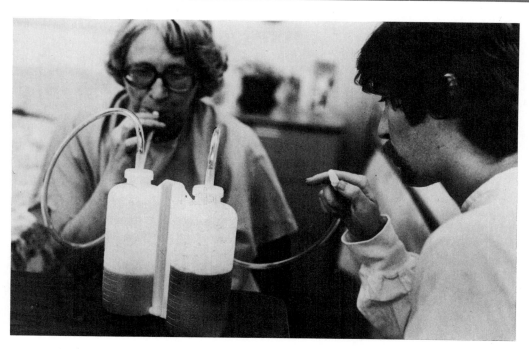

Illustration 17.4
A nurse instructs and supports a woman who has interference with oxygen uptake as she uses blow bottles. The procedure helps to increase an individual's alveolar expansion and strengthen muscles of respiration. *(Photo © Leonard Speier)*

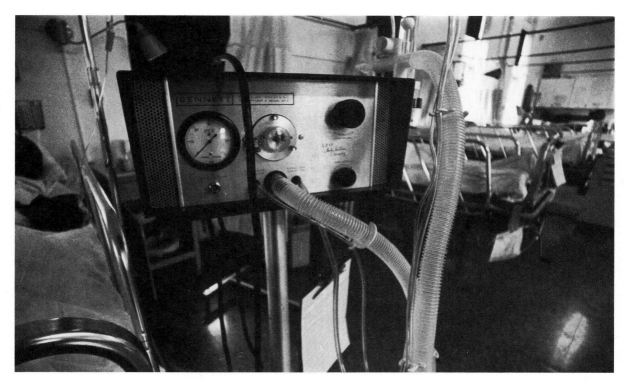

Illustration 17.5
The Bennett pressure breathing therapy unit aids gaseous exchange in the alveoli by providing
a certain concentration of oxygen under a specific positive pressure during inspiration. *(Photo
© Jan Lukas, from Photo Researchers)*

loosens secretions. Medications can also be supplied
▶ by **aerosol** using this technique.

A variety of machines can be used to give IPPB
treatments. These machines are attached to either an
oxygen or compressed air source (tank or wall outlet). When the gas source is oxygen, it is usually
mixed with room air to give a less than 100% concentration of oxygen. The mixing of gases that occurs
is regulated by an air-mix control mechanism found
on the unit. Regardless of the oxygen concentration
used, safety precautions related to the use of oxygen must be followed (Oxygen Therapy, page 428).
Illustration 17.5 shows a commonly used IPPB
machine.

The IPPB unit works by releasing a preset force
of air when the individual begins to inspire. When the
preset pressure is reached the machine automatically
stops air delivery, allowing for passive expiration.
Thus three major factors must be considered regardless of the type of machine used: (1) the effort required to trigger the unit (sensitivity), (2) the pressure
applied, and (3) the rate of gas flow. The sensitivity

setting is determined by the amount of effort the individual can or should apply as required by his or her
health state or therapeutic regimen. The pressure is
set according to the degree of lung inflation desired.
Lower pressures deliver a smaller volume of gas, thus
reducing the amount of lung inflation. The flow rate
is determined by the amount of pressure used and by
the length of time desired for the inspiratory phase.
For example, when the flow rate is increased, the gas
enters the lungs more rapidly. This causes the pressure to reach the preset level faster, thus ending the
inspiratory phase more quickly. Chart 17.15 outlines
the procedure for use of IPPB machines.

The use of IPPB therapy has recently come under
question because of the hazards it can produce and
because other interventions such as coughing, deep
breathing, and postural drainage can effectively replace it. (Chart 17.16)

Postural Drainage
When secretions decrease the alveolar surface
area and increase the distance across which gases

Chart 17.15
IPPB Treatment

TECHNIQUE	POINTS TO NOTE
Check orders for length of treatment, gauge settings, medications to be used.	Checking orders ensures proper treatment. Length of treatment is usually 15–20 minutes. Examples of medications: bronchodilators, mucolytic agents, surface-acting agents.
Check side effects of medications.	Allows for recognition.
Explain procedure.	As above.
Test machine by placing sterile gauze over mouthpiece and manually triggering machine.	Gauze acts to seal mouthpiece so pressures can be reached; pressure gauge will reach preset levels if machine is functioning properly.
Instill medication in nebulizer unit.	Nebulizer unit is cleaned before use. Medication should last for full treatment—if it does not, report to physician or respiratory therapist.
Place individual in semi-Fowler's or sitting position if tolerated.	As above.
Check pulse and respirations.	Having pretreatment values helps in assessing effectiveness, side effects of treatment, and/or medications used.
Instruct to:	
Tightly seal lips around mouthpiece	Closes the system so pressure can properly build.
Breathe through mouth, not nose (if unable to do this apply nose clip or have individual hold nose closed)	The negative inspiratory pressure within the mouth triggers machine.
Begin inspiration then allow pressure from machine to finish inspiration	Decreases effort. Allows for full inflation, aeration, and nebulization of lungs.
Hold breath for few seconds after machine cycles off	Allows for alveolar exchange of gases and medications.
Release seal around mouthpiece and exhale slowly	See breathing exercises.
Repeat procedure for time prescribed, allowing for rest periods as needed	As above.
Observe for change in pulse and respirations and any side effects throughout procedure and after treatment.	Changes in pulse and respiration may indicate adverse reactions to treatment. (See Chart 17.16 for Hazards of IPPB.) Side effects may necessitate stopping treatment.
Provide oral hygiene.	As above.

Note: Since treatment liquifies secretions, coughing may be stimulated and encouraged throughout IPPB treatment.

must diffuse, postural drainage may be ordered to mobilize and remove these secretions. Postural drainage utilizes gravity to drain secretions from the lower lobes of the lung. This is done by positioning the individual so that the upper lobes of the lung are in a dependent position in comparison to the lower lobes. Figure 17.11 illustrates some positions used in postural drainage.

Each position of postural drainage is maintained for approximately 5 to 10 minutes. The indi-

Chart 17.16
Hazards of IPPB

HAZARDS	SYMPTOMS
Decreased venous return or abolition of thoracic pump resulting in:	
Decreased cardiac output	Hypotension Tachycardia
Increased intracranial pressure	May complain of headache
Nausea	Nausea
Gastric insufflation	Gastric distension
Respiratory alkalosis secondary to hyperventilation	Tingling of extremities Dizziness
Depression of hypoxic drive In patients with COPD, check blood gases for hypercapnia ($PaCO_2 > 50$ mm Hg) with compensated pH ($7.35 - 7.40$) and low PaO_2 (<60 mm Hg).	Slowing of respiratory rate during treatment
Infection due to contaminated equipment	Elevated WBC and temperature Purulent sputum Positive sputum culture
Inadequate humidification	Thickening of secretions
Drug reactions	Tachycardia Hypotension Bronchospasm Anaphylaxis

From: Joseph Rau and Mary Rau, "To Breathe or Be Breathed: Understanding IPPB," American Journal of Nursing, 77(4):613, April, 1977. Copyright 1977 American Journal of Nursing Company. Reproduced with permission from the American Journal of Nursing.

vidual is encouraged to sit upright and cough between each position change. Postural drainage is usually carried out four times a day—when the individual awakens, before going to bed, and before lunch and dinner. It is never performed after a meal because of the possibility of vomiting and aspiration. If bronchodilators or humidification have been ordered for the individual, postural drainage will be most effective if performed after these treatments have been administered.

The choice of position will be determined by physician's orders, the individual's health state, and the area to be drained. Conditions such as lung abscesses or tumors, *pneumothorax, hemoptysis,* and pulmonary emboli may contraindicate the use of this treatment. The nurse can make the person as comfortable as possible by helping the individual avoid positions which produce dyspnea (e.g., head-down position), having him or her wear loose clothing, and providing support to the head and the extremities. At the completion of postural drainage the indivdiual is given oral hygiene to remove any secretions collected in the mouth and encouraged to rest for at least a half-hour.

Percussion and Vibration prior to Postural Drainage. Percussion and vibration may be ordered prior to or during postural drainage to loosen the secretions to be drained. Beland and Passos write that "this technique is often said to be based on the 'ketchup bottle' theory. In other words if you turn the bottle upside down and the ketchup does not come out, you pound on it, which is percussion, and you shake it which is vibration."[2]

In performing percussion, the chest wall is rhythmically clapped with a cupped hand. Effective clapping produces a hollow sound rather than a slapping sound. The degree of pressure applied should be individualized according to size, age, and general health state. Care is taken to avoid percussing over the spine, kidneys, liver, spleen, or incision to prevent injury to these areas. Percussion is done for approximately 1 minute, progressing in a cephalocaudal direction along the chest wall. Vibration follows percussion and is performed while the individual is exhaling.

Percussion and vibration may be ordered by themselves. These procedures are carried out for approximately 15 minutes with rest periods interspersed between each set. Effective, deep breathing and coughing is encouraged throughout to help raise the loosened secretions. Listening for changes in ad-

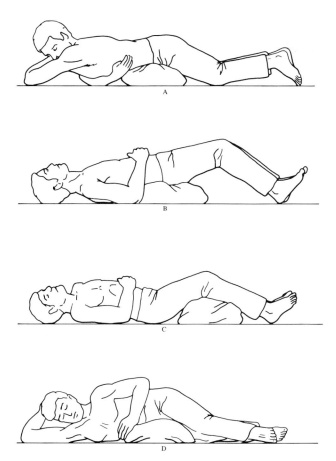

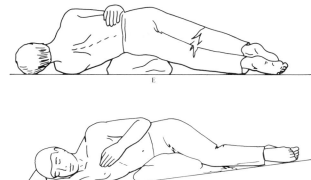

Figure 17.11

Positions for postural drainage. **A.** To drain lower lobes, individual lies face down with pillow under lower abdomen, and claps over lower ribs. **B.** Lying on one's back with a pillow under the hips drains the anterior chest. Clap over lower ribs. **C.** Lying on back, turned slightly to one side with pillow under knees, the anterior basal part of an individual's lower lobe is drained. Clap over lower ribs. **D.** An individual lying on his right side, pillow under lower abdomen, drains the left lower lobe. Clap over lower ribs. **E.** Lying on left side with pillow under lower abdomen drains right lower lobe. Clap over lower ribs. **F.** Lying on right side with pillow between hip bone and bottom ribs (feet higher than head) drains left middle lobe. Clap over left nipple area. NOTE: Clapping is always carried out along the rib cage to prevent damage to underlying structures.

ventitious sounds such as rales and rhonchi help evaluate the effectiveness of the procedures.

SUCTIONING

When secretions are particularly tenacious, the cough reflex depressed, or the individual otherwise incapable of bringing up secretions, mechanical removal of mucus through suctioning is necessary. **Suctioning** (Chart 17.17) is the application of a negative pressure to create a vacuum so that secretions move from an area of higher pressure (the airway) to a lower one (the suction collection bottle via the suction catheter). Suctioning may be done through the nose (nasopharyngeal), mouth (oropharyngeal), or trachea. Superficial suctioning clears secretions from the upper airway, while deep endotracheal suctioning clears secretions from the trachea and upper bronchi. No matter what route is used respiratory suctioning is a sterile procedure and therefore necessitates the use of sterile technique and equipment.

Indications that secretions are interfering with airway patency and gaseous exchange include gurgling or rattling respirations, rales, rhonchi, changes in pulse and respiratory rates, restlessness, and confusion. In short, any signs and symptoms of hypoxia help the nurse to assess the need for suctioning.

Equipment
The basic equipment needed for suctioning includes a sterile suction catheter, a suction setup, sterile water, and a sterile glove.

The Catheter. A pliable suction catheter is used to prevent injury to the mucous membrane lining of the airway and to increase ease of insertion along the respiratory tree. The catheter has an air vent to allow for control of the suction. The catheter tip is open-ended to help draw up secretions and prevent pushing any mucus or mucous plugs further down the respiratory tree. Catheters that are close tipped are never used as this type can force mucus along the airway. Some people find the use of side-opened catheters undesirable because of the possibili-ty of sucking in the mucosal lining of the respiratory tree as the catheter is withdrawn. Figure 17.12 shows commonly used open-ended catheters. Finally, the catheter should be the proper size. If the catheter is too large it will occlude the airway; if too small, sec-retions will not be able to pass through the opening. Common sizes in catheters for the adult are 12, 14, and 16 French (Fr), for children 10 Fr, and infants 5 and 8 Fr.

The Setup. The suction setup includes the suction machine itself, the collection bottle, and con-nective tubing. All connections should be tight to prevent dispersion of pressure. The suction machine creating the negative pressure may be either a porta-

---

Chart 17.17
Suctioning Technique

TECHNIQUE	POINTS TO NOTE
Explain procedure.	As above. Throughout procedure assess for signs of anxiety and intervene as necessary, as suctioning is an anxiety-producing situation.
General	

Assemble equipment:
  Catheter
  Tubing
  Collecting bottle
  Sterile glove
  Sterile water or saline
  Sterile container for water
	Make sure all connections are tight; collection bottle clean; equipment sterile; proper size catheter.
	Pour solution in container.
	Sterile water or saline acts as a lubricant and can be drawn through catheter to clear secretions.

If suctioning nasopharyngeally:
  Tongue blade
  Flashlight
	Aids in evaluating proper placement of catheter.

Position in semi-Fowler's or supine position with head slightly elevated and turned toward you.	Facilitates insertion and observation of catheter.
Check pulse, respiration, and chest sounds.	Provides base line for evaluation of effects of suctioning.
Note: Some authorities recommend administering 100% O_2 for approximately 5 minutes prior to suctioning, since suctioning draws out O_2, thus lowering PaO_2 levels.	
Adjust pressure valve to appropriate setting.	Setting determined by age, size, type, and amount of secretions.
Using sterile technique, glove dominant hand.	Dominant hand is used to manipulate sterile catheter. Other hand is used to manipulate nonsterile surfaces.
Test suction by placing tip of catheter in H_2O and observing pressure gauge and flow through catheter into collection bottle.	Equipment must be in working order to be effective. Maintain sterile technique.
Nasopharyngeal Suctioning	
With the catheter, measure distance from tip of the nose to tip of the ear.	Ensures catheter is inserted only as far as the pharynx.

(continued)

ble or wall unit. The force of suction used should be the lowest amount of negative pressure needed to remove secretions without causing undue trauma to the mucosal lining. Average pressure settings with the portable unit are 8–15 inches of mercury (in. Hg) for adults, 5–8 in. Hg for children, and 3–5 in. Hg. for infants. Wall unit settings are 110–150 mm Hg for adults, 100–110 mm Hg for children, and 60–100 mm Hg for infants. Illustration 17.6 shows the portable suction setup.

Oropharyngeal Suctioning
The procedure for oropharyngeal suctioning is the same as for nasopharyngeal, except the catheter is

Chart 17.17 (Cont.)
Suctioning Technique

TECHNIQUE	POINTS TO NOTE
Lubricate tip of catheter with H_2O.	Decreases resistance during insertion. Never use any lubricant which is not water soluble, e.g., oil based, as it can be aspirated into the lungs and become a focus of inflammation and block gaseous exchange.
With finger off air vent, gently insert catheter into one nostril, rotating the catheter in a downward direction along the floor of the nasal cavity.	Rotation decreases resistance and trauma, follows anatomical structure of nasal cavity. If gagging is produced, withdraw catheter to prevent vomiting and possible aspiration.
Stop insertion of catheter when distance measured is reached.	Prevents entering lower airway.
Check for placement of catheter by depressing tongue with tongue blade and shining flashlight into back of oral cavity.	Properly placed catheter will appear behind uvula.
Cover air vent with finger.	Seals system and starts negative pressure.
With rotating motion, remove catheter, applying suction for no more than 10 sec at a time.	Rotating catheter reduces trauma and helps clear secretions from all sides. Prolonged suction removes O_2 and may produce sudden death.
If any resistance is felt during suctioning, remove finger from air vent and withdraw catheter.	Prevents trauma of mucous membrane.
Rinse catheter.	Clears secretions and checks patency.
Repeat procedure for no longer than 3–5 minutes.	Repeating procedures helps clear airway. More than 3–5 minutes of suctioning removes excessive amounts of O_2 and reduces Pa_{O_2}.
Throughout procedure observe for signs and symptoms of hypoxia.	O_2 is being withdrawn with secretions, and this may result in O_2 deprivation.
Encourage deep breathing and coughing in between periods of suctioning.	Raises secretions so they can be removed.
Auscultate chest to evaluate effectiveness.	Change in chest sounds—rales, rhonchi—indicate movement of secretions.
Provide oral hygiene.	As above.
Discard used equipment and replace with unused sterile equipment.	Prevents contamination and maintains ready supply of equipment for next use.

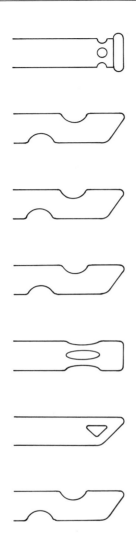

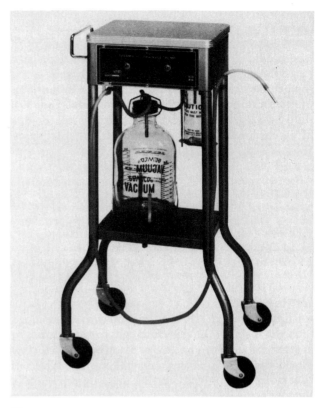

Illustration 17.6

A portable suction setup to remove mucus from an individual's airway. Secretions will move from the airway (area of higher pressure) to the collection bottle (area of lower pressure). *(Courtesy of Chemetron Medical Products, St. Louis, Missouri)*

Figure 17.12
Disposable suction catheter tip styles.

introduced through the mouth. To aid ease of insertion of the catheter, depress the tongue with a tongue blade as the catheter is introduced. Oropharyngeal suctioning is more likely to produce gagging and coughing than nasopharyngeal suctioning. The individual may also bite on the catheter, making further insertion difficult. If this occurs the jaw should be held open with the ungloved hand.

▶ **Note:** The same catheter is not used interchangeably for nasopharyngeal and oropharyngeal suctioning.

OXYGEN THERAPY

Oyxgen therapy is used to increase the amount of oxygen in the inspired air. Any condition which either actually or potentially leads to hypoxemia and/or hypoxia can indicate the need for oxygen therapy. Such conditions include chronic obstruction, inflammation, decreased ambient oxygen, respiratory depression, and cardiac insufficiency. The specific condition and blood gas levels will determine the concentration of oxygen to be used. However, in any condition which produces chronically high $PaCO_2$ levels (e.g., emphysema), only low concentrations of oxygen can be administered. This is true because long-term high $PaCO_2$ levels reduce the respiratory response to carbon dioxide. Thus, the secondary stimulus to respiration takes over (namely, lowered

▶ PaO_2 levels—the **hypoxic drive**). When PaO_2 is increased by the administration of high concentrations of oxygen, the stimulus to breathe is lost and apnea

▶ (lack of breathing) and **carbon dioxide narcosis** (unconscious state due to high $PaCO_2$ levels) occurs. Chart 17.18 outlines the common methods of administering oxygen, the concentration delivered by each and special points to note.

Chart 17.18
Methods of Administering Oxygen

METHOD	MAXIMUM O$_2$ (%)	FLOW (LITERS/MIN)	COMMENTS
Nasal catheter	30–40	6–8	Comfortable. Higher flows provide up to 40% oxygen, but can cause respiratory depression and drying of mucosa. Changed every 8 hr. Frequent nose care needed.
Nasal prongs	30–40	6–8	Comfortable. Higher flows provide up to 40% oxygen, but can cause respiratory depression and drying of mucosa. Easily displaced. Can cause skin breakdown if too tight.
T-piece	40–60	4–12	Provides enriched oxygen mixtures and humidification. Used most often in weaning patients from ventilator assistance before endotracheal tube is removed.
Face tent	30–55	4–8	Well tolerated. Good for supplying extra humidity. Moisture can cause skin irritation. Skin care necessary.

(continued)

Chart 17.18 (Cont.)
Methods of Administering Oxygen

METHOD	MAXIMUM O$_2$ (%)	FLOW (LITERS/MIN)	COMMENTS
Venturi masks	25–35	4–8	Mask well tolerated. Accurate concentrations delivered. Pressure from mask can cause skin breakdown. Frequent skin care necessary.
Mask without bag	35–45 45–55 55–65	6–8 10 10–12	Poorly tolerated. Significant CO$_2$ rebreathing possible at low flows. Highest percentages require tight mask fit. Pressure from mask can cause skin breakdown. Frequent skin care necessary.
Mask with bag	40–55 50–60 90+	6 8 8–12	Poorly tolerated. Significant CO$_2$ rebreathing possible at low flows. Highest percentage requires tight mask fit and a large bag. Pressure from mask can cause skin breakdown. Frequent skin care necessary.
Pressure-regulated ventilator	40–100	Direct from supply	Oxygen percent unpredictable.

(continued)

Chart 17.18 (Cont.)
Methods of Administering Oxygen

METHOD	MAXIMUM O_2 (%)	FLOW (LITERS/MIN)	COMMENTS
Volume-regulated ventilator	20—100	Direct from supply	Bennett MA1, Ohio 560 can be set to any desired percent.

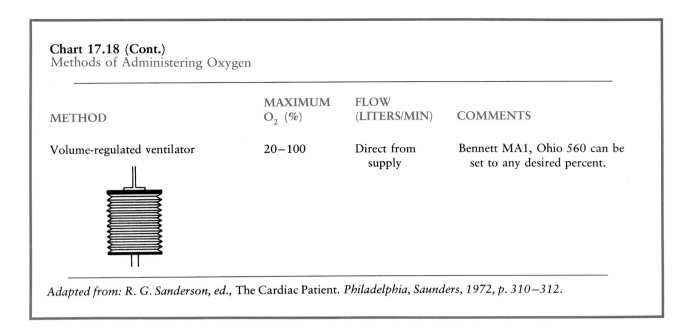

Adapted from: R. G. Sanderson, ed., The Cardiac Patient. *Philadelphia, Saunders, 1972, p. 310–312.*

Cautions

Oxygen is administered from a tank or piped-in wall unit. Regardless of its source, oxygen is hydrophilic and thus removes water from the tissues with which it comes in contact. Therefore, humidity must be supplied either by bubbling the oxygen through water immediately before administration or by vaporization. Consistent oral hygiene, including lubrication of lips, is a necessary part of nursing care for the individual receiving oxygen therapy. This is particularly true for mouth breathers, since the oral mucosa is directly exposed to the drying air.

Oxygen supports combustion, therefore caution must be taken to avoid using any highly flammable substance when oxygen therapy is being given. Among the items which must not be used are wool blankets, which can produce static electricity; cosmetics and lubricants which have an oil base; alcohol; electrical equipment such as call bells or electric beds, which can produce sparks; and open flames as with cigarettes and candles. Areas where oxygen is administered are indicated by posting large, easily read warning signs.

Individuals may feel that receiving oxygen therapy is an indication of critical illness. Whether or not it is in fact true, this feeling produces anxiety. The anxiety can often be reduced by explaining the rationale for the use of oxygen before and during its administration, in addition to employing other anxiety-reducing techniques previously discussed.

Equipment

Equipment needed for the administration of oxygen includes the specific administration device, connective tubing, humidification source, the oxygen flow meter, and the oxygen source. If a wall unit is used, the flow meter is plugged directly into the wall outlet. A humidification bottle filled with sterile distilled water is screwed onto the flow meter and the appropriate length of connecting tubing attached. The tubing should be long enough to allow the individual to turn in bed but not long enough to coil and kink. The administration device is then attached to the tubing. The flow meter is turned on and the oxygen is allowed to flow through the full length of the tubing. Bubbling in the water bottle will appear if the unit is functioning properly. The flow meter is turned off and the administration device is put on the individual. The flow meter is then adjusted to the prescribed flow rate.

If a tank is to be used as the source, the tank must first be "cracked." Cracking allows any dust particles to be blown away from the outlet. Cracking the cylinder is done by slightly opening the top tank valve until a hissing sound is heard and then closing it. Care is taken not to touch any of the tank connections with grease- or oil-based products. The oxygen level should also be checked by looking at the pressure gauge on the tank. Today these activities are frequently done by the respiratory therapist, but the nurse still needs to be aware of these procedures and to be able to perform them if necessary. The flow meter and humidifier is then screwed onto the tank connection and connective tubing attached. The nurse then proceeds as with the wall unit.

CLEARING AIRWAY OBSTRUCTION

Acute airway obstruction is easily confused with other causes of respiratory failure such as stroke and myocardial infarction; thus it is necessary to differentiate between these conditions. Choking on food is one of the most common causes of airway obstruction. While eating, a piece of food, especially meat, may become lodged in the victim's airway, resulting in either partial or complete obstruction. The victim usually clutches his or her throat, gasping for breath. If the obstruction is partial, a high, wheezing sound can be heard between coughs. Respirations, although difficult, may be seen. If the victim responds with a strong cough, he or she should be allowed to expel the food particle on his own. No attempt should be made to intervene at this point. Close observation is continued in the event of a change in the victim's respiratory status. However, the victim should be considered as having a complete obstruction and treated promptly if there are signs of respiratory deterioration such as a decrease in cough effectiveness, a shrill sound on inspiration, **stridor** (harsh, sharp sound on inspiration), or cyanosis. If the obstruction is complete, the victim will be unable to talk or breathe, rapidly becoming cyanotic and then collapsing.

Choking may be caused by talking and laughing while chewing and swallowing, decreased reflex action related to the consumption of alcohol, loose or poorly fitted dentures, edentulousness, poor chewing habits, gulping food, or generally "eating on the run."

Infants and children may easily fall victim to airway obstruction because of their natural inclination to put objects into their mouths, their moving about while eating, or their being given inappropriate food for their level of growth and development.

Treating Complete Obstruction

The treatment for complete airway obstruction consists of back blows, manual thrusts, and manual removal of the foreign body (see Charts 17.19 and 17.20). The back blow is a quick, sharp blow applied to the spine between the scapulae with the heel of the hand. This maneuver serves to raise the pressure along the respiratory tract rapidly, helping to dis-

lodge any foreign object. The manual thrust consists of a quick inward and upward pressure applied to the abdomen between the umbilicus and the sternum. It serves to force air out of the lungs by compressing the organs. As with the back blow, the pressure along the respiratory tract is raised, but in a lower, more sustained manner. The two maneuvers together are more effective than either one separately.

The manual removal of foreign objects with the index fingers is used to remove the particle dislodged but not expelled by the back blow and manual thrust.

If the victim is supine and unconscious, proceed as with a supine conscious victim after first attempting ventilation. Manual thrusts are replaced by chest thrusts if the victim is very heavy or pregnant.

Teaching

Because of the long-term nature of many of the interferences with oxygen uptake, the individual and the family and/or significant others will have to be taught intervention techniques for home use which will maintain a patent airway and promote gaseous exchange. In addition to learning the actual techniques, the individual and family and/or significant others will need basic assessment skills such as measuring respiratory patterns and determining respiratory adequacy, so that activities are matched with capabilities and limitations. The ability of family and/or significant others to assess subtle oxygen uptake interference and factors that may precipitate changes is vital to the success of a collaborative plan.

The techniques most often taught for home use are coughing and deep breathing, breathing exercises, postural drainage, respiratory hygiene measures, suctioning, and the use of IPPB and oxygen therapies.

Often the individual and the family and/or significant others will need to be aware of the effects that long-term interference with oxygen uptake will have on the home environment and personal interactions. For example, modifications in home humidification and filtering and greater accessibility of certain equipment and household facilities may be necessary in order to reduce respiratory effort. The nurse can play an important role in helping the individual and family and/or significant others to adjust to such changes. By providing concrete information and suggestions on how to assess and alleviate respiratory difficulty, the nurse can help reduce anxiety engendered by the home care situation. By providing an opportunity for the individual and the family and/or significant others to express their feelings and anxieties, the nurse assists in reducing anxiety.

In addition to teaching skills and counseling, the nurse may act as a resource person for referrals to appropriate agencies and services.

Individual and community teaching is geared toward prevention of interferences with oxygen uptake. Smoker education courses, environmental pollution hazards, and use of emergency techniques such as removal of airway obstruction are basic foci of preventive teaching.

Chart 17.19

Removal of Airway Obstruction in a Conscious Victim

TECHNIQUE	POINTS TO NOTE
Ask the victim to speak, looking and listening for respiration.	Establishes presence of complete obstruction.
If the victim cannot speak and respirations are absent, then, with the heel of one hand, administer four quick sharp blows to the spine between the victim's shoulder blades; the rescuer's other hand can be used to support the victim's chest.	See above text.
Stand behind the victim:	Best position for applying manual thrust.
Encircle the victim's waist with your arms	
Clench one hand into a fist and place, thumb-side in, between victim's umbilicus and sternum	Ensures effective pressure of manual thrust.
Clasp fist with other hand; forcefully press into victim's abdomen with four quick inward and upward thrusts.	
Repeat entire sequence until the obstruction is dislodged, or the victim becomes unconscious.	Death will ensue if airway is not cleared.
The above sequence should be repeated within 9–12 sec to prevent hypoxia.	

If the rescuer is smaller than the victim or the victim is supine, but conscious:

Place victim on side, facing you, with his chest against your knee.	Most effective position.
Lean over victim and administer four back blows.	As above.
Roll victim over onto back and kneel at victim's side, at hip level.	Most effective position. If victim is larger than the rescuer, rescuer may choose to straddle victim.
With one hand on top of the other, place the heel of your bottom hand between the victim's umbilicus and sternum.	As above.
Forcefully press into victim's abdomen with four quick upward thrusts.	As above.
Repeat entire sequence until the obstruction is dislodged or the victim becomes unconscious.	As above.

If the victim is an infant or small child who is conscious:

Place child face down in Trendelenburg position along your forearm.	Most effective position.
Deliver back blows as previously described.	As above.
	The age and size of the child will determine the inclusion of manual thrusts in the procedure.
	Manual thrusts are never performed on infants.

Chart 17.20
Removal of Airway Obstruction in an Unconcious Victim

TECHNIQUE	POINTS TO NOTE
1. Hyperextend the neck.	Opens airway by preventing the tongue from occluding air passage.
2. Attempt to ventilate with mouth-to-mouth breathing.	Provides oxygen supply. (Chapter 18 explains technique.)
3. If ventilation is not successful, reposition the head and attempt to ventilate again.	Airway may not have been adequately opened.
4. If the ventilation is still not successful: Administer 4 back blows Administer 4 manual thrusts Check for visibility of food particle by opening mouth with one hand; if visible or if you know choking was caused by food, then: Insert index finger of the other hand inside the cheek and deeply into the throat to the base of the tongue. With a hooking action, draw the foreign body into the mouth for removal.	See above. See above. Back blows and manual thrusts may have dislodged food particle. Do not place hand in mouth since individual may, as reflex, bite down. Hooking action prevents reaspiration of particle.
5. Attempt to ventilate victim.	Provides oxygen supply. After the removal of the foreign body, cardiopulmonary resuscitation may be necessary (Chap. 18).
If ventilation is unsuccessful, repeat step 4.	

EVALUATION

Evaluation of whether oxygen uptake needs are being met centers on the direction of change that has occurred in the person's ability to meet those needs and the effectiveness of nursing intervention.

Specific criteria for evaluating an individual's oxygen uptake needs include:

- How do the physiologic changes relate to changes in the oxygen uptake status? Psychologic changes? Environmental changes?
- Has the presenting respiratory pattern moved closer to the expected? Skin color? Position? Ease of respiratory effort? Adequacy of gaseous exchange? Behavioral responses? Environmental factors? Airway patency mechanisms? Physical exam? Diagnostic test results? Level of growth and development?
- What are the changes in the degree of oxygen uptake interference?
- What are the changes in coping with increased activity (changes in the individual and the family and/or significant others)? What are the changes in coping with limitations?
- What are the changes in knowledge about precipitating factors? Restrictions? Abilities? Therapies? Aseptic practices? Prevention?
- What skills have been acquired in utilizing devices? Carrying out exercises? Communicating oxygen uptake needs?
- What is the direction of change toward independence in coughing and deep breathing? Carrying out breathing exercises? Postural drainage? Using equipment?
- What are the changes in attitude toward oxygen uptake needs? Body image? Limitations? Respiratory hygiene? Exercises? Therapies?
- What are the changes in levels of anxiety concerning oxygen uptake needs? (Changes in the individual and family and/or significant others?)

RECORDING AND TEACHING–LEARNING ACTIVITIES

Teaching–Learning Topics

- The rationale for the therapeutic regimes.
- Methods to match capabilities with effort:
  how to make modifications in ADL based on level of growth and development;
  types of activities available to individual.
- Ways to structure the environment to facilitate meeting oxygen uptake needs.
- How to perform coughing and deep breathing, breathing exercises, postural drainage.
- How to use devices and do therapies in the home (e.g., IPPB, suctioning, tracheostomy care, oxygen).
- Importance of continuity of exercises and therapies.
- Aseptic techniques related to respiratory hygiene.
- Safety factors related to therapeutic regime (e.g., oxygen therapy, prevention of infection, suctioning).
- Ways to assess changes in ability to meet oxygen needs (e.g., behavior, physical).
- Preventive aspects (e.g., of airway obstruction, smoking, pollution, infection).
- Ways to modify personal habits which affect oxygen uptake (e.g., smoking, alcohol).
- How to use medications related to oxygen uptake.
- Rationale for continuity of care.
- Positions which ease respiratory effort and affect of posture on respiration.
- Factors which may precipitate respiratory distress.
- Methods to decrease anxiety related to oxygen.
- Ways to facilitate chest expansion (e.g., clothing).
- What the available resources are and how to use them.

Charting and Recording

Using appropriate oxygen uptake terms, objectively describe such factors as:

- Objective base-line data on the following: respiratory pattern, skin color, positions assumed with and without distress, ease of respiratory effort in relation to activity, what muscles are used for respiration at rest and with activity, level of growth and development, physical assessment, environmental factors, patency mechanisms, signs of respiratory interference.
- Objective and subjective changes that occur in the person's ability to meet oxygen uptake needs.
- Subjective assessment data on respiratory response to activity, positioning, any changes in sleep patterns.
- Objective and subjective data on behavioral responses related to oxygen needs.
- Attitudes towards interference and treatment.
- Subjective and objective reactions and responses to treatment.
- Schedule and methods of care.
- Teaching carried out.
- Discharge planning done.
- Interactions and responses of family and/or significant others.

Update Kardex concerning changes in goals and plans for meeting oxygen uptake needs.

Medications to Review

- bronchodilators: e.g., isoproterenol (Isuprel)
- mucolytic agents: e.g., acetylcysteine (Mucomyst)
- surface-acting agents: e.g., tyloxapol (Alevaire)
- CNS depressants: e.g., morphine
- CNS stimulants: e.g., dextroamphetamine (Dexedrine)
- expectorants: e.g., terpin hydrate
- antitussives: e.g., benzonatate (Tessalon)

Diets to Review

- high calorie
- high protein
- increased fluid
- high vitamin

CLINICAL APPLICATION: POSTOPERATIVE RESPIRATORY CARE

Many potential hazards of oxygen uptake are typically encountered in the postoperative individual.

Regardless of the surgery performed, factors such as personal habits, preoperative medications, general anesthetic agents, postoperative analgesics, pain, anxiety, and restrictions on movement create a situation which may threaten the individual's respiratory status.

Personal habits such as smoking, alcohol intake, or working in a highly polluted atmosphere decrease the body's resistance to respiratory infection, reduce gaseous diffusion through the buildup of secretions and limit lung expansion. These personal habits potentiate the effects of the other factors mentioned above in predisposing the individual to postoperative respiratory complications.

The common medications given to the person immediately before surgery include narcotics and anticholinergic agents. Narcotics—CNS depressants—depress the respiratory center, while anticholinergic agents decrease mucous membrane secretions. In addition, anticholinergic drugs relax the involuntary muscles, decreasing the gag and swallow reflexes. These effects are therapeutically desired during the operative phase; however, postoperatively they may add to the possibility of respiratory problems.

During the operative phase, several events occur which may further compromise respiratory adequacy. The general anesthesia given acts as a CNS depressant, thereby depressing respiration as well as irritating the mucous membranes, which, in turn pro-

---

Chart 17.21
Nursing Respiratory Management During the Operative Experience

PRESENTING BEHAVIOR	MECHANISM OF OCCURRENCE	NURSING INTERVENTION	RATIONALE FOR INTERVENTION
Increased secretions with increased viscosity and decreased mobilization.	Preoperative: Personal habits (e.g., smoking). Decreased ciliary movement. Irritation. Increase in goblet cells.	Encourage individual to stop smoking during immediate preoperative period (may also be long-term goal).	To prevent further damage to respiratory system.
	Debilitation Decreased mobilization of secretions. Decreased muscle tone.	Improve general health state through medical and nursing regime directed at specific cause of debilitation.	Positive health state decreases the incidence of postop respiratory complications.
		Teach coughing and deep breathing.	Helps reduce amount of secretions preop.
		Teach use of IPPB (if ordered).	Improves ventilation and mobilization of secretions.
		Teach how to turn and move.	Improves ventilation, mobilization of secretions, and muscle tone.
		Chart and report signs and symptoms of change in health state.	Provides baseline data, immediate treatment can be instituted.
	Poor hydration.	Increase fluid intake. Increase environmental humidity.	Thins secretions, helps mobilize secretions and improves general health state.

(continued)

duce excessive secretions and thus a possible site of infection. Intubation is necessary to facilitate introduction of anesthesia and oxygen and to help prevent laryngeal and bronchial spasms. Oxygen and other gases given to maintain oxygen supply also irritate the mucous membranes by their drying effects and cause additional mucous secretion. The prolonged immobility during surgery pools these secretions.

Pain, analgesics, and relative immobility affect respiratory functioning postoperatively. Pain often makes the person reluctant to turn frequently and to cough and deep breathe, all of which are necessary to overcome the effects of the pre- and intraoperative phases. Analgesics, particularly narcotics, add to the

situation. The fear of pain and the therapeutic regimen may also limit activity, which is necessary in mobilizing secretions and aerating the lungs.

A previously unrecognized upper respiratory infection or postoperative exposure to infection and a general debilitated health state may complicate the situation even further.

All of these factors can lead to respiratory difficulties and prolong the recuperative period. However, these complications can be prevented through careful nursing assessment, planning, and intervention throughout the entire operative experience. Chart 17.21 outlines the nursing respiratory management of the individual during the operative experience.

Chart 17.21 (Cont.)
Nursing Respiratory Management During the Operative Experience

PRESENTING BEHAVIOR	MECHANISM OF OCCURRENCE	NURSING INTERVENTION	RATIONALE FOR INTERVENTION
	Respiratory infection and pathology.	Observe for and report any signs and symptoms.	Immediate treatment can be instituted.
		Follow nursing and medical regimen for specific treatment.	Improves general health state and prevents post-op complications.
		Preoperative: Explain rationale for postoperative respiratory plan, e.g., coughing and deep breathing, IPPB, frequent turning and:	Individual learns better at times of decreased stress and without distraction of postoperative condition.
		Teach coughing and deep breathing.	Reduces anxiety by allowing individual to anticipate what will occur postoperatively.
		Teach use of IPPB.	Increases postoperative cooperation.
		Teach how to turn and move.	See above.
		Observe for upper respiratory infections.	
		Observe change in health state.	
		Evaluate hydration.	

(continued)

Chart 17.21 (Cont.)
Nursing Respiratory Management During the Operative Experience

PRESENTING BEHAVIOR	MECHANISM OF OCCURRENCE	NURSING INTERVENTION	RATIONALE FOR INTERVENTION
	Postoperative: Relative immobility. Results of intraoperative experience. Poor hydration.	Postoperative: Reinforce preoperative teaching.	Postoperative anxiety may cause a decrease in the amount of learning retained.
		Maintain a regular schedule of: Coughing Deep breathing Turning IPPB	Improves ventilation, mobilizes secretions, prevents pooling, and increases muscle tone.
		Splint incision.	Reduces pain of therapeutic measures.
		Maintain hydration.	Thins secretions.
		Observe for and report any signs of infection.	Immediate treatment can be instituted.
		Use analgesics with discretion and planning.	Postoperative analgesics may decrease respirations; proper timing of medication administration may decrease pain and anxiety, allowing individual to carry out activities.
		Carefully observe and report: Respiratory pattern. Breath sounds. Reactions to care.	Immediate treatment can be instituted if signs of problems appear, further complications can be prevented, gives information for evaluation of status.
		Maintain patent airway through coughing and deep breathing, turning, suctioning, etc.	Patent airway is necessary for respiratory adequacy.
		Encourage early ambulation and activity (as allowed).	Increases ventilation and muscle tone and mobilizes secretions.
		Encourage change in personal habits which negatively affect respiratory status.	Improves general health state, decreases chance of postoperative infection.

(continued)

Chart 17.21 (Cont.)
Nursing Respiratory Management During the Operative Experience

PRESENTING BEHAVIOR	MECHANISM OF OCCURRENCE	NURSING INTERVENTION	RATIONALE FOR INTERVENTION
		Relieve anxiety (see below).	Decreased anxiety allows individual to fully participate in activities, increases cooperation; anxiety is directly related to change in respiratory pattern; makes individual more comfortable.
Decreased lung expansion (hypoventilation).	Preoperative: Poor posture	Teach proper posture for age and condition.	Proper posture facilitates lung expansion.
	Restrictive clothing	Explain relationship between restrictive clothing and poor lung expansion.	Restrictive clothing limits lung expansion.
	Preexisting respiratory pathology	Follow nursing and medical regimen.	May help limit condition and prevent further complications.
	Debilitation	Increase health state.	Decreases postoperative respiratory complications.
	Postoperative, restricted chest movement due to: Pain	Relieve pain through proper positioning, decrease anxiety, and judicious use of medications.	Pain or fear of pain restricts lung expansion; pain may be relieved by nursing measures other than medication.
	Medications	Use with discretion.	Medications, by depressing CNS, may restrict lung expansion; proper timing of medications may allow individual to breathe more comfortably.
	Inactivity	Encourage turning, moving, early ambulation.	See above.
		Deep breathing exercises.	See above.
	Restrictive dressings	Check for and adjust dressings frequently.	Tight dressings restrict lung expansion.

(continued)

Chart 17.21 (Cont.)
Nursing Respiratory Management During the Operative Experience

PRESENTING BEHAVIOR	MECHANISM OF OCCURRENCE	NURSING INTERVENTION	RATIONALE FOR INTERVENTION
	Gaseous distention	Encourage activity. Administer medications and enemas as ordered (Chap. 20).	Measures which prevent gaseous distention, prevent gas from pushing on diaphragm, and restrict lung expansion.
	Anxiety	Preoperative teaching appropriate to physical symptoms. Check individual frequently.	Decreasing anxiety may allow individual to breath deeply and enhance lung expansion.
Inadequate gaseous exchange: Dyspnea Decreased PaO_2 levels Increased PCO_2 levels Behavioral responses (e.g., confusion, restlessness).	Preoperative: Increased secretions with increased viscosity and decreased mobilization (see 1 above) leading to: Decreased alveolar surface area and increased alveolar-capillary diffusion area Smoking, increasing blood carbon monoxide levels	Pre- and postoperative: All measures to treat increased secretions.	Same.
	Decreased environmental oxygen	Give oxygen and humidity (if ordered).	Increased available oxygen supply relieves dyspnea.
	Postoperative: Same. Hypoventilation (see Decreasing Lung Expansion above).	All measures to treat hypoventilation.	Same.
		Provide means of orienting individual in accordance with level of confusion and growth and development.	Increasing awareness of environment decreases confusion.
		Ensure safety of individual, e.g., side rails.	Protects individual from hurting himself or herself while confused or restless.
		Treat underlying cause of hypoxemia.	When O_2 uptake is sufficient, symptoms of confusion and restlessness abate.

(continued)

Chart 17.21 (Cont.)
Nursing Respiratory Management During the Operative Experience

PRESENTING BEHAVIOR	MECHANISM OF OCCURRENCE	NURSING INTERVENTION	RATIONALE FOR INTERVENTION
Anxiety.	Preoperative: Fear of unknown Fear of dying Fear of pain	Preoperative teaching: Explanation of expected postoperative course.	When individual knows what is expected and how to perform these activities, fear of the unknown decreases.
		Allow expression of feelings.	Enables individual to recognize fears and begin to problem solve, reassures individual that someone is interested in him or her.
		Clarify understanding of myths and misinformation related to surgery.	Accurate information decreases anxiety.
	Postoperative: Same as preoperative. Respiratory difficulty.	Provide comfort measures. Reinforce preoperative teaching.	When oxygen uptake needs are met sufficiently, anxiety decreases.
		Explain all procedures. Check individual frequently.	Increases confidence in care.
		Treat respiratory symptoms as above.	Same.
		Allow person to participate in planning of own care.	Increases feeling of control over situation.
		Allow expression of feelings.	As above.
		Note: Each person expresses anxiety in a unique way; intervention must therefore be individualized to the person and his or her situation.	

NOTES

1. William F. Ganong. *Review of Medical Physiology,* 8th ed. Los Altos, California, Lange Medical Publishers, 1977, p. 510.
2. Irene Beland and Joyce Passos. *Clinical Nursing,* 3rd ed. New York, Macmillan, 1975, p. 415.

SELECTED REFERENCES

Bates, Barbara. *A Guide to Physical Examination.* Philadelphia, Lippincott, 1974.
Beland, Irene and Passos, Joyce. *Clinical Nursing,* 3rd ed. New York, Macmillan, 1975.
Dison, Norma. *Clinical Nursing Techniques.* St. Louis,

Mosby, 1975.

Felton, Cynthia. "Hypoxemia and Oral Temperatures." *American Journal of Nursing,* 78:56, January, 1978.

French, Ruth M. *Guide to Diagnostic Procedures*, 4th ed. New York, McGraw-Hill, 1975.

Ganong, William F. *Review of Medical Physiology,* 8th ed. Los Altos, California, Lange Medical Publications, 1977.

Garb, Solomon. *Laboratory Tests in Common Use,* 5th ed. New York, Springer, 1971.

Guyton, Arthur C. *Textbook of Medical Physiology.* Philadelphia, Saunders, 1971.

Heine, Emily, ed. *Assessing Vital Functions Accurately* (Nursing 77 Skill Series). Horsham, Pennsylvania, Intermed Communications, 1973.

Jensen, David. *The Principles of Physiology.* New York, Appleton, 1976.

Koepke, John A. *Guide to Clinical Laboratory Diagnosis.* New York, Appleton, 1969.

Luckman, Joan and Sorenson, Karen. *Medical-Surgical Nursing.* Philadelphia, Saunders, 1974.

Malkus, Bobby. "Respiratory Care at Home." *American Journal of Nursing,* 76:1789, November, 1976.

Malasanos, Lois, Barkauskas, Violet, Moss, Muriel, Stoltenberg-Allen, Kathryn. *Health Assessment.* St. Louis, Mosby, 1977.

Murray, Ruth and Zentner, Judith. *Nursing Assessment and Health Promotion.* Englewood Cliffs, N.J., Prentice-Hall, 1975.

O'Malley, Penny and Zankofski, Mary Ann. "Disposable Suction Catheters." *Nursing* 79, 9:70, May, 1979.

Sana, Josephine and Judge, Richard D. *Physical Appraisal Methods in Nursing Practice.* Boston, Little, Brown, 1975.

Tilkien, Sarko M. and Conover, Mary H. *Clinical Implications of Laboratory Tests.* St. Louis, Mosby, 1975.

Wade, Jacqueline F. *Respiratory Nursing Care.* St. Louis, Mosby, 1977.

Waldron, Mary Webb. "Oxygen Transport." *American Journal of Nursing,* 79:272, February, 1979.

Widmann, Frances K. *Goodale's Clinical Interpretation of Laboratory Tests.* Philadelphia, Davis, 1973.

Wood, Lucille A. and Rambo, Beverly J., eds. *Nursing Skills for Allied Health Services.* Philadelphia, Saunders, 1977.

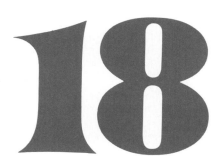

Clay lies still, but blood's a rover;
Breath's a ware that will not keep.
Up, lad: when the journey is over
There'll be time enough to sleep.
  —A. E. Housman, "Reveille"

OXYGEN TRANSPORT AND UTILIZATION AND WASTE PRODUCT REMOVAL

PRINCIPLES RELATED TO OXYGEN TRANSPORT AND UTILIZATION, AND WASTE PRODUCT REMOVAL

Any interference with O_2 uptake will cause an interference with O_2 transport and utilization.

Any interference with O_2 transport and utilization will alter O_2 uptake.

Adequate tissue perfusion is necessary for the survival of cells.

Cardiac output, tissue perfusion, and cardiac intake are related to:
1. efficiency of the pump (heart)
2. degree of resistance to blood flow
3. viscosity of the blood
4. amount of circulating blood
5. amount of area to be perfused
6. metabolic rate

The efficiency of the pump is related to:
1. strength of the myocardial muscles
    a. coronary blood supply
    b. muscle tone
    c. muscle size

2. electrical conduction
3. autonomic nervous system innervation
4. electrolyte content of the blood

The degree of resistance to blood flow is related to:
1. elasticity of the blood vessels
2. degree of vasoconstriction or vasodilation
3. autonomic nervous system innervation to the blood vessels
4. resistance of tissues surrounding blood vessels
5. force of gravity
6. emotional state

Viscosity of the blood is related to:
1. number of blood cells present
2. amount of plasma present
3. extracellular regulatory mechanisms
    The more concentrated a solution, the higher its viscosity.

Amount of circulating blood is related to:
1. hydration of the individual

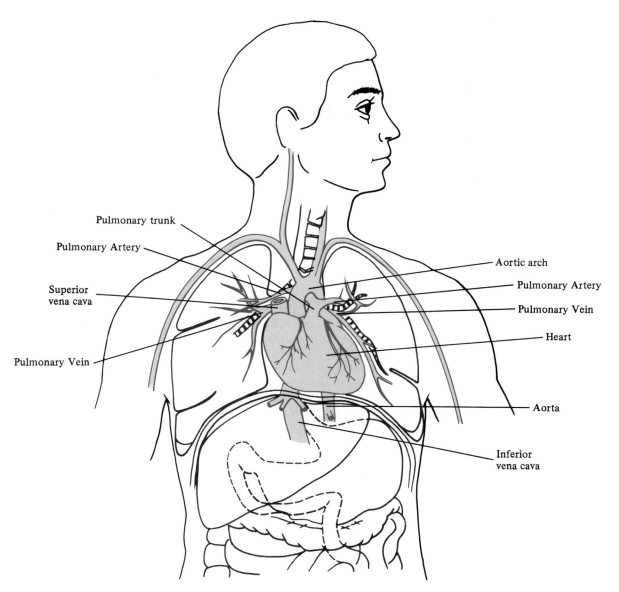

Figure 18.1
The heart and the major blood vessels in its circulation.

2. tissue demands
3. integrity of the closed system
4. amount of area to be diffused
5. extracellular regulatory mechanisms
6. blood-forming tissue (hematopoietic)
   activity

Amount of area to be perfused is related to:
1. stature
2. amount of adipose tissue
3. capillary–tissue diffusion area

Metabolic rate is related to:
1. activity
   a. increased activity increases metabolic
      rate
   b. decreased activity decreases metabolic
      rate
2. tissue demands (e.g., infection increases
   metabolic rate)
3. hormonal supply
4. emotions
5. hypothalamic regulating mechanisms

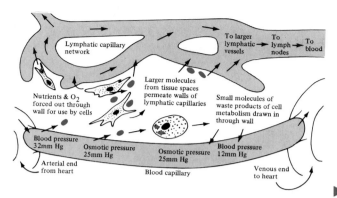

Figure 18.2
The diffusion of blood components.

Metabolic rate is *directly* related to:
1. heart rate
2. blood pressure
3. heat production

Movement of O_2 into the cells and removal of CO_2 from the cells is related to:
1. hydrostatic pressure
2. diffusion area
3. cell permeability
4. partial pressure of the gases
5. number of circulating red blood cells
6. hemoglobin level

Blood pressure is related to:
1. efficiency of the pump
2. degree of resistance to blood flow
    a. elasticity
    b. peripheral resistance
3. viscosity of the blood
4. amount of circulating blood
5. amount of tissue are to be perfused
6. metabolic rate
7. exercise
    a. increased exercise increases blood pressure
    b. decreased exercise decreases blood pressure
8. position
9. emotion
10. pain

Anxiety increases pulse rate.

Pain affects heart rate.
1. superficial pain usually increases heart rate by stimulating the sympathetic nervous system
2. deep pain usually decreases heart rate through parasympathetic nervous system control

Thermoregulatory centers in the hypothalamus control heat loss and conservation.

The ultimate goal of oxygen uptake is to provide adequate perfusion of oxygen to all body cells. **Perfusion** is the term used to describe the nourishment of cells by oxygen and other nutrients and the removal of by-products of cellular metabolism. Without adequate nourishment, cell metabolism cannot occur. Cells become hypoxic, necrose, and die. Also, with inadequate perfusion, waste products build up and the cells become toxic. Thus maintenance of an intact circulatory system is vital to life.

In a positive health state the body has several regulatory mechanisms which interact to maintain perfusion at adequate levels throughout the body. These mechanisms form the basis of assessment for oxygen transport and utilization, and waste removal.

ASSESSMENT

Tissue Perfusion

Nursing assessment of the adequacy of tissue perfusion begins with observation of the general behavior and appearance of the individual, as well as tolerance to activity. Behaviors characteristic of an interference with oxygen uptake can also reflect a disturbance in oxygen transport and utilization. Oxygen deprivation is the basic problem in both situations. An alteration in respiratory pattern will usually accompany inadequate perfusion, since the body attempts to bring in more air to supply oxygen to the vital organs.

When tissue perfusion is adequate, the individual appears "healthy." He is well hydrated, his skin is smooth, resilient, and translucent. The nails are also translucent, and the hair is glossy. The individual's energy levels are more than sufficient to carry out his activities of daily living.

The individual's overall tolerance to activity and stressors also depends on the state of tissue perfusion.

If tissue perfusion does not supply the cells with sufficient oxygen and nutrients and remove by-products of metabolism in adequate amounts, fatigue develops. Furthermore, if the perfusion deficit is severe and prolonged, organ function will be affected.

Often a decrease in tissue perfusion can be tolerated when the person is at rest and metabolic demands are few. However, when metabolic rate is increased through exercise, anxiety, infection, fever or any other type of stressor, signs of inadequate perfusion may appear. Changes in heart rate, blood pressure, and skin characteristics (e.g., color, temperature, and moisture) may indicate perfusion changes. If an area of the body is specifically affected by a decrease in perfusion, sensations such as pain, tingling, or numbness may be felt.

Being alert to such statements as "My foot feels like it is going to sleep all the time" or "Every little thing I do seems to be such an effort" may help the nurse to recognize early signs and symptoms of interferences with tissue perfusion. However, many of these presenting behaviors are not specific to cardiovascular pathology, but reflect the influence of other body subsystems on tissue perfusion. Thus these manifestations must be correlated with all other findings.

Nursing assessment of general tissue perfusion includes descriptions of:

- presenting behavioral pattern (e.g., anxiety, tension, confusion, restlessness)
- relationship between presenting behavioral pattern and usual pattern
- presenting tolerance to activity
- presenting pattern of fatigue
- ways fatigue are expressed
- metabolic demands (e.g., anxiety, fever, exercise)
- relationship of metabolic demands to adequacy of tissue perfusion
- changes in vital signs (pulse, blood pressure, respiration)
- changes in sensation in body part (pain, tingling, numbness)
- attitudes toward level of tolerance
- effect of behavior responses on family and/or significant others
- attitudes of family and/or significant others

The major components of tissue perfusion that are included in nursing assessment relate to the efficiency of the heart as a pumping mechanism, the degree of resistance to blood flow, the viscosity of the blood, the blood volume, the surface area to be perfused, and metabolic rate. The majority of these nursing assessments are indirect measurements of the adequacy of oxygen transport and utilization, and waste product removal. However, they do provide valuable information on which the nurse can plan to make a positive difference in the individual's health state.

Heart Rate, Rhythm, and Force

The first observations the nurse makes in assessing oxygen transport and utilization concern the efficient pumping action of the heart. Heart rate, rhythm, and amplitude give basic information about the heart's pumping ability. The three are related to an individual's age, sex, size, metabolic rate, tissue perfusion, blood pressure, drugs, pain, emotions, and level of wellness (Chart 18.1).

Heart rate is the speed at which the heart beats, and it is measured by the number of times the heart beats in a minute. As the left ventricle pumps blood into the aorta, a wave impulse is set up which moves the blood throughout the circulatory system. The rhythm of this wave reflects the regular pattern of ventricular contraction. The force (amplitude) of this wave mirrors the force of the contraction of the ventricles. These arterial contractions can be felt anywhere a superficial artery passes over a bone or firm body structure.

PULSE

Pulse is the term used for the wave phenomenon that occurs in arteries following ventricular contraction. Common arteries used and sites for measuring the pulse are listed in Chart 18.2.

Many times the pulse does not accurately indicate the activity of the heart. It can be distorted when the resistance of the arteries to blood flow is increased by the loss of elasticity of the vessel wall due to aging or pathology. Thus it is often desirable to measure heart activity directly at the apex of the heart.

The expected pulse is characterized as rhythmical (having equal intervals of time between beats), *full* (strong), and elastic (the springy feel of the arterial wall). Chart 18.3 describes common variations in rhythm, strength, and elasticity.

Nursing assessment of heart rate, rhythm, and force includes descriptions of:

- usual rate, rhythm, and force per minute
- presenting rate, rhythm, and force per minute
- relationship between presenting and usual
- factors influencing heart rate, rhythm, and force (e.g., activity, pain, anxiety)
- what the individual says about his heart rate, rhythm, force

Urine Output

Urine output is another parameter the nurse uses to assess tissue perfusion, because urine output is directly related to arterial pressure, which in turn is related to cardiac output. Therefore, when cardiac output drops, arterial pressure also drops and perfusion of the kidney decreases, with a resultant lowering of urinary output. For a complete discussion of urinary elimination, see Chapter 20.

Nursing assessment of urinary output includes descriptions of:

- amount
- changes in amount over time
- relationship to other circulatory findings (e.g., pulse, blood pressure)

Skin Color

Skin color is a gross index of tissue perfusion.

PALLOR

Pallor, a commonly reported change in skin color, is the loss of the underlying reddish hue of the skin due to superficial vasoconstriction or a deficiency in hemoglobin levels. With superficial vasoconstriction the skin usually feels cool to the touch. Vasoconstriction occurs as an attempt to conserve body heat when a person is exposed to a cold environment or when the sympathetic nervous system is stimulated during anxiety, with cigarette smoking, or in disease states (e.g., peripheral vascular disease). Pallor is also seen in any pathologic state that decreases the lumen of the superficial blood vessels (e.g., *arteriosclerosis*).

Chart 18.1
Factors Influencing Pulse

FACTOR	INFLUENCE ON PULSE
Age	Expected rate
Newborn	120–160
5 years	80–110
10 years	70–100
Adult	60–90
Sex	Females usually higher rate than males
Size	Rate inversely proportional to size
Metabolic rate	
↑ Metabolism	↑ Rate, ↑ force
↓ Metabolism	↓ Rate, ↓ force
Level of tissue perfusion	
↑ Perfusion	↑ Rate, ↑ force
↓ Perfusion	↓ Rate, ↓ force (Rate and force initially increase as compensatory mechanism)
Blood pressure	Blood pressure, heart rate, and respiration are directly proportional to each other
Pain	Superficial pain, ↑ rate Deep pain, ↓ rate
Emotions	Rate usually increases but can vary
Autonomic nervous system	
Sympathetic stimulation	↑ Rate, ↑ force
Parasympathetic stimulation	↓ Rate, ↓ force
Drugs	
CNS stimulants	↑ Rate
CNS depressants	↓ Rate
Cardiotonics	↓ Rate, ↑ force
Antiarrhythmics	help regulate rhythm
Vasodilators	↓ Rate, ↓ force
Vasoconstrictors	↑ Rate, ↑ force

Chart 18.2
Major Arteries and Sites Used in Measuring Arterial Pulse

ARTERY	SITE	POINTS TO NOTE
Temporal	Temple, where the temporal artery passes over the temporal bone	Can be felt in line with the top of the ear.
Carotid	Over the connective tissue of the neck between the sternocleidomastoid muscle and the trachea	The middle portion of the neck should be used for palpation to avoid occlusion of the carotid sinus. Do not palpate both carotid arteries at once, as this may cause syncope and vagal stimulation. It is easier to feel the pulse if the individual turns his or her head toward the side you are palpating. Best pulse to use if peripheral vascular shutdown is suspected. Carotid pulsations may be observed.
Brachial	Antecubital fossa, where brachial artery passes over ulna	Can be felt at the inner aspect of the elbow (little finger side). Used in taking blood pressure. Major site of catheter insertion for diagnostic tests.
Radial	Wrist, where radial artery passes over radius	Most commonly used site. Can be felt at the outer aspect of the forearm (thumb side).
Femoral	Hipbone, where femoral artery passes over the body of the ischium	Middle of the groin. Person should be in supine position. May be used as a site if peripheral shutdown is suspected. Often a site for drawing blood gases.
Popliteal	Popliteal fossa (back of the knee) where popliteal artery passes over the posterior articular surface of the femur	Can be felt best when knee is slightly flexed.
Posterior tibialis	Ankle, where posterior tibialis passes over the lateral malleolus	Calf should be at a right angle to the foot.
Dorsalis pedis	Dorsum of foot where dorsalis pedis artery passes over proximal phalanges between the first and second toe	Most often used after leg surgery and after application of leg casts. May be congenitally absent; if so, the tarsal artery over the proximal aspect of the foot can be palpated.
	The apical pulse is auscultated at the fifth intercostal interspace along the left midclavicular line	Can be heard below nipple line. Moving the breasts up or outward can aid in locating apical pulse. Site is known as point of maximal impulse (PMI) and if the chest is thinwalled or if there are abnormalities, a palpable or observable pulse may be present.

Chart 18.3

Common Variations in Pulse

TYPE	DESCRIPTION	TYPE	DESCRIPTION
Bigeminal pulse	A consistent irregularity in which two consecutive heartbeats are followed by a pause. May be caused by a drug overdose or electrolyte imbalance.	Palpitations	A conscious awareness of the heartbeat because of a change in the rate, rhythm, or force.
Bounding	Increased amplitude (force) of the pulse wave. May be seen in fever, anemia, or heart block (synonym: collapsing pulse).	Paradoxical pulse	Pulse which is stronger on exhalation and weaker on inhalation (opposite of usual). May accompany inflammatory compression of great vessels.
Bradycardia	Slow heart rate (below 50/minute) seen in digitalis (a cardiotonic drug) overdose and conduction problems.	Tachycardia	Increased pulse rate (usually above 100/minute) seen with anxiety, fever, disease state, or idiopathic.
Corrigan's pulse	An extremely bounding (and pounding) pulse characteristic of aortic valve insufficiency (synonym: water-hammer pulse).	Thready pulse	Weak and difficult to palpate. Seen in severe hemorrhage.
Dicrotic pulse	Two pulse waves for each heartbeat. Seen in nervous system depression.	Trigeminal pulse	A consistent irregularity in which three consecutive heartbeats are heard, followed by a pause. (Seen with heart block.)
Irregular pulse	Altered rhythm. Rhythm should be specifically described.	Wiry	A tense, hard pulse. May be seen with arteriosclerosis or atherosclerosis.

▶ Lowered hemoglobin levels or decreases in the number of red blood cells, as in **anemia,** will produce pallor as well. The pallor of anemia is best observed in the palpebral conjuctiva, as it is a superficially vascular area (Chap. 17). The mechanism here is the decrease in red-colored oxyhemoglobin.

Nursing assessment for pallor, as in other skin color assessment, must take into account the individual's usual skin tone. However, the light-skinned individual will usually appear whiter, and the dark-skinned individual, grayer or ashen. The creases in the palms of the hands are one of the best areas to check for pallor. With the individual's hands at heart level, the nurse looks for for the usual reddish tone of adquate oxygenation or the pallor indicative of a decrease in oxygenation. The palm creases are easy to assess because they reflect early changes in oxygen supply. The capillary filling test is another way to assess pallor (Chap. 17). These tests are useful for both light- and dark-skinned individuals. Consulting with family and/or significant others is an important way of obtaining baseline information about skin color and changes.

PERIPHERAL CYANOSIS

Another skin color change relating to O_2 transport and utilization is peripheral cyanosis. Peripheral cyanosis is the dusky blue-gray color found in the extremities as a result of decreased cardiac output or peripheral vascular changes. When vasoconstriction becomes prolonged or blood pools, the O_2 content of the hemoglobin decreases. This occurs because the surrounding cells continue to take up O_2 even though the blood flow is decreased and freshly oxygenated blood does not flow into the area. Chapter 17 discusses assessment of cyanosis.

▶ When vasodilation occurs, **erythema** appears. Erythema is the increased reddish color of the skin resulting from increased blood flow. Vasodilation takes place reflexively with embarrassment. It also occurs as an attempt to lose body heat when environmental temperatures are raised or the individual's metabolic rate is increased (e.g., fever, activity). Inflammation also causes vasodilation as a mechanism to bring more blood to an area to promote healing. Observation of erythema is often difficult in ruddy, sunburned, or dark-skinned individuals. Since vasodilation increases the skin temperatures, feeling for areas of warmth when erythema is suspected may be the best indication.

MOTTLING

▶ A final skin color change related to tissue perfusion that the nurse should be alert to is **mottling.** Mottling is blue-gray or purplish blotches usually seen in the peripheral limbs. Mottling is the result of a generalized peripheral vascular constriction due to decreased environmental temperature or severe illness.

Nursing assessment of skin color change includes descriptions of:

- usual skin color (including ethnic characteristics and areas of pigmentation)
- presenting skin color (including location)
- color of extremities, palms, nail beds, mucous membranes, etc.
- hemoglobin level
- presence of cyanosis (peripheral or central)
- factors related to skin color changes (e.g., environmental temperatures, habits, inflammation)
- relationships between skin color changes and tissue perfusion
- temperature of the skin

Peripheral Circulation

Tissue perfusion to the periphery can be determined by assessing the peripheral pulses, skin color and temperature, tissue hydration, and sensation.

PULSES

The pulses in the limbs reflect the force of the heartbeat and the degree of resistance as the wave travels from the heart to the periphery. Anything that increases vasoconstriction increases the resistance to blood flow. Vasoconstriction causes a decrease in the strength of the peripheral pulses. Obstruction to peripheral blood through severe vasoconstriction, thrombus formation, or severing of the vessel results in the absence of peripheral circulation and pulses. (Chart 18.2 lists common arteries used to measure peripheral pulses.) The nurse checks for the rate, rhythm, and force of peripheral pulses and may want to correlate them with the apical pulse. Any difference between the apical pulse and the peripheral
▶ pulse is known as a **pulse deficit.**

SKIN COLOR AND TEMPERATURE

Skin color and temperature and their relationship to vasoconstriction and vasodilation are discussed above. The skin may be dry and fragile in the presence of longstanding vasoconstriction or obstruction, since the amounts of oxygen and nutrients
▶ needed for healthy skin are decreased (**ischemia**). If untreated this will eventually lead to necrosis (death) of the tissues. Therefore, skin integrity is affected and skin breakdown appears.

TISSUE HYDRATION

If there is obstruction to venous return of blood from the periphery, blood will pool within the vessels. This causes an increase in hydrostatic pressure within the vessels and results in the movement of plasma from the blood into the interstitial spaces
▶ (**plasma shift**). The limb is swollen and the skin is
▶ tight, shiny, and pale (**edema**).

TISSUE SENSATION

A change in sensation in a limb may indicate a decrease in tissue perfusion. Pain, tingling, and numbness may be intermittent or continuous depending on the severity of the vasoconstriction and degree of necrosis. This is a subjective symptom that can be ascertained only through the individual's statements or through indirect observations such as reactions to pain and frequent flexing or massaging of the affected limb by the individual. In addition, a reduction of superficial hair and hypertrophied toenails may indicate a decrease in tissue perfusion.

Nursing assessment of peripheral circulation includes descriptions of:

- peripheral pulse rate, rhythm, and force
- pulse deficits
- presenting peripheral skin color, temperature, dryness, fragility, hair pattern, toenails
- their relationship to peripheral perfusion
- signs of skin necrosis and breakdown
- edema
- changes in peripheral sensations
- subjective statements of individual related to peripheral sensations
- actions reflecting changes in peripheral sensation (e.g., flexing limbs)
- attitudes and reactions to peripheral circulatory changes.

Blood Pressure

ARTERIAL PRESSURE

Arterial blood pressure measurement is a nursing assessment that reflects many facets of tissue perfusion. Arterial blood pressure measurement is determined by the force with which the heart pumps blood into the arteries against the resistance of the arterial wall. It rises to a maximum value during the systole, ▶ when the ventricles contract (**systolic pressure**) and falls to a minimum value during diastole, when the ▶ ventricles relax and fill with blood (**diastolic pressure**). Since the circulatory system is a closed one, arterial blood pressure is affected by the pumping ability of the heart, the elasticity of the arteries, the resistance of the circulatory system, the blood volume, and the blood viscosity. These factors, in turn, are influenced by age, size, general health state, medication, pain, activity, emotion, and position. Chart 18.4 details the relationship of these factors to blood pressure. Since so many influences affect blood pressure, no single reading is sufficient to establish baseline data.

The difference between the systolic and the dia-▶ tolic pressures is known as the **pulse pressure**. Pulse

pressure is determined by the stroke volume and the degree of blood vessel resistance and usually ranges from 40 to 60 mm Hg.

As Guyton[1] states:

In general, the greater the stroke volume output, the greater is the amount of blood that must be accommodated in the arterial tree with each heart beat, and therefore, the greater is the pressure rise during systole and the pressure fall during diastole, thus causing a greater pulse pressure.

On the other hand, the greater the compliance [reduced resistance] of the arterial system, the less will be the rise in pressure for a given stroke volume of blood pumped into the arteries. In effect, then, the pulse pressure is determined approximately by the ratio of *stroke volume output to compliance* of the arterial tree.

The arterial blood pressure can be directly measured by inserting a catheter attached to a manometer into an artery. One of the most common methods in use today is the Swanz-Ganz method. For an in-depth diccusion of this technique, the student is referred to a medical—surgical nursing text.

Arterial blood pressure is most commonly measured by the indirect method using a sphygmomanometer (blood pressure cuff). A sphygmomanometer is an instrument having a pressure gauge, a compression cuff (an inflatable rubber bladder enclosed in an inelastic covering), and a pressure source consisting of a pump bulb and pressure control valve. The pressure manometer can be either of the aneroid (displacing air) or mercury type (displacing a mercury column). Both types are read in millimeters of mercury (mm Hg).

Indirect blood pressure measurement is more than the mere recording of numbers. Values obtained from this technique not only help to assess tissue perfusion, and the effectiveness of medication, but can also be used to plan care around the individual's health state and his level of tolerance.

Nursing assessment of the arterial blood pressure includes descriptions of:

- presenting arterial blood pressure
- expected arterial blood pressure
- comparison between presenting and expected arterial blood pressure
- relationship of differences to tissue perfusion

Chart 18.4
Factors Influencing
Arterial Blood Pressure

FACTOR	INFLUENCE ON BLOOD PRESSURE (BP)	FACTOR	INFLUENCE ON BLOOD PRESSURE (BP)
Age	Expected BP	Location taken	BP in lower extremities slightly higher than in upper extremities
Newborn	Systolic: 60–80		
	Diastolic: 40–50		Variations of 5–10 mm Hg are common between right and left arms
5 years	Systolic: 90–110		
	Diastolic: 65		
10 years	Systolic: 95–110		
	Diastolic: 65–70	Cardiac output	
Adult	Systolic: 100–140	↑ Cardiac output	↑ BP
	Diastolic: 60–90	↓ Cardiac output	↓ BP
Size	BP directly proportional to size	Vasodilation	↓ BP
		Vasoconstriction	↑ BP
Metabolic rate		Viscosity	
↑ Activity	↑ BP	↑ Viscosity	↑ BP
↓ Activity	↓ BP	↓ Viscosity	↓ BP
Heart rate	BP, heart rate, and respiration are directly proportional to each other	Volume	
		↑ Volume	↑ BP
		↓ Volume	↓ BP
Pain	Superficial pain: ↑ BP	Drugs	
	Deep pain: ↓ BP	Antihypertensives	↓ BP
Emotions	Usually increased with anxiety and stress	Vasodilators	↓ BP
		CNS depressants	↓ BP
		Diuretics	↓ BP
Position	Increases slightly in movement from supine to standing	Vasoconstrictors	↑ BP
		CNS stimulants	↑ BP

- factors related to arterial blood pressure changes (e.g., anxiety, activity, obesity)
- presenting pulse pressure
- expected pulse pressure
- comparison between presenting and expected pulse pressures
- relationship of differences to tissue perfusion
- attitudes toward blood pressure
- knowledge of blood pressure

VENOUS PRESSURE

The second type of blood pressure the nurse assesses is venous pressure. Venous pressure is the force exerted by the blood as it returns to the heart. Venous pressure is significantly lower than arterial pressure, since venous return is a relatively passive process. Venous return depends on the pressure of blood in the right atrium of the heart (**central venous pressure—CVP**), the pumping action of the muscles surrounding the veins (**venous pump**), the integrity of the one-way valves of the veins, the decrease in thoracic pressure during inspiration (thoracic pump), and the competency of the pulmonary system.

A failure in any one of these mechanisms causes a decrease in venous return, with resultant pooling of blood, dilation of the veins (**venous engorgement**), and changes in hydrostatic pressure. These changes lead to dependent edema, buildup of waste products, increased possibility of thrombus formation, and reduced cardiac output. The absence of these changes is as significant as their presence in individuals who may have an alteration in venous return. All the nursing observations mentioned for assessing peripheral circulation apply here as well.

Nursing assessment of venous pressure includes descriptions of:

- peripheral pulse rate, rhythm, and force
- pulse deficits
- presenting peripheral skin color, temperature, dryness, fragility
- relationship to peripheral perfusion
- signs of skin necrosis and breakdown
- edema
- changes in peripheral sensations
- subjective statements by individual related to peripheral sensations
- actions reflecting changes in peripheral sensation (e.g., flexing limbs)
- attitudes and reactions to peripheral circulatory changes
- presenting CVP value
- expected CVP value
- comparison between presenting and expected CVP values
- factors related to changes in venous return

Position

The nurse assesses the effects of gravity on tissue perfusion by observing the influence of the position that the individual assumes.

EFFECT OF GRAVITY

Gravity influences venous return, cardiac output, and blood pressure. When an individual is in a standing or sitting position, the pressures in vessels lower than the heart are increased by the force of gravity, while the pressures in the vessels above the heart are lowered. When no pathology or prolonged inactivity is present, compensatory mechanisms such as vasoconstriction and vasodilation act to maintain cardiac output, venous return, and blood pressure within physiologic limits.

Frequent changes in position are necessary to

overcome the effects of gravity. Prolonged standing, sitting or lying has negative side effects on tissue perfusion. Such signs as dependent edema, a drop in blood pressure on standing (**orthostatic hypotension**), an increase in heart rate, changes in sensation in the extremities, skin color changes in the periphery, and dizziness may indicate that the individual's regulatory mechanisms are not able to compensate for the effect of gravity. Such subjective statements as "I feel so light-headed when I get up in the morning" or "When I stand in line at the checkout counter, my heart seems to race" may indicate perfusion problems related to position.

Nursing assessment of the effect of position on tissue perfusion includes descriptions of:

- presenting position
- duration of position
- tissue changes (e.g., skin color, dependent edema, decreased blood pressure)
- effects of position on cardiac output, venous return, blood pressure
- length of time individual can maintain position without changes in tissue perfusion
- duration of tissue perfusion changes
- influence of tissue perfusion changes on activities of daily living
- methods and/or devices which prevent tissue perfusion changes (e.g., oscillating bed, elevating legs)
- ways tissue perfusion changes are communicated (e.g., pain, dizziness)

Activity

Activity plays an important role in tissue perfusion by maintaining the tone of the heart muscles and the muscles of the venous pump. In addition, the direct effect of activity on metabolism is significant in its influence on oxygen uptake, heart rate, blood pressure, and body temperature.

METABOLIC EFFECTS

When metabolism is increased, the need for oxygen increases. The heart compensates by pumping faster to accommodate this need, and the blood pressure rises in response to the increased cardiac output. If the general health state is good, the increased demands can be met, the cardiac intake will equal cardiac output, and tissue perfusion will be adequate. After cessation of activity cardiac output and blood pressure will return within a few minutes to the usual resting values. However, if there is any interference with oxygen uptake, transport, or utilization or with waste product removal, fatigue and inadequate tissue perfusion result, leaving an oxygen deficit.

The nurse assesses the capabilities of the cardiovascular system by careful monitoring of pulse, blood pressure, and respiration (vital signs), endurance, and subjective reports of the individual.

Increased metabolism through activity results in increased heat production. The heat produced is dissipated through peripheral vasodilation, which leads to conduction, convection, and radiation of heat. Through parasympathetic innervation, the sweat glands increase their secretion and heat is lost by evaporation. The reverse mechanism occurs with a decrease in activity.

Changes in metabolism as a result of activity will directly influence basal temperature. In children the reaction is more pronounced than in adults due to children's immature temperature regulating mechanism and their greater muscle activity.

Body temperature changes can be assessed through temperature taking; observation of skin color, temperature, and moisture; involuntary muscle activity (e.g., shivering); and subjective statements and actions (e.g., curling up or putting on a sweater).

Nursing assessment of an individual's activity in relation to tissue perfusion includes descriptions of:

- presenting activity pattern
- usual activity pattern
- comparison between usual and presenting activity patterns
- relationship of changes to tissue perfusion
- adequacy of compensatory mechanisms
- time taken to return to resting values
- subjective statements and responses
- usual body temperature
- changes in body temperature
- signs of increased or decreased heat loss

Emotional Factors

Emotional factors such as anxiety, fear, and excite-

ment result in sympathetic nervous system stimulation. Tissue perfusion changes result from activation of the fight-or-flight mechanism. The degree to which the body can tolerate the changes in tissue perfusion without compromise to functioning is an important part of nursing assessment. The emotional situation can create a vicious cycle by its activation of the stress response, which results in such signs as increased pulse and blood pressure that can then lead to further anxiety, and in turn, to further sympathetic stimulation.

For example, the individual who complains of "palpitations" when angry may begin to worry about the possibility of heart disease because of the pulse changes. This worry, in turn, may increase the palpitations.

If the cardiovascular system is impaired in some way or the stressors prolonged, tissue perfusion will be inadequate. Observing the duration of signs, length of recovery, and the amount of fatigue produced help in assessing the impact of the emotional state on tissue perfusion.

Many people attach special significance to the heart and its functioning. It is viewed as the center of life and the seat of strong emotions such as love and hate. Common phrases such as "my heart stood still," "my heart is broken," "the heart of the matter," "my heart was in my mouth," and "hardhearted" reflect this emphasis. Thus any threat to the heart, real or perceived, produces increased anxiety and apprehension about survival, as well as threats to the individual's body image. Ascertaining the individual's attitudes and beliefs about the heart can often assist the nurse in determining what approach to use to help the individual cope in a positive way with anxiety about tissue perfusion changes.

Nursing assessment of the influence of the individual's emotional state on tissue perfusion includes descriptions of:

- signs and symptoms of tissue perfusion changes
- relationship of these changes to emotional state
- duration of signs
- length of recovery
- fatigue produced
- attitudes about the heart
- knowledge about tissue perfusion
- factors which precipitate emotional changes (e.g., interaction with family and/or significant others and their specific fears or worries)

- ways individual deals with changes in emotional state
- interferences with cardiovascular functioning
- changes in body image

Personal Habits

Smoking, dietary, and exercise habits are among those patterns which have been identified with changes in tissue perfusion.

SMOKING

Smoking constricts the peripheral blood vessels, leading to decreased blood supply to that area and to increased cardiac demands and arterial pressure. In addition, the stimulant nicotine (and perhaps caffeine as well) may produce changes in the conductivity of the heart.

DIET

High-calorie and high-fat diets increase weight and perfusion surface area, which necessitate an increase in cardiac output. And the increased area through which oxygen, nutrients, and waste products must diffuse is not matched by a proportional increase in vascularity. Obesity is usually accompanied
► by **hypertension** (elevated arterial blood pressure) and increased metabolic rate. High intake of triglycerides
► and sterols has been associated with **atherosclerosis** (buildup of fatty plaques on the walls of the blood vessels) which increases the resistance to blood flow.

Diets low in protein, vitamins, and minerals result in a deficiency of nutrients necessary for cell growth, maintenance, and repair, and for hemoglobin production, leading to difficulties in oxygen transport and utilization.

EXERCISE

Decreased exercise produces two types of detrimental effects on tissue perfusion. First, it results in decreased muscle tone, which interferes with the effectiveness of the heart-pumping mechanism and the venous pump. Second, it allows for the accumulation of fat, leading to obesity, since exercise is the main mechanism for burning fat in the body.

OTHER INFLUENCES

Culture, lifestyle patterns of family and/or significant others, anxiety, economics, and level of knowledge contribute to the individual's pattern of personal habits. Therefore, effective assessment and modification of personal habits must include the individual's family and/or significant others.

Nursing assessment of the influence of personal habits on tissue perfusion includes descriptions of:

- presenting habits
- their effects on tissue perfusion
- knowledge of effects (of individuals or family and/or significant others)
- understanding of effects held by individual and family and/or significant others
- their attitudes toward habits and effects
- factors which influence habits (e.g., lifestyle, culture)
- attitudes of family and/or significant others toward personal habits
- modification attempts

Interferences with Oxygen Transport and Utilization, and Waste Removal

Several types of interferences are responsible for inadequate tissue perfusion. The transport system may be affected by pump failure or interferences with the flow of blood. Any interference with the oxygen-carrying capabilities of the blood or cellular diffusion will affect the utilization of oxygen and nutrients. These interferences can affect waste removal. While these categories are useful for purposes of discussion, in reality they are all interdependent and a failure in one will either directly or indirectly affect the others.

PUMP FAILURE

Pump failure is the inability of the heart to move the blood through the circulatory system efficiently and effectively. It results in decreased cardiac output and all its accompanying sequelae. It can be caused by damage to the cardiac muscle, incompetent cardiac valves, and failure of the electrical conduction system of the heart.

Damage to the myocardium may occur when coronary circulation is decreased by occlusion, when inflammation or infection weakens the tissue, or by hypertension. Incompetent heart valves which allow back flow of blood can be caused by infection or congenital defects. The electrical conduction of the heart may be affected by an electrolyte imbalance, changes in the nervous supply to the myocardium, cardiac tissue damage and necrosis, and medications.

IMPAIRMENT OF BLOOD FLOW

Blood flow can be impeded by increased resistance of the vessels, increased viscosity of the blood, ▶ decreased venous return, and **hypotension** (decreased arterial blood pressure) or hypertension. Increased resistance to blood flow may stem from vasoconstriction or obstructions.

The blood can become more viscous in one of two ways. The plasma can shift from the blood vessel to the interstitial spaces because of dehydration, electrolyte imbalance, increased hydrostatic pressure within the vessel, or protein loss. See Figure 18.2. Or the number of red blood cells can increase in proportion to the amount of plasma present, as ▶ in **polycythemia** (increased production of red blood cells).

Decreased venous return is discussed on page 450.

Hypotension may be caused by blood loss, stress reaction, pump failure, reaction to toxins, or immobility. Hypotension decreases blood flow because the arterial pressure necessary to move the blood sufficiently is absent. Hypertension, on the other hand, can affect blood flow by increasing the resistance against which the blood must move. Hyperten- ▶ sion can result from obesity, **arteriosclerosis** (loss of elasticity of the vessel wall), atherosclerosis, and emotional factors. Although many factors have been associated with an increased incidence of hypertension, no actual cause may be apparent. Risk factors include genetic predisposition, race, hormonal balance, diet, and smoking. Neurologic damage may result in either hypertension or hypotension, depending on the area damaged.

Any alteration in the blood flow will, therefore, affect cardiac output, venous return, and cardiac intake, with their attendant changes in tissue perfusion.

OXYGEN-CARRYING CAPABILITY

The ability of the blood to carry sufficient amounts of oxygen to meet the body's metabolic needs is influenced by the level of hemoglobin, the number of circulating red blood cells, blood volume, or a change in the oxygenation system.

Hemoglobin, particularly oxyhemoglobin, must be available in order to carry oxygen to the cells. Decreased usable hemoglobin can be seen in anemias, hemorrhage, bone marrow depression, and genetic conditions (e.g., sickle cell anemia). Circulating red blood cells can be decreased in chemotherapy, hemorrhage, bone marrow depression, and anemias. Decreased volume can result from hemorrhage or plasma shift to the interstitial tissues. The oxygenation system may be affected by anatomic defects, oxygen uptake interferences (Chap. 17), or decreased pulmonary blood supply. Congenital defects and trauma may result in anatomic changes which shunt the blood back into the circulation before it can be oxygenated and the carbon dioxide removed. A decreased pulmonary blood supply can result from right-sided heart failure, impaired venous return, obstruction to pulmonary blood flow, or pulmonary hypertension.

CELLULAR DIFFUSION

The ability of oxygen and nutrients to move into the cells and waste products to move out of the cells is affected by the distance between the capillary and the cell. Any factor which increases the diffusion distance will interfere with utilization of oxygen and nutrients and removal of waste. Diffusion distance is increased by edema, tissue fibrosis, or accumulated adipose tissue.

Toxins such as cyanide also interfere with cellular diffusion by altering cell membrane permeability and the metabolic process of the cell.

Nursing assessment of interferences with tissue perfusion includes descriptions of:

- existing interferences
- effects of interference on tissue perfusion
- relationship of growth and development to interference
- relationship of interference to body image change

- relationship of interference to interaction with family and/or significant others
- assessment of interference by family and/or significant others
- conditions percipitating interference
- pertinent diagnostic test data
- attitude related to interference
- knowledge of interferences
- actions that relieve interferences

Physical Assessment

INSPECTION

Inspection begins with observation of the individual's skin color, response to activity, general health state, and appearance. These general impressions help focus the specific physical assessment for tissue perfusion. In addition, any subjective statements the individual may make concerning tissue perfusion is investigated through physical assessment.

The Extremities

The nurse then examines the extremities for adequacy of tissue perfusion. The fingernails are observed for thickening, color, and **clubbing**. Thickening of the nails may indicate inadequate circulation. The nail bed should be pink, firm, and relatively convex. The capillary filling test (Chap. 17) is done to note the time it takes for the capillaries to refill (immediate refilling is expected). If cyanosis is suspected, the test which differentiates peripheral from central cyanosis (Chap. 17) is carried out.

Clubbing is the increase, or flattening, of the angle between the base of the nail and the nail (Fig. 18.3). The expected angle is 160°. The tip of the finger becomes thicker and stubbier in clubbing and the nail bed softer. Clubbing accompanies chronic pulmonary and cardiac pathologies and may indicate a prolonged localized decrease in oxygenation.

The hands and arms are inspected for color, indicating the degree of vasoconstriction or vasodilation, edema, bilateral symmetry, hair pattern, and signs of skin necrosis. The location and description of any of these are noted. Edema of circulatory origin is usually bilateral, **pitting,** or dependent. Pitting is the depression of tissue left when moderate pressure is applied. The degree of pitting is measured on a five-point scale based on the degree of depression and the time it takes to return to the expected state. (Zero equals absence of edema; 4+ equals deep depression which takes several minutes to return to expected.) If edema is only in one extremity and not pitting, it may indicate a circulatory obstruction in that limb. The circumference of the two limbs is measured for a basis of comparison. The same area on each limb should be measured. (Illustration 18.1)

Skin necrosis may be indicated by ulcerated

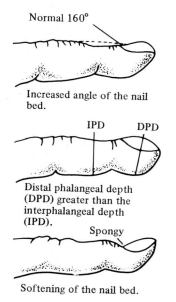

Normal 160°

Increased angle of the nail bed.

IPD   DPD

Distal phalangeal depth (DPD) greater than the interphalangeal depth (IPD).

Spongy

Softening of the nail bed.

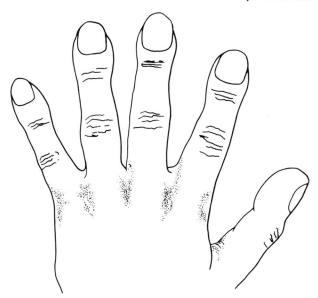

Figure 18.3
Clubbing of the fingers, thought to be caused by an interference in circulation.

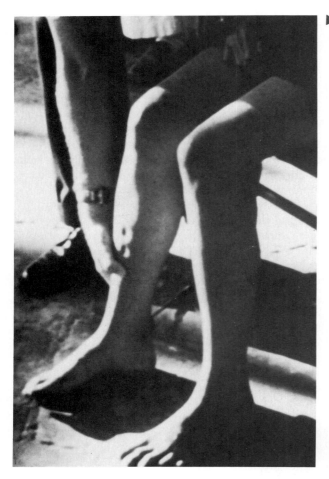

Illustration 18.1
Here, moderate pressure applied to the lower leg has left depressions in the tissue. These depressions, known as pitting edema, are due to circulatory interference. *(Photo © Lester V. Bergman and Assoc.)*

areas. The size, shape, distribution, color, smell, and any discharge from these areas should be noted.

Notation is made of bulging, tortuous, or pulsating blood vessels. Venous filling in the hands and arms can be observed by allowing the hands and arms to remain in a dependent position (below the level of the heart) for several seconds. The veins will bulge as they fill with blood. The hands and arms are then raised to heart level, and the vein should spontaneously return to the usual pattern. The time it takes for both filling and emptying is noted, as well as the changes in skin color. Expected filling time is within 10 sec. Increased filling time indicates an obstruction to venous flow.

The feet and legs are inspected in a similar man-

ner. In addition, the nurse observes for **varicosities** (outpuching and twisting of veins) and tests for the competency of venous valves. The Trendelenburg test is used to test for competency. The leg is raised above heart level for venous emptying. A tourniquet is then placed around the thigh and the individual is placed in a standing position. The vein should fill from below within 35 sec. The tourniquet is not left on for more than a minute. Distention of the veins after the removal of the tourniquet or filling from above may indicate failure of the valves. (Illustration 18.2)

The calves of the legs are tested for Homan's sign, which is diagnostic for thrombophlebitis. It is done by dorsiflexing the foot and observing for calf pain.

The Neck

After examining the extremities, the nurse inspects the neck for vein distention and pulsations. With the individual in a sitting position, veins are not distended and pulsations are usually not visible. With the individual in a supine position, the internal and external jugular veins fill, and pulsations can be seen. The pulsation of the jugular veins is wavelike and

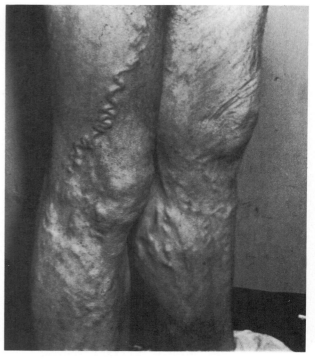

Illustration 18.2
Varicose veins. *(Photo © Lester V. Bergman & Assoc.)*

soft. It ceases when slight pressure is applied at the base of the neck above the clavicle. The pulsation will disappear as the individual rises to a sitting position. The presence of pulsations in the sitting position results from increased pressure in the right atrium. Venous distention in the sitting position also represents increased pressure in the right atrium.

The Chest

The chest is then observed for pulsations with the individual in both sitting and supine positions. The location and nature of any pulsations are noted. With the exception of very thin individuals, pulsations are not expected.

PALPATION

Palpation is done in conjunction with inspection. As the extremities are inspected, the nurse feels for skin temperature, using the back of the fingers, and takes the various pulses described in Chart 18.2. The nurse palpates any areas of swelling and any tortuous vessels and notes their flexibility and mobility.

The aortic valve area, the pulmonary valve area, the right ventricular area, the apical area, and the epigastric area are systematically palpated with the fingertips or palms for pulsations, **thrills** (vibratory sensation caused by abnormal blood flow) or **heaves** (an abnormal rising of the chest wall during systole). Thrills indicate heart murmurs resulting from the backflow of blood through the valves. Heaves result from hypertrophy of the ventricles.

The point of maximum impulse is identified. It is usually found at the apex of the heart.

PERCUSSION

Cardiac Borders

Percussion of the heart gives limited information but can be used to identify the boundaries of the heart. Using the same technique as in examining the lungs, the individual is placed in the supine position. The nurse percusses the third, fourth, and fifth interspaces moving from the left side to the midline. The change from resonance to dullness indicates the left cardiac border. The right border is difficult to percuss since it is covered by the sternum (Fig. 18.4). Ventricular hypertrophy will result in a distortion of the cardiac outline. When percussing the heart of women,

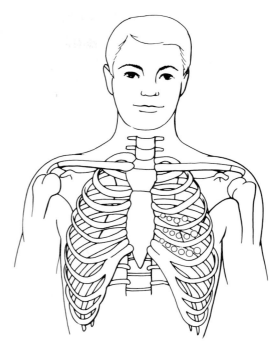

Figure 18.4
Cardiac borders. The size of the heart may be assessed by determining the cardiac borders. This is done by percussing the third, fourth, fifth interspaces indicated above by the rows of circles.

it is often necessary to move the breast upward during the procedure.

AUSCULTATION

Auscultation is used to measure blood pressure and identify heart sounds, heart murmurs, arrhythmias, and **bruits** (the rushing sound heard over an artery, reflecting a murmur).

Heart Sounds

Heart sounds are produced when the valves of the heart close during systole and diastole. When the mitral and tricuspid valves close just prior to ventricular contraction (systole), the first heart sound, S_1, is heard. This sound is the "lub" commonly referred to in the lub-dub sounds of the heart. S_2, the second heart sound, is heard when the aortic and pulmonic valves close prior to ventricular relaxation and filling (diastole) and is referred to as the "dup" sound. A third heart sound, S_3, is heard during the early stages of ventricular filling. It is more prominent in children and young adults than in older adults. S_4 is the sound of atrial contraction and is also not usually heard in adults. In auscultating the sounds, the diaphragm of the stethoscope is used to listen for S_1 and S_2. The bell of the stethoscope is pressed lightly against the chest wall to listen for S_3 and S_4 sounds. The ability to differentiate the basic heart sounds, S_1 and S_2, is necessary before it is possible to master other heart sounds such as murmurs, bruits, or pericardial friction rubs. Therefore, attention will be focused on the S_1 and and S_2 sounds, and the student is referred to a physical assessment text for the other sounds.

S_1 Sound.   Starting at the apex of the heart (mitral area), the student listens for the lub-dup. At this point the S_1 (lub) is louder. Concentrating on the S_1 sound, the student notes its strength as well as its placement in the cardiac cycle. The length of time between S_1 and S_2 (systole) is usually shorter than the time period between S_2 and S_1 (diastole). (Fig. 18.5) In tachycardia the diastolic interval approximates the systole interval.

After the S_1 sound has been heard clearly in the apical area, the student gradually and systematically moves the stethoscope to the tricuspid valve area, the aortic valve area, and then to the pulmonic valve

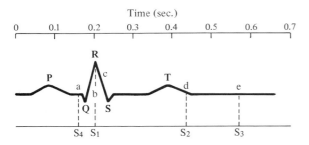

Figure 18.5
The relationship of heart sounds to the cardiac cycle: (b) as a result of increased ventricular pressure due to the beginning of ventricular systole, the mitral and tricuspid valves close, creating the first heart sound (S_1), or the "dub" sound; (c) with completion of ventricular contraction, ventricular pressure rises until all the ventricular blood is ejected, creating a drop in ventricular pressure which leads to (d) the aortic and pulmonic valve closing and the production of the second heart sound (S_2) or the "dup" sound; (e) period of diastole and rapid ventricular filling, the stage when S_3 (third heart sound) may be audible; (a) atrial contraction may be heard at this point (S_4), occurring immediately before the S_1 sound, and repeating the cycle.

area. The S_1 sound will diminish as the stethoscope is moved toward the aortic and pulmonic areas.

S_2 Sound.   Beginning in the aortic area the student now listens for the S_2 sounds. At this point the S_2 sound will be louder than the S_1 sound. Again, the strength and placement of the sound in the cardiac cycle is noted. The stethoscope is moved from the aortic valve area to the pulmonic valve area, mitral valve area, and then to the tricuspid area. The S_2 sound will diminish as the stethoscope is moved away from the aortic and pulmonic valve areas.

After the two sounds are clearly recognized separately, they are listened for together, proceeding in the same systematic order. In this way the rate and rhythm of the heartbeat can be ascertained. Irregularities of the heartbeat (**arrhythmias**) are described and noted. (Chart 18.3 lists common variations.)

Nursing assessment related to physical assessment of the cardiovascular subsystem includes descriptions of:

- Inspection
    general appearance
    skin color changes in the extremities
    thickening of nails
    clubbing
    capillary filling time
    edema
    symmetry of corresponding extremities
    signs of skin necrosis
    condition of the veins (e.g., bulging, tortuous, pulsations)
    venous filling
    varicosities
    valve competency
    calf pain (Homan's sign)
- palpation
    changes in skin temperatures
    pulses
    areas of swelling
    flexibility and mobility of vessels
    chest wall pulsations, thrills, and heaves
    location of point of maximum impulse (PMI)
- percussion
    cardiac borders
- auscultation
    blood pressure
    heart sounds (sequence, rate, rhythm)

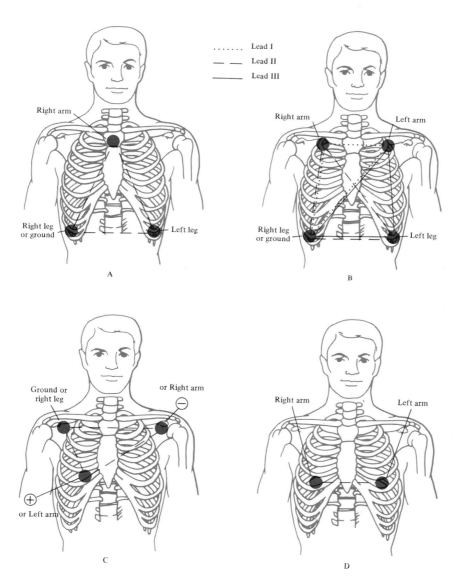

Figure 18.6
Placement and polarity of ECG leads.

Diagnostic Tests

Cardiovascular functioning may also be assessed by means of the electrocardiogram (ECG), blood tests, an angiogram, and stress tests.

THE ELECTROCARDIOGRAM

One of the major diagnostic tests for assessing cardiac function is the electrocardiogram (ECG). The ECG measures the electrical conductivity of the cardiac cycle. A full 12-lead ECG measures the electrical impulses from a variety of directions and is recorded on waxed, heat-sensitive graph paper. The most common lead taken is lead II (Fig. 18.7), which is the recording of electrical activity from the negative pole of the right arm to the positive pole of the left leg. Figure 18.6 illustrates the placement and polarity of leads I, II, and III. Electrical activity which flows toward a positive pole produces an ECG wave that is deflected above the base line. Flow toward a negative pole results in a downward deflection (Fig. 18.7).

Repolarization represents the resting phase of muscle tissue. Depolarization is the stimulation of muscle tissue. Both result from the shifting of ions across the muscle cell membrane. In Figure 18.7, the P wave represents atrial depolarization, the QRS complex represents ventricular depolarization, and the T wave is the ventricular repolarization. Each individual segment of the PQRST complex must occur within a specific timed sequence for efficient and effective cardiac function. Chart 18.5 and Figures 18.8 and 18.9 outline the expected time sequence of the PQRST complex.

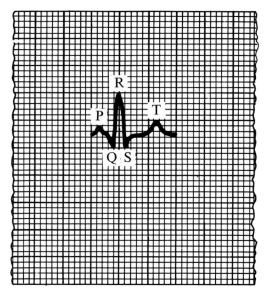

Figure 18.7
A Lead II ECG complex.

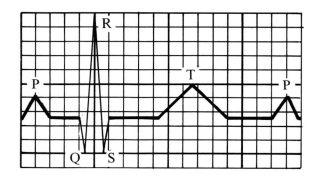

Figure 18.8
Expected time sequence of of an ECG. (Refer to Chart 18.5.)

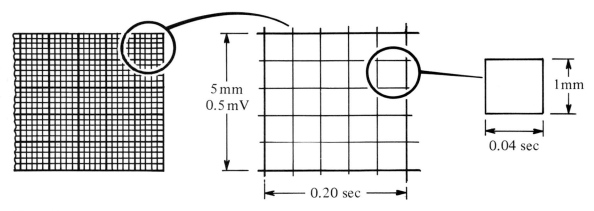

Figure 18.9
The time measurement represented by the graph paper on which an ECG is recorded.

Chart 18.5
Expected Time Sequence of ECG (Refer to Fig. 18.8)

CARDIAC CYCLE

ECG Sequence	Electrical Event	Mechanical Action	Heart Sounds
P wave (0.08–0.12 sec)	Depolarization of atria, impulse approaches AV node In AV node, slight delay in impulse conduction	Start of atrial contraction begins at peak of P wave Ventricles remain relaxed	4th heart sound
P-R segment (0.04–0.08 sec)	Stimulus traverses the His bundle, the ventricular conductive system, and starts into ventricular muscle	Conclusion of atrial contraction Atrioventricular valves remain open	
P-R interval (0.12–0.20 sec)	All above events	Atrial contraction	
QRS Complex (0.04–0.1 sec)	Orderly depolarization of ventricle: 1. midseptum, left to right 2. middle and lower free ventricular walls, endo- to epicardium 3. posterobasal or top portion, septum and left ventricular wall Repolarization of atria	Ventricular contraction begins at peak of R wave 1. atrioventricular valves close 2. isometric contraction of ventricles Beginning of atrial relaxation	1st heart sound
S-T segment (0.12 sec)	Most ventricular cells remain depolarized A few cells begin ventricular repolarization	3. opening of semilunar valves 4. rapid systolic ejection 5. ejection slows Atrial relaxation	
T wave (0.16 sec)	Repolarization of ventricle; generally agreed occurs in opposite direction of depolarization: 1. epicardium to endocardium 2. apex to base	Continued slowing of ejection: 6. closure of semilunar valves	2nd heart sound
Q-T interval (0.35–0.44 sec)	Ventricular depolarization and repolarization	Ventricular contraction	
T-P interval (variable)	Both atria and ventricle polarized	Isometric relaxation of ventricle Opening of atrioventricular valves Rapid ventricular filling Slow diastolic filling of ventricle	3rd heart sound

From: Una E. Westfall, "Electrical and Mechanical Events in the Cardiac Cycle." American Journal of Nursing, *76(2):231–235, February, 1976. Copyright 1976, American Journal of Nursing Company. Reproduced with permission from the* American Journal of Nursing.

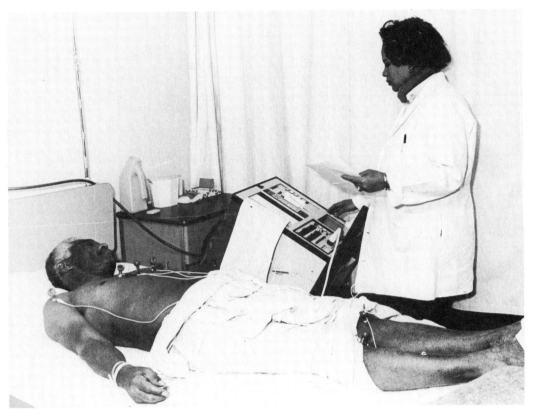

Illustration 18.3
Cardiac function may be assessed by means of an electrocardiogram which measures electrical impulses conducted during the cardiac cycle. This assessment is accomplished by placing leads at strategic points on the individual (precordial leads are those on the chest) and measuring the electrical activity that occurs between these various points. The impulses are recorded on a specially processed graph paper *(Photo by Martin M. Rotker, from Taurus Photos)*

Preparing the Individual

Preparation of the individual for an ECG includes explaining the purpose of the test and the method of proceeding. The procedure begins by removing all metal jewelry and restrictive clothing. The person is then placed in a supine position. The person should not be touching any metal objects such as side rails, since contact with any metal produces distortions in the ECG. The electrode leads are then applied to the chest and extremities. The electrodes may be applied by use of metal plates, self-adhesive tabs, or suction cups. A conductive paste placed between the electrode and the skin enhances the ECG reading. The precordial (chest) leads are moved in accordance with the direction of the polarity desired. The procedure is painless but requires the cooperation of the individual who must not move during ECG record-

ings, as doing so will distort the recording. (Illustration 18.3)

After the procedure is completed, any remaining conductive paste should be washed from the individual and from the equipment.

Electrocardiogram recordings are taken by qualified nurses, physicians, and technicians. Interpretation of ECG recordings requires knowledge and practice.

BLOOD STUDIES

Blood studies are another area of diagnostic significance in assessing tissue perfusion. The hematocrit, hemoglobin, red blood cell count, and reticulocyte count are basic tests for anemia and hemorrhage.

In performing these blood tests, no special prep-

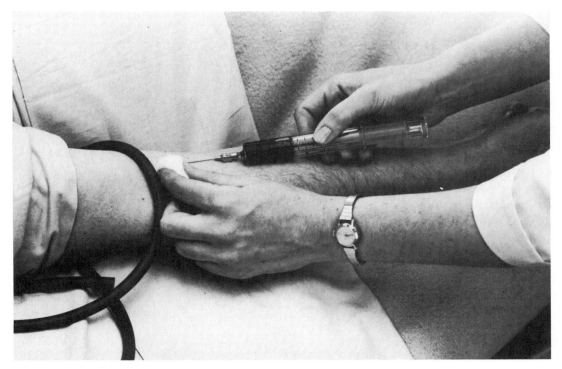

Illustration 18.4
The nurse withdraws blood into a syringe from an individual's arm. A tourniquet has been used to bulge the vein, facilitating the nurse's access to the vessels and the withdrawal of blood. *(Photo by Stan Levy, from Photo Researchers, Inc.)*

aration of the individual is necessary. Chart 18.6 gives the expected values for these tests. (Illustration 18.4)

Hematocrit

The hematocrit (Hct) is the ratio of the volume of red blood cells (RBCs) to the volume of blood and is expressed as a percentage (volume of RBCs/100 ml of blood). The hematocrit is elevated in such conditions as plasma shifts, plasma loss, burns, polycythemia, or whenever the RBC volume is increased in relation to blood volume. Any time the volume of blood increases in relation to RBC volume, the hematocrit is lowered, as in certain types of anemia (e.g., *pernicious* anemia) and chronic kidney inflammations (e.g., *nephritis*).

Hemoglobin

Hemoglobin (Hgb) is the weight (in grams) of hemoglobin per 100 ml of blood. Decreases in hemoglobin levels are seen in hemorrhage and anemias. Levels are increased in polycythemia.

RBC Count

The RBC count is the number of red blood cells present in one microliter (μl: 1/1000 of a cc and reported as a cubic millimeter, cu mm) of whole blood. Red blood cell counts are increased whenever there is an increased concentration of blood cells (e.g., plasma shift) or an increased production of RBCs (e.g., polycythemia). Decreased RBC counts are seen in hemorrhage and in some anemias. The RBC count may be a direct reflection of the efficiency of the bone marrow in producing RBCs.

Reticulocyte Cell Count

The reticulocyte cell count is the measurement of young RBCs (4 days old or younger). It indicates bone marrow efficiency. Reticulocyte cell counts are reported as the percentage of reticulocytes to 1000 RBCs. Bone marrow activity increases with an increase in the number of reticulocytes as a compensatory mechanism to blood loss or anemias. Reticulocytes decrease in number when the bone marrow activity is depressed.

TESTS FOR BLEEDING ABNORMALITY

Blood tests may be performed to assess the presence of bleeding abnormalities. This group of tests
► includes the platelet count, **coagulation time, pro-**
► **thrombin time** (PT), and **partial thromboplastin** time (PTT). (Chart 18.7)

Platelet Count

The platelet count is the number of thrombocytes per cu mm of blood. Whenever bone marrow production is increased, as in polycythemia, or when thrombocytes are released from the bone marrow, as in fractures, the platelet count will rise. A reduction in the platelet count is found in bone marrow depression (e.g., *aplastic anemia*) or suppression (e.g., toxic reaction to drugs) or in hemorrhage.

In all blood tests, the individual must be informed of their purpose and the procedure for collecting samples. Recognition of an individual's anxiety and fears accompanying venipuncture is particularly important. (See Chapter 7 for nursing implications of diagnostic blood tests.)

ANGIOGRAMS

Angiograms (x-ray visualization of the heart and blood vessels after the injection of a radiopaque dye) are frequently used to assess the patency of the heart chambers and the blood vessels.

STRESS TESTS

Stress tests (e.g., simulated stair climbing and treadmill running) are used to assess the cardiovascular response of the individual to activity. During these tests, portable ECG monitors are attached to the individual and vital signs are checked frequently. Stress tests are used not only to diagnose cardiovascular damage, but also to assess improvement in activity tolerance. (Illustration 18.5)

Chart 18.6
Expected Hematologic Findings

TEST	AGE	RANGE
Hct (%)	Adult	
	male	37–52
	female	35–45
	2 weeks	42–66
	1–6 years	33–42
	7–12 years	34–40
Hgb (g/100 ml)	Adult	
	male	14–18
	female	12–16
	2 weeks	13–20
	1–6 years	10–14
	7–12 years	11–16
RBC	Adult	
	male	4.5–6.5 million/cu mm
	female	4.0–5.6 million/cu mm
	Children	Similar to adults
Reticulocytes	All groups	0.5–1.5% of total RBC

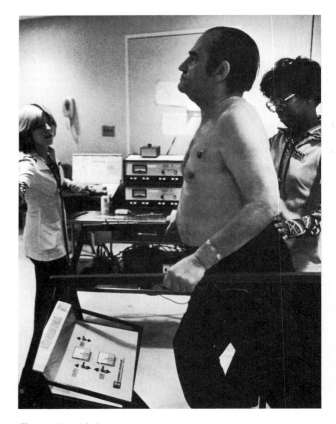

Illustration 18.5
As an individual walks on a treadmill, his response to the activity is measured on an electrocardiogram monitor. *(Photo by Mimi Forsyth, from Monkmeyer)*

Chart 18.7
Expected Blood Clotting Test Values

TEST	AGE	RANGE/MEAN
Platelet Count	All groups	150,000–450,000/cu mm
Coagulation Time	All groups	6–10 min (Lee White) 10–30 min (Howell)
PT Time	All groups	70–110% of control value (approx. 12–15 sec)
PTT Time	All groups	Variations widespread. Variations reported from 35–90 seconds. Values compared to control.

Nursing assessment of diagnostic tests related to tissue perfusion includes descriptions of:

- expected values
- presenting values
- relationship between expected and presenting values
- nursing implications of the test results
- relationship of interferences to test results
- special preparation needed
- posttest nursing care
- reactions to tests (of individual and family and/or significant others)
- attitudes toward tests
- level of understanding of the individual about tests

NURSING DIAGNOSIS

A 15-year-old Caucasian female, Ms. Aye, is brought to the clinic by her mother. The mother states she is worried about her daughter's extreme tiredness and lack of energy.

The nursing assessment that follows compares Ms. Aye's presenting (actual) behaviors that suggest inadequate tissue perfusion with those behaviors that the nurse would expect to find in a person of similar growth and development who is having no interference with perfusion. A physical assessment is included.

ASSESSMENT FACTOR	EXPECTED BEHAVIOR	ACTUAL BEHAVIOR
Behavioral pattern	Sleeps approximately 9 hours/night No regular naps during day High energy levels Actively participates in many activities	Sleeps 10–12 hours/night Takes nap after school States, "I just don't feel like doing anything." Recently quit cheerleading squad because "it took too much time and energy." Mother states, "I just can't understand it; she used to be in everything. I never could get her to slow down." Does not complete homework because she "can't stay awake."
Heart rate	80	96

(continued)

ASSESSMENT FACTOR	EXPECTED BEHAVIOR	ACTUAL BEHAVIOR
Heart rhythm	Regular	Regular
Force	Full	Bounding
Skin color—general	Light complexioned but pinkish tones, especially cheeks	Skin appears pale. Mother states, "She used to have such nice rosy cheeks."
Palpebral conjunctiva	Pink	Pale
Palms of hands	Pink	Pale
Skin condition	Translucent, "healthy glow," well hydrated	Dry, flaky, dull
Arterial blood pressure	120/80/70 mm Hg	100/70/60 mm Hg
Pulse pressure	40–60	40
Changes in peripheral sensation	None	None
Effect on position	Relatively little	"When I wait in line for a long time at the cafeteria, I feel dizzy sometimes."
Body temperature	98.6 F oral	99 F oral
Signs of heat loss	Dependent on environmental conditions	Diaphoretic upon exertion
Emotional factors	Self-critical, mood swings	"I really hate myself for being so lazy. My friends say I'm no fun anymore."
Change in body image	Time of body image changes Very much concerned with physical looks	See above "I'm turning into a limp noodle."
Ways individual deals with emotional changes	Unpredictable—dependent on basic interaction patterns	Mother states, "When she's not sleeping, she's crying. I just don't know what to do with her."
Personal habits		
Diet	Needs for age group: increased metabolic rate requires increased food intake (female, 1200–3000 calories) protein needs increase vitamin and mineral needs increase eating habits may be influenced by peer group, fad foods, body image	"Always dieting." Usual day's eating pattern: breakfast—none lunch—small green salad, diet soda after school—usually feels very hungry at this time and "cheats," e.g., ice cream cone, pizza or hamburger and french fries dinner—states, "My mother usually makes me eat some meat and vegetables." Drinks diet soda throughout evening but often "sneaks" cookies or candy

(continued)

ASSESSMENT FACTOR	EXPECTED BEHAVIOR	ACTUAL BEHAVIOR
Smoking	—	No
Exercise	See above	Walks one-half mile to and from school 15 minutes of calisthenics most evenings to help lose weight 1-hour gym period three times a week Goes dancing on Saturday nights Overall activity has decreased in the last three months because of "tiredness"
Physical Assessment		
Inspection		
Height, weight, build	Individual	5 ft, 3 in.; 115 lb, medium build
Nails	Smooth, pink, convex, firm	Slightly brittle
Hair	Glossy, flexible	Same
Skin color	See above	See above
Skin condition	See above	See above
Chest movement	No pulsations	None present
Palpation		
Heart rate, rhythm, force	See above	See above
Auscultation		
Arterial blood	See above	See above
Heart sounds	Loud and clear Regular S_1 and S_2 follow in sequence No murmurs or friction rubs	Same
Diagnostic Tests		
Hgb	12–16 g/100 ml	9.5 g/100 ml
Hct	35–45%	32%
RBC	4.0–5.6 million/cu mm	5 million/cu mm
Reticulocyte count	0.5–1.5% (of total RBC)	0.7%
Platelets	150,000–450,000/cu mm	290,000/cu mm
WBC with differential	5000–10,000/cu mm Neutrophils, 50–75% total WBC	7000/cu mm 56%
	Lymphocytes, 20–45% total WBC	37%
	Monocytes, 2–10% total WBC	4%
	Eosinophils, 0–6% total WBC	2.7%
	Basophils, 0–2% total WBC	0.3%

(continued)

ASSESSMENT FACTOR	EXPECTED BEHAVIOR	ACTUAL BEHAVIOR
Miscellaneous		
Menstruation	Onset: 11–17 years of age	Began menstruation 1½ years ago; pattern regular, moderate flow
Grade in school	Sophomore in high school	Same
Medical diagnosis	—	Iron deficiency anemia
Medical orders		Ferrous sulfate 150 mg, p.o., p.c. Return to clinic in 2 weeks.

Nursing diagnoses, in order of priority, might include:

- fatigue related to poor nutrition habits
- poor nutrition habits related to perceived negative body image
- increased hazard of infection related to nutritional deficiencies and lowered hemoglobin

PLANNING

Promoting adequate oxygen transport, utilization, and waste product removal is the major goal of planning. Promotion includes planning for the individual's foreseeable tissue perfusion needs as well as the immediate needs. Individuals who have been identified as being "at risk" for developing interferences with tissue perfusion will require health education about the effects of stressors, activity, diet, and other personal habits on tissue perfusion, as well as possible ways to modify habits. Since tissue perfusion is directly related to all body functioning, the effects on these systems must be considered in planning. Priorities of planning will focus on those factors that most compromise the functioning and survival of the individual.

In the situation of Ms. Aye, the plan for one nursing diagnosis listed above could be as follows:

NURSING DIAGNOSIS	GOALS	NURSING PLAN

Fatigue related to poor nutrition habits	Short-term
	Decreased fatigue within 2 weeks
	Gradual return to usual pattern of activity within 1 month
	Increased Hgb levels to promote adequate tissue perfusion within 2 weeks
	Increased iron and protein intake within 2 weeks
	Prevention of infection during period of low Hgb level
		1. Instruct in use of ferrous sulfate
		  a. How often to take
		  b. Benefits
		  c. Dosage limits
		  d. Rationale for taking after meals
		2. Explain relationship between dietary habits and fatigue.
		3. Give sample diets using popular foods
		  a. Weight charts
		  b. Diet diaries
		4. Explain relationship between rest and activity
		  a. Spacing of activities
		  b. Benefits
		  c. Ways in which activity and rest can be balanced
		5. Explain relationship between incidence of infection, decreased Hgb, and inadequate nutritional intake

(continued)

NURSING DIAGNOSIS	GOALS	NURSING PLAN

	Long-term
	   Modification of nutrition habits
	     consistent with level of growth
	     and development and activity
	   Return to usual pattern of activity
	   Prevent recurrence of decreased
	     Hgb levels
	   Prevent chronic fatigue
		1. Provide and explore options for
		   modifying nutrition habits, e.g.,
		   nutrition clinic, school nurse,
		   forming a peer group nutrition club
		2. All of above (to return to usual
		   patterns of activity and prevent
		   recurrences)

INTERVENTION

Pulse Measurement

One of the most frequent and valuable techniques for both assessing and evaluating tissue perfusion is measurement of the pulse. Pulse measurements not only give base-line information but also provide a means of evaluating response to activity, medications, and other therapeutic treatments. In measuring a pulse it is important to report rate, rhythm, and force as each component is only a part of the total picture. It is necessary to have a watch with a second hand in order to measure a pulse rate accurately. Chart 18.8 outlines the technique for pulse measurement. The same technique is used to palpate any pulse except where noted.

Chart 18.8
Palpating a Pulse

TECHNIQUE	POINTS TO NOTE
Explain procedure.	Decreases anxiety. Increases cooperation.
Position individual comfortably in either sitting or supine position. Position should be such that pulse site is accessible.	Uncomfortable positions may alter pulse or tense muscles so palpation is difficult. Femoral and lower extremity pulses require supine position. If taking respirations along with radial pulse, place arm across chest wall to facilitate measurement of respiratory pattern.
Place pads of first three fingers on artery to be palpated.	Use of three fingers increases surface area in contact with pulse site. Do not use thumb as it has its own pulse.
Clearly identify pulsation of artery by applying steady, moderate pressure.	Pressure should be even and sufficient to pick up all pulsations, without obliterating pulsations. Pulsations feel like a throbbing against fingers.
Count the number of pulsations in 30 sec and multiply by two. (If any irregularity is noted, count for full minute.)	Inaccuracies may result if counted for less than 30 sec, especially rhythm. Decreases chance of error.
Note rhythm, force, flexibility, and quality of vein wall.	Gives full assessment on evaluation information. Repeated practice is necessary to integrate all components.
Correlate with other findings.	Any one finding by itself is meaningless.

APICAL PULSE

If any irregularity in pulse has been noted or if the individual is being given a cardiotonic drug, (increases cardiac efficiency), an apical pulse is auscultated. Placing the diaphragm of the stethoscope on the point of maximal impulse at the apex of the heart, each S_1 and S_2 sequence is counted for a full minute. The rhythm and the intensity of the sounds is noted.

APICAL–PERIPHERAL PULSE

The apical and peripheral pulses are often taken simultaneously to evaluate conduction of the pulsation to the extremities. The apical–radial pulse is the most common pair taken. This procedure requires two people: one to take the apical pulse and the other to take the peripheral pulse. Both people start and stop counting pulsations at the same time. The pulses are taken for a full minute, and the results are compared for any deficits.

FETAL HEARTBEAT

Another pulse that is auscultated is the fetal heartbeat. A special stethoscope called a fetoscope is usually employed. The fetoscope utilizes bone as well as air conduction to facilitate hearing the best (Illustration 18.6). Chart 18.9 outlines the procedure.

Arterial Blood Pressure Measurement

Arterial blood pressure measurement, another skill used in assessment and evaluation, is accomplished through auscultation. Certain safeguards are followed to ensure accuracy of findings. These safeguards are outlined in Chart 18.10 along with the technique for auscultating arterial blood pressures.

NEWBORN'S BLOOD PRESSURE

Although not a routine procedure, a newborn's blood pressure may be measured by auscultation, palpation, or flushing. If by auscultation, both a leg and an arm are used for comparison. The flushing method is outlined in Chart 18.11.

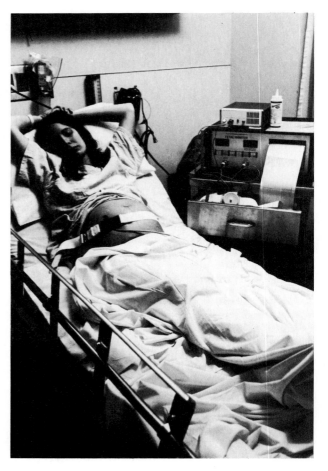

Illustration 18.6
The fetal heartbeat is auscultated by the fetoscope. This special type of stethoscope, placed on the side of the mother's abdomen, picks up the heartbeat along the fetus's vertebrae, the bone serving as the conductor of the sound. A fetal monitor records the vibrations. *(Photo by Sam Sweezy, from Stock, Boston)*

Promoting Venous Return

Promotion of venous return is a significant nursing intervention in maintaining adequate tissue perfusion. Several activities may prevent interferences and enhance venous return, for example, elevating the legs above heart level to help utilize the force of gravity in blood flow. This position helps to prevent pooling of blood and venous stasis. And when venous stasis or edema is already present, leg elevation can be therapeutic.

Chart 18.9
Auscultating the Fetal Heartbeat

TECHNIQUE	POINTS TO NOTE
Explain procedure to mother.	Same as Chart 18.8.
Locate the back of the fetus by palpating the sides of the abdomen of the mother and feeling for the "bumpy" prominences of the vertebrae.	Fetal heartbeat is best heard through fetus's back because fetal position prevents access to chest area.
Move fetoscope along the spinous process until fetal heartbeat is heard clearly.	If head is directed toward vaginal canal (presenting part), fetal pulse is usually felt below umbilicus. If buttocks is presenting part, fetal pulse usually felt above umbilicus.
Count pulsations for 30 sec while simultaneously palpating mother's radial pulse. Multiply by two.	Counting both pulses prevents mistaking mother's pulse for fetal pulse because the fetal pulse rate is higher than the mother's.
Note rate, rhythm, and intensity, and correlate with other findings.	Same as Chart 18.8.

Chart 18.10
Auscultating Arterial Blood Pressure: Safeguards and Technique

SAFEGUARDS AND TECHNIQUE	POINTS TO NOTE
Correct cuff width (cuff width should be 20% greater than half the circumference of the limb).	Too large a cuff gives falsely low readings. Too small a cuff gives falsely high readings.
Cuff should not be placed with any portion of it over a garment.	Muffles and disturbs sounds. Gives inaccurate values.
Middle of rubber bladder is centered proximal to and in line with palpated artery.	Allows for full transmission of sounds.
Cuff is placed approximately 1 in. above palpated artery site.	Allows for placement of stethoscope.
Cuff is wrapped smoothly and snugly.	Must be snug and smooth enough to ensure full, even transmission of sounds.
Aneroid gauge must be read directly from the front.	Reading gauge from sides will give false values.
Mercury gauge must be read at eye level with gauge on flat surface.	If read from top—falsely low values. If read from bottom—falsely high levels. Tilting gauge gives inaccurate readings.
Tubing must not be kinked or coiled.	Obstructs flow of air.
Limb is at heart level.	Limb above heart level gives falsely low values. Limb below heart level gives falsely high values. Arm is supported to maintain it at heart level.
Stethoscope is placed directly over palpated artery side.	Allows for full transmission of sounds.

(continued)

Chart 18.10 (Cont.)
Auscultating Arterial Blood Pressure: Safeguards and Technique

SAFEGUARDS AND TECHNIQUE	POINTS TO NOTE
For a one-time reading, do not reinflate while in middle of reading and wait at least 15 sec before reinflating.	Creates venous engorgement and inaccurate values. (If venous engorgement occurs, remove cuff and raise limb above heart level for 1–2 min before reapplying cuff.)
If repeated readings are necessary, wait at least five min between each inflation.	Prevents venous engorgement, capillary breakdown, and inaccurate values.
Explain procedure.	As above.
Inform individual of possible sensations of numbness or tingling.	Blood supply is temporarily decreased.
Position limb at heart level.	See above.
Choose appropriately sized cuff and check that cuff is fully deflated.	See above. Partial inflation distorts reading.
Close pressure valve by turning knob clockwise.	
Palpate artery site (most common site: brachial artery at antecubital fossa).	Ensures accurate placement of cuff.
If thigh is used, popliteal artery behind knee of calf is used, posterior tibialis behind ankle bone.	
Wrap cuff snugly and smoothly, with middle of rubber bladder in line with and approximately 1 in. proximal to palpated artery site.	As above.
Palpate artery site and place stethoscope directly over artery.	As above.
Steadily inflate rubber bladder 30 mm Hg above previous systolic pressure.	Prevents uneven application of pressure. Ensures proper occlusion of vessel and hearing all sounds.

(continued)

LEG AND FOOT MOVEMENT

The venous pump mechanism may be maintained and augmented by frequent movement of the legs and feet. Wiggling the toes or instructing the individual to "walk up" the footboard will activate the venous pump and help venous return. Individuals who stand in one position for any length of time are instructed to shift their weight from foot to foot or to move about in place to prevent venous stasis, dependent edema, muscle fatigue, and possible syncope. Passive and active range of motion exercises and frequent turning and positioning (Chap. 14) will also aid the venous pump and thus venous return.

ELASTIC STOCKINGS

Elastic (antiembolic) stockings or bandages may be ordered to supplement venous return by applying external compression on the blood vessels. They act as an external muscle pump. Elastic stockings or bandages may extend from the middle of the foot to below the knee or from the middle of the foot to below the groin. Figure 18.10 illustrates how they are applied. Care is taken to ensure that these devices do

---

Chart 18.10 (Cont.)
Auscultating Arterial Blood Pressure: Safeguards and Technique

---

TECHNIQUE	POINTS TO NOTE
Turn valve counterclockwise and release pressure slowly and steadily (2−3 mm Hg per heartbeat).	
Listen for sounds (Korotkoff sounds) and note values on gauge when they occur:	
First sound: systolic pressure	External pressure of cuff is equal to intra-arterial systolic pressure. Sound is a thumping, following pattern of heartbeat.
Auscultatory gap: 10−20 mm Hg; absence of sound between systolic and diastolic values	Most often occurs in hypertensive individuals. If not recognized, leads to inaccurate readings (low systolic or high diastolic).
Second sound: muffling of sound (may not always be present).	Change in intensity. Sounds becomes "blurry" (truer indication of intra-arterial diastolic pressure).
When sound no longer heard: diastolic pressure.	Represents minimum intrapressure and external pressures. Less than vessel pressure. Vessel is completely open.
Release pressure rapidly after diastolic.	Provides comfort for individual.
Remove cuff.	
Correlate values with other findings.	As above.

Note: If arterial blood pressure cannot be auscultated, the palpation method may be used. This same technique is used as above, except instead of using a stethoscope, the artery is palpated throughout the technique. Pulsations will be felt at the point of systolic pressure. Diastolic pressure cannot be determined by this method.

Chart 18.11
Newborn Blood Pressure Measurement by Flushing

TECHNIQUE	POINTS TO NOTE
Quiet child as much as possible.	Ensures accurate readings.
Measure and apply cuff as in Chart 18.8.	As above.
Raise limb above heart level until blanching occurs.	Decreases arterial flow. Promotes venous return. Prevents venous engorgement (massaging limb may help "milk" blood from veins).
Inflate cuff as in Chart 18.8.	As above.
Lower limb to heart level and slowly deflate cuff.	Causes venous engorgement. Opens arterial flow.
Note gauge value when the limb turns red (flushes).	Flushing occurs approximately midway between systolic and diastolic pressures as artery opens.

not obstruct circulation by impeding flow in the popliteal or femoral artery. They are applied smoothly and wrinkle free. Elastic stockings or bandages are applied before the person gets out of bed, since any venous stasis will be minimized by the effects of gravity in a supine position. The stockings or bandages are removed at least twice a day, and the leg is observed for any signs of skin irritation or breakdown or venous stasis.

LIMITING EXTERNAL PRESSURE

Individuals who are prone to poor venous return need to be particularly careful about crossing their legs at the ankles or knees or sitting with the popliteal space pressed against the side of a chair or bed. These actions will further alter hydrostatic pressure, venous return, and arterial flow to the lower extremities. Restrictive clothing such as circular garters, girdles,

How To Apply Stockings are not put on patient's legs like ordinary hosiery. If the stockings are gathered together in the typical "donut" fashion, the effect of the elastic material is multiplied many times and makes application difficult. By following these basic steps, T.E.D. Stockings are easily applied. CAUTION: DO NOT, UNDER ANY CIRCUMSTANCES, TURN DOWN TOP OF STOCKINGS. DO NOT COVER ANY PORTION OF THE KNEE.

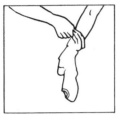

1. Insert hand into stocking as far as the heel pocket.

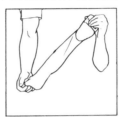

2. Grasp center of heel pocket and turn stocking inside out to heel area.

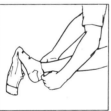

3. Carefully position stocking over foot and heel. Be sure patient's heel is centered in heel pocket.

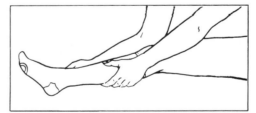

4. Pull stocking up and fit around ankle and calf, working up to final position. (Top of stocking is positioned approximately 1"-2" below bottom of knee cap.) Make sure heel and toe are positioned correctly. Smooth out any excess material between top of stocking and ankle with palms of hands. Pull toe section forward to smooth ankle and instep area and allow for patient toe comfort.

5. Patients should be instructed as to proper positioning of stocking to insure that the patient will not reposition the stockings incorrectly.

Figure 18.10
Application of elastic (anti-embolic) stockings. To apply external compression of the blood vessels in an individual's leg, thus aiding venous return, elastic stockings may be used. They are put on an individual before he gets out of bed and removed at least twice during the day so that the legs may be checked for signs of skin irritation and venous stasis. In applying the stocking, the nurse first turns it inside out, but only to the heel area (steps 1 and 2). Then the stocking is positioned carefully over foot and heel (step 3), and the fabric is centered and smoothed. The stocking is then pulled up (step 4), again being corked smoothly, to 1-2 inches below the knee. The knee-length stockings do not cover the knee to help prevent an interference in circulation in the popliteal and demoral arteries. *(Courtesy of Kendall Hospital Products, Boston, Massachussetts)*

socks, or stockings with elasticized tops are avoided for the same reasons.

Health Teaching

Health teaching is a major nursing intervention in helping to promote oxygen transport and utilization and waste product removal. The nurse counsels the individual about the effects of such things as smoking, diet, and activity on tissue perfusion.

PREVENTION AND ALTERATION

Education which is focused on the prevention of negative health behaviors is as important as that which is directed toward modifying existing negative health behaviors. The nurse must recognize that many personal habits are long standing and often meet needs that may not be obvious. Therefore, the principles of learning and the change process must followed if more positive health habits are to be incorporated into the individual's behavior. The family and/or significant others will have great influence over the individual's desire and ability to change.

Individuals who have interferences with tissue perfusion will need to alter their activity and rest patterns if they are to meet their oxygen needs. Oftentimes, as a therapeutic measure, bed rest is ordered to decrease tissue perfusion demands until there is an increased ability to meet the needs. People who have had bed rest ordered for them may not see the relationship between rest and tissue perfusion needs. Explanations are necessary if the person is to accept restrictions on activity. Any changes in body image, feelings of independence, and self-worth must be explored with the individual and nursing intervention individualized according to the specific needs of the person.

Ways in which the individual can match capabilities with limitations should be explored with the individual and family and/or significant others. Breaking up activity periods with rest periods, stopping when fatigue is first experienced, or organizing activity schedules and work spaces are just a few of the options available to the individual to conserve his or her energy.

Promoting Mental Rest

Rest is not only physical but also psychologic. A person may physically rest but expend a great amount of energy worrying about many things. Poorly planned activity schedules which do not consider the interactions of the individual's family and/or significant others or his or her personal preferences and style of coping often place more stress on the individual's tissue perfusion needs than would any physical activity.

Cardiopulmonary Resuscitation

Cardiopulmonary resuscitation (CPR), an emergency intervention, is used when there is a sudden cessation or severe diminution of heart and/or respiratory activity. CPR is used for **cardiac arrest** (sudden cessation of heartbeat), **circulatory collapse** (cardiac activity is decreased to the point where tissue perfusion is not sufficient for vital functioning), and respiratory arrest. These conditions result from damage to the myocardium, electrical shock, drowning, suffocation, neurologic damage, or drug reactions. Basic CPR is instituted with no delays and requires no equipment. (Fig. 18.11)

UNWITNESSED CPR

Chart 18.12 outlines the procedure for unwitnessed resuscitation, when there is a delay between time of collapse and starting CPR.

CPR is continued until the person is revived, advanced life support is initiated, or the rescuer is completely exhausted. Advanced life support involves the continuation of CPR but with medications and more definitive treatment. For discussion of advanced life support the student is referred to a medical–surgical text.

WITNESSED CPR

If an arrest has been witnessed, that is, the rescuer observes the event and is able to institute treatment immediately, the basic procedure for CPR is modified. The airway is opened as the carotid pulse is palpated. If a pulse is absent, one **precordial thump** is administered. A precordial thump is a forceful, sharp blow to the midsternum with the lateral aspect of a closed fist. The thump is started from 8 to 12 inches

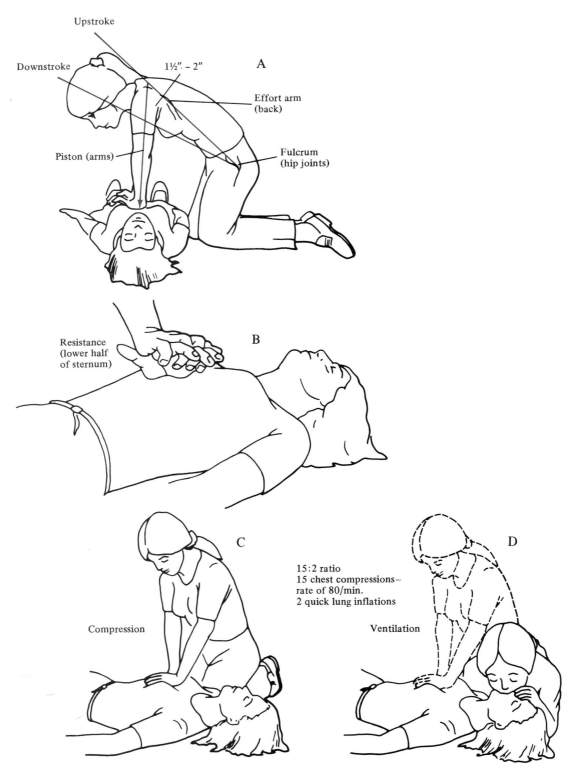

Figure 18.11

Proper positioning for cardiopulmonary resuscitation.

Chart 18.12
Unwitnessed Cardiopulmonary Resuscitation

TECHNIQUE	POINTS TO NOTE
Determine unconsciousness by shaking individual and/or speaking to him or her.	Establishes need for CPR.
Send for help while placing individual on back on hard surface.	Help may be necessary to sustain life by advanced treatment. Efforts are dispersed if CPR not done on hard surface.
Kneel alongside individual's head and shoulders.	Optimum position for performing procedure.
Open airway by hyperextending the neck: Push forehead back with one hand and Lift under the neck with the other hand.	Brings glottis in line with trachea and brings jaw foreward to prevent tongue from falling back and occluding airway.
Check for breathing by: Putting ear over individual's nose and mouth Listening and feeling for respirations.	Opening airway may be sufficient to reestablish breathing. If airway obstruction is suspected, start treatment for removal of obstructions in unconscious individuals (see Chap. 17).
Administer four ventilations by: Pinching off nose with hand from forehead Completely cover individual's mouth with your own, making sure there is a tight seal and Blow in 4 times while observing for rise of individual's chest.	Provides immediate air supply; seals airway, creating closed system. Ventilations are rapid and full. Observing chest establishes success of ventilation. If abdomen is rising, airway is not completely opened and air is forced into abdomen.
Check carotid pulse; if no pulse, administer four chest compressions by:	Evaluates need for cardiac compressions. Entire procedure up to and including this point should take no longer than 30 sec.
	Forces blood through body:
Locating xiphoid process and measuring two finger widths up	Avoids breaking off xiphoid process during procedure.
Place palm of one hand above site located and the other palm on top of first	Point of optimal compression. Make sure fingers are not touching chest wall to prevent force from palms being dispersed.
Apply sufficient pressure to depress sternum $1\frac{1}{2}$ to 2 in. by rocking body forward, with shoulders over heart, and keeping arms straight. (See Fig. 18.12 for proper positioning).	If pressure insufficient blood will not be pumped. Obese people require more pressure than thin people. Rocking helps to use force of whole body in applying pressure, as does keeping arms straight.
Check for return of respirations and carotid pulse.	Checks need for continuing CPR.
If pulse and respirations are still absent continue ventilation and chest compression at a 2:15 ratio (2 ventilations for every 15 compressions). If there are two rescuers, one does the ventilations while the other intersperses the compressions at a 1:5 ratio.	Ratio ensures adequate oxygenation for vital functioning. Ventilations and compressions must be administered in a steady, even rate with no delays or interruptions.

above the chest. The purpose of a thump is to provide a stimulus to the heart, and it may spontaneously start the heart beating. The carotid ·pulse is then checked again. If the pulse is still absent, CPR is instituted as outlined in Chart 18.12.

CPR FOR A CHILD

If an infant or child needs to be resuscitated, the basic procedure is the same. However, chest compressions and ventilations are modified according to the size of the child. With an infant compressions are given with one or two fingers, while with a child the heel of only one hand is used. Ventilations for an infant are given by using the air from the mouth only, in order to administer just "puffs" of air. The depth of ventilation increases proportionately to age and lung size.

MASTERING CPR

Repeated practice in simulated CPR situations is carried out before attempting actual resuscitation. CPR practice is done on a model, never on a person. Even after the skill has been mastered, repeated practice is important to retain dexterity and coordination.

EVALUATION

Evaluation of oxygen transport and utilization, and waste product removal centers on (1) the direction of change that has occurred in the person's ability to meet tissue perfusion needs, (2) the effects of other subsystems on tissue perfusion, and (3) the influence of intervention (whether specifically directed toward the cardiovascular system or not) on tissue perfusion.

Specific criteria for evaluating changes that have occurred in an individual's tissue perfusion needs include:

- How do physiologic changes (in other subsystems as well as in the cardiovascular system) influence tissue perfusion? Psychologic changes? Environmental changes?
- What is the relationship between the presenting pattern of tissue perfusion and the oxygen needs?

- Has the presenting tissue perfusion pattern (e.g., pulse rate, rhythm, force, blood pressure, urine output, skin color, diagnostic test values, and tolerance to activity) moved closer to the expected?
- What factors may account for changes in tissue perfusion?
- What are the changes in the degree of tissue perfusion interferences?
- What are the effects of tissue perfusion changes on other body subsystems?
- Are there changes in knowledge about the influence of personal habits on tissue perfusion?
- Are there changes in attitudes toward tissue perfusion and the effects of personal habits on it?
- Are there modifications in personal habits?
- Are there changes in attitudes toward tissue perfusion, related limitations, and treatments?
- Are there changes in attitudes by the family and/or significant others toward the individual's tissue perfusion needs? Changes in personal habits? Limitations? Treatments?
- What are the changes in the level of anxiety toward tissue perfusion needs?

RECORDING AND TEACHING–LEARNING ACTIVITIES

Teaching–Learning Topics

- the rationale for therapeutic regimes
- methods to match capabilities with limitations
- how to make modifications in ADL based on level of growth and development
- types of activities available to individual
- ways to structure the environment to facilitate meeting oxygen transport and utilization, and removal of waste products
- ways available to modify personal habits which affect tissue perfusion (e.g., diet, smoking, activity)
- measures to prevent compromise of tissue perfusion
- application of elastic stockings
- how to take pulse and blood pressure
- factors which impede venous return and how to eliminate these factors
- factors which have an effect on pumping ability of the heart and how to modify them
- methods to reduce anxiety
- factors which affect pulse and blood pressure

Charting and Recording

Using appropriate tissue perfusion terms, objectively describe such factors as:

- objective base-line data on appearance; tolerance to activity; heart rate, rhythm, and force; urine output; skin color; peripheral circulation; blood pressure; effects of position; anxiety; personal habits; level of growth and development; interferences; physical assessment
- objective and subjective data on changes in the individual's ability to meet tissue perfusion needs
- subjective data on heart rate, rhythm, and force and blood pressure in response to stress and activity
- attitudes toward tissue perfusion needs
- responses to treatments that answer the need
- schedule and methods of care
- teaching carried out
- discharge planning done
- interactions and responses of family and/or significant others
- update Kardex concerning changes in goals and plans for meeting oxygen transport and utilization needs and removing waste produces

Medications to Review

- cardiotonics, e.g., digoxin
- antihypertensives, e.g., methyldopa (Aldomet)
- antiarrhythmic drugs, e.g., quinidine
- vasodilators
    local, e.g., nitroglycerine
    peripheral, e.g., cyclospasmol
- vasoconstrictors, e.g., levarterenol (Levophed)
- hematopoietic drugs, e.g., ferrous sulfate
- whole blood and its constituents, e.g., plasma, packed cells
- anticoagulants, e.g., heparin, warfarin (Coumadin)
- antilipemics, e.g., clofibrate (Atronmid S)
- CNS depressants, e.g., diazepam (Valium)

Diets to Review

- low sodium
- low fat
- low cholesterol
- high protein
- high iron

CLINICAL APPLICATION: CARE OF THE INDIVIDUAL RECEIVING A BLOOD TRANSFUSION

Blood transfusion is often necessary to increase circulating blood volume (e.g., in hemorrhage), to increase the number of red blood cells (e.g., with severe anemia), to increase the number of platelets and other clotting factors (e.g., in leukemia), and to replace lost plasma proteins (e.g., in burns). Blood transfusion is the infusion of whole blood or its constituents into an individual's vein. In determining the need for and the type of transfusion, the physician will assess such factors as hemoglobin level, hematocrit, RBC count, platelet count, degree of blood loss, general health state, and their effects on tissue perfusion.

Today whole blood is used less often for transfusion than in the past. Through clinical use it has been found that whole blood supplies the individual with extra volume and blood components which he may not need or be able to handle. Therefore, **packed cells** (blood cells without the plasma), platelets, or plasma proteins are given, depending on the specific need.

Informing the Individual

The individual who is to receive a blood transfusion may have many fears and misconceptions concerning the procedure. The individual may assume that the need for a transfusion means he or she is critically ill or near death. This is not always the case, but regardless of the severity of the situation, the individual needs an opportunity to ventilate his or her feelings and fears. Some individuals may mistakenly believe that by receiving someone else's blood they will take on the donor's characteristics. Clarifying this and other misconceptions is an important nursing intervention. Individuals whose religious beliefs preclude receiving a transfusion are provided with an opportunity to explore all the options available to them and be accepted regardless of the choice made. As with any other treatment, the individuals are informed as to the nature of the procedure, the time it will take, and the reasons for it.

Safety Precautions

While institutions may vary in the actual performance of the procedure, certain steps are followed to insure the safety of the individual. Prior to the actual transfusion, a blood test, known as a type-and-cross

Chart 18.13
Common Transfusion Reactions

REACTION	PRESENTING BEHAVIOR	MECHANISM OF OCCURRENCE
Allergic reactions	Fever, chills, erythema, urticaria, nausea, vomiting, respiratory distress, headache, edema, itching	Unknown; thought to be an antibody–antigen reaction
Febrile (pyrogenic) reactions	Fever, chills, restlessness, flushing, lumbar pain, malaise, headache	Contamination of blood by bacteria
Hemolytic reactions	Fever, chills, backache, tachycardia, chest pain, nausea, vomiting, apprehension, hypotension, oliguria, anuria, jaundice, moderate cyanosis, hemoglobinemia, hemoglobinuria	Antibody–antigen reaction
Circulatory overload	Pulmonary congestion, cyanosis, dyspnea, stertorous breathing, cough, frothy sputum, hemoptysis, tachycardia	Transfusion is administered too rapidly or is greater than the heart can handle
Disease transmission (e.g., serum hepatitis, malaria, syphilis)	Depends on causative agent	Contamination of blood by blood-borne bacteria or viruses

match, is done to determine the individual's blood type, antibody pattern, and the compatibility of his or her blood with the donor's. If an intravenous (IV) infusion is not already in progress, then it will be necessary to start one (Chap. 21). Typically, a Y setup is used for blood transfusion. Commonly, physiologic (isotonic) saline is infused immediately before and after the transfusion; however, Ringer's lactate may also be used. Dextrose is never used because it causes hemolysis. Vital signs, including temperature, are taken prior to, during, and after the procedure. An antihistamine may be ordered prior to the transfusion to minimize the possibility of allergic reactions.

Administering the Blood

When the transfusion is to be started a check is made between the individual's name and identification number and that name and number appearing on the label of the blood container. There are usually specific forms for this, which are then attached to the individual's chart. To prevent spoiling, blood is kept refrigerated until it is administered.

Blood is administered in units. A unit of blood equals 500 cc, and a unit of packed cells equals 250 cc. One unit of blood is usually transfused over a 1-hour period unless the physician orders otherwise. During the procedure the vital signs are monitored frequently, and the individual is carefully observed for any adverse reactions. Chart 18.13 outlines these adverse reactions.

If a reaction occurs, the transfusion is stopped, the saline started, and the physician notified. The individual's vital signs, particularly temperature, are taken, and a urine specimen is sent to the laboratory for a hemoglobin test. The remaining blood from the transfusion is returned to the blood bank for testing.

At the conclusion of the procedure, the individual is made comfortable and the treatment charted.

NOTES

1. Arthur C. Guyton. *Textbook of Medical Physiology,* 4th ed. Philadelphia, Saunders, 1971, p. 220.

SELECTED REFERENCES

Bates, Barbara. *A Guide to Physical Examination.* Philadelphia, Lippincott, 1974.

Beland, Irene and Passos, Joyce. *Clinical Nursing,* 3rd ed. New York, Macmillan, 1975.

"Blood Therapy." *American Journal of Nursing* (Special Feature), 79:925, May, 1979.

"Congenital Cardiac Defects—A Special Feature." *American Journal of Nursing,* 78:256, February, 1978.

"Controlling High Blood Pressure." *American Journal of Nursing,* 78:824, May, 1978.

"Correcting Common Errors in Blood Pressure Measurement." *American Journal of Nursing,* 65:134, October, 1965.

Clausen, Joy P., Flook, Margaret H., and Ford, Boonie. New York, McGraw-Hill, 1977.

Dison, Norma. *Clinical Nursing Techniques.* St. Louis, Mosby, 1975.

French, Ruth M. *Guide to Diagnostic Procedures,* 4th ed. New York, McGraw-Hill, 1975.

Ganong, William F. *Review of Medical Physiology,* 8th ed. Los Altos, California, Lange Medical Publications, 1977.

Garb, Solomon. *Laboratory Tests in Common Use,* 5th ed. New York, Springer, 1971.

Gildea, Joan. "Techniques of Cardiopulmonary Resuscitation in Infants." *American Journal of Nursing,* 78:265, February, 1978.

Guyton, Arthur C. *Textbook of Medical Physiology.* Philadelphia, Saunders, 1971.

Hart, Romaine. "What to Do When You're Number 1: A Review of CPR for Adults." *Nursing 79,* 9:54, February, 1979.

Heine, Emily, ed. *Assessing Vital Functions Accurately* (Nursing 77 Skillbook Series). Horsham, Pennsylvania, Intermed Communications, 1973.

Jenson, David. *The Principles of Physiology.* New York, Appleton, 1976.

Koepke, John A. *Guide to Clinical Laboratory Diagnosis.* New York, Appleton, 1969.

Luckman, Joan and Sorenson, Karen. *Medical-Surgical Nursing.* Philadelphia, Saunders, 1974.

Miller, Karen. "Assessing Peripheral Perfusion." *American Journal of Nursing,* 78:1673, October, 1978.

Moody, Linda. "Primer for Pulmonary Hygiene." *American Journal of Nursing,* 77:104, January, 1977.

Murray, Ruth and Zentner, Judith. *Nursing Assessment and Health Promotion.* Englewood Cliffs, N.J., Prentice-Hall, 1975.

Malasanos, Lois, Barkauskas, Violet, Moss, Muriel, and Stoltenberg-Allen, Kathryn. *Health Assessment.* St. Louis, Mosby, 1977.

McConnell, Edwina. "Fitting Antiembolism Stockings." *Nursing 78,* 8:67, September, 1978.

Passman, Jerome and Drummond, Constance D. *The EKG—Basic Techniques for Interpretation.* New York, McGraw-Hill, 1976.

"Pulses in Physical Assessment: A Programmed Unit. *American Journal of Nursing* (Supplement), 79:115,

Rau, Joseph and Rau, Mary. "To Breathe or Be Breathed: Understanding IPPB." *American Journal of Nursing,* 77:613, April, 1977.

Sana, Josephine and Judge, Richard. *Physical Appraisal Methods in Nursing Practice.* Boston, Little, Brown, 1975.

Stright, Patricia and Soukeep, Sister Maurita. "How to Hear It Right: Evaluating and Choosing a Stethoscope." *American Journal of Nursing,* 77:1477, September, 1977.

Tilkien, Sarko M. and Conover, Mary H. *Clinical Implications of Laboratory Tests.* St. Louis, Mosby, 1975.

Ungvarski, Peter J., Argondizzo, Nina T., and Boos, Patricia K. "CPR: Current Practice Revisited." *American Journal of Nursing,* 75:236, February, 1975.

Van Meter, Margaret and Lavine, Peter G. *Reading EKG's Correctly* (Nursing 77 Skillbook Series). Horsham, Pennsylvania, Intermed Communications, 1975.

Warren, Freda, "Getting a Quick Reading on an Infant's Blood Pressure." *Nursing 75,* 5:13, April, 1975.

Westfall, Una. "Electrical and Mechanical Events in the Cardiac Cycle." *American Journal of Nursing,* 76:231, February, 1976.

Widmann, Frances K. *Goodale's Clinical Interpretation of Laboratory Tests.* Philadelphia, Davis, 1973.

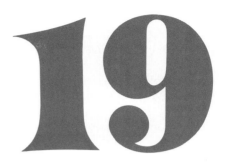

*Tell me what you eat and
I will tell you what you are.*
Anthelme Brillat-Savarin

NUTRITIONAL INTAKE

PRINCIPLES RELATED TO NUTRITIONAL INTAKE

Cellular processes require adequate amounts of protein, carbohydrates, fats, vitamins, minerals, and water for (1) tissue maintenance and repair, (2) energy, and (3) synthesis of hormones, antibodies, enzymes, and tissue.

Carbohydrates provide the most immediate sources of energy for the body.

Carbohydrates are used for energy before other nutrients, conserving protein for its vital functions.

Carbohydrates are necessary for the proper breakdown and deposition of fats.

Intake of excessive amounts of carbohydrates leads to a buildup of fat deposits in the body.

Insulin is necessary for the transport of glucose across the cell membrane.

Depletion of carbohydrate stores occurs within 24–48 hours.

Fats (lipids) provide the most concentrated source of energy for the body.

Fats are broken down by hydrolysis into fatty acids and glycerol.

Fatty acids are broken down into ketone acids.

The metabolism of fats is regulated by such hormones as insulin, glucocorticoids, corticotropin, growth hormones, thyroxine, epinephrine, and norepinephrine.

Fats are necessary for the absorption of the fat-soluble vitamins: A, D, E, K.

Fat is stored as adipose tissue in the subcutaneous level of the skin and surrounding major organs.

Fats help maintain the structural integrity of the cell and help to control the permeability of the cell.

The myelin sheath which insulates some nerves is composed, in part, of fat.

Fats help to protect tissue from trauma.

Fats are utilized in blood clotting as an essential component for thromboplastin.

Fats provide a reserve supply of phosphate ions.

Depletion of fat stores occurs within 5–6 weeks.

Cholesterol is a derived lipid which is used to form bile salts, steroid hormones, and provitamin D.

Cholesterol plays a role in preventing water evaporation from the skin.

Proteins are necessary for building, maintaining, and repairing body tissue.

Proteins are necessary to synthesize the nucleoproteins, antibodies, hormones, enzymes, hemoglobin, and plasma proteins.

Proteins help maintain fluid balance by regulating oncotic pressure.

Proteins provide energy when other sources are unavailable.

Proteins help maintain the pH balance of the blood by acting as buffer systems.

Amino acids make up proteins.

Essential amino acids are those which cannot be produced by the body and must be supplied in the diet.

Since amino acids cannot be stored in the body, daily intake of protein is necessary.

Protein metabolism is regulated by the growth hormones, glucocorticoids, testosterone, and thyroxine.

Adequate supplies of protein are necessary to maintain nitrogen balance.

A negative nitrogen balance results when protein is used for energy needs.

Metabolism results in the production of energy, which is measured in kilocalories.

► A kilocalorie (kcal) is the unit of measure which reflects the amount of energy necessary to raise 1 kilogram of water 1 degree centigrade.

One gram of protein yields approximately 4 kcal.

One gram of carbohydrate yields approximately 4 kcal.

One gram of fat yields approximately 9 kcal.

Water is an important constituent of the body, serving to maintain internal temperature and acting as the medium for chemical reactions.

Nausea and vomiting are reflexes.

Reflex centers for nausea and vomiting are located in the medulla oblongata.

Appetite is controlled, in part, by centers in the cerebral cortex.

Hunger, feeding, and satiety centers are located in the hypothalamus.

Food preferences and patterns are learned behaviors.

Nutritional patterns and habits are difficult to change.

Undereating and overeating may be coping reactions.

All processes of ingestion, digestion, and metabolism can be influenced by the psychosocial state of the individual.

Changing energy needs and health states require diet modifications.

Energy needs can be met successfully only when there is a continuous supply of oxygen and an adequate supply of nutrients for cellular processes. Cellular processes require a sufficient amount of carbohydrate, proteins, fats, vitamins, minerals, and water for metabolism and catabolism. Nutrition is the process
► of ingestion (the taking in of food), digestion (the breakdown and absorption of food substances),
► anabolism (the buildup of body tissue and sub-
► stances), catabolism (the breakdown of food, body tissues, and substances to release energy), absorption (the transfer of substances from the gastrointestinal
► tract into the tissues), and utilization (the process by

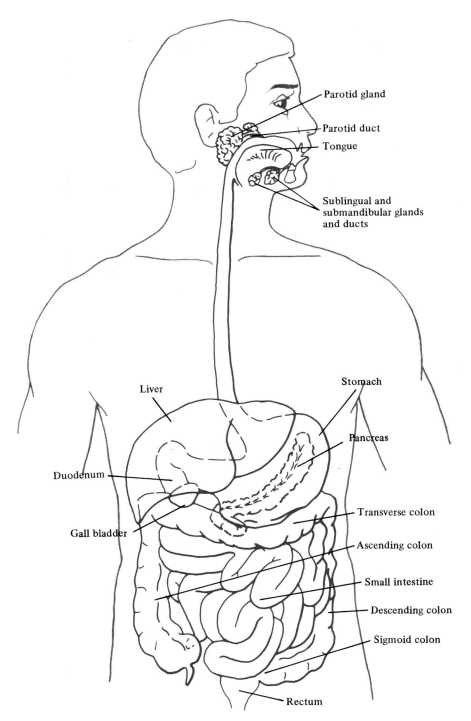

Figure 19.1
The subsystem for digestion.

which substances are used by the body). **Metabolism** consists of the processes of anabolism, catabolism, and absorption. Without the proper balance of these nutrients all aspects of the individual's life—physiologic, physical, psychologic, and cognitive—are negatively affected. Nutrients are found in **food**—which is any substance, solid or liquid, which is necessary for life. (Illustration 19.1)

Since no one food contains all, or even most, of these nutrients, the intake of any one food group does not necessarily result in good nutrition. The diversity of taste, lack of public knowledge, the variety of meanings food has, and the stratification of purchasing power are among the factors which create a national picture of marginal nutrition. Thus nursing care involves the assessment of, planning for, and intervening with not only those individuals with overt nutritional defects, but with any individual who enters the health care system.

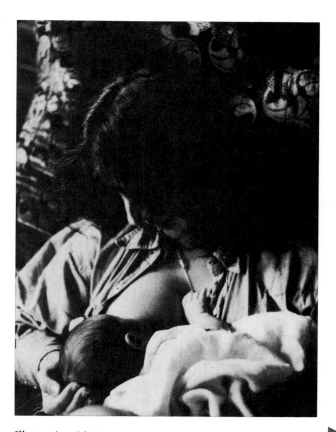

Illustration 19.1

A newborn seeks out his mother's breast and responsively sucks to receive nourishment. *(Photo © Leonard Speier)*

ASSESSMENT

Basic Four Food Groups

Assessment of nutritional status begins with identifying the intake needs of the individual. Each person ▶ requires a balance of the **basic four food groups** in his daily diet. The basic four are a categorization of the foods which provide the basic nutrients. They are (1) the milk group; (2) the meat, fish, and poultry group; (3) the fruit and vegetable group; and (4) the bread and cereal group. Chart 19.1 outlines the nutrients in the four basic food groups.

At each level of growth and development, requirements for these nutrients differ. Growth patterns, activity levels, developmental tasks, and pregnancy and lactation are factors that affect the demands of the body. Chart 19.2 outlines the specific nutritional requirements at various levels of growth and development. (Illustration 19.2)

Nursing assessment of an individual's intake of the basic four includes descriptions of:

- knowledge of nutrients and their relationship to well-being
- knowledge of the food groups
- knowledge of nutrients provided by the food groups
- knowledge of foods and portions within a food group
- nutrient requirements at present level of growth and development
- whether nutrient needs are being met for present level of growth and development

Factors Influencing Food Intake

PHYSICAL STATUS

The physical status of the individual plays a major part in determining his ability to ingest food.

The Oral Cavity

The condition of the oral cavity influences the ability of the individual to bite, masticate, and swal-
▶ low food. The presence or absence (**edentulousness**) of teeth and the condition of existing teeth often determine the types of food the individual is able to in-

Chart 19.1
Basic Four Food Groups

FOOD GROUP RECOMMENDED NUMBER OF SERVINGS

	Child	Teenager	Adult	Pregnant Woman	Lactating Woman
Milk	3	4	2	4	4
1 cup milk, yogurt, OR					
Calcium equivalent:					
1½ slices (1½ oz) cheddar cheese*					
1 cup pudding					
1¾ cups ice cream					
2 cups cottage cheese*					
Meat	2	2	2	3	2
2 ounces cooked, lean meat, fish, poultry, OR					
Protein equivalent:					
2 eggs					
2 slices (2 oz) cheddar cheese*					
½ cup cottage cheese*					
1 cup dried beans, peas					
4 tbsp peanut butter					
Fruit-Vegetable	4	4	4	4	4
½ cup cooked or juice					
1 cup raw					
Portion commonly served, such as a medium-size apple or banana					
Grain, whole grain, fortified, enriched	4	4	4	4	4
1 slice bread					
1 cup ready-to-eat cereal					
½ cup cooked cereal, pasta, grits					

The recommended servings from the Four Food Groups for adults supply about 1200 calories. The chart above gives recommendations for the number and size of servings for several categories of people.
*Count cheese as serving of milk OR meal, not both simultaneously.
"Others" complement but do not replace foods from the Four Food Groups. Amounts should be determined by individual caloric needs.
Copyright © 1977, 4th Edition, National Dairy Council, Rosemont, Illinois 60018. All rights reserved.

gest. Dentures that are loose or poor fitting often result in irritation of the gums and partial mastication of food. The condition of the gums and mucous membranes of the oral cavity may also interfere with chewing. Dryness of the mouth prevents the wetting of food and the beginning digestive processes and also hinders swallowing. Excessive mucous secretions alter taste and decrease appetite. Intact motor control of the tongue is necessary to move food around the mouth and toward the pharynx for swallowing.

Infants require a strong sucking reflex for food ingestion. Regardless of their age, all individuals require an intact swallow reflex. Food should not be offered to any individual whose swallow reflex is depressed or absent.

Debilitation

The degree of debilitation of the individual influences his desire and ability to eat. Often the person may have a desire to eat but not the strength to

Chart 19.1. B.
Nutrients—Sources and Functions

NUTRIENT	IMPORTANT SOURCES	SOME MAJOR PHYSIOLOGIC FUNCTIONS		
		Provide energy	Build and maintain body cells	Regulate body processes
Protein	Meat, poultry, fish; dried beans and peas; egg; cheese; milk.	Supplies 4 Calories per gram.	Constitutes part of the structure of every cell, such as muscle, blood, and bone; supports growth and maintains healthy body cells.	Constitutes part of enzymes, some hormones and body fluids, and antibodies that increase resistance to infection.
Carbohydrate	Cereal; potatoes; dried beans; corn; bread; sugar.	Supplies 4 Calories per gram. Major source of energy for central nervous system.	Supplies energy so protein can be used for growth and maintenance of body cells.	Unrefined products supply fiber—complex carbohydrates in fruits, vegetables, and whole grains—for regular elimination.
Fat	Shortening, oil; butter, margarine; salad dressing; sausages.	Supplies 9 Calories per gram.	Constitutes part of the structure of every cell. Supplies essential fatty acids.	Provides and carries fat-soluble vitamins (A, D, E, and K). Assists in fat utilization.
Vitamin A (Retinol)	Liver; carrots; sweet potatoes; greens; butter, margarine.		Assists formation and maintenance of skin and mucous membranes that line body cavities and tracts, such as nasal passages and intestinal tract, thus increasing resistance to infection.	Functions in visual processes and forms visual purple, thus promoting healthy eye tissues and eye adaptation in dim light.
Vitamin C (Ascorbic Acid)	Broccoli; orange; grapefruit; papaya; mango; strawberries.		Forms cementing substances, such as collagen, that hold body cells together, thus strengthening blood vessels, hastening healing of wounds and bones, and increasing resistance to infection.	Aids utilization of iron.
Thiamin (B$_1$)	Lean pork; nuts;	Aids in utilization of energy.		Functions as part of a

Nutrient	Important Sources	Provide Energy	Build and Maintain Body Cells / Regulate Body Processes
	fortified cereal products.		coenzyme to promote the utilization of carbohydrate. Promotes normal appetite. Contributes to normal functioning of nervous system.
Riboflavin (B₂)	Liver; milk, yogurt, cottage cheese.	Aids in utilization of energy.	Functions as part of a coenzyme in the production of energy within body cells. Promotes healthy skin, eyes, and clear vision.
Niacin	Liver; meat, poultry, fish; peanuts; fortified cereal products.	Aids in utilization of energy.	Functions as part of a coenzyme in fat synthesis, tissue respiration, and utilization of carbohydrate. Promotes healthy skin, nerves, and digestive tract. Aids digestion and fosters normal appetite.
Calcium	Milk, yogurt; cheese; sardines and salmon with bones; collard, kale, mustard, and turnip greens.		Combines with other minerals within a protein framework to give structure and strength to bones and teeth. Assists in blood clotting. Functions in normal muscle contraction and relaxation, and normal nerve transmission.
Iron	Enriched farina; prune juice; liver; dried beans and peas; red meat.	Aids in utilization of energy.	Combines with protein to form hemoglobin, the red substance in blood that carries oxygen to and carbon dioxide from the cells. Prevents nutritional anemia and its accompanying fatigue. Increases resistance to infection.

Nutrients are chemical substances obtained from foods during digestion. They are needed to build and maintain body cells, regulate body processes, and supply energy. About 50 nutrients, including water, are needed daily for optimum health. If one obtains the proper amount of the 10 "leader" nutrients in the daily diet, the other 40 or so nutrients will likely be consumed in amounts sufficient to meet body needs. One's diet should include a variety of foods because no *single* food supplies all the 50 nutrients, and because many nutrients work together. When a nutrient is added or a nutritional claim is made, nutrition labeling regulations require listing the 10 leader nutrients on food packages. These nutrients appear in the chart above with food sources and some major physiologic functions.
Copyright © 1977, 4th Edition, National Dairy Council, Rosemont, Illinois 60018. All right reserved.

Chart 19.2
Recommended Daily Dietary Allowances, Revised 1980[1]

	Age (years)	Weight (kg)	Weight (lb)	Height (cm)	Height (in)	Protein (gm)	FAT-SOLUBLE VITAMINS Vitamin A Activity (μg RE)[2]	Vitamin D (μg αT.E.)[3]	Vitamin E Activity (μg aT.E.)[4]
Infants	0.0–0.5	6	13	60	24	kg × 2.2	420	10	3
	0.5–1.0	9	20	71	28	kg × 2.0	400	10	4
Children	1–3	13	29	90	35	23	400	10	5
	4–6	20	44	112	44	30	500	10	6
	7–10	28	62	132	52	34	700	10	7
Males	11–14	45	99	157	62	45	1000	10	8
	15–18	66	145	176	69	56	1000	10	10
	19–22	70	154	177	70	56	1000	7.5	10
	23–50	70	154	178	70	56	1000	5	10
	51+	70	154	178	70	56	1000	5	10
Females	11–14	46	101	157	62	46	800	10	8
	15–18	55	120	163	64	46	800	10	8
	19–22	55	120	163	64	44	800	7.5	8
	23–50	55	120	163	64	44	800	5	8
	51+	55	120	163	64	44	800	5	8
Pregnant						+30	200	+5	+2
Lactating						+20	400	+5	+3

WATER-SOLUBLE VITAMINS

	Age (years)	Vitamin C (mg)	Folacin[5] (μg)	Niacin (mg N.E.)[6]	Riboflavin (mg)	Thiamin (mg)	Vitamin B_6 (μg)	Vitamin B_{12} (μg)
Infants	0.0–0.5	35	30	6	0.4	0.3	0.3	0.5[7]
	0.5–1.0	35	45	8	0.6	0.5	0.6	1.5
Children	1–3	45	100	9	0.8	0.7	0.9	2.0
	4–6	45	200	11	1.0	0.9	1.3	2.5
	7–10	45	300	16	1.4	1.2	1.6	3.0
Males	11–14	50	400	18	1.6	1.4	1.8	3.0
	15–18	60	400	18	1.7	1.4	2.0	3.0
	19–22	60	400	19	1.7	1.5	2.2	3.0
	23–50	60	400	18	1.6	1.4	2.2	3.0
	51+	60	400	16	1.4	1.2	2.2	3.0
Females	11–14	50	400	15	1.3	1.1	1.8	3.0
	15–18	60	400	14	1.3	1.1	2.0	3.0
	19–22	60	400	14	1.3	1.1	2.0	3.0
	23–50	60	400	13	1.2	1.0	2.0	3.0
	51+	60	400	13	1.2	1.0	2.0	3.0
Pregnant		+20	+400	+2	+0.3	+0.4	+0.6	+1.0
Lactating		+40	+100	+5	+0.5	+0.5	+0.5	+1.0

(continued)

Chart 19.2 (Cont.)
Recommended Daily Dietary Allowances, Revised 1980[1]

	Age (years)	MINERALS					
		Calcium (mg)	Phosphorus (mg)	Iodine (μg)	Iron (mg)	Magnesium (mg)	Zinc (mg)
Infants	0.0–0.5	360	240	40	10	50	3
	0.5–1.0	540	360	50	15	70	5
Children	1–3	800	800	70	15	150	10
	4–6	800	800	90	10	200	10
	7–10	800	800	120	10	250	10
Males	11–14	1200	1200	150	18	350	15
	15–18	1200	1200	150	18	400	15
	19–22	800	800	150	10	350	15
	23–50	800	800	150	10	350	15
	51+	800	800	150	10	350	15
Females	11–14	1200	1200	150	18	300	15
	15–18	1200	1200	150	18	300	15
	19–22	800	800	150	18	300	15
	23–50	800	800	150	18	300	15
	51+	800	800	150	10	300	15
Pregnant		+400	+400	+25	—[8]	+150	+5
Lactating		+400	+400	+50	—[8]	+150	+15

[1]The allowances are intended to provide for individual variations among most normal persons as they live in the United States under usual environmental stresses. Diets should be based on a variety of common foods in order to provide other nutrients for which human requirements have been less well defined.

[2]Retinol equivalents. 1 Retinol equivalent = 1 μg retinol or 6 μg carotene.

[3]As cholecalciferol. 10μg cholecalciferol = 400 I.U. vitamin D.

[4]α tocopherol equivalents, 1 mg d-α-tocopherol = 1 αT.E.

[5]The folacin allowances refer to dietary sources as determined by *Lactobacillus casei* assay after treatment with enzymes ("conjugases") to make polyglutanyl forms of the vitamin available to the test organism.

[6]1 NE (niacin equivalent) is equal to 1 mg of niacin or 60 mg of dietary tryptophan.

[7]The RDA for vitamin B_{12} in infants is based on average concentration of the vitamin in human milk. The allowances after weaning are based on energy intake (as recommended by the American Academy of Pediatrics) and consideration of other factors such as intestinal absorption.

[8]The increased requirement during pregnancy cannot be met by the iron content of habitual American diets nor by the existing iron stores of many women; therefore the use of 30–60 mg of supplemental iron is recommended. Iron needs during lactation are not substantially different from those of nonpregnant women, but continued supplementation of the mother for 2–3 months after parturition is advisable in order to replenish stores depleted by pregnancy.

From Food and Nutrition Board, National Academy of Sciences—National Research Council. Reproduced with permission.

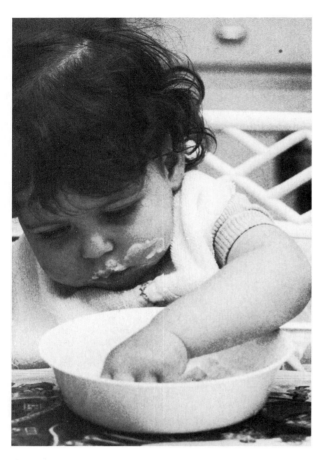

Illustration 19.2
A toddler's developing self-sufficiency at mealtime requires a lot of concentration and hard work! *(Photo © Peter Arnold, from Erika Stone)*

feed himself. The individual who is blind, has paralysis or **paresis** (muscle weakness) of the hands or face, flaccidity or spasticity of the extremities, or structural deformities of the arms, hands, or oral structures may have feeding difficulties and need someone's assistance or, perhaps, special devices to eat.

Nursing assessment of an individual's physical status and nutritional intake includes descriptions of:

- conditions of teeth—presence? absence? decay?
- chewing ability
- use of dentures
- condition and fit of dentures
- types of food individual has difficulty chewing? swallowing?

- condition of oral cavity and structures
- presence of swallow reflex
- quality of swallow reflex
- degree of debilitation
- relationship of debilitation to nutritional intake
- disabilities which interfere with nutritional intake
- assistance needed for feeding
- special devices needed for feeding

FOOD PATTERNS

The individual's food pattern is influenced to a great extent by his feelings about food. Food may mean such things as reward, punishment, comfort, or an activity of daily living. The meaning food has for an individual may result from parental use of food as a reward for good behavior, habitual consumption of certain foods during times of stress, forced feeding, withholding food as punishment, mealtime atmosphere, and the availability of food. A common expression related to the meaning of food is the saying "Some people eat to live; while others live to eat." (See Chart 19.3 and Illustration 19.3.)

Appetite and Hunger

Distinguishing between appetite and hunger is one way of determining whether an individual is meeting a physiologic need for food or a psychosocial one. **Hunger** is the body's response to stimuli in the feeding center of the hypothalamus and results in a seeking out of food. It is accompanied by stomach contractions, which are experienced as tight, gnawing sensations or hunger pangs. Decreased blood glucose levels often initiate this response. Restlessness, weakness, tension, or nausea may also accompany hunger states.

Appetite, on the other hand, while it may be combined with hunger, is often a subjective desire for a food or a food group. In part, appetite is regulated by the hypothalamus, but cerebral stimulation by smells, sights, or associations may increase or decrease appetite. When a person experiences a feeling of fullness after eating, centers in the brain inhibit the feeding center and a feeling of *satiety* results.

Helping individuals to identify and differentiate the feelings of hunger, appetite, and satiation may help them to modify their eating habits. Identifying those feelings with emotions associated with the intake of food further helps the person in changing food patterns.

Chart 19.3

Nutritional Patterns at Various Levels of Growth and Development

Infant	
newborn	Has several reflexes which aid in seeking out food and ingestion, i.e., rooting, sucking, swallowing. Pushes food out when placed on tip of tongue. Regurgitation common.
3–6 months	Birth reflexes diminish. Puts hands in mouth. Begins drinking from cup. Begins chewing. Solid foods can be introduced.
6–9 months	Begins to teethe. Feeds self finger foods. Holds own bottle. Begins weaning.
9–12 months	Eats with fingers. Reaches for foods. Attempts to use spoon.
Toddler (1–3 years)	Becomes self-sufficient in feeding. Still spills food frequently. Fussy eater. Food choice that of parents. Ritualistic in food patterns. Completes deciduous teeth. Periods of decreased food intake.
Preschooler (3–5 years)	Snacks are a necessity to compensate for increased activity. Finicky. Eating takes on social importance. Usually likes fruits, dislikes vegetables.
School age (6–12 years)	Develops table manners. Increases repertoire of foods liked. Hungriest time of day is after school. Becomes independent in seeking out food. School meals designed to provide ⅓ RDA.

School age (cont.)	Often too busy to stop to eat. Ideal time for nutrition teaching. Likes to eat with peers. Begins to develop permanent teeth.
Adolescent (12–18 years)	Faddish in food preferences. Girls have poorer nutrition than boys—frequently diet. Eat many meals outside home. Obesity frequent.
Young adult (18–40 years)	Lifestyle, occupation influence habits. Pregnancy and lactation increase dietary needs. Males have increased dietary needs over adolescence. Often eats on the run.
Middle adult (40–65 years)	Metabolism decreases 5–10% every 10 years. Dietary-related pathologies emerge. Eating a social activity. Physical activity often decreases. Weight gain frequent.
Older adult (65+ years)	Decreased enzyme secretion. Decreased nutrient absorption. Chronic diseases common. Alterations in taste and smell. Decreased gastrointestinal motility. Decreased social contacts may alter eating habits. Decreased physical activity. Fixed income may influence diet. Vitamin and mineral deficiencies common.

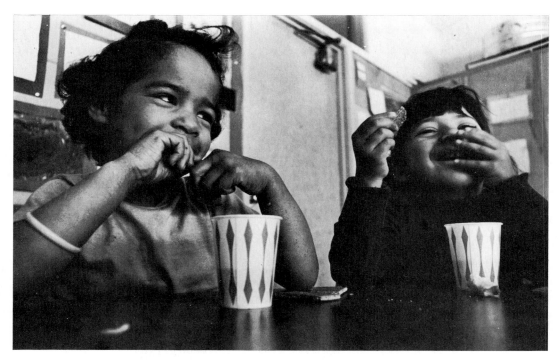

Illustration 19.3
New teeth, busy school days, and good friends influence the eating patterns of young school-age children. *(Photo by John Running, from Stock, Boston)*

Nursing assessment of the meanings of food intake for an individual includes descriptions of:

- what associations food has
- what generated these associations
- how they influence food patterns
- whether the individual can differentiate among hunger, appetite, and satiation
- what increases or decreases appetite

CULTURAL INFLUENCES

The culture individuals come from greatly affects both their food preferences and eating patterns.

Cultural Group

Although an individual's cultural group can give the nurse a general lead for assessment, it is not a hard and fast rule that all individuals follow the patterns of their culture. More commonly, in a diverse society such as the United States, individuals maintain certain ethnic and religious preferences while in-corporating foods from other cultures in their eating habits. Stereotypes of any kind can limit the insight and effectiveness of assessment. The ability of the individual's diet to meet the basic four requirements is the important factor, rather than adherence to any particular food habits. For example, the Mexican-American or vegetarian diet which uses beans, milk, and eggs can effectively meet protein requirements without having meat in the diet. (Illustration 19.4)

Geography

The geographic area in which individuals live plays a significant role in the types of foods they eat. The availability of meat and dairy products in the Midwest and North Central regions of the United States, seafood along the coastal areas, and the abundance of fruits and vegetables in the South and Southwest influence the eating habits and customs of many groups. Whether the individual lives in an urban, suburban, or rural area also affects food patterns. The rural person may have more cultivation and storage areas than the apartment dweller, while the urban resident may have a wider variety of foods from which to choose. These considerations are im-

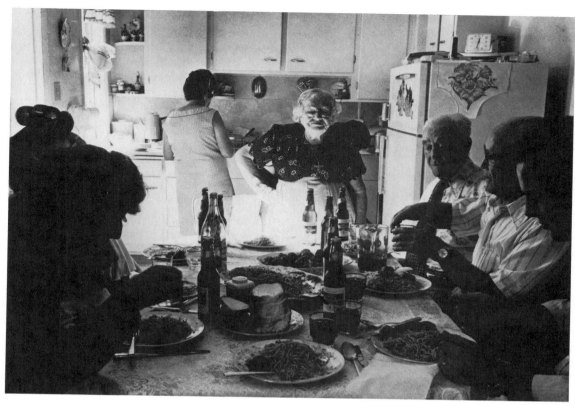

Illustration 19.4
Cultural influences help to determine the food preferences of individuals. Often these preferences do not include the basic four nutritional requirements; however, a person's pattern of eating from day to day—how he incorporates other foods with his "favorites"—will more significantly affect nutritional status. *(Photo © Karen R. Preuss, from Jeroboam)*

portant, not only in assessment, but also in the formulation of a plan that helps the individual take advantage of the food resources in his or her setting.

Nursing assessment of cultural and geographic influences on food intake includes descriptions of:

- the individual's cultural background, including religious beliefs and ethnic patterns
- how these beliefs influence food intake
- what proportion of the diet meets the requirements of the basic four
- the availability of culturally preferred foods
- the food benefits and disadvantage of the geographic location
- the relationship of the benefits and disadvantages to food intake

SOCIOECONOMIC FACTORS

Income Level

The income level of individuals and their family and/or significant others helps determine the types of food selected and the proportion of the food requirements which are met. Carbohydrate foods are usually the least expensive, while protein foods such as meat, fish, and poultry, and often fresh fruits and vegetables, are relatively high in cost.

A high income level, however, is not synonymous with a balanced diet, nor a low income with an inadequate one. The actual dollar income of the individual and the family and/or significant others is not necessarily an indication of their food buying power. The number of people to be fed, other fixed expenses, and supplemental food supplies such as gardens all affect the percentage of income which can be used for food. Increased consumer awareness has helped people to plan balanced meals with alternative food products such a soybean derivatives.

Prestige Foods

Certain foods have prestige value associated with them. Thus people may select them over other types with little consideration for their actual nutritional value. For instance, the woman who views milk as a prestige food may utilize the majority of her money budgeted for food on milk for her baby, to the exclusion of all other foods. Since milk has almost no iron, the infant and young child will develop iron deficiency anemia. Iron deficiency anemia in early childhood results in diminished physical and cognitive development, poor resistance to infection, and decreased energy levels. These infants and children may appear healthy because of "chubbiness"; however, they are lethargic and pale.

Knowledge of Nutrition

The individual's level of knowledge about what food combinations make a balanced diet, what foods are sources of nutrients, caloric needs, the relationship of nutrition to well-being, inexpensive alternatives to high-cost foods, and nutritious food preparation influence food habits and preferences. Like income, a knowledge of good nutrition does not guarantee a balanced diet. Habits, culture, preferences, lifestyle, and the availability of food may interfere with an individual's putting his or her knowledge into action.

Myths and Misconceptions

Myths and misconceptions can also interfere with the individual's meeting his or her energy needs in a nutritious way. Adages such as "a fat baby is a happy baby" and "the way to a man's heart is through his stomach" exemplify common attitudes toward nutrition. Even with high levels of knowledge, individuals may maintain inaccurate beliefs about nutrition from family or cultural traditions.

Nursing assessment of an individual's income and knowledge of nutrition includes descriptions of:

- income level and food buying power
- influence of income on dietary habits
- knowledge of alternatives to high-cost foods
- knowledge of balanced diet
- knowledge of sources of nutrients
- knowledge of relationship between level of growth and development and nutritional needs
- knowledge of nutritional food preparation
- myths and misconceptions held about nutrition
- degree to which nutrition knowledge is put into practice
- factors which interfere with putting nutrition knowledge into practice

EATING PATTERNS

The individual's patterns and habits of daily eating are important areas of nursing assessment in determining whether that individual is meeting energy needs. The times of day when meals are eaten, the number of meals, which meal is the main one of the day, food likes and dislikes, special diet requirements, the eating environment, and lifestyle comprise the individual's nutrition habits and patterns. They are influenced by the individual's culture, income, and level of knowledge. Food consumption is also affected by increased intake of "fast foods," weight consciousness, food fads, increased leisure time, and other changes in lifestyle. The effect these influences have on the individual and his or her nutrition intake is also included in assessing the individual's food habits and patterns.

Diet History

One method of ascertaining the individual's usual dietary eating habits is the diet history. In a diet history the individual lists total food intake for a typical day, including times and amounts. The individual lists the other characteristics of his or her eating pattern, such as emotional determinants of food intake and activity levels. Foods that distress the individual or to which he or she allergic are also noted.

Changing Inadequate Habits

Although habits and patterns may contribute to a poor nutritional state, the individual may not be willing or able to give up these habits and patterns. Thus the nurse must ascertain the individual's value of and commitment to these habits and patterns so that any necessary diet modifications can be planned around them. The influence of patterns and habits of the family and/or significant others on the individual's nutritional intake is also important. Their willingness or ability to change may greatly affect the flexibility of the individual to meet his or her energy needs: mealtimes may be fixed; the type of food available in the home may be limited; and knowledge of good nutrition, modifications, and food preparation may be inadequate. Therefore, the pattern of nutrition of the whole family and/or significant others system must be explored to give a complete picture of the nutritional pattern of the individual and to assist in bringing about changes in his or her diet.

Nursing assessment of nutritional habits and patterns includes descriptions of:

- usual daily pattern of intake
- times of day food is eaten? types? amounts?
- which meal is main meal of day
- food likes and dislikes
- eating environment
- special diet requirements
- relationship of lifestyle to food intake
- food allergies
- commitment to habits and patterns
- habits and patterns of family or significant others
- relationship of habits and patterns of family and/or significant others to individual's habits and patterns
- medications and methods used to aid digestion and nutrition intake
- influence of other medications on nutritional intake

ENERGY EXPENDITURE

The individual's energy expenditure provides additional meaningful data for assessing the nutritional status and energy needs of the individual.

BMR Determinants

▶ The energy expenditure of an individual at rest is called his **basal metabolic rate** (**BMR**). In order to meet the needs of an adult at rest, approximately 24 kcal/kg of body weight is needed each day. For example, if a person weights 58 kg (128 pounds), the number of kilocalories required at rest is 58 × 24, or 1392 kcal. However, individuals do not remain at rest throughout the day and need additional kilocalories for such daily activities as eating, dressing, cleaning, sewing, walking, and working. The BMR is influenced by level of growth and development, sex, body build, body surface area, physical exercise, environmental temperatures, present state of nutrition, and fever and disease processes. (Illustration 19.5. A–B)

Growth and Development. The energy expenditure of the individual is affected by his or her level of growth and development, since energy needs are increased during the periods of rapid growth such as toddlerhood and decreased with the reduced muscle tone and mass of later years. Concomitant with

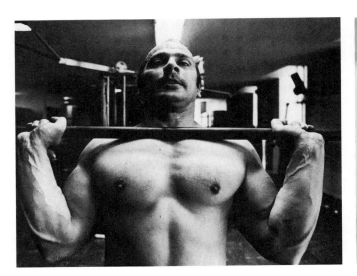 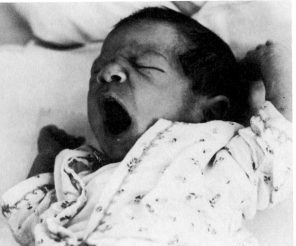

Illustration 19.5
Level of growth and development, body surface area, body composition, and physical activity are among the factors to consider when assessing whether an individual's intake of calories and nutrients is sufficient. (*Left photo © Ray Ellis, from Photo Researchers. Right photo by Anna Kaufman Moon, from Stock, Boston*)

certain developmental stages are increased or decreased activity levels which account for changing energy needs. Pregnancy, especially during the last three months, and lactation increase energy needs.

Sex.   Women have a 5 to 10% lower BMR than men of comparable height and weight. The exact cause is not known; however, factors such as percentage of adipose tissue and hormonal production contribute to this decrease in energy expenditure.

Body Surface.   Body surface, which includes weight, height, and build, directly influences the BMR. The greater the body surface area, the higher the BMR. However, this is greatly affected by the composition of the body. Adipose tissue consumes less oxygen than muscle tissue; thus the person with a high percentage of adipose tissue expends less energy

than the muscular person of the same height and weight.

Physical Activity.   The extent and intensity of physical activity greatly influence the BMR. Activities can be classified as sedentary, light, moderate, rigorous, or strenuous. The more strenuous the activity the greater the energy expenditure. Also, the larger the person, the greater the energy expenditure for any given activity. Chart 19.4 illustrates examples of various activity classifications and their energy expenditures.

Environmental Temperature.   In an attempt to maintain body temperature as a result of changes in environmental temperature, energy expenditure increases or decreases. Thus in warmer climates, metabolic rates are decreased to promote heat loss,

---

Chart 19.4
Activity Classifications and Their Energy Expenditures

TYPE OF ACTIVITY	KILOCALORIES PER HOUR*
Sedentary Reading; writing; eating; watching television or movies; listening to the radio; sewing; playing cards; typing; and miscellaneous office work and other activities done while sitting that require little or no arm movement	80–100
Light Preparing and cooking food; doing dishes; dusting; hand washing small articles of clothing; ironing; walking slowly; personal care; miscellaneous office work and other activities done while standing that require some arm movement; and rapid typing and other activities done while sitting that are more strenuous	110–160
Moderate Making beds; mopping and scrubbing; sweeping; light polishing and waxing; laundering by machine; light gardening and carpentry work; walking moderately fast; other activities done while standing that require moderate arm movement; and activities done while sitting that require more vigorous arm movement	170–240
Vigorous Heavy scrubbing and waxing; hand washing large articles of clothing; hanging out clothes; stripping beds; other heavy work; walking fast; bowling; golfing; and gardening	250–350
Strenuous Swimming; playing tennis; running; bicycling; dancing; skiing; and playing football	350 and more

*Lower figures apply to women, higher figures to men. The figures include the metabolism at rest as well as for the activity.
From: Corinne H. Robinson and Marilyn R. Lawler. Normal and Therapeutic Nutrition, *15th ed. New York, Macmillan, 1977, p. 97. Copyright © 1977 Macmillan Publishing Co., Inc.*

while in colder climates, metabolic rates are increased to conserve heat.

Nutrition. The ingestion, digestion, absorption, and utilization of food produces energy. This is known as the *specific dynamic action of food*. Protein produces several times more energy than fats and carbohydrates. Six to ten percent of the energy needs of the individual are met in this way.

The present state of nutrition may influence the BMR of an individual. In severe states of malnutrition, the BMR is reduced as a result of increased catabolism of body tissue.

Disease Process. Whenever body temperature increases, as with infection and stress, the BMR increases. For every one degree Fahrenheit that the body temperature rises, the BMR is raised approximately 7%. Other pathologic states, such as neoplasms and endocrine imbalances, also influence the BMR. Chart 19.5 gives some examples of the influence of disease on the BMR.

Sufficient Caloric Intake

When assessing the adequacy of an individual's food intake, it is necessary to determine whether the caloric and nutrient intake are sufficient to meet the

Chart 19.5
Conditions Altering Basal Metabolic Rate

CONDITION	INCREASE	POSSIBLE INCREASE	DECREASE	POSSIBLE DECREASE
Increased physical activity	X			
Pregnancy	X			
Fever	X			
Endocrine disorders:				
Hyperthyroidism	X			
Hypersecretion of pituitary gland		X		
Cushing's syndrome		X		
Tumors of adrenal glands		X		
Blood diseases:				
Leukemia (most often)	X			
Pernicious anemia		X		
Essential hypertension		X		
Myocardial stress	X			
Diabetes insipidus		X		
Shock			X	
Malnutrition			X	
Anemia (Severe)				X
Chronic Arthritis				X
Peptic Ulcer				X
Nephrotic syndrome (lipid nephrosis)			X	
Endocrine disorders:				
Hypothyroidism			X	
Addison's disease				X
Hypopituitarism				X
Nervous system diseases:				
Schizophrenia				X
Psychoneurosis				X
Autonomic imbalance (vagotonia)				X

From: Rosanne B. Howard and Nancie H. Herbold. Nutrition in Clinical Care. *New York, McGraw-Hill, 1978, p. 168.*

energy expenditures of the individual at that time. Insufficient calorie and nutrient intake results in malnutrition, while excessive intake results in **obesity**. If caloric intake is excessive while nutrient intake is deficient, the individual will become obese and malnourished at the same time. Chart 19.6 lists the sequelae of obesity and malnutrition.

Nursing assessment of an individual's energy expenditure includes descriptions of:

- the approximate BMR (number of kilograms of body weight times 24 kcal)
- factors which increase BMR (e.g., work patterns, exercise levels, stress, illness)
- factors which decrease BMR (e.g., presenting nutritional state, climate, body surface)
- relationship of food intake to energy expenditure
- relationship of activities of daily living to energy needs and expenditure
- whether caloric and nutrient intake are sufficient, deficient, or excessive
- how caloric and nutrient intake influence level of wellness
- rate of weight gain or loss; voluntary or involuntary
- effects of malnutrition and obesity on body image

IATROGENIC FACTORS

The influence of hospitalization on meeting nutritional needs is an often overlooked assessment area. Butterworth states that the following factors can lead to **iatrogenic malnutrition** (induced by the health care regimen and setting):

1 failure to record height and weight
2 rotation of staff at frequent intervals
3 diffusion of responsibility for patient care
4 prolonged use of glucose and saline intravenous feedings
5 failure to observe patients' food intake
6 withholding meals because of diagnostic tests
7 use of tube-feedings in inadequate amounts, of uncertain composition, and under unsanitary conditions
8 ignorance of the composition of vitamin mixtures and other nutritional products
9 failure to recognize increased nutritional needs due to injury or illness
10 performance of surgical procedures without first

Chart 19.6
Sequelae of Obesity and Malnutrition

OBESITY	MALNUTRITION
Decreased basal metabolic rate	Decreased energy levels
Decreased healing and tissue repair	Decreased healing and tissue repair
Hypertension	Depleted protein stores
Cardiac overload	Muscle wasting
Predisposition to atherosclerosis, diabetes, cerebral vascular accidents, gall bladder disease	Increased susceptibility to infection
Decreased blood supply to organs	Poor cognitive development and functioning
Compression of organs	Sensory loss
Increased mortality rate	Altered growth and development
Increased severity of gout, arthritis, surgery	Softening of bones
Stress on all body organs	Thyroid, parotid, liver, heart, and tongue hypertrophy
Psychological distress	Pallor
Altered pancreatic function	Anemia
Abnormal menstrual cycles and amennorrhea	Brittle hair and nails
Impaired release of growth hormone	Sunken, dull eyes
Increased secretion of adrenal steroids	Skin breakdown
Impaired venous return	Superficial hemorrhage Abnormal menstrual cycles and amennorrhea

making certain that the patient is optimally nourished, and failure to give the body nutritional support after surgery

11 failure to appreciate the role of nutrition in the prevention of and recovery from infection; the unwarranted reliance on antibiotics

12 lack of communication and interaction between physician and dietitian. As staff professionals, dietitians should be concerned with the nutritional health of every hospital patient

13 delay of nutritional support until the patient is in an advanced state of depletion, which is sometimes irreversible

14 limited availability of laboratory tests to assess nutritional status; failure to use those that are available.[1]

Thus not only must the individual's previous habits and home environment be assessed, but also the effects of the health care environment on his or her nutritional state.

Interferences with Nutrition

Any factor that interferes with ingestion, digestion, or utilization of nutrients can negatively alter the individual's nutritional state. These interferences may not always be directly related to the gastrointestinal system, but may be sequelae of other pathologic processes. Chart 19.7 summarizes conditions resulting in nutritional failure.

Three of the most common interferences with nutrition are anorexia, nausea, and vomiting.

ANOREXIA

▶ **Anorexia** is the loss of appetite and may be the result of a pathologic process, pain, stress and anxiety, unpleasant smells or sights, drugs, or nausea. Anorexia is a subjective feeling but can be objectively observed by such indications as decreased intake, reports of the individual, weight loss, or disinterest in favorite foods.

Chart 19.7
Conditions Resulting in Nutritional Failure

1. Inadequate intake—quantity
   Mechanical feeding problems or
      undeveloped feeding skills
   Anorexia (due to emotional problems,
      disease process, drugs)

2. Inadequate intake—quality
   Education of parents or caretaker
   Institutionalized setting
   Poor food habits
   Allergies

3. Increased metabolism
   Fever
   Infections
   Malignancy
   Hyperthyroidism
   Athetosis
   Surgery, stress, burns

4. Increased loss
   Vomiting
   Diarrhea
   Decreased food transit time through the gut

5. Defective utilization
   Metabolic diseases (aminoacidopathies,
      galactosemia, lipidoses)
   Disturbed metabolic states (hepatic
      insufficiency, renal tubular acidosis,
      nephrogenic diabetes insipidus, adrenal
      cortical hyperplasia with salt loss)
   Drug interference with nutrients

6. Defective absorption
   Intrinsic disease states (regional enteritis,
      Hirschsprung's disease)
   Exogenous states (intestinal parasitosis,
      celiac disease, surgical removal of the
      small bowel)
   Drugs

7. Defects in the function of major organ
   systems
   Severe congenital heart disease
   Severe chest disease
   Severe liver disease
   Kidney disease
   Brain damage

8. Excessive food or vitamin intake
   Obesity
   Vitamin intoxication—fat-soluble vitamins

From: Rosanne B. Howard and Nancie H. Herbold. Nutrition in Clinical Care. *New York, McGraw-Hill, 1978, p. 301.*

NAUSEA

▶ **Nausea** is the subjective feeling of being "sick to one's stomach." It often precedes vomiting and may induce anorexia. Many things may cause nausea, among which are pathologic processes (e.g., influenza), drugs, other stressors, and anxiety, irritating foods, pain, motion, and hunger.

VOMITING

▶ **Vomiting,** or **emesis,** is the reflex action which empties the stomach upward through the esophagus rather than downward through the intestines. Emesis is caused by the same factors that cause nausea. In addition, neurologic damage and structural defects such as pyloric stenosis induce vomiting.

When an individual vomits, the nurse notes the frequency, amount, color, consistency, and odor; the individual's reaction; the precipitating factors; and the sequence of events. Chart 19.8 lists and describes types of vomitus.

Nursing assessment of interferences with nutrition includes descriptions of:

- effect of the interferences on the amount of intake
- effect of interferences on the quality of intake
- effect on metabolism
- losses of intake (e.g., vomiting, increased intestinal motility)
- effect of the interferences on digestion
- effect on absorption
- effect on utilization
- pathologies in other than the gastrointestinal system which interfere with nutrition
- relationship of interferences with the state of well-being
- precipitating factors of interferences
- sequence of events
- duration of interferences
- attitudes toward interference (of individual, family and/or significant others)
- methods of coping with interferences (by individual, family and/or significant others)
- knowledge about interferences (individual's, family/significant others')
- therapeutic regimen for interferences
- effectiveness of therapeutic regimen for interferences

Chart 19.8
Types and Descriptions of Vomitus

TYPE	DESCRIPTION
Bilious	Greenish-yellow, contains bile; seen after continuous vomiting
Black	Nongranular, brown or black mixture of blood and stomach contents
Coffee-ground	Black or brown, granular mixture of blood and gastric contents; seen in hemorrhagic disorders of the gastrointestinal tract
Cyclic	Recurrent periods of vomiting
Dry	Retching, heaving, nonproductive vomiting attempts
Hematemesis	Vomiting of blood—may be bright red if fresh blood; brown or black if blood is partially broken down (old blood)
Partially digested food	Vomitus containing food which has been incompletely digested
Pernicious	Long-term, continuous, severe; may be life threatening; seen in pregnancy
Projectile	Forceful emission of stomach contents; seen in neurologic disease and pyloric stenosis
Reflex	Caused by irritation of pharynx as in coughing, suctioning, irritating chemicals, stress
Stercoraceous (fecal)	Vomitus containing fecal matter; seen in intestinal obstruction, structural defects
Undigested food	Vomitus containing food which has not been acted on by gastric juices

Physical Assessment

Inspection, percussion, palpation and auscultation are the techniques used to examine the individual's nutritional status.

INSPECTION

General

General inspection plays a significant role in the physical assessment of the individual for nutritional adequacy. The condition of the hair, its luster, texture, and flexibility; the skin, its turgor, texture, and state of hydration; and the eyes, their clarity and state of hydration are all indications of nutritional state. The general appearance of the individual's state of nutrition—i.e., well nourished, undernourished, or obese—and the distribution of body fat are also noted. The individual's height and weight are recorded and comparison made with expected measurements. Body build and stature are noted. Three types of body build are usually identified: asthenic (ectomorph)—slim, tall, and sinewy with a small frame; sthenic (mesomorph)—muscular with medium frame, height, weight; and pyknic (endomorph)—stocky with a short, broad frame and tendency to be overweight.

Oral Cavity

Specific inspection begins with observation of the mouth and oral cavity. Dentures are removed before inspecting the oral cavity. Chart 19.9 summarizes the inspection of the mouth and oral cavity.

Anterior Neck

The anterior neck is observed for bulges with the head erect, slightly extended, and with the individual swallowing water. The thyroid should not be visible in any of these positions.

The Abdomen

The abdomen is observed for scars, masses, or bulging, pulsations, peristalsis, distension, symmetry, vessel patterns, striae, and color. **Striae** are the lines caused by the stretching of the skin. New striae are pinkish or bluish, while older ones are whitish or silvery. Abdominal respiratory movements may be noted in adults (particularly in males) and children under seven. Visible peristalsis or pulsations are usually absent. However, the abdomen must be observed for several minutes to see if peristalsis is present. (Peristalsis may be visible in very thin people.) The vessel pattern should be barely distinguishable and the abdomen symmetrical without bulges or masses.

Figure 19.2 shows the abdominal areas that are points of reference during inspection. Chart 19.10 lists the underlying anatomic structures within those areas.

PALPATION

The Trachea

The trachea is palpated for position. It is usually found midline between the insertion points of the sternocleidomastoid muscles. Palpation of the trachea can be done by placing the thumb and forefinger on either side of the trachea just above the suprasternal notch or by palpating one side of the trachea with the forefinger and then the other, just above the suprasternal notch.

Thyroid Area

The thyroid area is palpated for size, shape, consistency, symmetry, tenderness, and presence of nodules or masses. The thyroid is usually not palpable, but the isthmus may be felt in thin-necked people as a line of tissue over the trachea in the midneck region.

Two methods are used to palpate the thyroid: the posterior method and the anterior method. The posterior method is performed with the individual in a sitting position, neck slightly flexed for relaxation, and the nurse standing behind. Placing the first two fingers of each hand on corresponding sides of the middle of the trachea, the nurse palpates for the isthmus and lateral lobes of the thyroid. The individual is asked to swallow while the nurse palpates. Swallowing causes the thyroid tissue to move upward, thus facilitating recognition. While palpating the lateral lobes, the nurse asks the individual to turn his or her slightly flexed head in the direction of the lobe being examined. The nurse moves the thyroid cartilage in the same direction and carefully palpates. The process is reversed for the opposite lobes.

The anterior method is performed with the individual again in a sitting position with neck slightly flexed. The nurse stands in front of the individual and uses the first two fingers of each hand to palpate the isthmus and to feel its rise as the individual swallows. The fingers are then moved to the side of the thyroid and the lobes are palpated in the above manner.

Chart 19.9
Inspection of the Mouth and Oral Cavity

REGIONS	FUNCTIONS	NORMAL CHARACTERISTICS	ASSESSMENT GUIDELINES
Lips	Speech Oral intake Control of secretions Contribute to facial expression	Pink, smooth, soft Exposed portion: dry, vermilion, usually marked by slight superficial vertical wrinkling Inside lips: grayish red	Color, form, position, function, texture asymmetry, chapping, cracking of the mucosa, irritations at the corners or angles of the mouth, congenital or acquired defects
Teeth	Mastication	White enamel surface; no debris, film, or hard deposits Number: 32 (full adult dentition) Number: 20 (deciduous)	Color, number, caries, size, discoloration, occlusion, notched or peglike, bridges, alveolar swelling
Gums	Supporting structure Mastication	Pale, coral-pink, firm, slightly stippled surface (like an orange), attached to teeth and projecting to fill interdental space as papillae	Color, form, density, retraction of gingival margin, pus in margins, inflammation, spongy or bleeding gums, localized gingival swelling
Tongue	Speech Mastication Taste Swallowing	*Dorsal:* moist, glistening coating, muscular; four types of papillae include: filiform (most important and numerous), fungiform (grayish-red), foliate (located along the lateral portion of the posterior of the tongue), vallate papillae (form a V near the back of the tongue) *Ventral:* pink, smooth, shows large veins	Color, size, texture, papillae cleanliness, moisture, voluntary or involuntary movements, deviation from midline, restricted protrusion, tenderness, position Varicose veins
Buccal mucosa (cheeks)	Mastication Houses parotid gland	Grayish-red color; may be crossed by fine grayish ridges where it settles between rows of teeth when the mouth is closed; the parotid gland emits a clear secretion	Color, texture, parotid gland, ulcer, melanin deposits, vesicles, neoplasms, cysts or swelling of parotid gland, ductal orifice

(continued)

Swallow Reflex

The swallow reflex is tested by touching the posterior wall of the pharynx with an applicator tip or tongue blade. If the reflex is present the person will gag. Once a gag reflex is established the nurse can further evaluate the swallow reflex by having the individual take sips of water and then observing the individual swallow. (**Note:** no fluids are given unless a gag reflex is present.)

Sucking Reflex

The sucking reflex is tested in infants by touching their lips with an applicator or nipple. To test for strength of the sucking reflex, the nurse gently but firmly attempts to pull the nipple away from the baby's mouth.

The Abdomen

Palpation of the abdomen is done after ausculta-

Chart 19.9 (Cont.)
Inspection of the Mouth and Oral Cavity

REGIONS	FUNCTIONS	NORMAL CHARACTERISTICS	ASSESSMENT GUIDELINES
Hard palate	Mastication Houses mucous glands	Pale pink, immovable, moist underlying bony process of the maxilla; no debris; irregular; rugae running transversely; orifices of ducts of mucous glands in the posterior part of hard palate; midline, hard swelling is a common variation	Color, texture, glands, ductal orifices; ducts may look like red dots in heavy smokers (nicotine stomatitis); swelling; rugae
Soft palate	Swallowing Speech Houses mucous glands	Pink, muscular; has abundant submucosal accessory salivary glands; shows fine vessels under the mucosa	Color, texture, glands, ulcers, fungal infections, inflammation
Breath odors	Manifestation of condition of mouth, oral intake, systemic disease, lung disease	Absent or sweet	*Fetid:* infections of oral cavity, poor oral hygiene, putrefactive disease of the lung *Acetone:* diabetic acidosis *Ammonia:* renal failure *Musty:* liver disease
Floor of the mouth	Supporting structures Houses submaxillary gland, sublingual gland, lymph nodes	Pale, coral pink, loose tissue Submaxillary glands emit a clear mucous secretion Submental and submaxillary lymph nodes	Neoplasms here are sometimes detectable only by palpation; cysts of sublingual glands; sublingual and submaxillary ductal orifices; lymph nodes are palpated for swelling

From: Josephine Sana and Richard Judge. Physical Assessment Methods in Nursing Practice. *Boston, Little, Brown, 1975, pp. 100–101.*

tion and percussion to prevent distortion of sounds by manipulation. Three types of palpation are used: light, moderate, and deep.

Light Palpation.   Light palpation uses the pads of the fingertips to explore areas of tenderness, muscle guarding, large masses, and distended organs. With the individual supine and in a relaxed position, the nurse stands at the side of the individual and lightly palpates all quadrants.

Moderate Palpation.   Moderate palpation uses the side of the hand to examine organs such as the liver and spleen which move on respiration. These organs are first examined with the individual breathing in a usual pattern and then while he or she takes deep breaths.

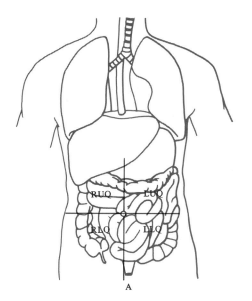

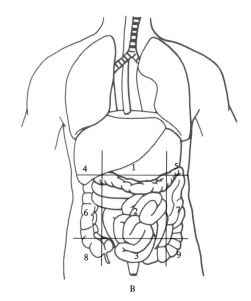

Figure 19.2

A. Abdominal quadrants: RUQ, right upper quadrant; RLQ, right lower quadrant; LUQ, left upper quadrant; LLQ, left lower quadrant. **B.** Regions within the abdomen and underlying structures: (1) epigastric, (2) umbilical, (3) hypogastric or suprapubic, (4) right hypochandriac, (5) left hypochandriac, (6) right lumbar, (7) left lumbar, (8) right inguinal, (9) left inguinal.

Deep Palpation. Deep palpation uses the palmar surfaces of the fingers to press into the abdomen to identify deep masses or organs.

Any masses should be described in terms of size, shape, mobility, location, and tenderness. Rebound tenderness can be determined by slowly pushing down on an area of the abdomen and then quickly releasing. The tenderness occurs on the withdrawal of the fingers rather than on insertion.

Bimanual Technique. Bimanual manipulation technique can be used with the obese person or to evaluate organs while they are stationary. One hand is used to fix the organ, while the other palpates it.

The Liver

The liver is not usually palpable, but to determine presence of enlargement, the nurse places her left hand under the reclining individual below the 11th and 12th ribs. The right hand is placed on the upper right quadrant where liver dullness was heard (see Percussion), with the fingers parallel to the individual's right side. Upward pressure is applied by the left hand to move the liver upward to the right hand.

The individual is asked to take a deep breath. With inspiration, an attempt is made to feel the liver as it slips under the fingers of the right hand. The liver edge feels firm, distinct, and continuous.

The liver should not be tender on palpation. Tenderness is not usually found and is indicative of inflammation. If the liver is not palpable, this technique is repeated with deeper palpation. Tenderness can be elicited when the liver is not palpable by the nurse placing one hand flat on the right rib cage and striking it with the ulnar surface of the fist of the other hand.

Other Organs

The gallbladder, stomach, and pancreas are usually not palpable. The spleen, although not usually palpable, may be detected when it is enlarged. In palpating the spleen, the left hand is placed under the lower left rib cage, while the right hand is placed on the abdomen just below the left costal margin. The individual is asked to take a deep breath, and the end of the spleen may be felt as the diaphragm pushes it downward. Notation is made of the size, shape, and location of the spleen in relation to the costal border and the umbilicus.

Chart 19.10

Abdominal Areas and Underlying Anatomical Structures

RIGHT UPPER QUADRANT

Liver and gallbladder
Pylorus
Duodenum
Head of pancreas
Right adrenal gland
Portion of right kidney
Hepatic flexure of colon
Portions of ascending and transverse colon

LEFT UPPER QUADRANT

Left lobe of liver
Spleen
Stomach
Body of pancreas
Left adrenal gland
Portion of left kidney
Splenic flexure of colon
Portions of transverse and descending colon

RIGHT LOWER QUADRANT

Lower pole of right kidney
Cecum and appendix
Portion of ascending colon
Bladder (if distended)
Ovary and salpinx
Uterus (if enlarged)
Right spermatic cord
Right ureter

LEFT LOWER QUADRANT

Lower pole of left kidney
Sigmoid colon
Portion of descending colon
Bladder (if distended)
Ovary and salpinx
Uterus (if enlarged)
Left spermatic cord
Left ureter

RIGHT HYPOCHONDRIAC

Right lobe of liver
Gallbladder
Portion of duodenum
Hepatic flexure of colon
Portion of right kidney
Suprarenal gland

EPIGASTRIC

Pyloric end of stomach
Duodenum
Pancreas
Portion of liver

LEFT HYPOCHONDRIAC

Stomach
Spleen
Tail of pancreas
Splenic flexure of colon
Upper pole of left kidney
Suprarenal gland

RIGHT LUMBAR

Ascending colon
Lower half of right kidney
Portion of duodenum and jejunum

UMBILICAL

Omentum
Mesentary
Lower part of duodenum
Jejunum and ileum

LEFT LUMBAR

Descending colon
Lower half of left kidney
Portions of jejunum and ileum

RIGHT INGUINAL

Cecum
Appendix
Lower end of ileum
Right ureter
Right spermatic cord
Right ovary

HYPOGASTRIC

Ileum
Bladder
Uterus (in pregnancy)

LEFT INGUINAL

Sigmoid colon
Left ureter
Left spermatic cord
Left ovary

PERCUSSION

Abdominal percussion helps to identify organ size and determine the presence or absence of fluid, gas, or masses. The quadrants are systematically percussed for signs of tympany and dullness.

The Liver

The size of the liver is defined by percussing upwards from a tympanic area below the umbilicus at the right midclavicular line to the point where the first dull percussion note is heard. This point is marked with a grease pencil. The upper border of the liver is ascertained by percussing downward from an area of resonance in the lung along the right midclavicular line until the first dull percussion note is heard. This point is generally between the fifth and seventh interspace and is also marked with the grease pencil. The distance between the two marks is then measured. The usual span is from 6 to 12 cm and is greater in men than women and in tall versus short persons. A span greater than 11 cm is suggestive of hepatomegaly.

These measurements can also be taken along the anterior axillary line and the midsternal line. The span along the midsternal line ranges from 4 to 8 cm. Liver dullness may shift downward by 2–3 cm when percussed on inspiration and upward when the individual holds a breath after expiration.

The Spleen

It may be possible to identify splenic dullness behind the midclavicular line between the 9th and 11th ribs. This dullness can be obliterated by gastric and colonic air. However, an increased area of dullness generally indicates splenic enlargement.

Abdominal Distension

Any abdominal distension (an increase in abdominal diameter) should be evaluated for presence of gas or fluid. Fluid produces a dull percussion note, while gas produces a tympanic note. An area of tympany may be noted in the lower left anterior rib cage and is known as the gastric air bubble.

AUSCULTATION

Thyroid

If the thyroid is enlarged, it is auscultated for a bruit (a blowing or brushing sound) with the bell of the stethoscope.

Abdomen

Auscultation of the abdomen is carried out before percussion and palpation. Using the diaphragm, the nurse places the stethoscope slightly below and to the right of the umbilicus. The usual sounds heard are rumbling and low pitch. When no sounds seem to be present, the nurse listens for at least 5 minutes before concluding that bowel sounds are absent. Either an increase or decrease in bowel sounds may indicate pathology, as does a change in pitch or pattern.

Nursing assessment related to the physical assessment of nutritional intake includes descriptions of:

- Inspection
  general appearance (e.g., hair, nails, health state, skin, eyes, state of nutrition)
    height, weight, body build
    oral cavity
    lips
    teeth
    gums
    tongue
    buccal mucosa
    hard and soft palate
    odors
    floor of the mouth
  thyroid gland
  abdominal characteristics
- Palpation
  position of trachea
  characteristics of thyroid gland
  presence of gag and swallow reflexes
  presence and quality of sucking reflex (in infants)
  presence and location of tenderness, masses, and organ borders in abdomen
- Percussion
  areas of tympany and dullness
  organ borders
- Auscultation
  location and patterns of sounds

Diagnostic Tests

Diagnostic assessment of nutritional status includes testing the structure and function of the gastrointestinal tract. In addition, metabolic by-products are assayed in the blood and urine to provide information about the efficiency of the nutritional process.

UPPER GASTROINTESTINAL SERIES

The most common visualization test done is the upper gastrointestinal series. The individual swallows a radiopaque medium (barium sulfate) and x-rays are taken as it moves through the esophagus, stomach, and small intestines. The test indicates: the continuity of the mucus lining; motility of the tract; patency of the cardiac and pyloric sphincters; any areas of stenosis, dilatation, or outpouching; encroachment of organs, masses, or tumors; and outline of the right atrium of the heart.

Preparation

The individual is usually N.P.O. (receives nothing by mouth) for 8–10 hours prior to an upper gastrointestinal series. He or she may also receive laxatives and/or enemas to assist in evacuating the intestines. The individual who is marginal or deficient in nutritional status may be further compromised by these preparations. Thus the nurse must assess the individual's ability to withstand the preparation.

The barium sulfate is distasteful to many people due to its chalky taste and thickness. Therefore, it is necessary for the individual, who may be nauseated, to understand the necessity for ingesting the barium. During the procedure the individual may have to assume a variety of positions to facilitate flow of the barium and the accuracy of the x-rays.

As with any diagnostic test, providing information about procedure and what is expected from the person increases cooperation and decreases anxiety. A light meal should be available after the procedure, and the individual should be encouraged to rest on completion of the test.

GALLBLADDER SERIES

The gallbladder series (cholecystogram) entails the ingestion of an iodine-based radiopaque substance (teleopaque) 10 hours before the test. The x-rays are taken of the gallbladder, common bile duct, and cystic duct throughout their emptying process. This is done to detect the presence of obstructions such as calculi in the bile drainage system. The individual is N.P.O. from the ingestion of the dye

until the procedure is completed (approximately 10–12 hours).

Posttest care is the same as for the upper gastrointestinal series. Both tests are frequently carried out without the hospitalization of the individual.

GASTRIC ANALYSIS

Samples of gastric secretions and contents may be aspirated from the stomach for analysis. A nasogastric tube is inserted (see Intervention) into the stomach and the contents of the stomach are removed with a syringe. The contents are examined for acidity, cytology, enzymes, and food content. The individual may or may not by N.P.O. depending on the purpose of the test.

PANCREATIC TESTS

The ability of the pancreas to secrete insulin and transport glucose across cell membranes is tested in a variety of ways. The tests include fasting blood sugar (FBS), glucose tolerance test (GTT), and urinalysis.

Fasting Blood Sugar

The FBS consists of taking a sample of venous blood from the individual after he has been fasting for 8–10 hours. The blood is then analyzed for glucose content. Expected values range from 60 mg/dl of blood to 120 mg/dl of blood. Values above 120 mg/dl may indicate diabetes mellitus.

Glucose Tolerance Test

The glucose tolerance test reflects the utilization of glucose by the body. The individual receives a high-carbohydrate diet (150–300 g per day) for three days preceding the test. He then fasts for 8 to 10 hours. A fasting blood sugar test is drawn and a high dose of carbohydrate is ingested (approximately 50–100 g). No other food is taken until the test is completed. Blood samples are then drawn at three consecutive hourly intervals and tested for glucose content. The upper limits for expected values are:

- FBS: 120 mg/dl
- after 1 hour: 185–195 mg/dl
- after 2 hours: 140 mg/dl
- after 3 hours: 120–125 mg/dl

Urine specimens may be collected along with the

blood samples to establish the renal threshold for glucose.

The individual may dislike fasting and being repeatedly "stuck" with needles. The nurse can increase cooperation and reduce anxiety by explaining the diagnostic value of the procedure before and during the test. Diversionary activities may help to channel the individual's attention throughout the long procedure.

Urinalysis

Analysis of the urine for the presence of glucose and acetone is a common nursing assessment. The diabetic individual will need to be taught this procedure for regulation of his or her dietary and insulin intake. Figure 19.3 and 19.4 outlines the procedure for testing urine for glucose and acetone. Reagent strips are also available for testing for glucose and acetone.

Figure 19.3
Procedure for Testing Glucose in Urine

PROCEDURES

AMERICAN HOSPITAL FORMULARY SERVICE CATEGORY NUMBER 36 88
For accurate test results, always use special Clinitest Droppers and Test Tubes.

1 Collect urine in clean receptacle. With dropper in upright position, place 5 drops urine in test tube. Rinse dropper and place 10 drops of water in test tube.

2 Drop 1 Clinitest Tablet into test tube. Watch while reaction takes place. Do not shake test tube during reaction nor for 15 seconds after boiling inside test tube has stopped.

3 At end of 15-second waiting period, shake test tube gently and compare with color chart.

Testing urine to establish glucose utilization in the body. Any of several methods may be used to test for excess sugar and acetone in the urine. The tests employ tablets or reagent strips. In the Ames test (using 5 drops of urine) the quantity of sugar in the urine is determined by the color of the urine-water-tablet solution at the end of 15 seconds. Six shades may occur, ranging from dark blue to orange, and indicate percentages of sugar in the urine—from zero percent (negative) to 2 percent, and reported on a 0 to 4+ scale. If the color changes occur more rapidly than the 15-second period described above and end in a dark greenish-brown (rather than the orange indicating 2 percent), it may be recorded that the urine contains more than 2 percent sugar. The chart provided with the test to determine the quantity of acetone in the urine defines amounts as small, moderate, or large, according to the color change that has occurred in the tablet. The color ranges from unchanged to deep purple. *(Courtesy of Ames Division, Miles Laboratories, Inc.)*

INTERPRETATION OF TEST

Negative
No sugar (glucose)—the liquid will be blue at the end of a waiting period of 15 seconds. The whitish sediment that may form has no bearing on the test.

Positive
Sugar present—the liquid will change color. The more sugar, the greater the change and the more rapidly it occurs.

The amount of sugar is determined by comparing the color of the solution in the test tube with the Color Chart* at the end of the 15-second waiting period. Color changes developing after the 15-second waiting period should be disregarded.

Important
Careful observance of the solution in the test tube while reaction takes place and during the 15-second waiting period is necessary to detect rapid *"pass-through"* color changes caused by amounts of sugar over 2%. Should the color rapidly *"pass-through"* bright orange to a dark brown or greenish-brown, record as over 2% sugar without comparing final color development with the Color Chart.

---

*Color Charts come with the Clinitest Tablets and only this chart should be used.
Adapted with permission from Ames Division, Miles Laboratory, Inc.

Figure 19.4

Testing for Ketones in Urine

PROCEDURE: FOLLOW EXACTLY

1 Remove tablet from bottle and recap promptly. Place tablet on clean, dry, white paper.

2 Put one drop of urine, serum, plasma or whole blood directly on top of tablet.

3 For urine testing—compare color of tablet to Color Chart at *thirty seconds* after application of specimen.

For serum or plasma testing—compare color of tablet to Color Chart at *two minutes* after application of specimen.

For whole blood testing, *ten minutes* after application of specimen—*remove clotted blood* from tablet and compare color of tablet to Color Chart.

Quality Control

For best results, quality control checks can readily be made each time a new bottle is opened by using a negative and positive control as knowns. The negative gives confidence that no "false positives" are obtained. The positive control gives confidence that the tablets are properly reacting with positive specimens. When testing with commercial controls for routine urinalysis, observe color of tablet for entire 30 second period. Any purple color during this period should be considered positive. In addition, a negative and a positive should be hidden in each batch of urines tested throughout the day. These results plotted on the usual quality control chart provide evidence that the proper handling and testing procedures are being followed in the laboratory. Urinalysis is considered to be slipping out of control if a negative urine is called positive more than 5% of the time and/or if a positive reaction is called negative more than 5% of the time. Each laboratory should establish its own goals for adequate standards of performance. If continued unsatisfactory performance is obtained, the personnel involved may need further training, or closer supervision may be required.

Results

Test results are recorded as negative if no purple color is apparent on the tablet at the appropriate reading time. Positive results are recorded as small, moderate or large on comparison with the Color Chart. No calculations are necessary.

Limitations of the Procedure

Improper handling of the product to allow moisture absorption will adversely affect results.

Expected Values

Ketones are not found in blood or urine under normal conditions of carbohydrate metabolism.

Specific Performance Characteristics

Reagent tablets will detect as little as 5 mg of acetoacetic acid/100 ml in urine. They are specific for the detection of acetoacetic acid and acetone. It is about 10 times more sensitive to acetoacetic acid than acetone and will not react with betahydroxybutyric acid. In urine, the small color block corresponds to approximately 10 mg acetoacetic acid/100 ml, the moderate color block to 30–40 mg/100 ml, and the large color block to approximately 80–100 mg/100 ml.[4] The lower limit of detection in serum, plasma or whole blood is approximately 10 mg acetoacetic acid per 100 ml.

SUMMARY AND EXPLANATION

Commercial testing kits, containing a reagent tablet composed of several ingredients, are primarily used to test for the presence of ketones (acetoacetic acid and acetone) in urine. Serum, plasma or whole blood may also be tested with the tablet for the presence of ketones. The presence of ketone bodies is important in the evaluation of carbohydrate metabolism. The test is based on the nitroprusside reaction with ketone bodies to give a purple color. Combining the active ingredients into a tablet form, commercial tablets were first made available in 1949 and have been described in various publications.[1,2,3]

Equipment required for the test include the reagent tablet, a dropper and a clean, white piece of paper. The procedure is easy to perform and gives reliable answers if attention is given to recapping the bottle promptly and storing the material at temperatures under 30°C (86°F), but not in a refrigerator.

Chemical Principles

Acetoacetic acid or acetone in urine or blood will form a colored complex with nitroprusside in the presence of glycine. Buffers provide the optimum pH for this reaction.

(continued)

Figure 19.4 (Cont.)
Testing for Ketones in Urine

Reactive Ingredients
1 part sodium nitroprusside, 9 parts glycine plus buffer, filler and binder.

Warnings and Precautions
Reagent tablets are for *in vitro* diagnostic use.

Storage and Handling
Reagent tablets have prolonged stability in the unopened container if stored at temperatures below 30°C (86°F). Once they are opened, stability is highly dependent on exposure to moisture. The bottle must be recapped promptly after removing a tablet. Tablets should be used on a regular basis and not stored for an extended period of time after the bottle is opened.

Important Note
When a drop of urine is put onto a tablet, the drop should be absorbed within 30 seconds. If absorption takes longer than 30 seconds, the tablets have been exposed to moisture and may not give good results.

Protection
Avoid exposure to light, heat and moisture to guard against altered reagent reactivity. Deterioration may be noted by tan-to-brown discoloration or darkening of the tablet. If this is evident, or when test results are questionable or inconsistent with expected findings the following steps are recommended:
  1) Confirm that product is within expiration date shown on label.
  2) Check performance against known positive control material. If proper result is not ob-

tained, discard and retest with fresh product.
(NOTE: As with all laboratory tests, definitive diagnostic or therapeutic decisions should not be based on any single result or method.)

Specimen Collection and Preparation
Use fresh specimens. When necessary, the specimen may be refrigerated. Preservatives do not prevent the deterioration of urine ketones. The preservative 8-hydroxyquinoline may cause false positives. Other preservatives when used as directed do not affect the test.

Interfering Substances
Urines containing bromsulfalein or very high quantities of phenylketones may give false positive results, as will urines preserved with 8-hydroxyquinoline. L-dopa metabolites may give an atypical reaction which could be interpreted as a positive result.

1. Free, H. M., Smeby, R. R., Cook, M. H., and Free, A. H.: A comparative study of qualitative tests for ketones in urine and serum. *Clin. Chem.* 4:323, 1958.
2. Riekers, H. and Miale, J. B.: Ketonuria: an evaluation of tests and some clinical implications. *Amer. J. Clin. Path.* 30:530, 1958.
3. Levinson, S. A., MacFate, J. H.: *Clinical Laboratory Diagnosis,* 7th ed., London, Lea & Febiger, 1969, p. 588.
4. Free, A. H. and Free, H. M.: Nature of nitroprusside reactive material in urine in ketosis. *Amer. J. Clin. Path.* 30:7, 1958.
Adapted with permission from Ames Division, Miles Laboratories, Inc.

OTHER TESTS

A variety of procedures is available for testing for inborn errors of metabolism such as phenylketonuria and cystic fibrosis. The student is referred to a pediatric textbook for explanation of these pathologies and the appropriate diagnostic tests. Other tests which may be carried out to assess the individual's nutritional status include hemoglobin and hematocrit (Chap. 18), electrolyte (Chap. 21), and serum enzyme (Chap. 18) tests.

Nursing assessment of diagnostic tests re-

lated to nutritional needs should include descriptions of:

- expected values
- presenting values
- the relationship between expected and presenting values
- nursing implications of the test results
- relationship of interferences to test results
- special preparation needed
- posttest nursing care
- reactions to tests
- attitudes toward tests

- level of understanding of individual and family and/or significant others about tests

NURSING DIAGNOSIS

Mr. Dee is an 83-year-old male and a resident of a nursing home. He has been sick in bed for two days with a temperature of 101 F. He has been refusing to eat and is only drinking three or four cups of tea a day.

The nursing assessment that follows compares Mr. Dee's presenting (actual) behaviors that suggest inadequacies in his nutritional processes with the behaviors that the nurse would expect to find in a person of similar growth and development who is having no interference with his nutrition.

A physical assessment is included.

ASSESSMENT FACTOR	EXPECTED BEHAVIOR	ACTUAL BEHAVIOR
Knowledge of nutrients and relation to well-being	A balance of carbohydrates, fats, minerals, proteins, and vitamins are necessary to maintain health	Same
Knowledge of food groups	Knows basic four	Same
Knowledge of nutrients provided by food group	Knows the major nutrient type in each food group	Same
Knowledge of food and portions in a food group	Basic understanding of the foods most commonly used by the individual, the nutrients they contain, and average portions	Same
Nutrient requirements of present level of growth and development	For males over 51 years of age, approximately 5 ft, 9 in. and 154 lb, the requirements are: Kcal: 2050 Protein: 56 g Vitamin A: 1000 IU Vitamin D: 200 IU Vitamin E: 10 × T.E. Ascorbic acid: 60 mg Folacin: 400 μg Niacin: 16 mg Riboflavin: 1.4 mg Thiamin: 1.2 mg Vitamin B$_6$: 2.2 mg Vitamin B$_{12}$: 3 μg Calcium: 800 mg Phosphorus: 800 mg Iodine: 150 μg Iron: 10 mg Magnesium: 350 mg Zinc: 15 mg	When not ill, the intake is higher in calories, lower in protein, lower in vitamin A than recommended daily allowances (RDA). Ht: 5 ft. 8 in. Wt: 160 lb Past 3 days: no nutritional intake except 100 oz. of tea (3000 cc) for 3-day total
Relationship of present nutrition to energy needs at level of growth and development	—	Totally inadequate in view of absence of intake and fever
Condition of teeth	Full set of 32 teeth	Well-fitting upper and lower dentures

(continued)

ASSESSMENT FACTOR	EXPECTED BEHAVIOR	ACTUAL BEHAVIOR
Chewing ability	Can properly chew all foods	Same. At present states, "I ache so much that even chewing hurts."
Condition of oral cavity	Intact with functional structures	Same
Swallow reflex	Present and able to control all food swallowed	Same. States that it "hurts to swallow."
Degree of debilitation	None	Weak, weight loss of 5 lb in last 3 days, "feels shaky."
Relationship of nutritional intake to debilitation	—	"I don't have enough strength to eat."
Assistance needed for feeding	None	When not ill none; at present needs help holding cup up to mouth
Associations of food	—	"I don't want anything heavy on my stomach."
Where associations generated from	—	"Growing up, my mother used to say 'feed a cold and starve a fever,' and so she only gave us tea when we were sick. It's certainly worked all these years."
What increases and decreases appetite	—	"Smell of food makes me sick to my stomach." "Boy, would I like some homemade strawberry ice cream."
Cultural background	—	First-generation American Hungarian Eastern Orthodox religion, eats no meats on Fridays, Holy days or Lent likes sausage, all pork products, lamb, noodles, breads, and rich desserts; favorite foods, however, are pizza and ice cream
Availability of culturally preferred foods	—	Foods not available at nursing home; family brings them weekends and holidays
Knowledge of nutritional food preparation	—	Not applicable, foods prepared by nursing home dietary staff
Knowledge of relationship between level of growth and development and nutritional needs	Nutrient intake varies with level of growth and development	"I'm an old man and I'm entitled to eat what I want."
Myths and misconceptions	—	See above

(continued)

ASSESSMENT FACTOR	EXPECTED BEHAVIOR	ACTUAL BEHAVIOR
Degree to which nutrition knowledge is put into practice	—	Eats all meals but snacks on high carbohydrate foods
Factors which interfere with putting nutrition knowledge into practice	—	Institutionalization
Usual daily pattern of intake	—	Breakfast, 8:15 a.m. Lunch, 12 noon Dinner, 5:30 p.m. Snack, 8 p.m. Frequent snacks interspersed on own
Food likes and dislikes	—	Likes: see above; dislikes: cabbage, "makes me gassy of late."
Eating environment	—	Eats in communal dining room; enjoys other people who sit at his table; thinks food is attractively served and portions sufficient
Special dietary requirements	None	Same
Allergies	None	Same
Approximate BMR	—	1747.2 kcal, base line
Factors which increase BMR	—	Usual: square dancing, painting, pushing wheelchairs for other residents; at present: fever— 21% increase in BMR needs
Factors which decrease BMR	—	At present on bed rest
Relationship of food intake to energy expenditure	—	Usual intake slightly outweighs energy expenditure; at present, energy expenditure far exceeds intake; caloric and nutrient deficit in all areas
Rate of weight loss	—	Lost 5 lb in past 3 days; loss involuntary
Influence of hospitalization on meeting nutritional needs	None	No laboratory facilities available to evaluate nutritional status
Interferences with nutrition	—	Anorexia, nausea when food is brought into room, body aches, weakness
Relationship of interference to state of well-being	—	Is becoming dehydrated, involuntary weight loss, weakness, decreased resistance to infection
Precipitating factors of interference	—	Onset of "viral flu" 3 days ago

(continued)

ASSESSMENT FACTOR	EXPECTED BEHAVIOR	ACTUAL BEHAVIOR
Attitudes toward interference	—	"My mother died of the flu in the 1918 epidemic. I hope history isn't going to repeat itself."
Coping methods of family and/or significant others	—	Visits have increased to once a day
Physical Assessment		
Inspection:		
Mouth	Moist	Dry
Lips	Smooth, pink and soft	Cracked, dry
Gums	Moist	Dry
Tongue	Muscular, glistening	White coating
Buccal mucosa	Moist	Dry
Breath odor	Absent, sweet	Fetid
Eyes	Clear, moist	Slightly sunken, itchy
Skin	Dry, resilient	Flaky, moist, tenting when pinched
Auscultation:		
Bowel sounds	Present	Same, slow
BP	120/80/70	140/92/88
Resp.	14–20 minute	20, regular, even
	No adventitious sounds	Same
Palpation		
Abdomen	Soft, with no masses or tenderness	Same
Pulse	76 regular, full	92 regular, full
Diagnostic tests		None available
Medical diagnosis		Viral flu
Medical Orders		Full fluid diet
		Calorie and protein supplement 8 oz, t.i.d.
		Aspirin 10 gr, q4h, p.r.n. for temp over 101 F, Rectal
		Bed rest
		Cough and deep breath
		Intravenous (IV) 1000 cc dextrose 5% in water (D5W) q8h with 20 mEq of potassium chloride (KCl) and vitamins B and C (2 cc)
		Intake and output
Effectiveness of therapeutic regime	—	Refusing oral intake, IV started and in progress 5 hours

Resulting nursing diagnoses, in order of priority, might include:

- dehydration related to increased BMR requirements and decreased intake
- increased body temperature related to inflammatory response
- increased potential for hazards of immobility related to decreased activity and weakness
- increased energy needs related to increased body temperature
- sudden weight loss related to decreased intake
- inadequate intake of nutrients related to nausea, weakness, and muscular aches
- fear of dying related to present illness and family history

PLANNING

To balance nutritional intake with energy expenditure is the major focus of planning. Maintaining this balance necessitates planning for increasing level of knowledge about nutrition of the individual and the family and/or significant others, as well as assisting them to modify nutritional patterns and habits. An awareness of the effects of pathologic states, surgery, and other interferences with nutritional intake enables the nurse to plan interventions that will promote, maintain, and restore nutritional adequacy. Any dietary change must be considered within the context of the person's culture, preferences, income, habits, and patterns.

In the situation of Mr. Dee, the plan for one nursing diagnosis listed above could be as shown below.

NURSING DIAGNOSIS	GOALS	PLAN

Increased energy needs related to increased body temperature	*Short term:*
	1. Decrease energy expenditure within 12 hours
		1. Explain need for energy conservation
		
		2. Explore methods for energy conservation
		
		3. Devise plan with individual to:
		  a. Assist with activities of daily living
		  b. Decrease environmental stimuli
		  c. Balance rest with activity
		  d. Provide increased comfort

	2. Decrease body temperature within 24 hours	1. Take temperature q2h
		
		2. Administer aspirin q4h for temperature above 101 F
		
		3. Regulate IV to run at 2 cc or 32 gtt per minute
		
		4. Offer strawberry ice cream q2h while awake
		
		5. Offer 2 oz of calorie and protein supplement every hour on the half-hour between 8 A.M. and 8:30 P.M.
		
		6. Promote evaporation by:
		  a. Keeping clothing dry
		  b. Keeping skin clean and dry
		  c. Maintain environmental temperature at 72–74 F and a relative humidity of 40–50%

(continued)

NURSING DIAGNOSIS	GOAL	PLAN
	3. Meet energy needs within 48 hours	1. As above
		2. Explore with individual misconceptions about food intake during illness
		3. Assist with feeding
		4. Ask family to bring in favorite fluids
		5. Administer vitamins B and C and KCl via IV
	Intermediate:	
	1. Make up energy deficits within 1 week	1. As above
		2. Consult with physician re changing diet as tolerated
	2. Temperature maintained at expected for 1 week	1. As above
		2. Reduce contact with individuals with infectious processes

INTERVENTION

Nutrition Education

Nutrition education is a major nursing intervention. Its aim is to help the individual and the family and/or significant others to change inadequate nutritional habits and support and maintain those habits which are positive. Through assessment the nurse establishes a profile of the individual's knowledge base, attitudes, preferences, and lifestyle related to nutrition. This profile reflects areas of strength and weakness.

The nurse's responsibility for nutrition education is not limited to the hospitalized individual or the individual with overt nutritional interference. Nutrition education is carried out in a variety of settings, such as the clinic, home, school, community organizations, and occupational settings. (Illustration 19.6)

The nutrition teaching performed by the nurse falls into two general categories: basic nutrition education and nutrition reeducation.

BASIC NUTRITION EDUCATION

Basic nutrition education includes all situations where the individual has no preexisting nutrition patterns or information. Examples of this are the school-child, the woman who is pregnant for the first time,

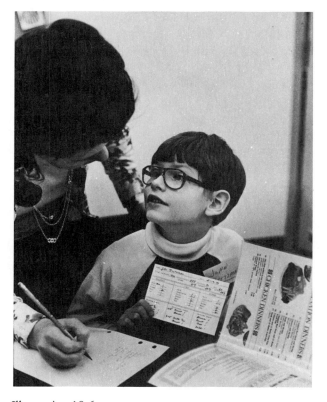

Illustration 19.6
The nurse often works with school children to help establish adequate nutritional patterns. Nutrition education follows the nurse's assessment of the child's knowledge base, lifestyle, and food preferences. *(Photo © Bob Adelman)*

the newly formed family or living unit, the family with a new child, or the person who is preparing his or her own meals for the first time.

This type of education centers around assisting the person to plan a dietary pattern based on the information provided by the nurse. Information the nurse provides includes such topics as how to shop economically, nutritious food planning and preparation, food requirements, and food portions.

NUTRITION REEDUCATION

Nutrition reeducation is for individuals who have longstanding nutritional patterns which must be modified because of nutritional deficits or interferences. Individuals who have physiologic structural changes, special diets to help control pathologic processes, malnutrition, or obesity are included in this group. Several therapeutic diets are outlined in the Appendix.

Nutrition reeducation focuses on helping the individual to modify and change dietary patterns. The nurse attempts to accomplish this in the context of the individual's changing needs, cultural preferences, likes and dislikes, and dietary and functional restrictions.

THE GENERAL PROCESS

Many methods are available to the nurse in carrying out nutrition teaching plans. Posters, charts, pamphlets, simulation games, films, and diet-analysis forms are just a few of the techniques that can be utlized.

Nutrition education is a lifelong process which begins with teaching the parents of the newborn to establish nutritious eating habits for their child, continues with teaching the schoolage child about the judicious use of "junk food," and extends through teaching middle-aged and older adults to modify their caloric intake with changing energy expenditure. While nutrition education is a nursing responsibility, the nurse also acts as a resource person to direct the individual to nutrition experts and services when appropriate.

Assisting the Individual to Eat

Some individuals may need assistance with eating because of age, motor dysfunctions, debilitation, loss of vision, or structural defects. They may need either to be fed or to be helped in feeding themselves.

GENERAL GUIDELINES

Certain general guidelines are applicable in any situation when assisting someone to eat. They are listed below.

When feeding or assisting with feeding an individual, the nurse:

1 allows sufficient time for tasting, chewing, and swallowing
2 creates a relaxed, unhurried environment by allowing enough time for the procedure and engaging in conversation
3 gives the individual an opportunity to clean mouth, wash hands, and empty bladder before and after eating
4 makes the eating environment as physically pleasant as possible by covering drainage, removing bad odors, etc.
5 assumes a comfortable position, usually sitting, within reach of the individual, food, and utensils
6 serves food at the proper temperature
7 allows the individual to choose the order of feeding
8 cuts food into bite-size bits when necessary
9 gives moderately sized spoonfuls and forkfuls
10 does not prop infants when feeding, but holds them
11 places individual in a position which facilitates swallowing, enhances comfort, and fits within the therapeutic regimen
12 introduces food at the front of the mouth, not to the side or area of paralysis
13 does not chop, grind, or mash food for the nurse's own convenience but allows the individual sufficient time to chew, swallow, and rest between bites
14 allows toddlers and children to manipulate fingerfoods
15 encourages the individual to assist whenever possible
16 never gives food or fluid to an individual whose swallow reflex is diminished or absent
17 opens all containers and utensil packages and pours all liquids
18 butters bread, toast, etc.
19 adds condiments according to preference and special diet requirements

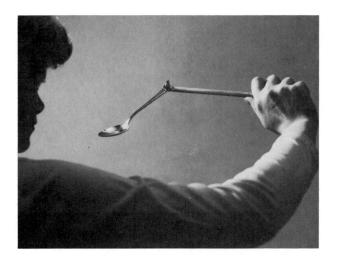

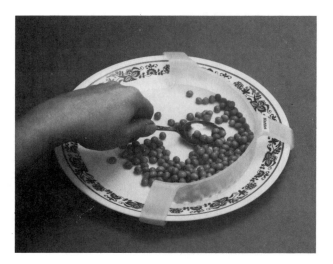

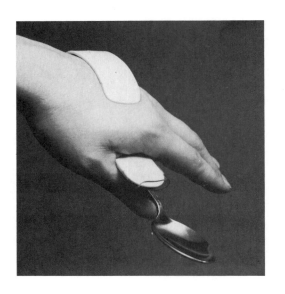

Illustration 19.7
Assistive eating devices make self-feeding possible for individuals with temporary or permanent disabilities. *(Courtesy of Park Surgical Co., Inc., Brooklyn, N.Y. © Bel-Art Products, 1979)*

20 places food and utensils within easy reach of the individual

HELPING BLIND PERSONS

When feeding individuals who are blind, a routine of placing food and utensils in the same position every meal is established. The most commonly used approach for this is to position food and utensils according to the hours of a clock. For example, meat would always be at 12 o'clock, potatoes or starches at 3 o'clock, and vegetables at 6 o'clock.

ASSISTIVE DEVICES

Assistive devices are available for individuals with eating disabilities. Illustrations 19.7. A–C show some of these devices. These devices may be purchased ready-made, specially designed for the individual, or improvised by the nurse. The type of aid depends on the length of time the individual will need the device, financial resources of the individual, and the nurse's creativity. When individuals with disabilities are admitted to the hospital, the nurse should ascertain what devices they use at home and ask to have them brought in.

Alleviating Nausea, Vomiting, and Anorexia

TREATING THE CAUSE

Alleviating the underlying causes and/or pathophysiology of nausea, vomiting, or anorexia is one of the major nursing interventions for individuals whose nutritional intake is interfered with by these conditions. Often treating a concurrent pathology will relieve the interferences. For example, the person with constipation may be nauseated, and thus promoting defecation will eliminate the nausea.

MODIFYING ENVIRONMENT

Since environmental conditions may potentiate the individual's nausea and vomiting and induce anorexia, modifying the environment may help alleviate them. Eliminating unpleasant odors or sights and maintaining appropriate temperature and ventilation are ways that the environment can be positively modified. Providing an atmosphere which is calm and unhurried is conducive to better food intake and less discomfort.

PRESENTING FOOD ATTRACTIVELY

How food is presented to the individual is another important factor to consider. Small, frequent feedings are often more palatable to the nauseated or anorexic individual than large, more widely spaced meals. Foods that the person likes and desires at that particular time are offered. Within the institutional setting, foods brought in by family and/or significant others may increase appetite and be more appealing to the individual. Serving foods at their appropriate temperature and consistency adds to their appeal. Often, avoiding spicy or fatty foods may also decrease nausea.

RELIEVING PAIN AND ANXIETY

Relieving pain, anxiety, or activity which may contribute to nausea, vomiting, or anorexia will increase food intake and feelings of well-being. Activities which may be painful or aesthetically distasteful are spaced so that they do not occur around mealtimes. Any measure which increases the individual's comfort and general feelings of well-being will decrease nausea and increase the individual's appetite.

USING ANTIEMETICS

Obtaining orders for antiemetics and using them when the individual first complains of nausea is an important adjunct to care. Oftentimes waiting until the person is extremely nauseated or about to vomit undermines the therapeutic value of these medications. At the same time, this increases the individual's anxiety and decrease his or her trust in the efficacy of treatment. (Other medications the individual is receiving may have nausea, vomiting, and anorexia as side effects and must be considered in the total picture for relief of these interferences.) Giving antiemetics at least one-half hour before meals may also help to increase appetite. Individuals who are able to eat without attendant nausea and vomiting are more likely to continue eating than those individuals who are faced with them each time they attempt to eat. Oral administration of antiemetics may be self-defeating, as they may produce nausea. Thus careful consideration of the route of administration is necessary.

OTHER SPECIAL CONSIDERATIONS

The individual who is nauseated or vomiting may be helped by instructing him or her to take slow, deep breaths. When vomiting is present the individual is positioned so that aspiration of the vomitus is prevented. Placing the head to the side in a slight dependent position helps. Noting the sequence of events that caused the vomiting, as well as the characteristics of the vomitus, is also important.

Provision of mouthcare after an individual vomits or when a person is nauseated promotes comfort and reduces the possibility of further nausea and vomiting. Withholding foods and fluids may also be necessary. Individuals who are vomiting are losing fluids and electrolytes and are thus prone to dehydration and metabolic alkalosis. (Chap. 21). Replacement of lost nutrients through parenteral routes may be necessary if nausea, vomiting, or anorexia is severe enough to compromise the individual's nutritional status.

Using Alternate Feeding Methods

Nasogastric tubes may be used to feed the individual when the oral cavity or esophagus needs to be bypassed as a result of trauma or surgery, when the swallow reflex is absent or diminished, and when the individual is too debilitated or confused to take food by mouth. Nasogastric tubes are also utilized to instill medications directly into the stomach, to remove stomach contents for analysis, or for decompression. Decompression is the removal of food, fluid, secretions, and gas by means of negative pressure. **Gastric gavage** is the term used for feeding with a nasogastric tube and **gastric lavage** is the term used for removing stomach contents through a nasogastric tube.

Chart 19.11
Insertion of a Nasogastric Tube

TECHNIQUE	POINTS TO NOTE

Collect equipment:
  Nasogastric tube
  Water-soluble lubricant
  Clamp
  Towel
  Emesis basin
  Adhesive tape
  Syringe
  Stethoscope
	Readily available equipment saves time and helps ensure organized carrying out of procedure. If rubber tubes are used, a bowl of ice is needed to chill the tube, making it less flexible. Disposable plastic tubes should be used whenever possible for ease of insertion and to prevent tissue trauma.

Explain procedure to individual.	Anxiety is lessened when individual is aware of what is expected of him or her and why it is necessary. Information increases cooperation.
Explain mouth breathing and swallowing techniques during insertion.	Mouth breathing reduces possibility of nausea and vomiting during insertion of tube. Swallowing moves tube.
Set up a communication signal if individual feels that he or she is choking or has pain during procedure.	Individual will have more control over situation and feel less panic if he or she should start to gag.
Position individual in high Fowler's position with neck hyperextended, if condition permits.	High Fowler's position permits gravity to aid insertion and decreases chance of aspiration. Hyperextension decreases resistance of pathway.
Place towel across chest and under head.	Prevents secretions from getting on individual or bed.
Measure tube from the tip of the nose to the earlobe and from earlobe to tip of xiphoid process, and mark.	Ensures sufficient length to pass through to stomach.
Clear nostril of secretions.	Facilitates insertion.
Lubricate tube with water-soluble lubricant.	Facilitates insertion by decreasing resistance, prevents tissue trauma. Oil-based lubricants are never used, as they may act as foreign bodies and set up an inflammatory process.
Slowly and gently insert tube into the nostril in a backward and downward motion until it reaches the back of the nasopharynx, at which point the individual will gag.	Prevents trauma and reduces stimulation of vomit and gag reflexes. Follow contour of nasopharyngeal cavity. Gagging results from irritation of pharynx and fauces.
Stop insertion until gagging ends.	

(continued)

GAVAGE FEEDING

Nasogastric tubes may be inserted through either the oropharyngeal cavity or the nasopharyngeal cavity (Chart 19.11). They may be left in place for long periods or removed and replaced as necessary (e.g., with each feeding). A Levin tube is the most com-

monly used nasogastric tube. (Chapter 21 describes intubation tubes.)

Gavage feeding of the individual is described in Chart 19.12 and Figure 19.5. Whenever feeding an individual by this method, the same guidelines previously mentioned for feeding any other individual are followed.

Chart 19.11 (Cont.)

Insertion of a Nasogastric Tube

TECHNIQUE	POINTS TO NOTE
Instruct individual to resume usual head position, i.e., extension.	Facilitates insertion by straightening out passageway.
If the individual is allowed fluids by mouth, instruct him or her to take small sips of water. Continue insertion of tube.	Swallowing facilitates movement of tube.
If individual is not allowed fluids, instruct him or her to keep swallowing as tube continues to be inserted.	As above.
If resistance is met, remove tube, repeat procedure.	Prevents tissue trauma.
Observe for signs of respiratory distress, i.e., wheezing, coughing, gasping, cyanosis. If present, remove tube immediately.	If tube is in trachea or lungs, individual will experience respiratory distress.
Once tube is inserted to area marked off by measurements, check for placement of tube by injecting 5 cc of air into tube while simultaneously auscultating epigastrium with a stethoscope.	Measurements show approximate distance to stomach. A soft popping sound is heard when tube is in stomach. (An alternative method for checking placement in stomach is to aspirate a small amount of stomach contents.)
If placement of tube cannot be determined in stomach, remove tube immediately and repeat procedure of placement.	May be in lungs.
If placement is determined, securely tape tube to nose and cheek, following the natural line of the tube.	Prevents pulling out of tube, irritation of nasopharyngeal passage, and continued passage of tube.
Clamp or plug tube tightly.	Prevents passage of air into stomach and leakage of stomach contents out of the tube. Nasogastric tube may also be attached to intermittent suction (Chap. 20).
Remove equipment and make individual comfortable.	Aesthetically pleasing and prevents irritation and infection.
Nasal and mouth care should be carried out as often as needed.	Long-term intubation may result in irritations and ulcerations, infection of the nasopharyngeal passages, esophagus, and stomach and loss of muscle tone necessary for swallowing. Thus tubes should be removed periodically and reinserted in opposite nostril.
Chart and record procedure.	

GASTROSTOMY AND JEJUNOSTOMY

Feeding tubes are occasionally inserted directly into the stomach (gastrostomy) or jejunum (jejunostomy). This is done when the esophagus is occluded or for convenience if long-term gastric feeding is necessary. These procedures for feeding are similar to nasogastric feedings. The skin area around the tube should be kept clean and free of any leakage, as gastric juices will ulcerate the skin.

These procedures, including insertion and feeding, may be taught to the individual or family and/or significant others and carried out independently by them.

Chart 19.12
Gavage Feeding

TECHNIQUE	POINTS TO NOTE
Explain procedure.	Anxiety is lessened when individual is aware of what is expected and why it is necessary. Information increases cooperation.

Obtain equipment:
  Funnel or bulb syringe
  Water
  Ordered feeding
  Stethoscope
	Readily available equipment saves time and helps ensure organized carrying out of procedure.

Check type and amount of feeding.	Ensures proper nutrition and prevents overload.
Warm feeding to room temperature.	Feedings are usually kept in refrigerator. Heating of formula is not necessary, as passage along tube performs this function.
Position individual in comfortable sitting position if not medically contraindicated.	Prevents aspiration, regurgitation, and pneumonitis and simulates usual eating position.
Reclamp and attach funnel for feeding.	Prevents air from entering stomach. Some agencies require checking stomach contents before beginning feeding to prevent overload.
Unclamp tube and check for placement of tube, as above.	Ensures that feeding goes into stomach.
Reclamp and attach funnel for feeding.	Prevents air from entering stomach. Some agencies require checking stomach contents before beginning feeding to prevent overload.
Unclamp and instill approximately 15–30 cc of water through tube.	Clears and ensures patency of tubing. Once fluid has been added to the tube, the fluid level should not fall below neck of funnel to prevent air from getting into tubing and thus into stomach.
Instill feeding slowly and regulate flow by raising and lowering funnel.	Feedings should take 10–20 minutes. Too rapid instillation of feedings results in nausea, vomiting, and diarrhea. Gravity is used to instill feeding and not pressure. If feeding is too high in carbohydrates, diarrhea may result. More protein and fats will need to be added to formula to prevent this.
Instill 15–30 cc of water and clamp.	Clears tube, maintains patency, and prevents growth of microorganisms along tube. Clamping prevents air from entering and fluid from leaking.
Instruct individual to rest in a sitting position for at least 15 minutes.	Prevents aspiration.
Chart and record procedure.	

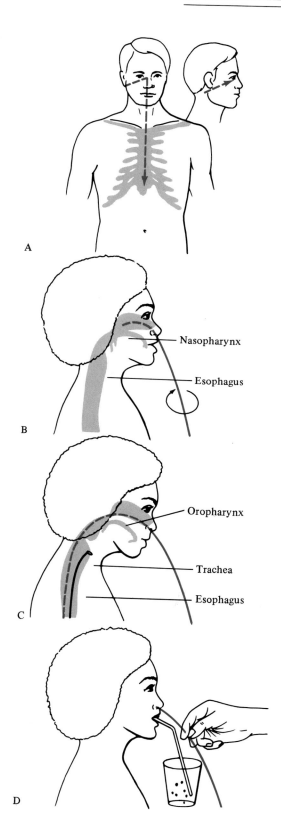

Figure 19.5
Inserting, maintaining, and removing a nasogastric tube.

A. To measure an amount of tubing sufficient to reach the individual's stomach, put the tip of the tubing at the individual's earlobe and extend the tubing to the bridge of the nose and down to the xiphoid process, or from the tip of the nose to the earlobe and then to the xiphoid process. Mark the tubing with tape where it meets the xiphoid—that point indicating the approximate amount of tubing necessary to reach the stomach.

B. Coil the first 5 inches (12.5 cm.) of tubing tightly around the fingers so that it will curve slightly when unwound. This will aid insertion of the tube. Apply a water-soluble lubricant to the first 3 or 4 inches (7.5 to 10 cm.) of tubing and insert it slowly, passing it backward along the floor of the nasal passage toward the individual's ear, not the nose, until it passes around the corner of the nasopharyngeal junction and points toward the esophagus. If resistance is met, remove tubing, relubricate it, and begin again.

C. Once tubing is pointed toward the esophagus, have the individual drop his or her head forward in order to close the trachea and open the esophagus. Then, advance the tube into the esophagus.

D. To help prevent the individual's gagging or choking during insertion of the tube, have the individual sip water through a straw or suck on ice chips. If water is contraindicated for the individual, have the individual dry swallow or suck air through a straw.

(continued)

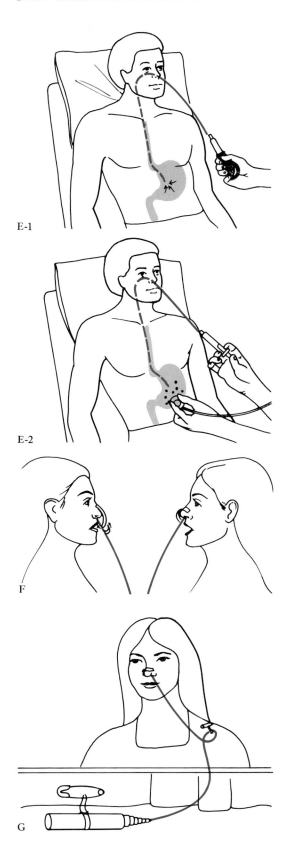

Figure 19.5 (Cont.)

E. When tubing has been inserted to the mark made during tube measurement (**A** above), test to see that the tube is in the stomach, not the trachea. Attach a bulb syringe (**E–1**) or 50-ml catheter-tip syringe (**E–2**) to the exposed end of the tube and apply gentle suction. If stomach contents are aspirated, the tube is in the correct place. If stomach contents are not aspirated, insert the tube a bit further to make sure that when first inserted it was not above the fluid level in the stomach. Another way to check the tube's position is to insert 15 cc of air through the tube, using a syringe. Auscultate the individual's epigastric region with a stethoscope and listen for a "whoosh" of air entering the stomach. If it can not be determined that the tubing is in the stomach, remove tube at once and repeat insertion procedure from beginning.

F. When the nasogastric tube is determined to be in place in the stomach, it is anchored at the nose in such a way that will prevent pressure from the tubing on the nostril. One way that this is done is to use a strip of *hypo-allergenic* tape about 1.5 inches (3.7 cm.) long. The tape should be 1 inch (2.5 cm.) wide. Split the tape lengthwise from one end for about 1 inch and attach the unsplit end to the individual's nose. Wrap the split ends in opposite directions around the tubing. *Note:* To prevent skin irritation, use the least amount of tape possible and preferably hypoallergenic tape. Another method of securing the tube to the individual's nose is to use a black silk suture or narrow piece of cloth tape. Loop the suture or tape around the tube below the nostril and attach it to the tip of the nose with a small hypoallergenic tape tab. Securing the tubing this way allows it to move when the individual swallows, thus promoting his or her comfort.

G. To minimize the tube's dragging, loop a rubber band around the tube in a slip knot and attach the band to the shoulder of the individual's clothing with a safety pin. If suction equipment is being used, attach its tubing to the individual's bedsheet in the same manner.

(continued)

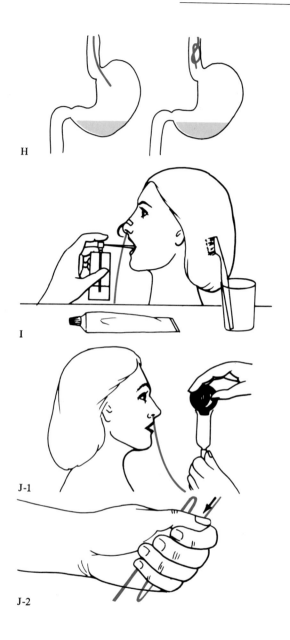

H

I

J-1

J-2

Figure 19.5 (Cont.)

H. Part of the care required for an individual while a naso-gastric tube is inserted is to prevent it from irritating the mucosa of the individual's gastrointestinal tract. Extra mucus is usually secreted by the body to protect itself from the tubing, but gently rotating the tube, each day or more often if necessary, will also help prevent the tube from adhering to the GI tract. Another necessity in caring for this individual is to be sure of the tube's continued proper placement in the stomach. If when irrigating the tube fluid flows freely into the individual but there is no return, the nurse may suspect that the tubing has slipped back above the fluid level in the stomach or curled itself in the esophagus. These two conditions may usually be corrected by retracting or advancing the tube 1 or 2 inches (2.5 or 5 cm.). *Note:* Do not advance tubing if the physician has positioned it as part of a specific procedure. Check with the physician before taking any action. If in irrigating the tubing, fluid does not pass through easily and the tube does not drain, the sucking ports may be obstructed or the tube curled in the stomach. In such a case, rotate tube and pull it back 1 or 2 inches, then try again to irrigate the tube.

I. The individual with a nasogastric tube inserted may develop a dry mouth, coated tongue, and cracked lips because he or she is mouth breathing and secreting less saliva due to not eating. Encourage the individual to brush the teeth and tongue regularly (using soft brush), massage the gums, and occasionally to rinse the mouth with a nonastringent substance or mist it with water from a spray bottle. *Note:* Avoid frequent rinsing or spraying because it could lead to an electrolyte imbalance. The individual may chew gum or suck hard candy if his condition permits. For individuals with severe discomfort, the physician may order anesthetic lozenges or spray.

J. To remove the tubing, have the individual in an upright position, place a towel across his or her chest, carefully remove the tape that has secured the tube, and rotate the tubing to ascertain that it moves freely. Flush the tube with irrigating solution (J-1). Ask the individual to take a deep breath and hold it, during which time the nurse clamps the tube securely (J-2) and lets the fluid flow out, slowly but steadily. Feed the liquid into a towel, out of the individual's slight if possible.

Continuous instillations of feedings or medications may be desired. This can be accomplished through a Kangaroo tube feeding set. (Illustration 19.8)

HYPERALIMENTATION

A method of feeding which totally bypasses the gastrointestinal tract is **hyperalimentation,** or **total parenteral nutrition.** With this method, amino acids, glucose, electrolytes, minerals, and vitamin solutions are instilled into the venous system. Large veins such as the superior vena cava or the jugular are used. This technique is used when the entire gastrointestinal tract needs to be bypassed or when long-term feeding is necessary. Figure 19.6 shows the setup for hyperalimentation.

Individuals on hyperalimentation therapy are prone to infection and fluid, electrolyte, and glucose disturbances because of the route of administration and type of solutions used. Strict sterile technique is utilized at all times when preparing and manipulating equipment and solutions. The individual is observed

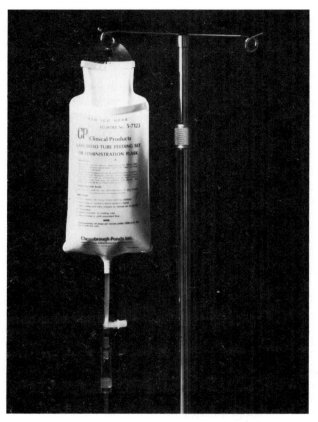

Illustration 19.8
A Kangaroo tube feeding; it is one alternate feeding method that bypasses the upper gastrointestinal tract. *(Courtesy of Chesebrough-Pond's, Inc. Hospital Products Division, Greenwich, Ct. 06830)*

for both local and systemic signs and symptoms of infection. Frequent serum glucose and electrolyte determinations are done to monitor the individual's status and make modifications in treatment. The individual is also observed for signs and symptoms of circulatory overload, dehydration, and electrolyte imbalance (Chap. 21). In addition, the possible complications of any type of intravenous therapy can occur and thus need to be monitored to prevent their occurrence and/or sequelae. Mouth care and other comfort measures are instituted to promote well-being.

INTRAVENOUS FEEDINGS

Intravenous feedings can be used to supply glucose, electrolytes, water, medications, and water-soluble vitamins. However, routine feedings through superficial veins do not supply needed protein and

fats. Thus long-term intravenous therapy is not adequate for maintaining or restoring nutritional status. (See Chapter 21 for a complete discussion of intravenous therapy.)

The nutritional content of intravenous feedings can be calculated. To calculate nutritional content one needs to know that a gram of metabolized glucose produces 4 kcal of energy and that each milliliter of fluid weighs one gram. Therefore, 1000 ml of 10% glucose and water solution yields 400 kcal. This is figured out by first determining the amount of glucose in the solution. In the example above, there are 100 g of glucose (10% of 1000). Total kilocalories are found by multiplying the amount of glucose (in grams) by 4 kcal/g. In the above example, 100 g of glucose times 4 kcal equals 400 kcal. The amount of protein in a hyperalimentation solution is derived in a similar manner.

EVALUATION

Evaluation of nutritional intake and energy needs centers on the direction of change in the person's ability to adequately balance nutritional intake with energy expenditure. Other important evaluation factors are: (1) the nutritional modifications that are required to maintain the individual's nutritional well-being, (2) the effectiveness of intervention, and (3) the influences of nutritional status on other body systems (and vice versa).

Specific criteria for evaluating an individual's energy needs and nutritional intake include:

- How do physiologic changes (in other subsystems as well as the gastrointestinal subsystem) influence energy intake? Psychologic changes? Environmental changes?
- What is the relationship between the presenting nutritional pattern and nutritional needs?
- Has the presenting nutritional pattern (e.g., caloric intake, nutrient intake, physical activity) moved closer to the expected?
- What factors may account for changes in nutritional pattern?
- What are the changes in the degree of nutritional interferences?
- What are the effects of nutritional pattern changes on body subsystems?

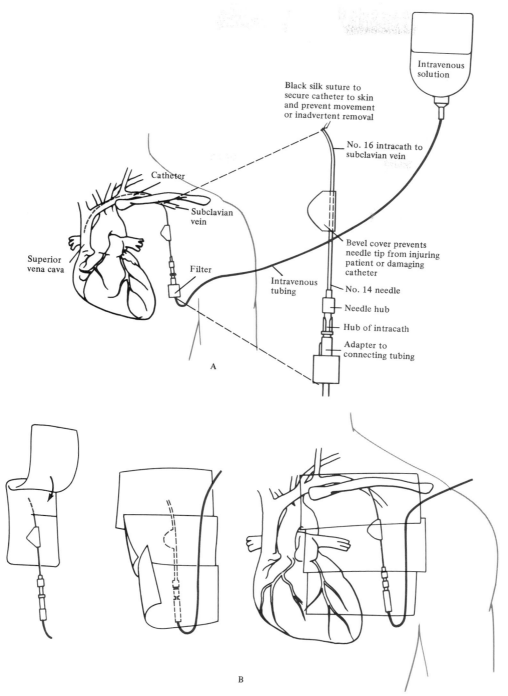

Figure 19.6
Hyperalimentation set-up and dressing. Hyperalimentation is used to maintain an individual's nutrition when the entire gastrointestinal tract needs to be bypassed in feeding. Insertion of the catheter, done by the physician, is a sterile procedure. The subclavian vein is usually used for insertion because of the large volume of blood, which will quickly dilute the intravenous solution. The catheter is then threaded through the innominate vein into the superior vena cava. The jugular vein is preferred for insertion in infants. **A.** Placement of the catheter in subclavian vein, the intracatheter and needle parts (closeup is at right), and tubing coming from intravenous solution. **B.** Application of air-occlusive dressing over intracatheter to protect against infection.

- Are there changes in knowledge (of individual, family and/or significant others) about the influence of nutritional habits on well-being? Nutritional needs? Level of growth and development? Food preparation? Meal planning, etc.?
- Are there changes in knowledge concerning accommodating cultural nutritional patterns to diet modifications?
- Are there changes in attitudes toward nutritional pattern and the effects of personal habits (individual, family and/or significant others)?
- Are there modifications of personal habits (individual, family and/or significant others)?
- What skills have been acquired in meal planning, budgeting, food preparation?
- What skills have been acquired in feeding techniques (e.g., infant feedings, nasogastric feedings)?

RECORDING AND TEACHING–LEARNING ACTIVITIES

Teaching–Learning Topics

- information about basic four
- rationale for therapeutic regimens
- methods to match nutritional intake with energy expenditure
- how to make modifications in nutritional pattern based on level of growth and development, culture, preferences, lifestyle, dietary needs
- ways to modify environment to facilitate meeting energy needs
- how to perform feeding techniques
- how to budget, plan, and shop for nutritious food
- low-cost food alternatives
- importance of continuity of good nutritional pattern
- different nutritional intake patterns at various levels of growth and development
- ways to assess changes in ability to meet nutritional needs, e.g., behavior, physical
- preventive aspects, e.g., balanced meals, balanced intake, and energy expenditure
- ways to modify personal habits which affect meeting nutritional needs

- available nutritional resources and how to use them
- how to modify nutritional pattern according to interference

Charting

Using appropriate nutritional terms, objectively describe such factors as:

- objective base-line data on nutritional status, habits, preferences, interferences, level of growth and development, level of nutritional knowledge, physical assessment, balance between food intake and energy expenditure, environmental factors, cultural factors, level of knowledge
- objective and subjective changes that occur in the person's ability to meet energy needs
- subjective assessment data on changes in nutritional intake and energy expenditure
- objective and subjective data on behavioral responses related to nutritional needs
- attitudes toward interference and treatments
- subjective and objective reactions and responses to treatment
- schedule and methods of care
- teaching carried out
- discharge planning done
- interactions, responses, and attitudes of family and/or significant others
- degree of change in adequacy of nutritional patterns
- update Kardex on nutritional needs

Medications to Review

- antacids. e.g., aluminum hydroxide
- anticholinergic drugs, e.g., propantheline (Pro-Banthine)
- corticosteroids, e.g., hydrocortisone
- gastrointestinal antibiotics, e.g., neomycin
- antidiarrheal agents, e.g., diphenoxylate (Lomotil)
- antiemetics, e.g., trimethobenzamide (Tigan)
- sedatives, e.g., phenobarbital

Diets to Review

See Appendix.

NOTES

1. Charles Butterworth, Jr. "The Skeleton in the Hospital Closet." *Nutrition Today*, 2:8, March-April, 1974.

SELECTED REFERENCES

Baker, Dorothy I. "Hyperalimentation at Home." *American Journal of Nursing*, 74:1826, October, 1974.

Bates, Barbara. *A Guide to Physical Examination.* Philadelphia, Lippincott, 1974.

Borgen, Linda. "Total Parenteral Nutrition in Adults." *American Journal of Nursing*, 78:224, Feburary, 1978.

Buckly, John E., Addicks, Connie L., and Maniglia, John. "Feeding Patients with Dysphagia." *Nursing Forums* 15:69, 1976.

Butterworth, Charles E. "The Skeleton in the Hospital Closet." *Nutrition Today*, 2:4, March-April, 1974.

Caly, Joan C. "Assessing Adult Nutrition." *American Journal of Nursing*, 77:1605, October, 1977.

Colley, Rita and Wilson, Jeanne "Meeting Patients' Nutritional Needs With Hyperalimentation." *Nursing 79*, 9:76, May, 1979.

Feingold, Ben F. "Hyperkinesis and Learning Disabilities Linked to Artificial Food Flavors and Colors." *American Journal of Nursing*, 75:797, May, 1975.

Griggs, Barbara A. and Hoppe, Mary C. "Update: Nasogastric Tube Feedings." *American Journal of Nursing*, 79:481, March, 1979.

"Helping People Eat for Health" (A Symposium). *American Journal of Nursing*, 77:1605, October, 1977.

Hill, Martha. "Helping the Hypertensive Control Sodium Intake." *American Journal of Nursing*, 79:906, May, 1979.

Howard, Rosanne Beatric and Herbold, Nancie Harvey. *Nutrition in Clinical Care.* New York, McGraw-Hill, 1978.

Keithley, Joyce K. "Proper Nutritional Assessment Can Prevent Hospital Malnutrition." *Nursing 79*, 9:68, February, 1979.

Lambert, Martin. "Drug and Diet Interactions." *American Journal of Nursing*, 75:402, March, 1975.

Malasanos, Lois Barkavskas, Violet, Moss, Muriel, Stoltenberg-Allen, Kathryn. *Health Assessment.* St. Louis, Mosby, 1977.

Mallison, Mary. "Updating the Cholesterol Controversy: Verdict—Diet Does Count." *American Journal of Nursing*, 78:1681, October, 1978.

Markersbery, Barbara and Wong, Wendy. "Helping People Eat for Health: Points for Maternity Patients." *American Journal of Nursing*, 77:1612, October, 1977.

Meiling, Richard L. "The Institutional System." *Nutrition Today*, July-August: 34, 1974.

Nursing 79 (in consultation with Robert L. Lavine). "How to Recognize . . . and What to do About . . . Hypoglycemia." *Nursing 79*, 9:52, April, 1979.

Nursing 79 (in consultation with Edwina A. McConnell). "Ten Problems with Nasogastric Tubes . . . and How to Solve Them." *Nursing 79*, 9:78, April, 1979.

Robinson, Corinne H. and Lawler, Marilyn R. *Normal and Therapeutic Nutrition*, 15th ed. New York, Macmillan, 1977.

Rose, James C. "Nutritional Problems in Radiotherapy Patients." *American Journal of Nursing*, 8:1194, July, 1978.

Sana, Josephine and Judge, Richard. *Physical Appraisal Methods in Nursing Practice.* Boston, Little, Brown, 1975.

Williams, Eleanor R. "Making Vegetarian Diets Nutritious." *American Journal of Nursing*, 75:2168, December, 1975.

What goes in must come out.
—Colloquial saying

20

ELIMINATION AND OUTPUT

PRINCIPLES RELATED TO ELIMINATION OUTPUT

Bowel evacuation occurs through the contraction and relaxation of the involuntary muscles of the intestinal wall (peristalsis).

The defecation reflex results from stimulation of the intestine by feces.

The duodenal colic and gastrocolic reflexes initiate movement of the intestine when food is released into the intestine from the stomach.

The duodenal colic and gastrocolic reflexes initiate movement of the bowels.

Defecation is a voluntary act learned in childhood.

The movement of the small intestine is much more rapid than that of the large intestine.

Feces contain bacteria, food residue, bile pigments, mucus, inorganic salts, epithelial cells, and water.

Movement of the bowel is mainly controlled by innervation from the spinal cord.

The main functions of the intestines are completion of the process of digestion, absorption of water, and elimination of waste products.

The urinary bladder is made of elastic, smooth muscle which will expand to store up to 4000 cc of urine in adults.

The urinary tract is a closed, continuous, sterile system.

Urine is produced by the kidneys at a rate of 30–50 cc an hour.

The amount of urine produced is directly proportional to fluid intake.

The amount of urine produced by the kidneys is influenced by the blood flow to the kidneys, antidiuretic hormones, state of hydration, fluid and electrolyte balance, and hydrostatic pressure.

Micturition is under voluntary control.

Urine contains water, nitrogen, urea, electrolytes, inorganic salts, and pigment.

Micturition is mainly controlled by innervation from the spinal cord.

Many bowel and bladder patterns are culturally determined.

Stress produces changes in bowel and bladder patterns.

Bowel and bladder control are major contributors to positive self-esteem.

The processes of energy intake and metabolism result in the production of heat and metabolic by-products. For maintenance of well-being, some of this heat must be dissipated and by-products eliminated. These losses occur via the skin, kidneys, intestinal tract, and respiratory system. When any one of the routes of elimination is impaired, waste products and heat build up and survival is threatened. In pathologic states, fluids and heat can be lost through artificial openings and drainage from body cavities (Chap. 21). These losses, if not monitored and compensated for, also threaten life.

The nurse's role in meeting elimination needs includes assessing losses, promoting those elimination processes which support well-being, decreasing detrimental losses, and helping to compensate for imbalances between intake and output. Using his or her knowledge of the expected functioning and the sequelae of detrimental output—both excessive losses and deficient elimination—the nurse can assist the individual to promote, maintain, and restore the internal environment of the body.

ASSESSMENT

The nurse assesses losses from the urinary and intestinal tracts, and, when present, pathology related losses. The factors which influence the individual's elimination pattern make up the first area the nurse assesses.

Factors Influencing Elimination Pattern

Each individual has a unique elimination pattern. These patterns are learned in early childhood and reflect the type of bladder and bowel training, cultural background, and general style of his or her early family life. Bladder- and bowel-training techniques cover the full spectrum from strictly scheduled and rigid programs to flexible patterns of "when the

child's ready, he'll learn." These approaches lead to the individual's attitudes about elimination, flexibility of schedule, and the significance of elimination in his or her daily life. (Illustration 20.1)

CULTURAL INFLUENCES

Different cultures place varying emphasis on circumstances under which elimination occurs. The degree of privacy required, the frequency, the attitude toward odors and sounds of elimination, and methods used to promote elimination are just a few factors which can be culturally determined. Some cultures, that of the United States, for example, put a high value on complete privacy for elimination, along with separation of the sexes. Others, such as the Turkish, carry out elimination in communal and mixed-sex settings.

EARLY LIFESTYLE

Elimination patterns are also influenced by early family lifestyle. The availability of facilities, the number of people using a bathroom, and family habits all contribute to the individual's elimination pattern.

These early childhood influences are often carried throughout life, affecting the individual's adult elimination habits. The individual's presenting elimination habits also reflect diet, level of activity, muscle tone, level of growth and development, emotional state, lifestyle, elimination interferences, and the medications or assistive devices he or she uses.

DIET

Diet plays a major role in determining bladder and bowel function. The amount, color, and concentration of urine depend greatly on the amount of fluid taken in—both as solid and liquid foods. The proportions of nutrients (particularly proteins and sodium) ingested and the efficiency of digestion and metabolism also regulate the urine output. For example, a high fluid intake much in excess of the body's metabolic requirements will result in a high urinary output.

The amount of bulk in the diet, the fluid intake, and the ingestion of irritating food affect the amount, frequency, color, consistency, and odor of feces. Bulk

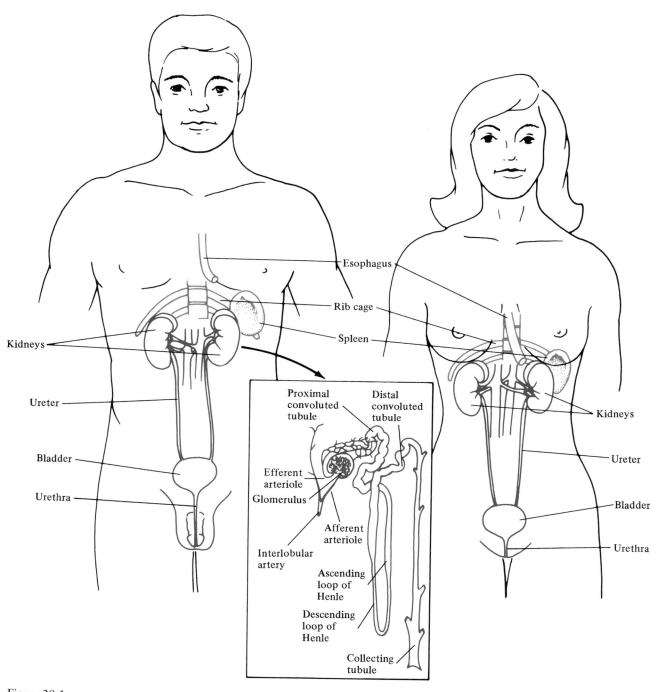

Figure 20.1
The urinary subsystem. An enlarged rendering (inset) shows the anatomy of the nephron.

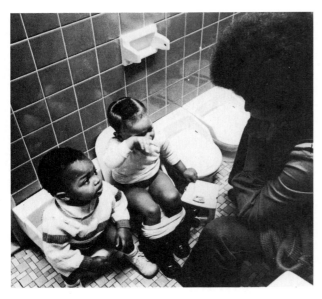

Illustration 20.1
A child is ready for toilet training between the ages of 15 months and 3 years. The pattern of elimination that the individual learns during this early period is one that he or she will continue to demonstrate. *(Photo © Joel Gordon, 1979)*

foods high in cellulose such as fresh vegetables and fruits leave a metabolic residue in the colon. The amount of residue in the colon determines when the defecation reflex will occur. The type and amount of bacteria present in the intestine in part determine the degree to which the cellulose is broken down. Diets high in bulk will result in large amounts of residue remaining in the colon, with a resultant stimulation of the defecation reflex.

Water constitutes approximately 75% of feces. Thus an increase or decrease in the amount of water available for the production of feces will result in a change in consistency. The longer the feces stay in the intestine, the drier they become, since water is constantly being reabsorbed from the bowel.

If a person has a consistently low-bulk diet, the time required to build up sufficient residue for initiation of the defecation reflex is increased. Thus the feces stay in the bowel a longer period and water is removed. The feces are therefore harder and drier and have difficulty moving along the intestinal tract, leading to **constipation.**

If, however, the evacuation of the bowel is speeded up by irritating foods, inflammation, drugs, or structural or functional defects, little water is reabsorbed, and watery, nonformed feces result (**diarrhea**).

The amount of bacteria in ingested food affects the consistency, color, and frequency of feces. As previously noted, bacteria are responsible for the degree of cellulose breakdown. In addition, certain bacteria irritate the intestinal mucosa, resulting in changes in function. Bacterial processes which work on food residues account, in part, for the odor of the feces.

ACTIVITY

The level of activity the individual engages in is significant in maintaining the muscles necessary for the processes of elimination. Bladder elimination requires good bladder tone, intact, functional internal and external uretheral sphincters, and perineal muscle. Inactivity due to debilitation, paralysis, sedentary lifestyle, and disease pathologies may result in a weakening of these muscles and improper emptying of the bladder. Loss of muscle tone also occurs in chronic overdistention of the bladder as a result of failure to urinate when stimulation occurs, as well as with structural defects and inflammation.

Emptying of the intestines results from bowel tone, contraction of the internal and external anal sphincters, and tone of the perineal muscles. The same factors contribute to the loss of tone in the muscles needed for defecation as with urination.

GROWTH AND DEVELOPMENT

The level of growth and development determines many facets of the elimination pattern. Chart 20.1 outlines elimination patterns at different levels of growth and development.

ANXIETY AND STRESS

Increased anxiety and stress in the individual can result in elimination patterns changing in any direction. Such stressors as changes in environment, illness, hospitalization, and occupational tensions can cause extremes in increased or decreased urination and defecation. Many people, however, have an inconsistent pattern which is usual for them. The nurse needs to differeniate between usual patterns and those which deviate from the expected. Changes in elimination as a result of stressors are connected to the alteration in neurohormonal function initiated by the stress response.

Chart 20.1
Elimination Patterns at Different Levels of Growth and Development

STAGE	PATTERN
Neonate (0–1 month)	First bowel elimination within first 24 hours of life. Meconium—dark green, tarry. Urinates within first 2 days of life.
Infant (1–14 months)	Defecates 4–6 times a day. If breast fed, feces are pasty, loose, and yellow. If milk fed, feces are firmer and darker yellow. Feces become more formed and fewer in number as the infant begins solid food. Urinates 5–40 times a day, depending on such factors as fluid intake, environmental temperature. Urine dilute and odorless.
Toddler (15 months–3 years)	Begins toilet training. Exact age depends on muscle tone and myelination of nerve tracts. Involuntary night urination (enuresis) continues.
Preschooler (3–5 years)	Has almost complete voluntary control of elimination. However, will have "accidents" when stressed or involved in activities.
Schoolage (6–12 years)	Complete elimination control. Urinary output approximately 1000 cc per day. Defecation follows adult patterns.
Adolescent (13–18 years)	Adult patterns of elimination.
Young adult (18–45 years)	Pregnant women may have frequent constipation and frequency of urination. Expected pattern: defecation, individual; urination, 4–6 times daily.
Middle age (45–65 years)	Continuation of patterns. Increasing periods of constipation as diet changes and activity and muscle tone decrease.
Old age (65+ years)	Peristaltic action decreases nutrition absorption—dietary and muscular changes contribute to change in pattern. Loss in functional nephrons cause increased frequency of urination. Urinary retention common. Sphincter reflexes decreased.

PRESENT LIFESTYLE

The individual's lifestyle affects his or her pattern of elimination in many ways. Questions such as "Do you take time out from your schedule to urinate or defecate when the stimulation occurs?" "What are the facilities available for elimination?" and "Are you able to maintain a regular schedule for elimination?" will help the nurse assess the effect of the individual's lifestyle on his or her elimination patterns. (Illustrations 20.2. A–B)

Nursing assessment of the influences on an individual's elimination pattern includes descriptions of:

- cultural influences
- relationship of toilet training to present elimination pattern
- amount of fluid intake
- amount of bulk in diet
- foods which increase or decrease elimination
- frequency of constipation or diarrhea
- factors which contribute to and alleviate constipation and diarrhea
- activity level and muscle tone
- influence of activity level on elimination
- interferences with activity
- relationship of growth and development to elimination patterns—expected, presenting
- relationship of stressors to elimination patterns

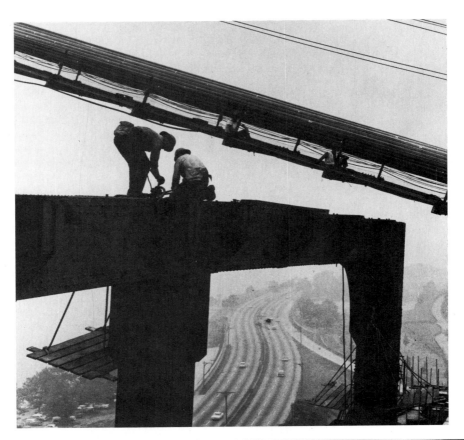

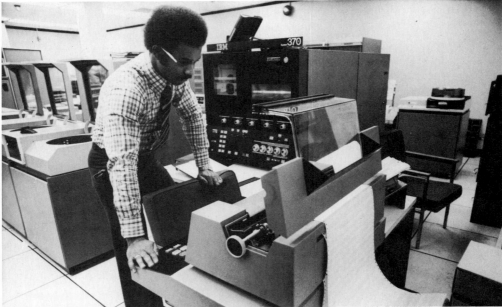

Illustration 20.2
Different kinds of lifestyles influence what patterns of elimination an individual develops. For example, depending upon the accessibility of toilet facilities where a person works, the stimulation to defecate or urinate may have to be ignored. *(Top photo by Bruce Davidson, © Magnum Photos, Inc. Bottom photo © Joel Gordon, 1979)*

- stress factors which initiate changes in elimination patterns
- lifestyle factors which influence elimination
- attitudes toward elimination (of individual, of family and/or significant others)
- knowledge about elimination and the effects of elimination on well-being (of individual, of family and/or significant others)
- beliefs about elimination (of family and/or significant others)

Patterns of Elimination

The second area of elimination that the nurse assesses is the individual's patterns and habits. The urination (**voiding**) pattern of the individual includes how often and at what times of day voiding takes place, the amount with each voiding, and any discomfort felt on urination or when attempting to urinate. Chart 20.2 defines terms used to describe urination patterns.

CHARACTERISTICS OF URINE

The nurse also needs to assess the characteristics of the urine, including its color, concentration, odor, pH, and clarity. Chart 20.3 outlines the expected characteristics of urine and some common variations.

DEFECATION PATTERN

The defecation pattern of the individual includes the frequency of defecation, the amount of feces (**stool**) with each defecation, and any discomfort felt on defecation or when attempting to defecate.

CHARACTERISTICS OF FECES

The nurse also assesses the characteristics of the feces: amount, color, consistency, odor, and constituents. Chart 20.4 outlines the expected characteristics of feces and some common variations.

REGULATION OF PATTERN

The nurse also determines methods by which the individual promotes or maintains his or her elimination patterns. Foods, medications, scheduling, and privacy are among the ways individuals regulate their elimination patterns.

Nursing assessment of elimination patterns includes a description of:

- frequency of elimination (bowel and bladder)
- factors increasing or decreasing frequency
- amount of elimination
- discomfort on elimination
- factors precipitating and alleviating discomfort
- the characteristics of urine and feces
- any variations from expected
- methods which promote, maintain, and restore elimination

Interferences with Elimination

Interferences of both bladder and bowel elimination fall within three general categories: inflammation, obstruction, and mechanical defects or failures.

INFLAMMATION

Inflammations of the bowel and bladder can result from local or systemic infection, trauma, chemical injury, the stress response, or a secondary response to obstructions or mechanical failure.

Inflammations of the bladder are characterized by frequency, urgency, dysuria, burning, intermittent fever, and lethargy. If inflammation is severe enough, prolonged, or untreated, it can lead to permanent kidney damage and life-threatening renal failure.

Examples of urinary tract inflammations are cystitis (inflammation of the bladder), nephrotic syndrome (autoimmune renal response), and pyelonephritis (bacterial infection of renal pelvis).

Bowel inflammation is typified by diarrhea, fever, dehydration, and fluid and electrolyte imbalance. Intestinal inflammation can lead to malabsorption, malnutrition, weight loss, mechanical failure, intestinal hemorrhage, intestinal perforation (rupture of bowel with spilling of intestinal contents into the peritoneal cavity), and, if severe enough, death.

Bowel inflammations can result from bacteria, viruses, or parasites, as well as from those conditions listed previously. Types of bowel inflammation include ulcerative colitis, appendicitis, diverticulitis, dysentery, and trichinosis.

OBSTRUCTION

Tumors and **strictures** are obstructions common to both the urinary and intestinal tracts. In addition,

Chart 20.2
Terms Describing Urination Pattern

TERM	DESCRIPTION	TERM	DESCRIPTION
Albuminuria	Presence of albumin in the urine; results from renal dysfunction		brown; color depends on amount present or length of time blood has been in urinary tract; results from trauma, blood diacnsis, lesions of urinary tract
Anisuria	A repeated cycle of excessive urination followed by decreased urination	Incontinence	Loss of urinary control; results from neurologic damage, loss of muscle tone, and other stresses
Anuria (suppression)	Lack of urine production; results from renal dysfunction	Micturition	Urination
Bradyuria	Slow urination; results from urinary tract obstructions	Nocturia	Voiding during the night; may be excessive; results from obstructions, inflammation, drinking fluids before bedtime
Burning	Burning sensation on urination; results from inflammation of the urinary system		
Diuresis	Excessive urination; results from diabetes mellitus, medications, anxiety, large fluid intake	Oliguria	Decreased urinary production; results from renal dysfunction
		Polyuria	Same as diuresis
Dysuria	Pain or difficulty with urination; results from inflammation of the urinary tract	Proteinuria	Presence of protein in the urine; results from renal dysfunction
		Pyuria	Pus in the urine; results from infections of the urinary tract
Enuresis	Involuntary urination; results from stress, muscle atony, pressure from laughing or coughing (commonly used to describe bedwetting)	Residual	More than 50 cc urine which remains in the bladder after voiding; results from obstruction, loss of muscle tone
Frequency	Increased number of urinations; results from inflammation, stress, pregnancy	Stranguria	Painful and intermittent urination; results from inflammations of the urinary tract
Glycosuria	Glucose in the urine; results from diabetes mellitus	Urgency	Feeling of immediate need to urinate; results from inflammation
Hematuria	Blood in urine; may be bright red, pink, or		

Chart 20.3
Expected Characteristics of Urine and Variations

CHARACTERISTIC	EXPECTED	VARIATION
Amount	1000–1500 cc per day	
Color	Yellow to amber, depending on concentration	Pale—dilute urine or diabetes insipidus Milky—fat globules Reddish—blood, food, drugs Green—bile pigment Brown/black—poisoning, hemorrhage
Concentration	Specific gravity 1.003–1.030. Specific gravity (SG) is inversely proportional to volume	
Odor	Spicy fragrance; may smell like ammonia after standing	Sweet—acetone Fishy—cystitis Fecal—connection between intestinal and urinary tracts New-mown hay—diabetes
pH	4.5–8.0, usually slightly acidic	
Clarity	Clear, transparent; may turn cloudy on standing due to precipitation of mucus	Turbid—pus

Chart 20.4
Expected Characteristics of Feces and Variations

CHARACTERISTIC	EXPECTED	VARIATION
Amount	Individual, depending on intake and capacity of intestines	Any decrease or increase from usual pattern
Frequency	1–3 days	Any change from usual pattern
Color	Brownish	Clay colored—absence of bile Black or tarry—gastrointestinal bleeding, iron supplements Bright red—lower intestinal bleeding
Consistency	Firm and formed	Water—malabsorption Dry, hard—increased water absorption in intestines; dehydration Steatorous—fatty; malabsorption of fats Flattened—rectal obstruction Greasy—jaundice
Odor	Individual, depending on diet and intestinal flora	Depends on disease
Constituents	Mucous threads—partially digested food	Foreign objects that have been ingested Parasites

► **calculi** (precipitations of minerals) can obstruct the urinary system. Obstructions can result in distension of the system proximal to the obstruction, pooling of urine or feces, infection, backflow of urine or feces, diarrhea, constipation or impaction, tissue necrosis,

► **gangrene** (death of tissue related to inadequate blood supply; results from bacterial invasion of area), pain, shock, and death. Examples include pyloric stenosis, carcinoma of the colon, bladder, or prostate, and renal calculi.

MECHANICAL DEFECTS

Mechanical defects and failure result when a functional failure occurs either in a part of or in the entire urinary or intestinal system. This can be caused by congenital anamolies, genetic defects, trauma, infection, or obstruction. The resulting pathology will be determined by the exact nature of the failure and is the same as with inflammation and obstruction. Examples of mechanical defects include malabsorption diseases (e.g., cystic fibrosis and celiac disease),

► intestinal **adhesions, diverticula,** paralytic ileus, and hydroureter.

Certain elimination interferences are commonly found within different stages of growth and development. Chart 20.5 lists some of these interferences.

Nursing assessment of interferences with elimination includes descriptions of:

- type of interference
- signs and symptoms
- sequelae of interference
- precipitating factors
- attitude toward interference
- knowledge about interference
- therapeutic regimen
- relationship of interference to level of growth and development
- effects on energy intake and expenditure
- relationship of interferences to body image changes
- effect of interference on family and/or significant others

Physical Assessment

Examination of the gastrointestinal and urinary systems is carried out in conjunction with the physical assessment of the abdomen (Chap. 19), and the same methods are used. The assessments described below are also made.

INSPECTION

The external urinary meatus is examined for swelling, lesions, redness, discharge, and position. In women this is done by parting the labia minora. In an uncircumcised male, the prepuce is retracted. Gentle manipulation of the meatus should not produce pain or discomfort. The expected findings are a light pink color with no tenderness or swelling. Clear mucous drainage may sometimes be present.

Anus

The anus is observed for varicosities, fissures, redness, lesions, nodules, and masses. Asking the individual to bear down as the nurse observes aids in the detection of hemorrhoids. Expected findings are no varicosities, fissures, masses, or redness. The individual is asked whether he or she has any discomfort during urination or fecal elimination.

PALPATION

Kidney

To palpate the left kidney, the individual is supine and the nurse stands on the right side of the individual and reaches across, placing her left hand under the left posterior rib cage. She presses upward with her left hand to move the kidney forward. Using the right palmar surface of her hand, the nurse deeply palpates, for the kidney is usually not palpable. It may, however, be felt as a soft, rounded mass on inspiration. The procedure is reversed for the right kidney.

Bladder

The bladder, unless filled with urine, is not palpable. The nurses places a hand above the symphysis pubis and palpates for a smooth, round, slightly hard mass. The nurse notes how many centimeters the bladder is elevated above the symphysis pubis.

Rectum

To palpate the rectum, the nurse uses a lubricated rubber glove or finger cot. In women this procedure is usually done after the vaginal examination, with the individual in a lithotomy position. However, the knee-chest, a leaning over position, or supine left

Chart 20.5
Common Interferences in Elimination at Various Levels of Growth and Development

STAGE OF GROWTH AND DEVELOPMENT	INTERFERENCE	EXAMPLE
Neonate (0–1 month)	Mechanical	Intestinal: Imperforate anus Congenital megacolon Hirshsprung's disease Meconium ileus Urinary: Hypospadias
Infant (1–14 months)	Inflammation	Intestinal: Intestinal infection Salmonella Urinary: Pyelonephritis
	Obstructions	Intestinal: Pyloric obstructions
	Mechanical	Intestinal: Intussusception Celiac disease Cystic fibrosis Prolapse of rectum and sigmoid colon Megacolon
Toddler (15 months–3 years)	Inflammation	Intestinal: Parasites Infection Urinary: Nephotic syndrome
	Obstruction	Urinary: Wilm's tumor
Preschooler (3–5 years)	Inflammation	Intestinal: Infections
	Mechanical	Urinary: Trauma Acute glomerulonephritis
Schoolage (6–12 years)	Inflammatory	Intestinal: Duodenal ulcer Urinary: Infection
	Mechanical	Intestinal: Meckel's diverticulum Urinary: Enuresis Infections

(continued)

Chart 20.5 (Cont.)
Common Interferences in Elimination at Various Levels of Growth and Development

STAGE OF GROWTH AND DEVELOPMENT	INTERFERENCE	EXAMPLE
Adolescent (13–18 years)	Inflammatory	Intestinal: Ulcerative colitis
Young adult (18–45 years)	Inflammatory	Intestinal: Ulcerative colitis Ulcers Urinary: Urinary tract infection
	Mechanical	Intestinal: Hemorrhoids
Middle adult (45–65 years)	Inflammatory	Intestinal: Ulcer Diverticulitis Spastic colon
	Obstruction	Intestinal: Tumors Urinary: Tumors Calculi
	Mechanical	Intestinal: Diverticulosis
Older adult (65+ years)	Inflammatory	Intestinal: Diverticulitis
	Obstructions	Intestinal: Tumors Urinary: Tumors Calculi
	Mechanical	Intestinal: Diverticulosis Adhesions

lateral position may be used for both males and females.

The individual is instructed to bear down as in defecation. The index finger is inserted gently but firmly. The individual may feel the desire to defecate at this point. The individual is asked to tighten the anal sphincter for determination of sphincter tone.

The rectal walls are then palpated in a slow, circular motion for nodules, irritation, and tenderness. The finger is then removed and feces remaining on the glove or finger cot can be tested for possible occult (hidden) blood or for parasites. Examination of the prostate in males and of the tip of the uterus in females is usually done during the rectal examination (Chap. 24).

Diagnostic Tests

URINE EXAMINATION

Examination of the urine is done through microscopic and chemical analyses.

Midstream Specimen

To obtain a urine specimen, the individual cleanses the perineal area or the tip of the penis, moving from front to back. The individual is asked to void a small amount into the toilet or bedpan and then to void into a clean specimen cup (midstream), finishing into the toilet or bedpan.

Sterile Specimen

A sterile specimen is obtained for culture and sensitivity. Sterile specimens are obtained in a similar manner as a midstream; however, care is taken to avoid contaminating the sterile container and the meatus, particularly in women, after cleansing. A sterile catheter may be used to obtain urine specimens, but this should be avoided unless no other means for urine collection is available. The urine specimen is tightly capped and labeled. It is sent to the laboratory as soon as possible, since leaving it standing may alter test results. (Illustration 20.3)

Tests

The urine is examined for color, clarity, transparency, specific gravity, and presence of expected and unexpected constituents (e.g., glucose, protein, pus, red blood cells).

FECES EXAMINATION

Feces can be examined for ova and parasites and for occult blood. Testing for occult blood may be done by the nurse or the specimen may be sent to the laboratory. Special kits are available for performing the test for occult blood.

Obtaining a Specimen

Specimens can be obtained by having the individual defecate in a bedpan and using a clean tongue blade to remove and place the specimen in the appropriate container. If the individual uses the toilet, first lay down some toilet paper in the bowel so that the feces will float on the paper; obtaining the specimen in this way will be easier. A bedpan is preferable, however, because the chance of contamination of feces by urine is decreased. Specimens for ova and parasites are sent to the lab immediately, or kept at

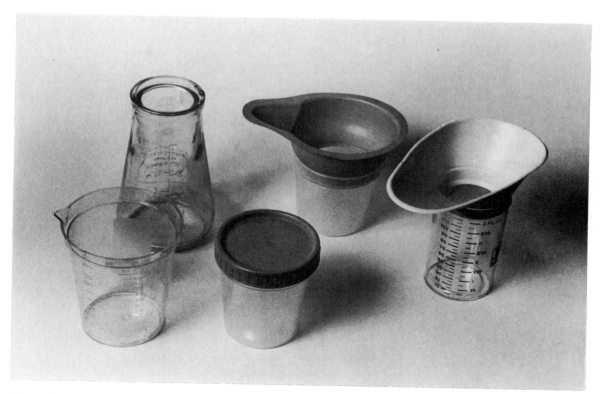

Illustration 20.3
Urine containers (*Photo © Leonard Speier, 1979*)

body temperature, to decrease the chance that the parasites, if any, will be killed by cool temperatures.

VISUALIZATION OF THE BLADDER, RECTUM, SIGMOID COLON

Other tests used are cystoscopy, visualization of the bladder; proctoscopy, visualization of the rectum; and sigmoidoscopy, visualization of the sigmoid colon.

Both proctoscopy and sigmoidoscopy entail insertion of a warm, lubricated cylinder into the intestine. The individual is usually given enemas and laxatives prior to the procedure to cleanse the intestines. The person is usually placed in a knee-chest or lithotomy position and told to breathe deeply through his or her mouth as the scope is inserted. The walls of the intestine are observed as the scope is removed. Air may be injected into the bowel to facilitate visualization, and biopsies may also be taken.

Postprocedural care involves allowing the individual to rest, as the procedure is a tiring one. Observations are made later for bleeding on defecation and irritation of the anal sphincter. Since the bowel has been manipulated, the possibility of perforation of the bowel exists. Thus the individual is observed for signs of **peritonitis** such as nausea, vomiting, absence of bowel sounds, fever, abdominal pain, high white blood cell count, shock, and boardlike abdomen.

Cystoscopy is the insertion of a tube into the bladder through the meatus and urethra while the individual is in a lithotomy position. Fluid is usually injected into the bladder to increase visualization. The ureters and kidneys may also be catheterized at this time, as well as biopsies taken and bladder stones crushed and removed. Sedatives may be given prior to the procedure.

The individual may experience difficulty in voiding after the procedure, and the urine may be pink tinged. Observation for gross hematuria is made and reported if present, as are signs of peritonitis. Forced fluids, lower abdominal heat applications, analgesics, and urinary antiseptics may be prescribed for the individual to relieve posttest discomfort.

These procedures are often embarrassing and uncomfortable for the individual. Explanations of the procedure and its purpose, the individual's role in it, and the feelings he or she may experience (e.g., desire to void or defecate) are important to increase cooperation and decrease anxiety. Careful draping of the individual during the procedure may help alleviate some of the embarrassment he or she may experience.

VISUALIZATION OF LOWER BOWEL

Barium enemas are performed for indirect visualization of the lower bowel. A radiopaque substance (barium) is injected into the intestine through the rectum, and x-rays are then taken of the area. Prior to and after the procedure, the individual is given enemas and/or laxatives to cleanse the bowel. The individual is N.P.O. for 8 to 10 hours prior to the procedure, as with the upper gastrointestinal series. The individual may be nutritionally and physically exhausted following this procedure and should be allowed to rest and eat then. Feces will be chalky white until all the barium has been expelled. The individual is observed for constipation and impaction.

VISUALIZATION OF KIDNEYS

Intravenous pyelograms allow visualization of the kidneys. A radiopaque iodine-based dye is injected into a vein and x-rays are taken as the dye moves through the renal system. Laxatives are given the night before to cleanse the bowel and so prevent x-ray distortion. The individual is usually allowed a light breakfast before the procedure. Some nausea and hot flashes may be experienced with the injection of the dye. Otherwise it is a painless procedure. The individual will be required, however, to remain quiet while the procedure is carried out. Posttest precautions include observation for allergic reactions and inflammation at the site where the dye was injected.

X-rays of the kidney, ureters, and bladder (KUB) are frequently done. Observations are made for masses and distortion of organ shapes. No special pre- or posttest care is necessary.

BLOOD TESTS FOR RENAL FUNCTION

Blood tests commonly performed for assessing renal function and catabolism are the blood urea nitrogen test (BUN), nonprotein nitrogen test (NPN), and creatinine test.

Blood Urea Nitrogen
The BUN measures the amount of nitrogen in the form of urea present in the blood. Expected levels are 5–25 mg/dl of blood.

Nonprotein Nitrogen

The NPN shows the amount of nitrogen in the blood which is not in the form of protein. Expected levels are 25–40 mg/dl of blood.

Creatinine

The creatinine test assesses the amount of creatine in the blood. Together with the amount excreted in the urine, the renal threshold can be calculated. The renal threshold is the level of concentration at which a substance is excreted by the kidney. The expected blood values are 0.8–1.4 mg/dl of blood; the expected urine values are 0.8–1.9 g per 24 hours.

Chart 20.6
Procedure for Measuring Specific Gravity

---

1. Be familiar with the equipment used to test the specific gravity of urine:
   a. The apparatus consists of two parts—the cylinder to contain the urine and the urinometer.
   b. Note that the urinometer is calibrated in units of 0.001, beginning with 1.000 at the top and progressing downward to 1.060. A urinometer is read from top to bottom.
   c. New urinometers should be checked for accuracy against distilled water before use, and rechecked from time to time thereafter—even a slight discrepancy can be significant.
2. The urine sample must be fresh.
3. The urine sample must be well mixed—remember, the specific gravity test measures solute concentration and a uniform solution must be used to yield an accurate reading.
4. The cylinder should be three quarters full with urine.
5. After the urinometer is placed in the cylinder, it is given a gentle spin with the thumb and forefinger to prevent it from adhering to the cylinder's sides.
6. Should there be an insufficient amount of urine to float the urinometer, the reading cannot be made. In such an event, *q.n.s.* (quantity not sufficient) is charted.
7. To read specific gravity, it is necessary that the urinometer be at eye level. It is read by imagining a line where the lower portion of the meniscus crosses the scale on the urinometer.

Adapted from: Norma Matheny and W. D. Snively. Nurses Handbook of Fluid Balance. Philadelphia, Lippincott, 1974, pp. 69–70.

A variety of tests is done to determine the renal threshold for various medications, nutrients, chemicals, and electrolytes. The student is referred to a medical–surgical nursing text for an explanation of the procedures.

SPECIFIC GRAVITY OF URINE

The specific gravity of the urine indicates the degree concentration of the urine and is based on a comparison between the specific gravity of distilled water and the urine. Chart 20.6 along with Fig. 20.2 outlines the procedures for measuring specific gravity of urine. This measurement is done for the individual with burns, renal and cardiovascular disease, febrile states, and general surgical conditions.

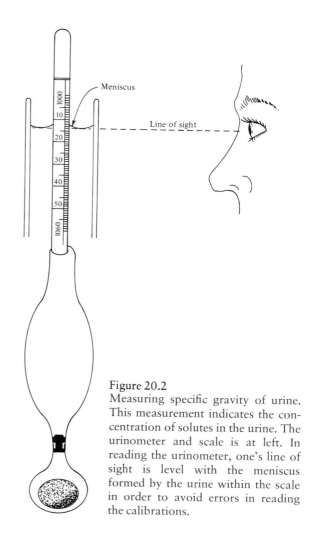

Figure 20.2
Measuring specific gravity of urine. This measurement indicates the concentration of solutes in the urine. The urinometer and scale is at left. In reading the urinometer, one's line of sight is level with the meniscus formed by the urine within the scale in order to avoid errors in reading the calibrations.

NURSING DIAGNOSIS

Ms. Ex, 27 years old and pregnant (36 weeks gestation), comes to the prenatal clinic for her routine checkup. Her pregnancy is progressing well, but she complains of persistent constipation.

The nursing assessment that follows compares Ms. Ex's presenting behaviors related to elimination patterns with those behaviors that the nurse would expect to find in a person of similar growth and development (36th week of gestation) who has no disturbance with elimination. A physical assessment is included.

ASSESSMENT FACTOR	EXPECTED BEHAVIOR	PRESENTING BEHAVIOR
Diet	Fluid: 6–8 glasses per day	Five glasses; states she is not much of a drinker
	Breads and cereals: 4 servings	Breads and cereal: 4 servings
	Fruits and vegetables: 4 servings (vitamin C rich, 1 svg.; leafy green veg., 2 svgs.; other, 1 svg.)	Fruits and vegetables: 2 servings "Lettuce prices have gone way out of sight lately."
Exercise	Continue with usual activities unless contraindicated by complications of pregnancy	"I've been just sitting around waiting the last couple of weeks. I feel too slow and heavy to do much moving around."
Influence of growth and development on bowel pattern	In last 3 months of pregnancy, constipation is common because of pressure of enlarged uterus on intestines	—
Increased stress and anxiety	Increased physiologic and psychologic stress during pregnancy	Very much excited over birth of baby but can't wait until it's over
Effects of lifestyle on elimination	—	Eats three regular meals a day; facilities adequate; income level moderate but sufficient for meeting basic needs
Pattern	Individual	Prior to constipation went every other day; soft, formed, brown stool. Now goes once every 3–4 days with feelings of pressure and desire to defecate. Stool: dry, small pieces
Methods to promote and maintain elimination	—	Used to take laxative for occasional constipation, now afraid to take any medications because of pregnancy
Interferences	—	Third trimester pregnancy, slight pressure on intestine
Physical Assessment		
Uterus	Fundus of uterus may reach to just below xiphoid process at 40 weeks gestation	Fundus of uterus 5 cm below xiphoid process

(continued)

ASSESSMENT FACTOR	EXPECTED BEHAVIOR	PRESENTING BEHAVIOR
	Uterus mobile	Same
	Striae expected	Same
	L.O.A. (left side of fetus's head in the anterior position)	Same
Fetal heart beat	120–160/minute	136
Maternal heart beat	Up to 10 beats above nonpregnant state	82
Diagnostic tests	Urine protein: negative	Same
	Urine sugar and acetone: negative	Same

Resulting nursing diagnoses might include:

- constipation related to low fluid and bulk intake
- constipation related to decreased activity
- potential nutritional deficits related to low intake of fruits and vegetables

PLANNING

Planning for elimination includes promoting, maintaining, and restoring the individual's expected elimination patterns. Planning for intervention considers the influence of the level of growth and development, physiologic mechanisms, interferences, personal habits, and the individual's usual pattern.

In the situation of Ms. Ex, the plan for one of the nursing diagnoses listed above might look as follows:

NURSING DIAGNOSIS	GOALS	PLAN
Constipation related to low fluid and bulk intake	*Short term:* Increase fluid intake to 8 glasses per day within 2 days.	Review need for adequate fluid intake. Determine fluid preferences. Plan with individual a regular schedule of fluid intake.
	Increase fruit and vegetable intake to 4 servings per day within 2 days.	Review need for adequate amount of fruit and vegetable intake. Review fruits and vegetables high bulk.
	Decrease constipation within 4 days.	Devise plan with individual for increasing fruit and vegetable intake in meal plan. Discuss inexpensive alternatives to fruits (i.e., chicory, fruits in season).
	Long term: Prevent recurrence for remainder of pregnancy. Promote life-long adequate bowel habits.	Reinforce positive aspects of diet intake (e.g., breads and cereals). 1. As above 2. Determine methods which promote evacuation for individual. 3. Review physiologic mechanisms of bowel elimination. 4. Devise plan with individual for bowel evacuation schedule. *Long term:* As above

INTERVENTION

A Teaching Program

Promotion of bowel and bladder elimination focuses on teaching the individual positive elimination habits and reinforcing existing ones. Teaching stresses the importance of eliminating when the stimulus is felt; the role of diet and exercise in elimination; the judicious use of laxatives and enemas; and the significance of an unhurried, relaxed environment and regular elimination habits. Methods of scheduling elimination, increasing fluid and bulk intake and activity, and using physiologic mechanisms are provided for the individual.

PLANNING AN ELIMINATION SCHEDULE

The individual can plan an elimination schedule by recording his or her usual pattern for a week. This record should include the times of day he or she eliminates, the factors such as specific food intake which stimulates elimination (e.g., many people find coffee to have a laxative effect), and the conditions which enhance elimination. Once these are determined a regular schedule can be devised which fits into the daily routine.

ANALYZING DIET

Diet analysis for fluid and bulk intake assists the person to determine what stimulants to elimination are present in the diet and which are not. The nurse can help the person fit preferences with income and lifestyle to make up dietary deficits. Often, once aware of the influence of dietary intake in elimination, the individuals willingly adjust their diet to rid themselves of discomfort.

INCREASING EXERCISE

The effects of sedentary or decreased exercise patterns on elimination are also analyzed with the individual. Activities that are enjoyable and which can easily be incorporated into the individual's lifestyle are those which are most likely to be adopted. For example, walking up and down one flight of stairs instead of waiting for the elevator not only increases exercise but also saves time. (Illustration 20.4)

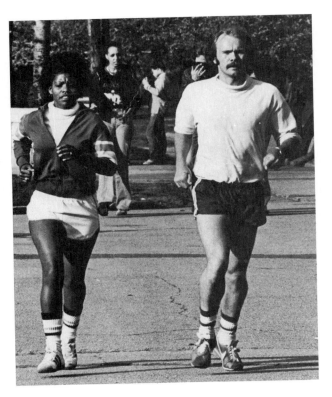

Illustration 20.4
Adequate exercise is necessary to maintain the muscles used in urination and defecation. The activities that a person enjoys are encouraged by the nurse when helping an individual to overcome the effects of a sedentary lifestyle. (Photo © Joel Gordon, 1979)

REALIZING NATURAL MECHANISMS

The nurse can teach the individual to benefit by the use of the naturally occurring physiologic mechanisms. Since food and fluids entering the stomach and intestines stimulate peristalsis (gastrocolic and duodenal-colic reflexes), the individual is taught to attempt defecation after meals. This technique is particularly effective in the morning, when the stomach is empty.

Evacuation can be enhanced by the assumption of a sitting position. Intra-abdominal pressure can be raised by the individual leaning slightly forward and with feet firmly placed on the ground. While this is important for all individuals, small children should have toilet chairs which allow their feet to completely reach the ground. The Valsalva maneuver, while increasing intra-abdominal pressure, should be avoided, since it increases intrathoracic pressure (Chap. 14). Finally, evacuating when the stimulus occurs aids in regular bowel and bladder elimination. If the stimulus is not heeded, the bowel or bladder will expand to accommodate the larger amounts of waste, and the desire to eliminate will be lost.

Assisting the Individual Confined to Bed

The individual who is confined to bed may need assistance using the bedpan or urinal.

DEFECATION

Chart 20.7 outlines the procedure for assisting the individual on and off the bedpan.

If the individual cannot sit up or assist, the bedpan may be placed by rolling the individual on his or her side (Chap. 14), placing the bedpan at the angle of the body and the bed, and rolling the individual onto the bedpan. Two people may also lift the indi-

---

Chart 20.7
Assisting the Individual On and Off a Bedpan

TECHNIQUE	POINTS TO NOTE
Obtain equipment: Bedpan, Bedpan cover, Toilet paper Soap, water, and towel	Assembled equipment helps insure organization.
Explain procedure.	Increases cooperation; decreases anxiety.
Provide privacy by closing curtains, closing door, etc.	Privacy maintains dignity of individual, increases elimination.
Raise head of bed slightly. Nurse faces side of bed so that nondominant hand is toward foot of bed and dominant hand is toward head of bed.	Gives individual support when raising buttocks.
Fold back covers.	Prevents them from hindering procedure.
Instruct to raise buttocks by digging heels into bed and pushing off with hands and arms as nurse lifts the buttocks with nondominant hand and slides warmed bedpan under individual with dominant hand.	Assists with raising buttocks. Bedpan warmed to prevent discomfort.
Position bedpan so it is centered and comfortable for individual.	Comfort enhances elimination.
Cover individual.	Maintains privacy.
Raise head of bed to high Fowler's if condition permits.	Position most conducive to elimination.
Instruct individual to flex knees and lean slightly forward.	Simulates physiologic position. (Raise side rails for individual to grasp for support.)
Place call bell and toilet paper within reach.	Allows individual method of communication; gives individual method of wiping perineum.
Leave immediate environment.	Increases privacy.
When individual is ready assist with wiping perineum if he or she is unable to do so unassisted.	Prevents skin irritation from fecal matter or urine.
Remove bedpan by reversing procedure.	
Assist individual with washing hands.	Increases comfort; decreases spread of microorganisms.
Measure and record output if necessary.	

vidual onto the bedpan. The individual is positioned in as close to the physiologic position as permitted.

If the individual can use a commode for elimination, the nurse uses the same methods as for assisting him or her to a chair (Chap. 14) and then positions the person for elimination. (Illustrations 20.5 and 20.6 show different types of bedpans, urinals, and commodes.)

URINATION

The nurse can utilize various techniques to help initiate voiding. They include placing the individual in the natural physiologic position, providing privacy, warming the bedpan, placing a hot-water bottle over the lower abdomen, running warm water over the perineum to relax muscles, running water in the sink, applying manual pressure over the bladder or digital pressure by the meatus, and forcing fluids.

Catheterization

▶ **Catherization** (the insertion of a sterile tube, using sterile techniques, into the urinary bladder) may be

ordered to remove residual urine left in the bladder after urination, to empty the bladder for surgical procedures, to prevent the contamination of wounds by urine, to empty the bladder when the individual cannot void, and for diagnostic procedures. Although catheterization is used to control incontinence with paralyzed individuals or individuals with structural failure, it should not be used in place of bladder retraining and scheduling.

TYPES OF CATHETERS

There are two main types of catheters, the indwelling (retention) catheter, which remains in place for a period of time, and the nonretention catheter, which is removed after the bladder is emptied. Urinary catheters are usually measured in the French (Fr) system—the smaller the number of the catheter, the smaller the lumen (e.g., a 14 Fr catheter is smaller than a 22 Fr catheter). Figure 20.3.A—F shows several different styles of catheters, and Figure 20.4.A shows a catheter in place. Chart 20.8 outlines the procedure for indwelling catheterization.

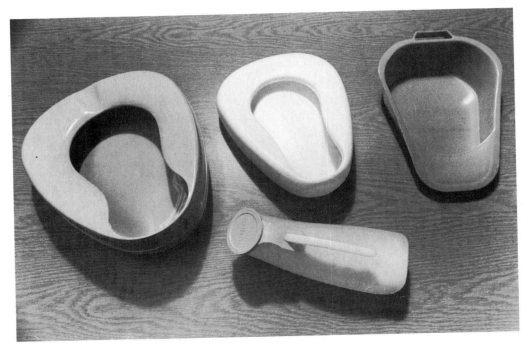

Illustration 20.5
Types of bedpans and a urinal *(Photo © Leonard Speier, 1979)*

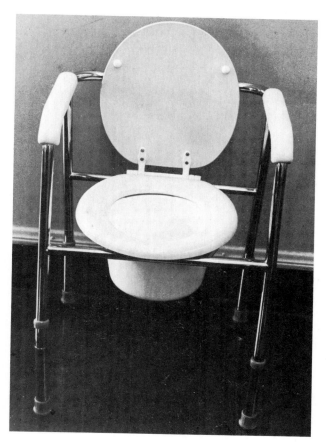

Illustration 20.6
A commode. *(Photo © Leonard Speier, 1979)*

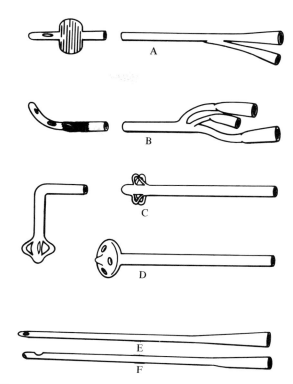

Figure 20.3
Self retaining catheters: **A.** Foley cathether; **B.** Three-way catheter; **C.** Melecot catheter; **D.** Pezzer catheter. Straight urinary catheters (not self-retaining): **E.** Round tip catheter; **F.** Whistle tip catheter.

PREVENTING INFECTION

The individual with an indwelling catheter requires special attention to prevent urinary tract infection. Fluids are forced (up to 3000 cc per 24 hours unless medically contraindicated) to keep the urine dilute and free of irritants; the drainage bag is kept below the level of the bladder and the tubing free of kinks; the system remains closed as much as possible; and the catheter must be kept clean.

The catheter can be cleansed by cleaning the perineum and labia or penis with soap and water (using backward strokes) and washing the catheter proximal to the meatus with antiseptic solution. This is done at least twice a day and more often as necessary. During the cleansing procedure, the meatus is observed for redness, discharge, and inflammation. Family and/or significant others are taught this method if the individual is to have the catheter in the home situation.

OBTAINING A SPECIMEN

To obtain a urine specimen from an indwelling catheter, the nurse needs a syringe, a needle, an antiseptic swab, and a clamp. Twenty to thirty minutes before the specimen is to be collected, the catheter is clamped above the junction between the water inflow valve and the drainage tube. The urine will collect in the bladder. At collection time, the nurse cleans the side of the urine drainage tube above the clamp (or in the collection window) with the antiseptic swab and inserts the needle at this point. The nurse then withdraws the desired amount of urine, opens the clamp, and allows the urine to flow as usual. The urine is injected into the appropriate specimen container. This method keeps the system closed, thus helping to prevent microorganisms from entering the urinary tract. The specimen that is collected is a sterile one and can be used for all types of urine testing. (Figure 20.4.A–C)

Chart 20.8
Indwelling Catheterization*

TECHNIQUE	POINTS TO NOTE
Check orders for type of catheterization.	Insures use of proper catheter.

Collect equipment:
  Sterile gloves
  Sterile catheter (usually 14–16 F for women, 16–20 F for men; size determined by size of urethra)
  Sterile cotton balls
  Sterile forceps
  Antiseptic solution
  Syringe and needle (syringe size will depend on size of inflatable balloon on catheter; usually 5–30 cc)
  Collection bag
  Tape
  Garbage bag
  Sterile drape
  Underpads
  Light
  2 sterile towels
  Water-soluble lubricant
  (All equipment may be available in a sterile package.)
	Insures organization of technique and helps maintain sterility.

Explain procedure.	Reduces anxiety; increases cooperation.
Provide privacy.	Maintains dignity of the individual.
Clean perineum and meatus thoroughly with soap and water.	Removes secretions, excretion, and surface flora.

Place underpad under buttocks.
Position individual:
  female—lithotomy position
  male—supine
	Provides best position for visualization and insertion. It may be necessary to have another staff member assist in supporting individual's legs.

Place light so it is directed on meatus.	Provides ease of reach for equipment.

If the individual is cooperative and able to maintain position, set up sterile field:
  females—between legs
  males—alongside thighs
Otherwise set up sterile field on clean bedside stand.
	Prevents contamination of equipment if individual is restless.

Open all equipment using sterile technique and place on field.	Organizes equipment; maintains sterility.
Fill syringe with appropriate amount of sterile water and place alongside sterile field.	Increases organization.
Put on sterile gloves, maintaining sterile technique.	Maintains sterile conditions.
Pour antiseptic solution on sterile cotton balls.	
Using nondominant hand, open outer and inner labia in females; grasp penis at right angle to plane of body in males.	Exposes area for cleaning.

(continued)

556

Chart 20.8 (Cont.)
Indwelling Catheterization*

TECHNIQUE

With dominant hand, pick up a sterile cotton ball
  with forceps:
    females—using a firm motion, wipe one side of the
      meatus from front to back, discard cotton ball;
      repeat for other side and middle; do not let labia
      close after cleaning; keep nondominant hand in
      place.
    males—retract foreskin of penis if present; wipe
      meatus using circular motion from center out.

Carefully observe for opening of meatus.

Lubricate catheter (distal 3–4 in.).

Instruct individual to breathe deeply. With dominant
  hand gently insert catheter into meatus using a
  rotating motion:
  females—until urine begins draining (approximately
    2–3 in.).
  males—until resistance of the internal urinary
    sphincter; stop and wait until sphincter relaxes,
    then continue insertion until urine begins to flow
    (approximately 6–8 in.).

Do Not Force Catheter.
Insert catheter another 2 in. after urine begins to
  flow.

Remove nondominant hand and connect drainage
  bag; pick up syringe.†

Connect syringe tip to water inflow valve on
  catheter.
Inject sterile water.

Pull gently on catheter. If stable, secure catheter to
  thigh with tape.

Place drainage below level of bladder, free of kinks.

Remove equipment.

Position individual.

Chart

POINTS TO NOTE

Cotton balls should not drip solution, which will
  contaminate field.
Cleans meatus.
Firm stroke in middle helps visualize meatus.
Prevents contamination after cleaning.

Cleans meatus; do not force foreskin.

A clear view aids in proper insertion.

Hold end of catheter in hand to prevent
  contamination. Lubrication reduces resistance, aids
  in insertion.

Reposition if in urethra but no flow of urine, e.g.,
  turning, sitting up slightly.

In males, internal sphincter contracts when
  stimulated.

Prevents balloon from being inflated in urethra.

Hold catheter in place to prevent it from slipping out.

Inflates balloon to secure catheter.

Assures placement.
Allow room for movement. In males, follow angle of
  penis and individual's preference. Replace retracted
  foreskin to prevent irritation and infection.

Prevents backflow and blockage; bag should not
  touch floor to avoid contamination.

Increases comfort.

Provides permanent record.

Note: Do not remove more than 750 cc at one time, to prevent shock, as rapid removal of large amounts of
  fluid from a body cavity causes pressure changes and fluid moves from vascular circulation.

*For a non-retention catheterization, the procedure is the same except that the balloon is not filled and the catheter
is removed after emptying the bladder.
†If specimens are to be collected, the end of the catheter is placed in a sterile container until the needed amount of
urine is collected. Then the catheter is connected to the drainage bag.

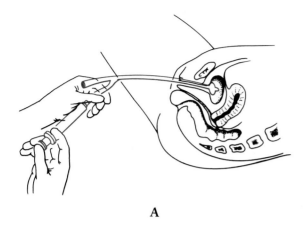

A

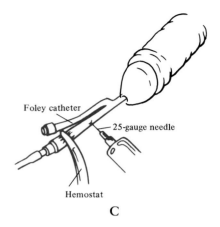

C

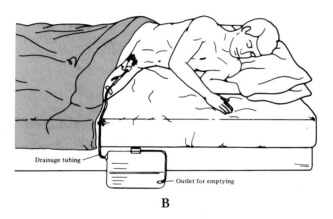

B

Figure 20.4
A. Correct technique for collecting a urine specimen from an individual with an indwelling catheter. **B.** Closed drainage system. An indwelling catheter is drained by means of gravitational force into a closed draining system. The drainage tubing is sealed in the collection container to lessen the chance of contamination in the setup, thus decreasing the likelihood of infection in the urinary tract of the individual. Most closed systems have disposable drainage bags and tubing. The tubing is not allowed to kink or touch the floor. **C.** Obtaining sterile urine specimen from a catheter. Approximately one-half hour before urine specimen is to be collected a clamp, or hemostat, is placed above the juncture of the water inflow valve and the drainage tubing in order to close off the catheter. When specimen is to be taken, the tubing is cleaned with an antiseptic solution. A 25-gauge needle is inserted into the tubing where it was cleaned, the sterile specimen is removed, and the clamp released to open the drainage tubing.

IRRIGATING THE INDWELLING CATHETER

Irrigation of the indwelling catheter may be ordered to remove particles which would block the flow of urine. Frequent, unnecessary irrigation, however, predisposes the individual to urinary tract infection. Some catheters have a built-in irrigating tube. To irrigate the catheter the nurse needs a sterile irrigating set containing a bulb syringe, a solution container, antiseptic swabs, and sterile irrigating solution (usually normal saline).

Using sterile technique, the nurse opens the irrigating set and pours the solution into the container. The catheter is disconnected from the drainage tube.

The drainage is capped with a sterile cover and placed on a clean surface. The end of the catheter is wiped with the antiseptic swab. Then 30 cc of irrigating solution (unless otherwise ordered) is drawn up in the bulb syringe. The tip of the syringe is inserted into the end of the catheter, and the solution slowly and gently instilled. The syringe is removed, and the irrigating solution is allowed to drain by gravity into a sterile basin. The procedure is then repeated according to agency policy and physician's orders. The amounts of solution instilled and returned are carefully noted. The catheter end is reconnected to the drainage tubing. Care is taken throughout the procedure to see that no part of the catheter, syringe, solution, or drainage tube is contaminated.

Care of the Individual with Diarrhea

The nursing care of the individual with diarrhea focuses on maintenance of nutrition, prevention of skin breakdown, comfort, and slowing intestinal motility. Individuals with diarrhea are losing fluids and electrolytes (Na^+, K^+, and Cl^-), and they are not getting the full benefit of food absorption. The individual is often weak and debilitated; thus safety precautions such as side rails and assistance in ambulation may be necessary. Infants and children are especially prone to dehydration and electrolyte imbalance as a result of diarrhea. (See Chap. 21 for discussion of fluids and electrolytes.)

DIET AND MEDICATION

Diets high in calories, protein, vitamins, and minerals are planned. Foods which are known by the individual to cause intestinal irritation are avoided. Intestinal motility is often slowed by eating a nonirritating diet and using antidiarrheal medications or sedatives. The individual usually receives antidiarrheal medications after each bowel movement.

SKIN CARE

The individual's skin is cleansed after each bowel movement to protect it from irritation and breakdown. Application of oil-based ointments or powder may reduce the irritation and protect the skin. Sitting in a warm tub or basin of water (Sitz baths) relieves inflammation and soothes the skin.

OBSERVING FECES

The nurse notes the frequency, amount, color, odor, and consistency of each bowel movement. The presence of loose, watery stools is carefully assessed, as they not only indicate diarrhea, but may also result from the seepage of stool around intestinal obstructions or fecal impaction.

Fecal Impactions

Fecal impactions may result from constipation or intestinal malabsorption problems. A **fecal impaction** is the presence of hard, dry stool in the lower intestine that occurs when water has been absorbed from the stool. The individual experiences a fullness in the rectum and the desire to defecate but is usually unable to expel fecal material. The impaction is usually removed by means of digital extraction and/or oil-retention enemas. Agency policy varies as to whether the nurse or the physician removes an impaction.

The individual is taught the significance of diet, regular bowel habits, and exercise in preventing future impaction.

DIGITAL REMOVAL

Digital removal is accomplished by placing the individual in a left-sided lying position (Sim's position) if permitted. The nurse inserts a well-lubricated gloved index finger into the individual's rectum and gently attempts to break up the impaction and remove the pieces by hooking the finger.

Administering Enemas

Enemas are used to empty the lower intestine of fecal material and to instill medications. The individual is taught not to rely on frequent enemas or laxatives as a regular means of bowel evacuation. (*Laxatives* are oral bowel cleansers.) Chart 20.9 lists common enemas and laxatives. Chart 20.10 outlines the procedure for giving an enema. (Figure 20.5)

Relieving Gaseous Distension

Individuals who have gaseous distension of the lower intestine (**flatulence**) may be relieved by the insertion of a rectal tube into the rectum. The tube is lubricated and inserted in the same manner as an enema tube; however, no solution is used. The tube is left in place approximately 20 minutes at a time.

The Incontinent Individual

Incontinence is the loss of bowel and/or bladder control as a result of loss of muscle tone, neurologic damage, stress, or inability to perceive physiologic signals for urination or defecation. Incontinence is usually embarrassing and a threat to the self-esteem of the individual. Negative feelings are often rein-

Chart 20.9
Commonly Used Enemas and Laxatives

TYPE	DESCRIPTION
Tap water enema	Distends the rectum, stimulating peristalsis.
Saline enema	Draws water into colon and produces increased pressure, stimulation, and peristalsis.
Soap suds enema	Irritates and stimulates colon.
Oil enema	Lubricates and softens fecal matter.
Irritant enemas	Cause localized irritation of intestinal wall, resulting in peristalsis.
Bulk-increasing laxatives	Increase fecal volume and result in stimulation.
Lubricant laxatives	Lubricate and soften fecal material.
Irritant laxatives	Cause localized irritation of intestinal wall, resulting in peristalsis.
Saline laxatives	Help retain water in intestine and draw water into colon, producing increased pressure, stimulation, and peristalsis.
Stool softeners	Wetting agents, act as detergents and mix with and soften stool.

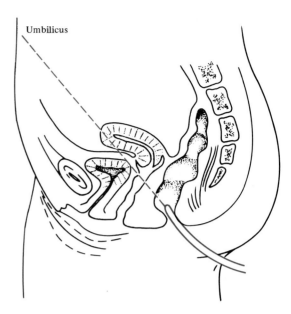

Figure 20.5

Insertion of rectal tube. A rectal tube is inserted through the anus. Point the tip in the direction of the umbilicus. Whether the tube is inserted to give an enema or to relieve flatulence, its tip is lubricated to ease passage and to avoid injury to the wall of the rectum. The tube is not inserted further than approximately 2–3 inches (5–7.5 cm.) in order to prevent intestinal damge.

at all times. Urine or feces left on the skin cause skin irritation and breakdown, are uncomfortable, and produce embarrassing odors.

RETRAINING

Bladder and bowel retraining can be effective in the majority of incontinent individuals. The nurse should note the times of day and type of each incontinency. Situations which produce incontinence such as coughing, ambulating, or food intake should also be noted. Once a pattern of incontinence has been established, the individual can be placed on the bedpan or taken to the commode or toilet when incontinence is most likely to occur.

Exercising the abdominal and perineal muscles assists the individual to increase muscle tone. Contracting and then relaxing these muscles is one method of increasing tone. If an indwelling catheter is to be removed, it can be clamped for increasingly long intervals for several days prior to removal.

forced by the attitudes of family and/or significant others and the health team members caring for the individual. The adult who is incontinent is not to be treated like a child and made to feel guilty about his or her actions. Use of diapers or any facsimile on adults are avoided. Children who are incontinent should not be punished or treated as though they were "bad."

The incontinent individual is kept clean and dry

Chart 20.10
Procedure for Enema

TECHNIQUE	POINTS TO NOTE
Check orders for amount and type of solution.	Insures proper amount and type.

Collect equipment:
  Prepackaged commercial enemas or enema set
    containing a solution container with tubing
  Lubricant
  Rectal tube if not attached to tubing
  Clamp
  Underpads
  Bedpan if individual unable to use commode or
    toilet
	Insures organization of procedure.

Mix solution if necessary: usually 500–1000 cc for adults unless it is to be retained, then 100–200 cc. (Infants, 250; toddlers, 500.)	Aids organization, decreases individual's waiting time. Use of too much solution causes damage to the bowel; too little results in ineffectual cleansing. Amount depends on size and age of person and purpose of enema.
Solution should be between 105–110 F. (Infants and children, 100 F.)	Prevents chilling or burning. Check temperature using a thermometer.
Explain procedure.	Increases cooperation; decreases anxiety.
Fill container with solution and allow it to run through to reduce air bubbles.	Prevents added air from getting into intestine.
Place pads under individual.	Prevents contamination of individual and bedding.
Place individual in left lateral position if permitted. (Supine position or sitting position can be used.)	Follows route of intestine.
Lubricate tip of tube, 2–3 in.	Eases insertion, prevents trauma.
Insert tube into rectum slowly in a rotating motion.	Eases insertion, prevents trauma.
Instruct individual to take deep breaths during insertion and to attempt to hold solution.	Enemas are more effective if solution is held approximately 20 minutes.
When tube is inserted (approx. 4–5 in. in adults; 2–3 in. in children), open clamp and slowly allow fluid to enter intestine. (Speed of instillation can be increased or decreased by raising or lowering container—container should never be raised more than 24 in. above the level of the rectum.)	If clamp is opened before tube is fully inserted, solution will flow out. Fast instillation causes cramping and may traumatize intestine. If cramping or discomfort occurs, clamp tubing; allow individual to rest; lower container to decrease flow when resuming instillation.
Clamp tubing and remove from rectum.	Prevents solution from dripping on individual or bedding.
Position on bedpan or assist to bathroom.	Allows for evacuation.
Remove from bedpan or toilet and position comfortably.	Increases comfort.
Chart results.	Provides record of procedure and results.

When the clamp is released, the individual is instructed to push out the urine as if voiding. This helps to regain the tone lost while the indwelling catheter is in place.

Withholding fluids after dinner is one way to decrease nighttime incontinence. Awakening the individual periodically during the night to offer the bedpan or remind him or her to use the toilet may also decrease nocturnal enuresis. (However, if this method is overused, it may drastically interfere with normal sleep patterns.)

EVALUATION

Evaluation for elimination focuses on the direction of change in the ability to eliminate adequately waste products via the urinary and intestinal tracts. Modification of elimination patterns, the effectiveness of nursing interventions, and the influences of elimination status on other body subsystems and vice versa are other important evaluation factors.

Specific criteria for evaluating an individual's elimination needs include:

- How do physiologic changes (in the gastrointestinal and urinary subsystems as well as others) influence elimination? Psychologic changes? Environmental changes?
- What is the relationship between presenting elimination patterns and elimination needs?
- Has the presenting elimination pattern moved closer to the expected?
- What factors may account for changes in elimination patterns?
- What are the changes in degree of interferences with elimination?
- What are the effects of changes of elimination patterns on body subsystems?
- Are there changes in knowledge (of individual, of family and/or significant others) about the influence of elimination habits on well-being? Elimination needs? Level of growth and development?
- Are there modifications of personal elimination habits?
- What skills have been acquired to assist elimination (e.g., colostomy and catheter care, enemas)?

RECORDING AND TEACHING–LEARNING ACTIVITIES

Teaching–Learning Topics

- rationale for therapeutic regimen
- special techniques (e.g., catheter care, colostomy care, enemas, care of incontinent person)
- elimination patterns at various levels of growth and development
- ways to promote, maintain, and restore elimination
- importance of exercise, diet, fluid intake, regular elimination patterns, etc., in maintaining elimination
- ways to modify personal habits which affect elimination needs
- ways to assess changes in elimination pattern
- use of physiologic mechanisms to promote elimination
- how to modify elimination pattern according to interferences

Charting

Using appropriate elimination terms, objectively describe such factors as:

- objective base-line data on elimination status, habits, preferences, interferences, level of knowledge, environmental factors, cultural factors, balance between elimination and elimination needs, level of growth and development, physical assessment
- objective and subjective changes that occur in the person's ability to meet elimination needs
- subjective assessment of changes in elimination habits and needs
- objective and subjective data on behavioral responses related to elimination needs
- attitudes toward interferences and treatments
- subjective and objective reactions and responses to treatment
- schedule and methods of care
- teachings carried out
- discharge planning done
- family and/or significant others interactions, responses, and attitudes
- degree of change in adequacy of elimination pattern

- terms individual uses for elimination patterns
- update Kardex on elimination needs

Diets to Review

- high residue (bulk)
- low residue
- bland

Medications to Review

- bulk-increasing laxatives, e.g., psyllium hydrophilic mucilloid (Metamucil)
- lubricant laxatives, e.g., mineral oil
- irritant laxatives, e.g., cascara sagrada
- saline laxatives, e.g., milk of magnesia
- stool softeners, e.g., dioctyle sodium sulfosuccinate (Colace)
- antidiarrheal drugs, e.g., Kaopectate, diphenoxylate (Lomotil)
- antispasmodics, e.g., donnatol
- antiflatulent drugs, e.g., simethicone
- diuretics, e.g., furosemide (Lasix)
- urine-acidifying agents, e.g., ammonium chloride
- urine-alkalizing agents, e.g., sodium citrate
- irrigating solutions, e.g., acetic acid

CLINICAL APPLICATION: THE INDIVIDUAL WITH A COLOSTOMY

A frequently seen alteration in the route of fecal elimination is the colostomy. The nurse encounters individuals with colostomies in the home and clinic setting, as well as in acute hospital settings. This alteration causes physical, physiologic, and psychosocial changes. Therefore, an understanding of these changes and the impact on the individual and the family and/or significant others is necessary for the nurse to intervene effectively in assisting the individual to maximize his or her level of wellness.

▶ A **colostomy** is a surgical opening in the abdomen to which a portion of resected bowel has been attached. It creates a direct conduit for elimination of
▶ fecal matter. A portion of the bowel called the **stoma** protrudes externally. Colostomies can be either temporary or permanent.

Temporary Colostomies

Temporary colostomies are performed when a portion of the bowel is inflamed or traumatized. The bowel is transected, and the portion proximate to the damaged area is brought to the abdominal surface and functions as the route of elimination. The damaged portion and the area distal to it are also brought to the abdominal surface, not to perform any physiologic function but so that healing can occur. This is known as a double-barreled colostomy. Once healing has occurred, the ends of the bowel are anastomosed (reattached) and the abdominal openings closed.

Another type of temporary colostomy is the loop colostomy. A loop of bowel is brought to the abdominal surface and partially transected. The loop is held at the surface by a glass rod which is slipped under the loop at a right angle to the bowel. Figure 20.6 shows the double-barrel and loop colostomies.

Permanent Colostomies

Permanent colostomies are performed when damage to the bowel is irreparable or when pathologic processes such as carcinoma invade the intestine. Permanent colostomies are usually single barreled, with only the functional portion brought to the abdominal surface. When the colostomy is necessitated by an invasive process such as carcinoma, the distal portion of the intestine is removed through an incision in the perineum (abdominal–perineal resection). Otherwise, the nonfunctional portion is left in place and allowed to atrophy. Figure 20.6 shows single-stoma and double-stoma colostomies.

Types of Stool

The type of stool which is produced and the degree of voluntary control the individual has over the elimination process depend on the site of the colostomies. If the colostomy has been performed in the ascending colon, the resulting stool is watery, and there is no voluntary control; if performed in the proximal transverse colon, the stool is semiliquid, and there is little voluntary control; in the distal transverse colon it is more formed, and some control may be obtained; if performed in the sigmoid or descending colon the stool is semiformed or formed, and voluntary control is possible. Individuals with no voluntary control

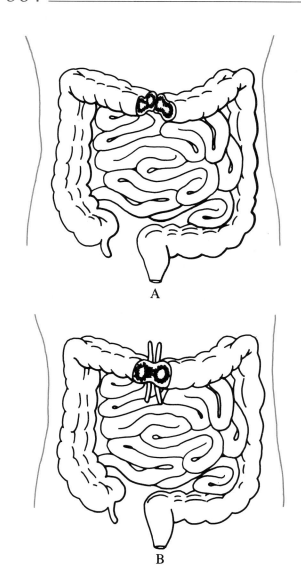

A

B

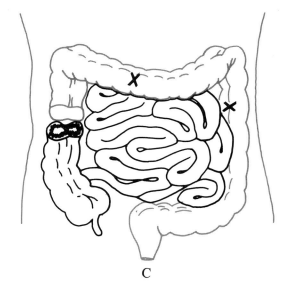

C

Figure 20.6
Colostomies. A. Double barrel colostomy; B. Loop ostomy; C. Single stoma colostomy (and ascending colostomy is illustrated; X's show locations of transverse and descending, or sigmoid, colostomies).

noise, odor, and attention. The individual with a colostomy fears that his bowel elimination is obvious to all with whom he comes in contact.

The individual also fears rejection by family and/or significant others, physical unattractiveness, sexual undesirability, and inability to perform sexually. Individuals who have any type of colostomy other than an abdominal–perineal resection will have no resulting physical interferences with sexual performance, although the psychologic stressors induced by the colostomy may interfere with sexual performance.

Grieving and Loss

Concomitant with these threats and fears, the individual will be moving through the grieving and loss process (Chap. 25), as will the family and/or significant others. The family and/or significant others may also experience fear that they will hurt the individual or be embarrassed by or unable to face the future with him or her.

Each person and his or her family and/or significant others must be assessed individually and counseled according to personal needs. Dissemination of accurate information, while not erasing fears

must wear a collection device at all times, while those with regulated voluntary control often wear only a small dressing over the stoma.

The Individual's Self-Esteem

The individual with a colostomy is often faced with a severe assault on his self-esteem and body image (Chap. 22). Bowel control is a significant value in American society, indicating independence and control of one's own body. In addition, bowel elimination frequently has negative, "dirty" connotations. It is only to be carried out in private with minimal completely, may allow the person more options and reduce misconceptions. Self-help groups such as the ostomy club may assist the individual and the family and/or significant others through this period.

Preoperative Management

Preoperative management of the individual undergoing a colostomy includes explaining the nature of the surgery, exploration of the effects it will and will not have on a lifestyle, dealing with the fears he or she has, and preparing the person physically. The family and/or significant others are included in these discussions.

Physical preparation involves routine laboratory tests, bowel preparation—including enemas, laxatives, and intestinal antimicrobial drugs—and restoring any nutritional deficits. These individuals are often in a poor nutritional state as a result of long-term intestinal dysfunction.

Postoperative Care

Postoperatively, the stoma is red and swollen as a result of surgical manipulation. It is observed for excoriation, bleeding, or signs of bulging. The stoma will shrink over a period of weeks until it reaches its expected size. Since the intestine itself has no pain sensors, subjective pain reports from the individual cannot be relied on to assess the status of the intestine.

The individual will have a nasogastric tube and be N.P.O. until bowel sounds are heard. Once peristalsis has returned, he or she will be on a low-residue, bland diet to promote rest and healing of the intestine. Intravenous therapy will be ongoing during this time. The individual is observed for fluid and electrolyte imbalance and signs of nutritional deficiences. The stoma is kept clean and covered with either a dressing or a collection bag. The drainage will be mucoid and blood tinged, but no signs of frank bleeding should be present. Fecal drainage will appear until food intake and peristalsis are resumed.

Irrigations

Irrigations of the intestine are not begun until approximately 5 days postoperatively. The physician will order when the first irrigation is to take place and

the type and amount of fluid to be used. Some temporary colostomies and those in the ascending and beginning transverse colon are not irrigated. The principles of a colostomy irrigation are the same as those for an enema. Fluid is instilled through the stoma into the intestine to stimulate peristalsis of the bowel and to flush out fecal material. The first irrigations are usually done with the individual in bed, but as soon as strength has returned, they are done with the individual sitting on the toilet.

When irrigating a double colostomy, care must be taken not to irrigate the distal portion of the bowel. This portion is not functioning for elimination and often can be damaged by the instillation of fluid. The position of the two stomas can be deceptive, so it is best to check the position with the physician.

The individual and family and/or significant others are taught to irrigate the colostomy at home. Initially, many individuals avoid looking at the stoma. The nurse is aware of clues from the individual which indicate a readiness to begin taking on responsibility. Statements such as "How does it look today" or "Exactly what are you doing" may be such indications. Every effort is made for the individual to view and begin the care of the colostomy before he or she goes home. Ostomy companies provide charts and anatomic models which can be used for pre- and postoperative teaching.

Irrigations are scheduled at the time of day which best fits into the lifestyle of the individual and the family and/or significant others. The best choice is after a meal, preferably breakfast, and at a time when the bathroom will be free for 30–45 minutes.

EQUIPMENT

A variety of equipment is available for colostomy irrigation. The equipment used will depend on the type the individual is taught to use in the hospital, the preference of the physician and of the individual, and finances. Whatever equipment is used, the basic components are a container to hold the solution, tubing, a clamp, and a colon tube. If the bulb syringe method is used, a bulb syringe and a solution holder are necessary. Figures 20.7 and 20.8 show some of the commonly used equipment and methods for using the Hollister® irrigation sets.

Many individuals with descending colon colostomies will eventually gain enough control and predictability over evacuation that irrigations and collec-

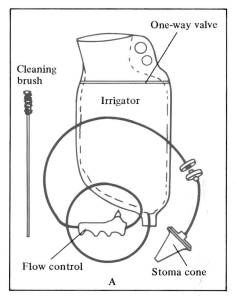
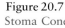

(continued)

Figure 20.7
Stoma Cone irrigation (open method). The following procedure for irrigating a colostomy will serve as a guide for the nurse in teaching an individual with a colostomy to provide self-care. *(Adapted with permission from Hollister® Stoma Cone Irrigation, copyright © 1975 Hollister Incorporated, Chicago, Illinois)*

A. Check to see that equipment or stoma cone irrigation is complete: irrigator, stoma cone, flow control, and cleaning brush. Fill the irrigator with water, first making sure that the flow control is completely closed. Use lukewarm water in the amount specified by the physician. Hang the filled irrigator so the bottom of it will be no higher than shoulder level when the individual sits down for the irrigation.

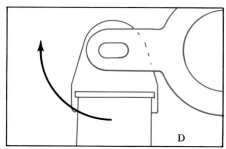

B. Pick up the stoma cone and make sure that the tube leading from it is pushed into the cone as far as it will go. The connector on the end of this tube mates with a similar connector on the tube leading from the irrigator. Push the fittings together and twist until a distinct "snap is felt."

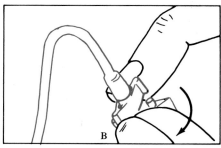

C. Gently pull a disposable stoma irrigator drain apart at the top until the blue metallic closure strip bends slightly. This will make it easy to insert the stoma cone through the open top of the drain.

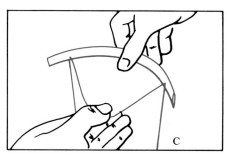

D. Fasten one end of the belt to the gasket of the irrigator drain and rotate belt into position. Buttons on belt should point away from the body.

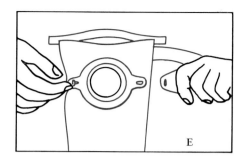

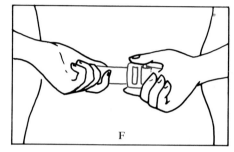

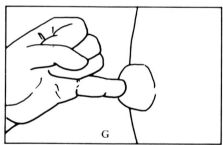

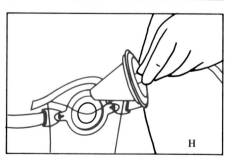

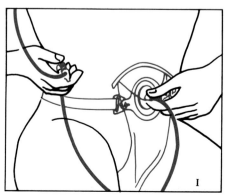

Figure 20.7 (Cont.)

E. Holding the gasket away from the stoma, wrap belt around body with soft side touching skin. Fasten loose end of belt to gasket and position gasket so it's centered around the stoma.

F. Adjust belt by moving the plastic slide adjuster. Belt should be as snug as possible, to prevent leakage. The individual sits on the toilet or on a chair next to the toilet and lets the open end of the irrigator drain hang down into the bowl.

G. If the doctor recommends dilating the stoma before irrigation: Put on the dilator glove and apply a small amount of stoma lubricant to the little finger. Gently insert gloved finger into the stoma and use a massaging motion to relax the muscles. As the opening enlarges, repeat with larger fingers for maximum dilation. If dilation is not recommended, simply apply lubricant to the stoma opening. Just before irrigating, open the flow control and let a little water run through the stoma cone into the toilet in order to drive air out of the tubing. Use of lubricant on the stoma cone is optional.

H. Insert the stoma cone and its connecting tube through the opening in the top of the irrigator drain and on into the stoma. The physician will specify how much pressure to apply when inserting the cone into the stoma; gentle pressure should be sufficient. The doctor will also specify at what angle to insert the cone so that it follows the natural course of the colon.

I. Holding the stoma cone snugly in the stoma, open the flow control and let water flow into the colon. The rate of flow may be adjusted by changing the setting of the flow control or by raising or lowering the irrigator itself. If the individual experiences cramps, it's usually because the water's running in too fast or the water's too cold. Reduce or stop the flow of water until cramps subside. When the prescribed amount of water has entered the colon, it should remain there from 5 to 15 minutes. The amount of time required varies from person to person. When the water has remained in the colon for the proper amount of time, remove the cone from the stoma and bring it out through the open top of the irrigator drain.

(continued)

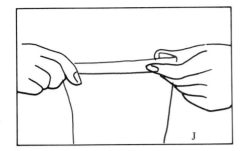

Figure 20.7 (Cont.)

J. Straighten the blue metallic closure strip. Rotating it outward, fold it twice around the top of the drain. Then fold the metal strip toward the body so it seals shut the top of the drain. After the initial return of water, it will take up to half an hour for the colon to fully empty. Gently massaging the abdomen often helps to stimulate the discharge.

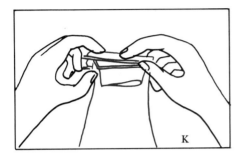

K. A drainable bag clamp seals the bottom of the irrigator drain to give the individual freedom to move about during the time between initial return and completed discharge. When the discharge is complete, unhook the belt and remove the irrigator drain. Clean the area around the stoma and dry carefully. Until the individual is well-regulated, a Hollister stoma bag may be applied in case there is any discharge between irrigations.

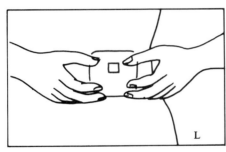

L. The Hollister stoma cap is an after-irrigation cover that is used for a regulated colostomy. About the size and weight of a folded handkerchief, it has a filter disc that deodorizes any escaping gas. The Stoma Cap will absorb any mucus or other occasional secretions.

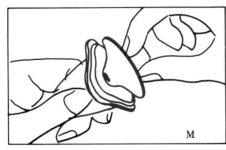

M. To clean the stoma cone, remove the connecting tube, then pop the backing disc off the cone by squeezing the sides. A cleaning brush is provided with each Hollister irrigator kit. The stoma irrigator drain should not be discarded into a toilet or into a septic sewerage system, and should be rinsed thoroughly before discarding into any public garbage collector. Or, the drain may be cleaned for re-use.

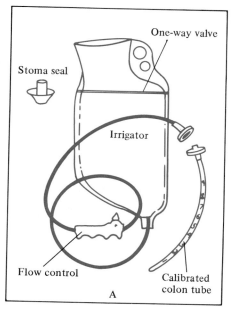

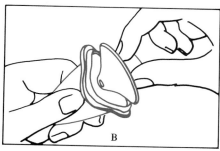

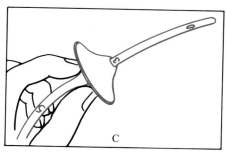

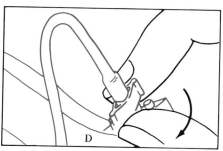

Figure 20.8
Colon tube irrigation (open method). The following procedure for irrigating a colostomy will serve as a guide for the nurse in teaching an individual with a colostomy to provide self-care. (*Adapted with permission from* Colon Tube Irrigation, *Copyright © 1975 Hollister Incorporated, Chicago, Illinois*)

A. Check to see that equipment for colon tube irrigation is complete: irrigator, stoma seal, flow control, and calibrated colon tube. Fill the irrigator with water, first making sure that the flow control is completely closed. Use lukewarm water in the amount specified by the physician. Hang the filled irrigator so the bottom of it will be no higher than shoulder level when the individual sits down to irrigate.

B. Pull the tube out of the back of the stoma cone and lay this tube aside; use the calibrated colon tube instead. The cone iself is in two parts. Pop the backing disc off the cone by squeezing the sides. This disc becomes a stoma seal when irrigating with the colon tube.

C. Push the calibrated colon tube through the back of the stoma seal disc, so the convex surface of the disc faces the tip of the colon tube. Slide disc along tube until its front (point) is at the marking that corresponds to the number of inches that the physician specified for the tube to be inserted into the colon. The doctor should also indicate at what angle to insert the tube so that the natural course of the colon will be followed.

D. The connector on the end of the colon tube mates with a similar connector on the tube leading from the irrigator. Push the fittings together and twist until a distinct "snap" is felt. If the doctor recommends dilating the stoma before irrigation: Put on the dilator glove and apply a small amount of Hollister stoma lubricant to the little finger. Gently insert gloved finger into the stoma and use a massaging motion to relax the muscles. As the opening enlarges, repeat with larger fingers for maximum dilation. If dilation is not recommended, simply apply lubricant to the stoma opening before inserting colon tube. See illustration 20.8 G.

(continued)

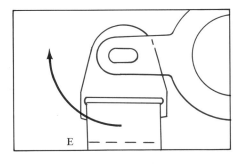

Figure 20.8 (Cont.)
E. Remove the belt and a disposable stoma irrigator drain from the box. Fasten one end of the belt to the gasket on the irrigator drain and rotate belt into position. Buttons on belt should point away from the body.

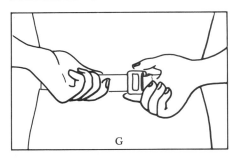

F. Holding the gasket away from the stoma, wrap belt around body with soft side touching skin. Fasten loose end of belt to gasket and position gasket so it's centered around the stoma.

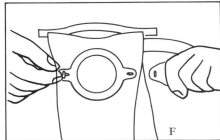

G. Adjust belt by moving the plastic slide adjuster. Belt should be as snug as possible to prevent leakage. The individual should sit on the toilet or on a chair next to the toilet and let the open end of the irrigator drain hang down into the bowl.

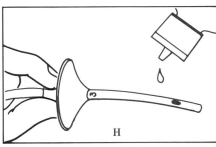

H. Hold the end of the colon tube over the toilet, open the flow control, and let a small amount of water flow in order to drive air out of the tubing. Close the flow control and coat the end of the colon tube with stoma lubricant (optional).

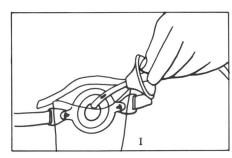

I. Pass the colon tube through the open top of the irrigator drain and very gently begin inserting it into the stoma. Proceed slowly and carefully until the point marked by the stoma seal is reached. **Do not force the colon tube.** If resistance is met, pull out a bit, release a little water, and wait a short time for the water to act. Then try again. If several attempts fail, stop and inform the doctor.

(continued)

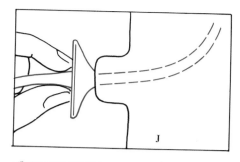

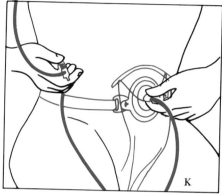

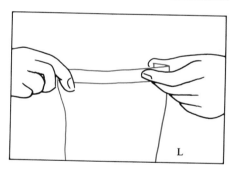

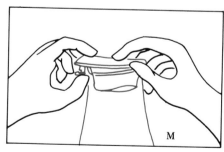

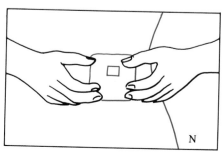

Figure 20.8 (Cont.)

J. When the colon tube is inserted to the recommended depth, the stoma seal will be pressing against the stoma. Hold it there firmly. This will keep water from flowing out before it can act on fecal matter and stimulate bowel motion.

REMEMBER:
Never force the tube into the colon.

K. Open the flow control and let water flow into the colon. Adjust the flow rate either by changing the setting of the flow control or by raising or lowering the irrigator itself. If the individual experiences cramps, it's usually because the water's running in too fast or the water's too cold. Reduce or stop the flow until cramps subside. When the prescribed amount of water has entered the colon, it should remain there from 5 to 15 minutes. The amount of time required varies from person to person.

L. The blue closure strip at the top of the irrigator drain is for sealing it closed when water and intestinal contents begin returning. As soon as the colon tube is removed from the stoma, fold the closure strip outward and downward two turns around the top of the drain. Then fold the metal strip toward the body so it seals shut the top of the drain. After the initial return, it will take up to half an hour for the colon to fully empty. Gently massaging the abdomen often helps to stimulate the discharge.

M. A drainable bag clamp seals the bottom of the irrigator drain. This will give the individual freedom to move about during the time between initial return and completed discharge. When the discharge is complete, unhook the belt and remove the irrigator drain. Clean the area around the stoma and dry carefully. Until the individual is well-regulated, a stoma bag may be applied in case there is any discharge between irrigations.

N. A stoma cap is an after-irrigation cover for a regulated colostomy. About the size and weight of a folded handkerchief, it has a filter that deodorizes any escaping gas. The cap will absorb mucus or other occasional secretions that flow from an otherwise-regulated colostomy. The stoma irrigator drain should not be discarded into a toilet or into a septic sewerage system, and should be rinsed thoroughly before discarding into any public garbage collector. Or, the drain may be reused along with the rest of the equipment.

(continued)

tion bags will not be necessary. However, they should have this equipment available in case it is needed.

Skin Care

Skin care is another major factor in the care of the individual. The skin and the stoma are kept clean from fecal material. Fecal material and intestinal secretions will result in excoriation of the tissue. Usually, frequent washing with soap and water is sufficient. A snugly fitting collection bag also prevents secretions from getting onto the skin. The opening of the collection bag is readjusted as the stoma shrinks. Figure 20.9 demonstrates the application of the Hollister® Karaya Seal Drainable Stoma Bag. Many other types of drainage bags, both disposable and reusable, are available and can be modified according to the individual's needs.

Diet

Diet plays an important role in the control of flatus and the consistency and odor of feces. Foods which are known to have caused gas or intestinal irritation prior to surgery should be avoided. The individual adds new foods to the diet, one at a time, to test their effects. In most cases, a full, regular diet can be enjoyed by the individual with colostomy.

Pre-Illness State

Once healing has occurred and the individual has regained his or her strength, clothing, exercise, and other activities can return to the pre-illness state. Educational literature is available to the ostomate conerning these areas.

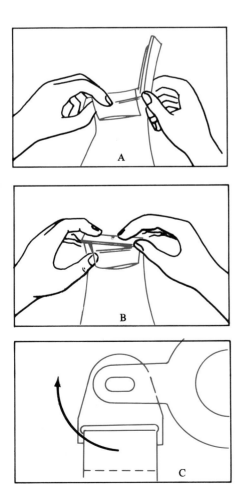

Figure 20.9

How to use the Hollister® Karaya Seal* Drainable Stoma Bag with or without adhesive square. NOTE: Instructions written in *italics* apply only to appliances with the adhesive square. You may skip over these if you are using the plain Karaya Seal appliance. Having the correct size stoma bag is essential. Measure the stoma before ordering. With a Karaya Seal appliance, the size stamped on the appliance refers to the gasket that holds the Karaya Seal Ring. The actual stoma opening in the ring is about a half-inch smaller. This overlap provides a snug, comfortable fit around the stoma. *(Adapted with permission from* How to Use the Hollister® Karaya Seal Drainable Stoma Bag, *copyright © 1974 Hollister Incorporated)*

A. Attach the plastic Drainable Bag Clamp to the stoma bag. Open the clamp by pressing the finger latch. Fold the bottom of the bag carefully around the thin, inner bar of the clamp. Be sure that the outer ends of the clamp are curving toward the inside (Karaya Seal) surface of the bag so that the clamp follows the curve of the body.

B. The bottom of the appliance should lie flat against the bar of the clamp, with no wrinkles. Fold only once. Close the clamp while holding bag firmly around the bar. Press the two parts of the clamp together until they latch securely. Test the security by trying to pull the clamp open. Thoroughly clean and dry the skin around the stoma. *Skin must be dry and free of any oily or soapy residue when using adhesive-square appliance.*

C. Some ostomates find it easier to fasten one end of the belt to the appliance gasket before putting the appliance over the stoma. Others recommend adhering the appliance firmly to the body *before* attaching the belt—particularly

(continued)

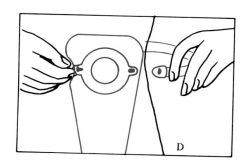

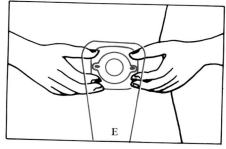

with an adhesive-square appliance. When the belt is attached, the buttons on the plastic fasteners should point away from the body. Peel the protective covering from the Karaya Seal Ring. *(But don't take the cover paper off the adhesive square.)* Hold the Karaya Seal Ring over the stoma to make sure it will fit snugly; it must be snug enough for adequate skin protection. The shape of the ring can be adjusted to some extent by warming it between the palms and then molding it with the fingers. Depressions in the skin or areas left exposed around an irregularly-shaped stoma should be protected with a layer of Hollister Karaya Paste.

D. If fitting an appliance without an adhesive square, simply press the Karaya Seal Ring firmly against the skin and finish attaching the belt. Moistening the Karaya Seal Ring slightly will make it tacky enough to hold the appliance in place while applying the adhesive or preparing to attach the belt. *With an adhesive appliance, remove the large center section of covering paper just before applying the bag to the body. The appliance may be held by the two narrow strips remaining along the sides, but do not press the adhesive to the skin until the Karaya Seal Ring is firmly in place and the appliance is hanging in the desired position.*

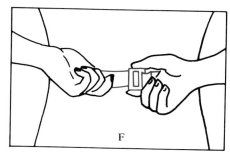

E. *With an adhesive-square appliance, first carefully smooth down the lower half of the adhesive patch. It must be pressed firmly against the skin and lie flat, without wrinkles. Apply the top half in the same manner. Then, remove the two remaining strips of paper and apply the sides of the adhesive patch to the skin.*

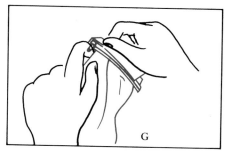

F. Adjust belt for proper fit by moving the plastic slide adjuster. Belt should be tighter when lying down than when standing. An individual may have more than one belt, and keep one adjusted for each position.

G. To empty, position appliance over toilet or other receptacle. Lift bottom of bag so contents are shifted away from clamped end. With one hand holding the bag near the clamp, use the other to push in the finger latch and release the clamp.

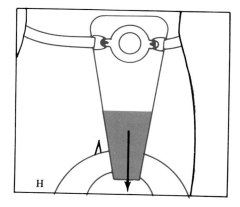

H. Allow bag to unfold downward and empty. Then, clean the outside with water and tissue and reseal as shown in A and B above. Premoistened towlettes, sold under a variety of names, are handy for cleaning the appliance when away from home. The Drainable Stoma Bag may be emptied as often as one likes. Length of wear depends on the condition of the Karaya Seal. Do not discard appliance into a sewage system. *Save* the reusable clamp.

*The Karaya Seal Ring is made from a naturally occurring gum, which will protect skin from excoriating digestive fluids, and each may vary in color. Also, the ring is softened by heat or moisture. The very properties that make karaya effective in protecting skin cause the Karaya Seal Ring to gradually break down in the presence of extremely liquid discharge. Storing Karaya Seal products in a cool, dry place will keep the seal firm prior to use. The dry indoor air of winter tends to make the Karaya Seal firmer and less tacky. Moistening the dry Karaya Seal Ring with a touch of warm water will provide the right amount of tackiness for good adhesion.

SELECTED REFERENCES

Altshuler, Anne, Butz, Marie, and Meyer, Jane. "Even Children Can Learn Self-Catheterization." *American Journal of Nursing,* 77:97, January, 1977.

Bass, Linda. "More Fiber—Less Constipation." *American Journal of Nursing,* 77:254, February, 1977.

Bates, Barbara. *A Guide to Physical Examination.* Philadelphia, Lippincott, 1974.

Black, Curtis D., Popovich, Nicholas, G., and Black, Marilyn C. "Drug Interactions in the Gastrointestinal Tract." *American Journal of Nursing,* 77:1426, September, 1977.

Blackwell, Ardith K. and Blackwell, William. "Relieving Gas Pains." *American Journal of Nursing,* 75:66, January, 1975.

Baum, Mary E. " 'I Want to Be Dry': The (Almost) Carefree Way to Conquer Urinary Incontinence." *Nursing 78,* 8:75 , February, 1978.

Chavigny, Katherine and Nunnally, Diane M. "A Comparison of Methods for Collecting Clean Catch Urine Specimens." *American Journal of Obstetrics and Gynecology,* 122:34, May, 1975.

Copeland, Lucia. "Chronic Diarrhea in Infancy." *American Journal of Nursing,* 77:451, March, 1977.

Conners, Melba. "Ostomy Care: A Personalized Approach." *American Journal of Nursing,* 74:1422, August, 1974.

Corman, Marvin L., Veidenheimer, Malcom C., and Coller, John A. "Cathartics." *American Journal of Nursing,* 75:273, February, 1975.

Cospor, Bonnie. "Physiological Colostomy." *American Journal of Nursing,* 75:2014, November, 1975.

Curtis, Christine. "Colonoscopy—The Nurse's Role." *American Journal of Nursing,* 75:430, March, 1975.

Degroot, Jane. "Urethral Catheterization." *Nursing 76,* 6:51, December, 1976.

———— and Kunin, Calvin. "Indwelling Catheters." *American Journal of Nursing,* 75:448, March, 1975.

Desautels, Robert E. "Managing the Urinary Catheter." *Geriatrics,* 22:67, September, 1974.

Dudas, Susan, ed. "Care of the Ostomy Patient." *Nursing Clinics of North America,* 2:389, September, 1976.

Eppink, Henrietta. "Catheterizing the Maternity Patient." *American Journal of Nursing,* 75:829, May, 1975.

Gross, Linda. "Ostomy Care: A Letter to Parents." *American Journal of Nursing,* 74:1427, August, 1974.

Habeeb, Majorie C. and Kallstrom, Mina D. "Bowel Program for Institutionalized Adults." *American Journal of Nursing,* 76:60, April, 1976.

Hogstel, Mildred. "How to Give a Safe and Successful Cleansing Enema." *American Journal of Nursing,* 77:816, May, 1977.

Juliani, Louise. "Assessing Renal Function." *Nursing 78,* 8:34, January, 1978.

Literte, Jean W. "Nursing Care of Patients with Intestinal Obstruction." *American Journal of Nursing,* 77:1003, June, 1977.

Malasanos, Lois, Barkavskas, Violet, Moss, Muriel, and Stoltenberg-Allen, Kathryn. *Healthy Assessment.* St. Louis, Mosby, 1977.

Sana, Josephine and Judge, Richard D. *Physical Appraisal Methods in Nursing Practice.* Boston, Little, Brown, 1975.

Watt, Rosemary C. "Colostomy Irrigation—Yes and No." *American Journal of Nursing,* 77:442, 1977.

The sea lies all around us . . . . In its mysterious past is encompassed all the dim origins of life and receives in the end, after, it may be, many transmutations, the dead husks of that same life. For all at last returns to the sea—the beginning and the end.

—Rachel Carson, The Sea Around Us

21

FLUID, ELECTROLYTE, AND ACID-BASE BALANCE

PRINCIPLES RELATED TO FLUID, ELECTROLYTE, AND ACID-BASE BALANCE

Fluids in the interstitial spaces, plasma, spinal cord, gastrointestinal tract, pleural cavity, and peritoneal cavity are extracellular (ECF).

Intracellular fluid (ICF) is the fluid found inside the cells.

Fluid balance is regulated by the kidneys, endocrine system, fluid intake, electrolyte concentration, the lungs, skin, and gastrointestinal tract.

The antidiuretic hormone (ADH) produced in the posterior pituitary is a major control of fluid balance.

The osmolarity of the ECF stimulates the hypothalamus to manufacture and relay the message to the posterior pituitary for release of ADH.

Diffusion is the movement of particles from an area of high concentration to an area of lower solute concentration.

Filtration is the movement of solute and solvent by hydrostatic pressure from areas of higher concentra-

tion and/or pressure to areas of lower concentration and/or pressure.

Osmosis is the movement of water across a semipermeable membrane from an area of lower *solute* concentration to an area of higher *solute* concentration.

Oncotic pressure is the drawing power of nondiffusible substances (e.g., plasma proteins) for water.

Insensible losses of water are those which occur through the lung and skin regardless of fluid intake or output.

Sensible losses of water are those which are regulated according to the availability of fluid in the body (i.e., urine, feces, sweat).

Sodium is the major cation in the extracellular fluid.

Potassium is the major cation in the intracellular fluid.

For fluid and electrolyte balance, the anions and cations in the extracellular fluid must equal one another and the anions and cations in the intracellular fluid must equal one another.

Aldosterone, produced in the adrenal cortex, plays a major role in sodium balance.

The kidneys are responsible for much of the electrolyte balance in the body.

An isotonic (isosmolar) solution exerts the same osmotic pressure as the fluid on the other side of the membrane and thus maintains equilibrium.

A hypotonic (hyposmolar) solution contains less solute than an isotonic solution. This reduces the osmotic pressure in the compartment where it is present, causing the fluid to move out of that compartment.

A hypertonic (hyperosmolar) solution contains a greater concentration of solute than an isotonic solution. This increases the osmotic pressure in the compartment where it is present, causing the fluid to move into that compartment.

Tonicity is controlled by fluid balance in the body and the excretion or reabsorption of electrolytes by the kidneys.

The pH of the blood is related to the hydrogen ion concentration of the blood.

The expected pH of the blood is 7.4, which is chemically slightly alkaline but is considered physiologically neutral. Thus any blood pH level below this value is considered acid, while any pH level above this value is considered alkaline.

A physiologic balance of water, electrolytes, acids, and bases is necessary to maintain an environment that is conducive to the metabolic processes which meet energy needs. In wellness, the regulatory mechanisms of the body compensate for shifts of fluids and electrolytes. For example, when water levels are low, the individual becomes thirsty and fluid is taken in; or when sodium intake is above that needed for physiologic processes, the excess is excreted in the urine. However, in pathologic states the compensatory mechanisms may not be sufficient, resulting in disturbances of electrolyte, fluid, and acid—base balances and a threat to survival. A knowledge of the fluid and electrolyte needs of the individual and the conditions which interfere with meeting these needs is essential for the nurse in order to help maintain the individual's fluid and electrolyte balance.

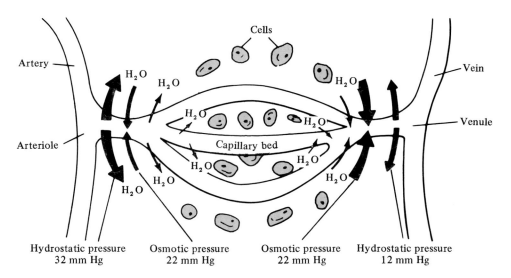

| Hydrostatic pressure | Osmotic pressure | Osmotic pressure | Hydrostatic pressure |
| 32 mm Hg | 22 mm Hg | 22 mm Hg | 12 mm Hg |

Figure 21.1

The relationship between osmotic and hydrostatic pressure is illustrated. The osmotic pressure attempts to draw water across a membrane moving from an area of lower solute concentration to an area of higher solute concentration. Hydrostatic pressure attempts to push solutes and solvents from areas of higher concentration and/or pressure to areas of lower concentration and/or pressure.

REGULATION OF FLUID, ELECTROLYTE, AND ACID–BASE BALANCE

Regulation of fluid, electrolyte and acid–base balance is dependent on unimpaired structure and function of all body subsystems, particularly the cardiovascular, urinary, respiratory, endocrine, gastrointestinal, and integumentary subsystems, as well as cellular integrity. Cardiac output is directly related to the blood supply of the kidneys and vice versa. The kidneys, in turn, help regulate the fluid, electrolyte, and acid–base content of the blood through excretion and reabsorption of these constituents. The respiratory subsystem, through its diffusion of gases and pattern of action, influences water and acid–base balance. The gastrointestinal tract helps control fluid, electrolyte, and acid–base intake, uptake, and elimination. The hormonal secretions of the endocrine subsystem—including aldosterone, ADH, and parathyroid hormone—play a major role in fluid and electrolyte balance. An intact integument helps control regulation necessary for metabolic processes and acts as a barrier to prevent fluid and electrolyte losses.

Water Balance

Water is the medium in which all the chemical reactions of the body take place. Water transports nutrients to and waste away from the cells, helps to maintain body temperature, acts as the modality in which the inorganic and organic constituents of body fluid are dissolved or suspended and maintains the pressure necessary for the transport of substances across cell membranes. Water is found in three body compartments—in the cell (intracellular), around the cells (interstitial), and in the vessels (intravascular—plasma). Extracellular fluid consists of the interstitial fluid and the intravascular fluid. Water balance is maintained through ingestion in food and fluids, production of water through oxidation, and loss of water through the kidneys, skin, respiration, and feces. Chart 21.1 outlines the balances between fluid intake and output.

The water composition of the body varies according to age, sex, electrolyte concentration, and amount of fat present. The more fat the body has, the smaller the percent of water contained in the body. Chart 21.2 compares these constituents in men, women, and infants. Infants have proportionately greater fluid needs than adults because they have

---

Chart 21.1
Balance Between Fluid Intake and Output

INTAKE (CC)	OUTPUT (CC)
Fluid intake: 1500	Sensible losses:
Fluid in food: 1000	Urine, 1600
Oxidation: 200	Insensible losses:
	Skin, 500
	Respiration, 500
	Feces, 100

---

higher metabolic rates, poorer concentration of urine by the kidneys, and a greater percentage of fluid in the interstitial spaces, which is easily lost. Infants require at least 125 cc of fluid per kilogram of body weight each day to compensate for these factors. The average adult, on the other hand, requires only 30–40 cc of fluid per kilogram of body weight each day. The obese person and the infant are more prone to fluid imbalance than other groups. The older adult may have difficulty maintaing fluid balance because of gastrointestinal tract malabsorption, cardiovascular insufficiency, changes in the ability of the kidney tubules to concentrate urine, and improper intake patterns.

REGULATORY MECHANISMS— THE HYPOTHALAMUS AND ADH

In wellness, fluid balance is controlled in two ways. The first is the thirst center in the hypothalamus. Activation of this center results in increased thirst, while deactivation results in water satiation. The second is the release or inhibition of the ADH by the posterior pituitary gland. Secretion of ADH results in the reabsorption of water by the kidney tubules. The hydrostatic and osmotic pressures help in regulating the movement of water from one compartment to another.

Electrolyte Balance

Electrolytes are substances which, when dissolved in water, decompose into ions, which are electrically charged. There are two types of electrolytes: those carrying a negative charge (**anions**) and those with a positive charge (**cations**). Chart 21.3 lists the electrolytes and their functions.

Chart 21.2
Relation of Body Water and Body Solids to Body Weight

MALE ADULTS	FEMALE ADULTS	INFANTS
The average body weight consists of approximately: 60% water* 40% fats and fat-free solids	The average body weight consists of approximately: 50% water 50% fats and fat-free solids	The average body weight consists of approximately: 77% water 23% fats and fat-free solids
Of the 60% body water, approximately: 45% is intracellular 15% is extracellular	Of the 50% body water, approximately: 35% is intracellular 15% is extracellular	Of the 77% body water, approximately: 48% is intracellular 29% is extracellular
Of the 15% extracellular, approximately: 11% is interstitial 4.5% is intravascular (Plasma)	Of the 15% extracellular, approximately: 10% is interstitial 4.3% is intravascular (Plasma)	Of the 29% extracellular, approximately: 25% is interstitial 4.1% is intravascular (Plasma)

*This figure varies with the amount of fat tissue present.
From: The Fundamentals of Body Water and Electrolytes. Copyright © 1967 *Travenol Laboratories, Inc., Deerfield, Illinois.*

Chart 21.3
Electrolytes, Chemical Symbols, and Functions

ELECTROLYTE	CHEMICAL SYMBOL	FUNCTION
Cations		
sodium	Na^+	Major extracellular cation; fluid balance; crystalloid osmotic pressure
potassium	K^+	Major intracellular cation; neuromuscular excitability; acid–base balance
calcium	Ca^{++}	Neuromuscular irritability; blood clotting; bone structures
magnesium	Mg^{++}	Enzyme systems
Anions		
chloride	Cl^-	Major extracellular anion; fluid balance; crystalloid osmotic pressure
bicarbonate	HCO_3^-	Acid–base balance
proteinates		Colloid osmotic pressure; acid–base balance
organic acids		Intermediary cellular metabolism
phosphates	HPO_4^{--}	Major intracellular anion
sulfate	SO_4^{--}	Protein metabolism

From: Violet R. Stroot, Carla A. Lee, and C. Ann Schaper. Fluids and Electrolytes: A Practical Approach. *Philadelphia, F. A. Davis, 1977, p. 7.*

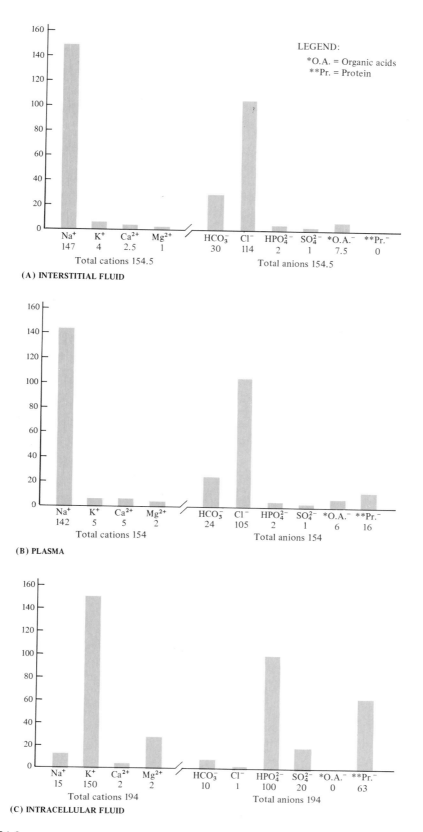

Figure 21.2
Electrolyte levels in body components. *(Reproduced with permission from* The Fundamentals of Body Water and Electrolytes. *Copyright © 1967, Travenol Laboratories, Inc., Deerfield, Illinois)*

After the first week of life, the individual attains fairly constant physiologic levels of electrolytes. (The premature infant, however, will often retain high electrolyte levels for several weeks after birth.) Figure 21.2 shows the electrolyte levels for the three body compartments. The infant, while maintaining electrolyte levels similar to the adult, has a more rapid turnover of electrolytes and thus needs more frequent replenishment.

Electrolytes are supplied through food and fluid intake. All the electrolytes are found in a wide variety of foods. However, certain foods have high concentrations of the major electrolytes. Chart 21.4 lists some of the foods with high electrolyte content.

REGULATORY MECHANISMS— EXCRETION AND CONSERVATION

The body has regulatory mechanisms which help conserve all electrolytes, except potassium, when intake is low or output is high. In the well state, the excretion or conservation of sodium by the renal tubules is regulated by the aldosterone and water levels in the body. Since each sodium ion excreted or reabsorbed in the kidney tubules is tied to a chloride

ion, the control mechanisms are the same for both. Calcium conservation or excretion is inversely related to phosphorus. As one increases, the other decreases and vice versa. The parathyroid hormone regulates the calcium/phosphorus ratio (i.e., increased parathyroid hormone results in increased serum calcium and decreased serum phosphorus). Calcium is excreted via the urine and the feces. (Illustration 21.1)

Acid–Base Balance

The pH of the extracellular fluid must be maintained within a range of 7.35–7.45 for metabolic processes and cellular functioning to occur. The slightly alkaline pH of extracellular fluid is controlled by chemical body buffers, the lungs, cells, and kidneys. These all act, in the well state, to preserve a plasma

---

Chart 21.4
Foods with High Electrolyte Content

ELECTRO-LYTE	FOOD
Sodium	buttermilk, cheese, pork products meats soaked in brine, smoked or salted meats, canned shellfish, canned vegetables, sauerkraut, olives, pickles, salted butter, mayonnaise, breads and cereals containing salt, potato chips, pretzels, canned soups, soft drinks, beer, seasonings containing salt
Potassium	concentrated meat broths, bananas, boiled meat, skim milk, orange and tomato juice, figs, prune juice, cantaloupe, legumes
Chlorides	usually in conjunction with sodium
Calcium	milk, cheese, ice cream, green leafy vegetables except, spinach, beet greens, and chard

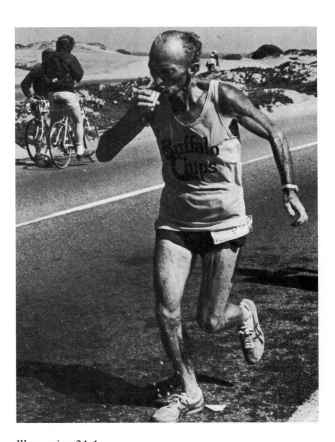

Illustration 21.1
Many mechanisms in the body work to maintain its fluid and electrolyte balance. For example, thirst is regulated by activation or deactivation of the hypothalamus, and the lungs help to control the balance by increasing or decreasing an individual's respiratory pattern. (*Photo by Bob Clay, from Jeroboam*)

bicarbonate/carbonic acid ratio of 20:1. The major chemical buffers are the plasma proteins, hemoglobin, and bicarbonate, which readily combine with acids or bases in the bloodstream to maintain the pH level. The function of the chemical buffers is to absorb excess hydrogen ions or to release hydrogen ions when a deficit is present.

The lungs act to regulate acid–base balance by increasing the respiratory pattern when carbonic acid has built up, thus releasing hydrogen ions and conserving bicarbonate. The opposite occurs when bicarbonate builds up.

When hydrogen ions build up in the extracellular fluids, the cells will increase their absorption of hydrogen ions. However, when hydrogen ions are depleted in the plasma, the cells will yield retained hydrogen ions.

The kidneys, while the slowest regulatory mechanism, are the most effective in maintaining overall acid–base balance. When hydrogen ions in the plasma are in excess, the kidneys excrete the hydrogen in the form of ammonium chloride and phosphoric acid and retain bicarbonate ions. And when hydrogen ions in the plasma are depleted, the kidneys retain the hydrogen ions while increasing the secretion of bicarbonate ions.

Response to Stress

A final factor which plays a part in the regulation of fluid, electrolytes, and acid–base balance is the body's response to stress. Prolonged physiologic or psychologic stressors result in the retention of sodium and chlorides, the excretion of potassium, and increased secretions of ADH. These responses are caused by the increased secretion of adrenocorticotropic hormone (ACTH) by the anterior pituitary. In response to this secretion, increased amounts of aldosterone, desoxycorticosterone, and hydrocortisone are produced. The overall stress response is a compensatory attempt by the body to maintain blood volume.

ASSESSMENT

Balance in Well State

When assessing the individual in the well state, the nurse looks at those factors which promote the maintenance of fluid, electrolyte, and acid–base balance. The nurse examines the fluid and electrolyte needs based on the individual's age, sex, degree of body fat, activity level, and environmental temperature to determine if the individual's intake is sufficient to meet his or her needs. Sudden environmental extremes such as prolonged heat waves will place unusual demands on the fluid and electrolyte (particularly sodium) needs of the individual. The infant, young child, and older adult are most susceptible to the effects of such changes.

When the well individual is undergoing periods of increased stressors, the nurse ascertains the effectiveness of compensatory mechanisms in maintaining fluid and electrolyte balance by observing for decreased urinary output. Since this is an expected response, the nurse explains the mechanism to the individual and no attempts should be made to counteract its effects.

The individual's fluid output, including urine, perspiration, and feces (their consistency denotes the amount of fluid lost), is compared with intake to assure a relative balance between the two. Although, on a day-to-day basis, there may not be an exact balance between intake and output, over time there will be a balance in the well individual.

Nursing assessment related to fluid, electrolyte, and acid–base balance in the well state includes descriptions of:

- the relationship of age, sex, degree of body fat, activity level, and environmental conditions to intake of fluid and electrolytes
- the relationship of these factors to intake and output
- the relationship of degree of stressors to intake and output
- subjective feelings related to fluid balance
- the relationship of personal or cultural habits on fluid, electrolyte, and acid–base balance

Interference with Fluid Balance

EXTRACELLULAR

Whenever there is a retention of fluid by the kidneys, an extracellular fluid excess occurs. This fluid reenters the vascular system, but soon much of it moves into the interstitial spaces since the pressure in the vascular system will be higher than in the sur-

---

Chart 21.5
Comparison of Intracellular and Extracellular Fluid Excesses

	INTRACELLULAR EXCESSES	EXTRACELLULAR EXCESSES
Signs and symptoms	Twitching, convulsions, changes in cognition, coma. Serum sodium levels reduced.	Excessive weight gain, hypertension, dyspnea, engorgement of neck veins, pitting edema, pulmonary edema, ascites.
Causes	Excessive water intake, hemorrhage, kidney disease, excessive tap water enemas.	Excessive administration of NaCl solutions intravenously, cardiac failure, kidney failure, cortisone therapy, liver disease.
Treatment	Restrict fluid intake.	Restrict fluid and sodium intake, diuretics.
Nursing actions	Monitor intake and output; observations of signs and symptoms.	Monitor intake and output, daily weights, observe for signs and symptoms; careful regulation of intravenous fluids.

rounding tissue. Chart 21.5 summarizes the process, results, and treatment of extracellular fluid excess.

A deficit in extracellular fluid results whenever fluid shifts to a third space or is lost from the body. A *third space* is any area where fluid collects (e.g., peritoneal cavity) but is unavailable for use by the body. Chart 21.6 summarizes the process, results, and treatment of extracellular fluid deficit.

INTRACELLULAR

Excesses and deficits can also occur in the intracellular compartment. When there is insufficient water intake or excessive water loss, fluid moves from within the cells to the extracellular compartments. This is an attempt by the body to maintain circulating blood volume and pressure to supply vital organs with oxygen, nutrients, and electrolytes.

Conversely, when there is prolonged extracellular fluid excess, some of the fluid will move into the intracellular spaces, resulting in a dilution of cellular solutes. This is an attempt by the body to prevent circulatory overload of the vascular system. Charts 21.5 and 21.6 summarize the processes, results, and treatments of intracellular excesses and deficits.

While the physiologic responses of these fluid shifts are the result of pathologic processes, they are attempts by the body to restore fluid and electrolyte balance and maintain vital processes.

Chart 21.6
Comparison of Intracellular and Extracellular Fluid Deficits

	INTRACELLULAR DEFICITS	EXTRACELLULAR DEFICITS
Signs and symptoms	Twitching, convulsions, oliguria, flushing, increased temperature. Increased serum sodium. Increased specific gravity of urine. Increased plasma proteins.	Decreased blood pressure, poor skin turgor, dry skin and mucous membranes, oliguria, nausea, anorexia, muscle weakness. Elevated hematocrit.
Causes	Insufficient fluid intake; excessive water losses.	Gastrointestinal tract losses, wound drainage, profuse sweating.
Treatment	Replacement of fluids.	Replacement of fluid with NaCl, treatment of underlying causes.
Nursing actions	Monitor intake and output; force fluids, observe for signs and symptoms.	Monitor intake and output, observe for signs and symptoms.

Nursing assessment related to fluid imbalance includes descriptions of:

- pathologic processes which may influence fluid balance (e.g., cardiac insufficiency, renal failure)
- treatment modalities (e.g., IV therapy, diuretics) which may influence fluid balance
- signs and symptoms of fluid imbalance (e.g., edema, oliguria, poor skin turgor, CNS irritation)
- the comparison between expected and actual serum electrolyte values, hematocrit, BUN, and specific gravity
- rapid changes in body weight
- comparison of intake and output records

Interference with Electrolyte Balance

SODIUM

Sodium deficits (**hyponatremia**) occur when there is either a dilution of the concentration of sodium ions or actual loss of sodium ions from the body. In the case of dilution, the number of sodium ions present in the body remains constant, but the amount of water in which the ions are dissolved increases. The serum sodium levels will decrease, since they are measurements of the proportion of sodium ions to water.

Dilution hyponatremia is the result of an increase in extracellular fluid caused by excessive water intake, retention of water through pathologic processes (e.g., renal failure, congestive heart failure), increased production of ADH, or the movement of fluid from the cells to the extracellular compartment (e.g., in diabetes mellitus). In all cases except the last, treatment is usually aimed at restricting fluid intake and promoting water output through the use of diuretics.

Actual loss of sodium ions from the body occurs in cases of vomiting, diarrhea, burns, overuse of diuretics (particularly with concurrent sodium intake restriction), draining from fistulas, and limited sodium intake (as in starvation). In most cases of actual sodium loss, there is a simultaneous loss of water. Treatment is geared at replacing sodium without further fluid imbalance.

When sodium is diluted or lost from the extracellular fluid, potassium moves from inside the cell to the extracellular compartments in an attempt to maintain electrical balance. The direction of fluid shifts will depend on whether there is extracellular fluid excess or deficit.

Sodium excess (**hypernatremia**) occurs when there is an increased concentration of sodium ions in the extracellular fluid. This results whenever more water is lost from the body than sodium (e.g., diaphoresis, polyuria), whenever there is an increased sodium intake without proportional increases in water or with the administration of hypertonic salt solutions, or whenever there is limited fluid intake.

Hypernatremia results in hypertonicity of the extracellular fluid. In an attempt to counteract this, water is drawn from the intracellular compartment. However, both the intracellular and extracellular compartments will consequently have high sodium concentrations.

CHLORIDE

The anion chloride is closely tied to the sodium, potassium, and bicarbonate ions. Sodium losses or gains usually result in chloride losses (**hypochloremia**) or gains (**hyperchloremia**). However, chloride losses or gains do not occur in a 1:1 ratio with sodium losses or gains, as sodium may bond with the bicarbonate ions rather than the chloride ions. As the bicarbonate ions in the body increase, the chloride ions decrease, and vice versa. Thus chlorides play a role in maintaining acid–base balance. In addition, chloride may bind with potassium and be excreted as potassium chloride. Therefore, potassium losses are often accompanied by chloride losses.

POTASSIUM

Potassium deficits (**hypokalemia**) result whenever there is renal or aldosterone production impairment, body fluid losses, activation of the stress response, insufficient intake, and with certain medications (e.g., potassium depleting diuretics). Any condition in which the body tends to retain sodium will result in potassium loss.

Hyperkalemia (potassium excess) occurs whenever the kidneys cannot excrete potassium (as in renal failure); whenever there is extensive cell damage, which releases potassium into the extracellular fluid; and in cases of inadequate production of aldosterone or excessive administration of intravenous potassium.

The symptoms of hypo- and hyperkalemia are very similar, and since serum potassium levels may not always immediately reflect potassium levels, electrocardiogram changes may be used to differentiate between the two in the early stages.

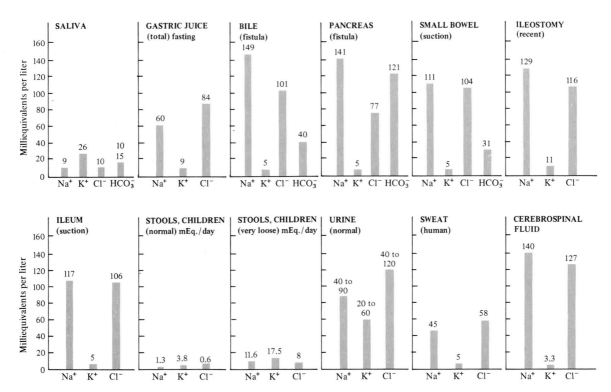

Figure 21.3
The electrolyte content of body fluids and secretions. *(Reproduced with permission from* The Fundamentals of Body Water and Electrolytes. *Copyright © Travenol Laboratories, Deerfield, Illinois)*

Correction of deficits is through replacement of potassium or prevention of its loss. Excess is treated by use of an exchange resin (hypertonic kayexalate), which increases absorption of potassium into the intestine, or by alkalizing the potassium with hypertonic sodium solutions.

CALCIUM

▶ Calcium deficits (**hypocalcemia**) may result from inadequate intake, diarrhea, wound drainage, parathyroid dysfunction, or metabolic disorders. Hypocalcemia results in bone and muscle depletion of calcium. Adequate amounts of vitamin D are necessary for calcium utilization. Treatment involves the replacement of calcium and/or vitamin D.

▶ **Hypercalcemia** (calcium excess) occurs with hypersecretion of the parathyroids, excessive vitamin D intake, or any condition which results in the movement of calcium from the bones in the bloodstream (e.g., prolonged immobilization). Treatment is centered on relief of the underlying cause.

DISTINGUISHING IMBALANCES

In all cases of electrolyte imbalance, the ultimate treatment is aimed at underlying causative pathology. Figure 21.3 shows the electrolyte composition of body secretions and excretions. Electrolyte imbalances influence all facets of the body's responses and frequently mimic one another. Differentiation is made through knowledge of the underlying pathology, treatments, diagnostic tests, and careful observation of the individual. Chart 21.7 outlines the signs and symptoms of electrolyte imbalance.

Nursing assessment related to electrolyte imbalance includes descriptions of:

● conditions which may precipitate electrolyte imbalance
● signs and symptoms of electrolyte imbalance
● serum electrolyte values compared with expected values
● effects of treatments instituted

Chart 25.7
Signs and Symptoms of Common Electrolyte Imbalances

SODIUM EXCESS

Increase in heart rate
Increase in body
  temperature
Hallucinations
Dry, sticky mucous
  membranes
Dry skin
Increase in blood
  pressure
Headache
Nausea and vomiting
Flushing of skin
Thirst
Oliguria
Increase in urine
  specific gravity
Poor skin turgor
Increase in serum
  sodium level

SODIUM DEFICIT

Thready, rapid pulse
Decrease in pulse
  volume with
  position change
Decrease in body
  temperature
Cold, clammy skin
Decrease in blood
  pressure
Orthostatic
  hypotension
Lethargy
Headache
Nausea and vomiting
Increase in anxiety
  level
Abdominal cramping
Muscle weakness
Tremors
Convulsions
Decrease in urine
  specific gravity
Decrease serum
  sodium level

CALCIUM EXCESS

Nausea and vomiting
Flank pain
Decrease in muscle
  tone
Loss of appetite
Thirst
Deep bone pain
Urinary calculi
Osteoporosis
Lethargy
Constipation
Increase in serum
  calcium level

CALCIUM DEFICIT

Crowinglike
  respirations
Voice changes
Tingling of fingers
  and toes
Muscle cramps
Numbness of
  extremities
Chvostek's sign
Carpopedal spasms
Tetany
Twitching
Increased risk of bone
  fracture
Decrease blood
  clotting
Decrease in serum
  calcium level

POTASSIUM EXCESS

Thready, slowed
  pulse
Shallow breathing
Decreased blood
  pressure
Restlessness
Irritability of muscle
Numbness and
  tingling of
  extremities
Nausea
Cardiac arrythmias
Oliguria
Flaccid paralysis
Diarrhea
Increase in serum
  potassium level

POTASSIUM DEFICIT

Thready, rapid pulse
Shallow breathing
Lethargy and apathy
Carphology
Loss of orientation
Speech difficulty
Abdominal cramping
Muscle cramps
Numbness of
  extremities
Nausea and vomiting
Decrease in muscle
  tone
Loss of appetite
Diarrhea
Cardiac arrhythmias
Decrease in blood
  pressure
Hypoactive reflexes
Decrease in serum
  potassium level

MAGNESIUM EXCESS

Decrease in heart rate
Decrease in blood
  pressure
Drowsiness and
  lethargy
Decrease in level of
  consciousness
Flushing of skin
Diaphoresis
Hyporeactive reflexes
Decrease in
  respiration
Increase in serum
  magnesium level

MAGNESIUM DEFICIT

Increase in heart rate
Increase in blood
  pressure
Depression
Carphology
Hallucinations
Loss of orientation
Hypersensitivity to
  sound
Convulsions
Insomnia
Tremors
Tetany
Twitching
Cardiac arrhythmias
Leg cramps
Decrease in serum
  magnesium level

Interference with Acid–Base Balance

Disturbances in fluid balance and electrolyte composition create alterations in the acid–balance, resulting in a change in the pH of the blood. Acidosis occurs when the pH of the blood goes below 7.35, and alkalosis occurs when it goes above 7.45. In acidosis there is an excess of hydrogen ions in the blood; in alkalosis, an excess of base. There are two types of acidosis and alkalosis—metabolic and respiratory.

METABOLIC DISTURBANCES

Metabolic acidosis and alkalosis are mainly the result of improper metabolism, resulting in either an excess or deficit in acid or base.

Acidosis

Metabolic acidosis occurs when metabolism is incomplete and an excess of acid end product results, increasing the hydrogen ion content in the blood. In an attempt to neutralize this excess acid, the circulating bicarbonate ions attach to the hydrogen ions and a relative deficit of base results. In other words, the 20:1 ratio of base to acid is altered.

Metabolic acidosis also occurs when there is an absolute loss of base from the body. This happens whenever intestinal elimination is drastically increased and the pancreatic secretions, which are high in base, are lost.

In an attempt to compensate for metabolic acidosis, the lungs hyperventilate to blow off hydrogen ions. This increase in respiratory rate results in an increased production of water and carbon dioxide by the lungs and a loss of hydrogen ions in the form of water.

Alkalosis

Metabolic alkalosis results when more alkali is taken in than can be neutralized by the available hydrogen ions, when acids are lost from the body through the gastrointestinal tract, or when potassium deficits result in the use of hydrogen ions in place of potassium. The lungs may again attempt to compensate for this imbalance through hypoventilation. Hypoventilation results in fewer hydrogen ions being lost from the body in the form of water.

RESPIRATORY DISTURBANCES

Respiratory acidosis and alkalosis result from an alteration in respiratory pattern.

Acidosis

When the respiratory pattern is decreased, carbon dioxide in the form of carbonic acid (H_2CO_3) is retained and **respiratory acidosis** results. The kidneys attempt to compensate by increasing excretion of hydrogen ions and reabsorbing bicarbonate ions.

Alkalosis

Respiratory alkalosis occurs when the respiratory pattern is increased and excessive amounts of carbonic acid are blown off in the form of carbon dioxide and water. The kidneys again attempt to compensate by reabsorbing hydrogen ions and increasing excretion of bicarbonate ions.

Charts 21.8 and 21.9 outline the process, sequelae, and treatments of acidotic and alkalotic states.

Nursing assessment related to acid–base imbalance includes descriptions of:

- conditions which may precipitate acidosis or alkalosis
- the type of acid–base imbalance
- compensatory mechanisms present
- pertinent lab values
- signs and symptoms of acidosis or alkalosis
- effects of therapies

Physical Assessment

Physical assessment of an individual in relation to fluid, electrolyte, and acid–base balance centers around observation of the state of hydration, mental status, identification of areas of losses such as fistulas and draining wounds, measurement of vital signs and weight, and testing for neuromuscular irritability. The specific physical assessment of body subsystems is determined by the underlying cause of imbalance and other factors in the individual's situation. The student is referred to Chapter 7 for specific techniques.

Diagnostic Tests

SERUM ELECTROLYTE LEVELS

Serum electrolyte levels are one of the major measurements done to determine the amount of electrolytes present in the blood. There is no readily

Chart 21.8

A Comparison of Metabolic Acidosis and Respiratory Acidosis

	METABOLIC ACIDOSIS	RESPIRATORY ACIDOSIS
Signs and symptoms	Nausea, vomiting, diarrhea, headache, changes in level of consciousness, muscle twitching, increased rate and depth of respirations, tremors, convulsions. Blood pH lowered. Serum CO_2 levels lowered. Plasma O_2 levels usually within normal limits serum potassium elevated, bicarbonate ion to carbonic acid ratio 8:1.	Shallow respirations, weakness, changes in level of consciousness, cardiac arrhythmias, e.g., tachycardia. Blood pH lowered. Plasma CO_2 increased. Plasma O_2 values can be normal or decreased, serum potassium increased, carbonic acid to bicarbonate ion ratio 13:1.
Causes	Renal insufficiency, ketoacidosis, starvation, hypoxia, diarrhea, severe infections.	Morphine and barbiturate overdoses, chronic organic pulmonary disease, CNS depression.
Treatment	Treat underlying pathology, administration of sodium bicarbonate (IV), maintain fluid balance at appropriate levels, increase carbohydrate intake for energy and conservation of fats and protein.	Treat underlying pathology, improve ventilation through IPPB, mechanical respiration.
Nursing actions	Monitor intake and output, seizure precautions, observe for signs and symptoms.	Maintain airway patency, promote increased ventilation through coughing, deep breathing, and exercise, observe for signs and symptoms.

Chart 21.9

A Comparison of Metabolic Alkalosis and Respiratory Alkalosis

	METABOLIC ALKALOSIS	RESPIRATORY ALKALOSIS
Signs and symptoms	Decreased respirations, tetany, convulsions, hyperactive reflexes, nausea, vomiting, diarrhea. Blood pH increased. Serum CO_2 increased. Serum potassium and chloride decreased. Plasma O_2 normal.	Rapid respirations, changes in level of consciousness, numbness. Blood pH increased. Plasma CO_2 decreased. Plasma O_2 normal. Alkaline urine. Serum potassium decreased.
Causes	Gastrointestinal tract loss, severe diuresis, Cushing's disease.	Hyperventilation, salicylate intoxication.
Treatment	Treat underlying cause, administration of NaCl (IV), potassium replacement.	Treatment of underlying pathology, rebreathing.
Nursing actions	Monitor intake and output. Promote diet high in chloride and potassium. Observe for signs and symptoms.	Promote rest, relieve anxiety, observe for signs and symptoms.

Chart 21.10

Expected Values Related to Fluid
Serum Electrolyte Balance

ELECTROLYTE	RANGE
Na	135–145 mEq/l. blood
Cl	95–105 mEq/l. blood
K	3.5–5.0 mEq/l. blood
Ca	4.5–5.8 mEq/l. blood
Mg	1.4–2.3 mEq/l. blood
P	2.5–4.5 mg
HCO₃	24–30 mEq/l. blood in
(Circulating	adults;
CO₂)	18–27 mEq/l. blood in
	children
Protein	14–19 mEq/l. blood
HPO₄	1.7–2.6 mEq/l. blood
Organic acids	
Lactic acid	0.9–1.9 mEq/l. blood
Total organic	2–10 mEq/l. blood
acids	

available direct way of measuring intracellular electrolyte levels, but the serum values do indirectly reflect those levels. Chart 21.10 lists the expected serum electrolytes ranges.

A complete battery of serum electrolyte tests requires approximately 10 ml of blood. This may seriously compromise the circulatory volume of the small infant (particularly if the tests are repeated within a short period of time); therefore, smaller amounts may

have to be used and special care must be taken so that specimens are not lost or spoiled and that testing is not unnecessarily repeated.

CARBON DIOXIDE COMBINING POWER

The carbon dioxide combining power test is one of the most useful in determining acid–base balance. This test is done by exposing the plasma of the blood to 7 percent carbon dioxide. When the plasma reaches a physiologic level of carbon dioxide, the amount of carbon dioxide is measured in the form bicarbonate. The expected value is 24–35 mEq/liter of blood. An increase of this value reflects metabolic alkalosis, while a decrease reflects metabolic acidosis.

NURSING DIAGNOSIS

A 10-month-old boy, Dee, is brought to the pediatric emergency room by this mother. She says he has had diarrhea for the past 24 hours.

The following nursing assessment compares the presenting (actual) behaviors of 10-month-old Dee that reflect a fluid, electrolyte, and acid–base imbalance with those behaviors that the nurse would expect to find in an infant of similar growth and development as Dee but who has no interference in fluid and electrolyte balance.

ASSESSMENT FACTOR	EXPECTED BEHAVIORS	PRESENTING BEHAVIORS
Number of stools	One to two	Five
Consistency of stools	Formed or semiformed	Watery. Mother states, "It's just running out of him."
Contributing factors	Infection; food irritation; increased intestinal motility	Mother states he had apple juice added to his diet the previous day. No other known contributing factor.
Activity level	Playful, active	Lethargic. "He just wants to be held."
Mood	Cheerful and friendly as long as with mother and/or significant others	Whining, crying
Thirst	—	Eagerly grabs for bottle and rapidly drinks contents.

(continued)

ASSESSMENT FACTOR	EXPECTED BEHAVIORS	PRESENTING BEHAVIORS
Temperature	99.6 F (rectal)	101 F (rectal)
Pulse	100 (approx.)	110
Respirations	20–40	32, regular
Mucous membranes	Well-hydrated, pink	Dry, pink
Fontanels		
Anterior	Closes 8–18 months	Closed
Posterior	Closes 2–3 months	Closed
Eyeballs	Not sunken	Same
Urine output	Frequent, copious	"I can't really tell because the diaper is wet from diarrhea."
Skin turgor	Resilient	Resilient
Weight	Triple birth weight	25 lb at doctor's visit last week; 24.0 lb at present
Neuromuscular status	No twitching; hand–mouth coordination; sits alone	Same
Diagnostic tests	—	None taken
Medical diagnosis	—	Diarrhea probably related to reaction to apple juice
Medical orders		1. No solid food except soda crackers until diarrhea stops × 2 days; then resume diet as tolerated 2. Coca-Cola as desired 3. Return to clinic if symptoms do not subside within 48 hours or if condition worsens

The resulting nursing diagnoses for this situation might include:

- mild isotonic dehydration related to intestinal irritation
- decreased energy level related to fluid and nutritional loss
- elevated temperature related to fluid loss

PLANNING

Planning for fluid, electrolyte, and acid–base imbalances focuses on directing intervention toward replacement of specific losses, prevention of further losses, treating the underlying pathologies, decreasing excesses, and prevention of further gains. Promotion of comfort, safety, and nutrition are also major planning goals.

The care plan for one of the nursing diagnoses listed above in the situation of 10-month-old Dee might look like that on page 590.

INTERVENTION

Treatment of underlying pathologies of fluid, electrolyte, and acid–base imbalance and prevention of their sequelae are the major thrust of nursing intervention.

Intake and Output Measurement

Whenever an individual has an alteration in fluid and electrolyte balance, his or her intake and output are monitored. Intake and output are monitored by

NURSING DIAGNOSIS	GOALS	PLAN

Mild isotonic dehydration related to intestinal irritation	*Short term:*
	
	Decreased number of stools within 24 hours
	
	Increased fluid intake to 175 ml/kg body weight/day
	
	(10.9 kg × 175 = 1908 ml) within 24 hours
	
	Mother to withhold apple juice until child is older
		1. Explain need for food restriction.
		
		2. Explain action of Coca-Cola
		  a. replaces fluid
		  b. replaces K^+
		  c. supplies glucose.
		
		3. Explain action of soda crackers
		  1. decreases hunger
		  2. supplies Na and Cl.
		
		4. Devise schedule of round-the-clock Coca-Cola intake
		
		5. Teach signs and symptoms of dehydration and ask for return to clinic if symptoms appear.
		
		6. Explore knowledge of introducing new foods.
		
		7. Reinforce areas of knowledge.
		
		8. Supplement other areas of knowledge as needed.

	Long term: Decreased irritation of intestines by food	As above 6–8.

measuring all fluids which are taken into the body and all fluid output. Measurements are recorded on an I & O sheet. Fluid intake includes all fluids taken in by mouth, parenterally, and through irrigation and tube feedings. Output includes urine output (through either a catheter or urination), drainage, hemorrhaging, vomitus, and liquid stool. Often the physician will order intake and output measurements, but the nurse can independently initiate this action whenever the nurse feels they should be evaluated. Indications for intake and output (I & O) measurement follow:

- diuretic therapy
- surgery
- removal of indwelling catheter
- IV therapy
- nasogastric therapy, gastrostomy or jejunostomy
- tube feeding
- stress states
- fever burns
- draining wounds
- cardiovascular disease
- renal disease
- urinary tract dysfunction
- hormonal imbalance
- neurologic dysfunction

- anorexia
- vomiting
- diarrhea
- dehydration/overhydration
- altered intake and output patterns
- hyperalimentation

Food such as ice cream, sherbert, gelatin, ice pops, ice chips, consommé, and cream soups are included in fluid intake.

Fluid intake is usually measured according to each specific agency's standard for the fluid volume of containers. However, in certain circumstances, it may be necessary to more accurately measure intake by use of graduated containers.

Output is measured in graduated containers. Sometimes when the individual is incontinent, has draining wounds, is hemorrhaging, or has vomited, output is estimated by weighing linen or pads or by stating the number of pads used. (Illustration 21.2)

I & O SHEETS

Whenever the person takes in or puts out fluid, it is recorded by amount, type, and time. Intake and

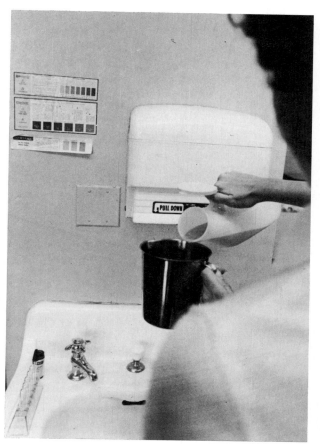

Illustration 21.2

The nurse pours urine from an individual's urinal into a graduated container so that a record may be kept of the person's urine output. *(Photo © Leonard Speier)*

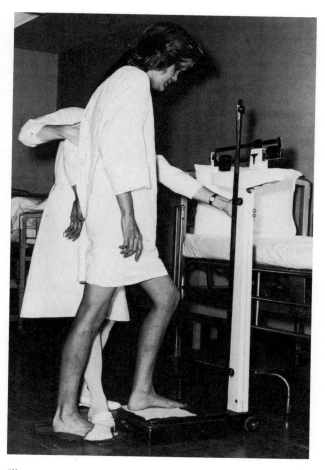

Illustration 21.3

An accurate measurement of intake and output may be obtained if an individual is weighed at the same time each day and with the same clothes on. A weight gain or loss of 0.5 kg within 24 hours indicates a water gain or loss. *(Photo from Lester V. Bergman & Assoc.)*

output is subtotaled at least every eight hours and a grand total is calculated every 24 hours. In this way the distribution of fluid throughout the day can be ascertained. This is particularly important with individuals who have fluid restrictions or who are having forced fluids. In such cases fluids can be scheduled throughout the day so that sleep patterns and individual preferences are not drastically interrupted. Fluid intake should be divided to accommodate meals, fluid with medication, IVs, and to prevent thirst. Figure 21.4 shows an example of an intake and output sheet.

The nurse alerts the individual and the family and/or significant others when an individual's intake and output are being measured so that they can report any fluid intake or output. They can be taught to measure and record I & O.

WEIGHING THE INDIVIDUAL

A person's weight directly reflects the amount of fluid retained by the tissues rather than simply indicating the amount of fluid ingested and eliminated. In addition, measuring of intake and output often doesn't account for losses through respiration, perspiration, and defecation. The individual is weighed at the same time each day preferably after voiding and before breakfast. This gives the individual's minimum daily weight which is not influenced by input for that particular time.

The person is weighed wearing the same type of clothing. A separate hospital gown can be kept for the individual for this purpose. Clothing can be weighed separately and their weight subtracted from the total weight. An unaccounted-for weight gain or loss of 0.5 kg within a 24-hour period is indicative of water gain or loss, not a sign of calorie intake changes. (Illustration 21.3)

Weighing is particularly useful in measuring intake and output in infants, small children, and incontinent individuals. In pathophysiologic conditions, such as metabolic and cardiovascular disorders,

weighing is necessary to accurately determine fluid balance changes. When fluid loss or gain is expected or desired, as in diuretic therapy, a baseline weight is important to determine the effectiveness of therapy. Frequently, weighing and measurement of intake and output are done in conjunction to give a complete picture of fluid intake, retention, and output. Movable stretcher scales are fequently used for individuals who are unable to stand or ambulate.

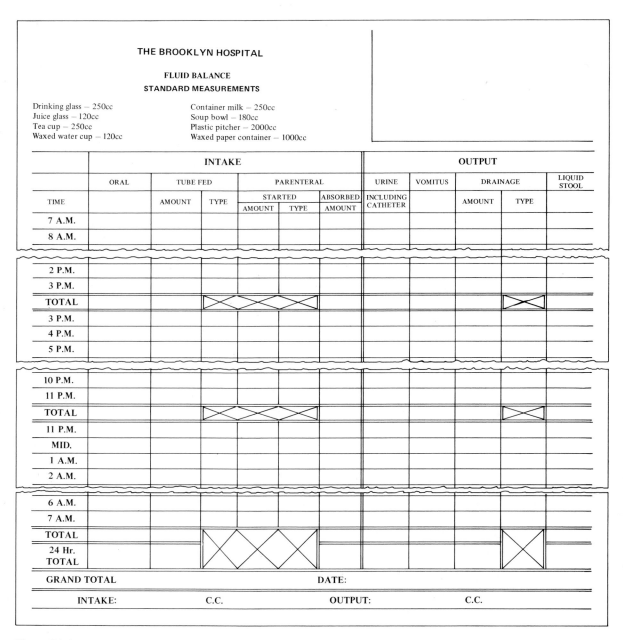

Figure 21.4
Intake and output sheet. *(Courtesy of The Brooklyn Hospital)*

Intravenous Therapy

Intravenous therapy is used to restore and maintain fluid and electrolyte balance, prevent fluid and electrolyte loss, and provide a route for administration of medications into the bloodstream. Although many health professionals view IV therapy as a means of maintaining nutrition, the actual nutritional value of routine IV therapy is minimal (Chap. 19).

INSERTION SITES

The veins of the forearm and dorsum of the hand are the most common insertion sites in adults, while the superficial veins in the temporal area of the skull are used with infants and small children. Inserting an IV is a sterile technique—sterile in order to prevent entry of pathogens into the bloodstream.

EQUIPMENT

Equipment needed for starting an IV is the prescribed IV solution, tubing with drip chamber, needle (straight or butterfly) or catheter, prepping antiseptic solution, tourniquet, IV pole, tape (preferably hypoallergenic), and an armboard. An armboard is used to immobilize the arm and prevent dislocation of the needle.

Figures 21.5–7 outline the procedures for preparing the IV solution and tubing, inserting the IV,

1. Remove overseal

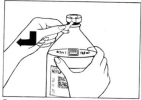

Downward, Clockwise. Grasp the tab. Remove the overseal by tearing downward *and to one side* (clockwise, when looking down on the bottle.)

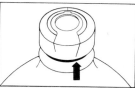

Note that Abbott cuts the tab farther along one side (arrow) than the other. Thus when you tear down and to one side, there's little chance of accidentally breaking off the tab.

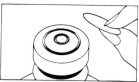

Now Lift Disk. Remove the metal disk to expose the rubber stopper.

2. Prepare Venoset

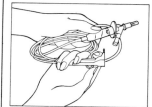

Close Clamp. Remove the Venoset from its carton, but leave it coiled for easy handling. Close flow control clamp, so air drawn into the bottle must enter through the filter.

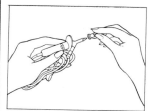

Expose Pin. Remove piercing pin cover, being careful to preserve sterility.

3. Attach Venoset

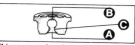

This cross section shows the inner channel (A) of the Abbo-Vac stopper. Note that only a thin upper portion (B) is to be pierced. A friction ring (C) holds piercing pin securely after penetration.

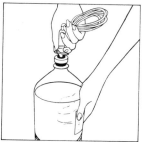

Insert Piercing Pin. in. Rest bottle on a firm surface. Hold as shown, with heel of your hand uppermost (this way you'll be able to invert the bottle without changing grip). Thrust piercing pin through bull's-eye. Do not twist or angle.

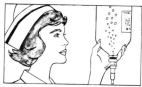

Invert Immediately. A low hiss indicates vacuum as the pin penetrates the rubber stopper. To establish proper level in drip chamber (half full) automatically, invert bottle without hesitation. Rising, filtered bubbles demonstrate vacuum. Discard any bottle without vacuum, unless vacuum was previously expended in adding supplemental medications.

4. Attach needle, and prime

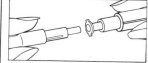

Maintaining Sterility. remove the covers from Venoset needle adapter and from needle hub. (Leave needle itself covered until ready for venipuncture.) Attach needle and uncoil tubing.

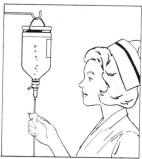

Open Flow Control Clamp. to clear air bubbles from tubing, then close the clamp. Check that drip chamber is half full. If necessary to increase level, squeeze chamber, to reduce level, close clamp, turn bottle upright and squeeze chamber.

Set is now ready for use.

I.V. sets should be changed within 24 hours.

HOW TO ATTACH THE VENOSET®

Figure 21.5
Preparing intravenous solution and tubing. *(Courtesy of Abbott Laboratories, Chicago, Illinois)*

RECOMMENDED PROCEDURES—

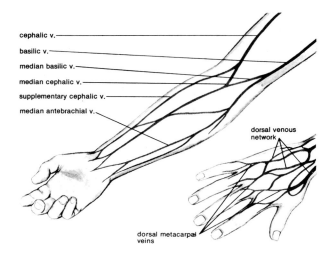

cephalic v.
basilic v.
median basilic v.
median cephalic v.
supplementary cephalic v.
median antebrachial v.

dorsal venous network

dorsal metacarpal veins

1. Vein selection and preparation. Although most superficial veins are suitable for I.V. infusion, those in the forearm are among the best. They are relatively straight, visible, and easily stabilized. They are preferred to those in the antecubital fossa for prolonged infusion because they don't interfere with elbow movement. Other suitable veins are located in the back of the hand and in the upper arm. Veins of the ankle and foot are generally least preferred because of the increased potential for thrombophlebitis and embolism. Veins showing marked varicosity at or above the injection site should not be used.

After selecting the vein, prepare the site. Apply a tourniquet, distend vein and thoroughly cleanse venipuncture site. The dorsum of the hand is well supplied with veins suitable for small and medium-size infusion sets. In the forearm, basilic, cephalic and median antebrachial veins offer convenient sites for larger infusion sets.

The Butterfly® Winged Infusion set:

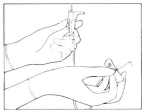

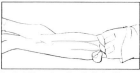

2. Prime set. Connect adapter of Butterfly set to administration set. Clear all air from tubing and needle by loosening clamp and expelling some fluid from open end of needle guard. Close clamp. Remove guard.

3. Stabilize vein. Steady limb with one hand. Stretch skin and anchor vein using slight thumb or finger pressure over skin surface just below injection site.

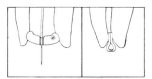

4. Grasp wings with bevel up, molded gauge number facing *up* on *left wing*. Squeeze wings firmly together.

The Abbocath-T®

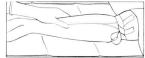

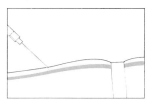

2. Stabilize vein. Steady limb with one hand, using slight thumb or finger pressure over skin surface just below injection site, to stretch and anchor vein.

4. Pierce skin. Holding needle at 45° angle to skin surface, firmly pierce skin and underlying tissue to reach but not penetrate vein.

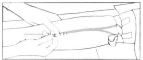

3. Remove needle guard and position needle tip slightly to one side of vein, about ½ inch below site selected for entering vein proper, bevel up. Point needle in direction of venous flow (toward shoulder). Note: Do not disengage needle and catheter prior to venipuncture as this can disrupt tip fit.

Figure 21.6

Inserting I.V. needle, and caring for injection site. *Courtesy of Abbott Laboratories, Chicago, Illinois. (continued)*

and calculating the flow rate of the IV. The IV tubing and bottle are changed at least every 24 hours, while catheters are changed every 48 hours, although this may be extended for individuals with few available veins.

CHANGING SOLUTION BOTTLES

IV bottles are changed whenever the solution runs out, when new IVs are ordered, when the bottle has been hanging for more than 24 hours, or whenever contamination is possible (e.g., when the IV system has been disconnected). When the solution in the hanging bottle is low, usually about 150 cc (the amount will depend on the flow rate), the nurse checks the physician's orders and prepares a new bot-

tle. The nurse takes the replacement bottle to the bedside and when the solution has reached the neck of the hanging bottle, closes the clamp on the tubing. The nurse then removes the hanging bottle from the hook, turns it right side up, and detaches the drip chamber and tubing, using aseptic technique. Care is taken not to squeeze the drip chamber. The drip chamber and tubing are now connected to the replacement bottle. This bottle is inverted and hung on the hook. The solution level in the drip chamber is adjusted and the clamp opened. The flow rate is regulated according to the amount of solution, the drip factor, and the time it is to run. The amount of fluid infused from the old bottle is recorded; the time of replacement and the amount and type of solution in the replacement bottle are also charted.

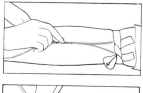

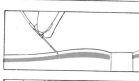

5. Position needle tip slightly to one side of vein, about ½ inch below site selected for entering vein proper. Point needle in direction of venous flow (toward shoulder).

6. Pierce skin. With needle at 45° angle above skin surface, firmly pierce skin and underlying tissue to reach, but not penetrate vein.

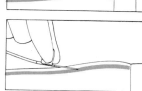

7. Lower needle shaft until almost flush with skin surface and move tip directly over vein. Then, pierce and enter vein carefully, verifying entry by flashback of blood into clear plastic tubing.

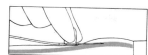

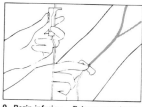

8. Advance needle. Cautiously move needle well into the vein, simultaneously lifting wings slightly upwards to avoid piercing opposite wall.

9. Begin infusion. . Release tourniquet. Release Butterfly wings and hold set flat against skin. Temporarily open administration set clamp to check for free flow, then partially close clamp.

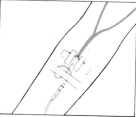

10. Anchor set. Tape each wing parallel to the needle and tape protective loop of tubing to the skin. For added security tape may also be applied across the wings at a 90° angle. Finally, adjust clamp to prescribed administration rate.

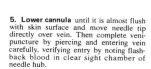

5. Lower cannula until it is almost flush with skin surface and move needle tip directly over vein. Then complete venipuncture by piercing and entering vein carefully, verifying entry by noting flashback blood in clear sight chamber of needle hub.

6. Lower : Abbocath-T ¼ inch to position plastic catheter inside lumen of vein.

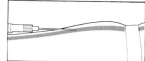

Advance ¼″

7. Advance catheter. Disengage catheter from needle hub and cautiously advance plastic cannula well into the vein. Hold needle hub firmly in place. *Do not advance needle.* (In the event of a tight fit between needle and catheter, grasp catheter hub firmly and rotate needle to loosen.)

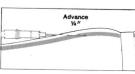

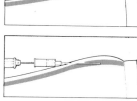

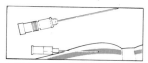

.8. Withdraw and discard needle when catheter is properly positioned in the vein.

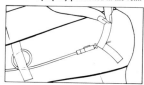

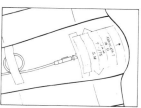

10. Apply sterile dressing, recording location of catheter tip, type of catheter, gauge size, date, time of insertion and your initials on taped surface. Change dressing daily, using aseptic technique.

9. Begin infusion. . Immediately attach a primed I.V. set to the exposed hub of the Abbocath-T catheter. Release tourniquet and open clamp on I.V. set to check for unimpeded flow. Tape catheter as shown, with chevron around cannula and hub. Cross tape and tape in a safety loop for added security.

Figure 21.6 (Cont.)

If the IV bottle is not changed before all the solution runs out of the drip chamber, air is introduced into the tubing. The above method is one way of preventing this. However, attaching a secondary bottle is another time-saving practice, if the IV solutions are compatible and the sequence of infusion is not important. Figure 21.8 illustrates how to set up a secondary system.

WITHDRAWING THE NEEDLE

To remove an IV needle or catheter, the nurse needs an antiseptic pad and a small dressing. The nurse explains the removal process to the individual, clamps off the tubing, and gently removes all dressings and tape from the insertion site. The nurse then places the antiseptic pad firmly over the point of insertion and withdraws the needle or catheter with a single, steady motion, keeping the needle parallel to the skin. Once the needle is removed, the nurse places firm pressure over the site with the antiseptic pad until any bleeding stops. The site is then dressed with a small bandage.

CARE OF THE INDIVIDUAL WITH AN IV

The individual who has an IV may feel restricted, uncomfortable, or frightened by the procedure. A

1. Calculate flow rate

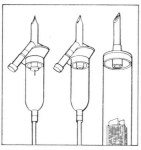

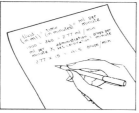

How much blood or solution does the patient need? Over what period of time? Be sure you have a physician's instructions for *both* of these variables.

Check calibration of I.V. set being used. Regular Abbott I.V. sets are calibrated at 15 drops per milliliter, Microdrip® sets at 60 drops, blood sets at 10 drops.

To find flow rate in milliliters per minute, divide total fluid volume (in milliliters) by total time of infusion (in minutes). To find drops per minute, multiply this figure by the calibration of the set.

®MICRODRIP–Drop-forming nozzle, Abbott.

2. Start infusion, adjust clamp

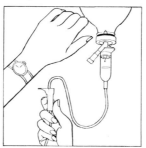

Release clamp on set slowly and adjust until proper drop count is established.

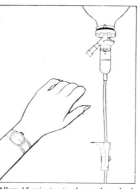

Allow 15 minutes to elapse, then check drop count again and readjust as necessary to maintain proper flow. Thereafter, check drop count every hour.

3. Watch for change!

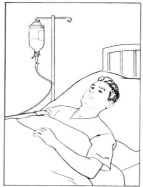

Check occasionally to see if patient has raised or lowered bed, or if I.V. stand has been repositioned. Any change in distance from venipuncture site to I.V. bottle will affect delivery of fluid. Flow rate will decrease if patient is raised or if bottle is lowered, increase if patient is lowered or if bottle is raised. When I.V. tubing is stretched or tugged, all manual flow control clamps may lose flow control effectiveness. Precautions such as anchoring the tubing below the clamp (as shown above) and using sets with tubing of sufficient length should be observed.

4. Check for free I.V. flow

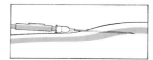

Slow flow: May mean that needle pathway is partly obstructed by blood clot, or solution has infiltrated the tissue surrounding the vein. Adjust position of needle inside vein. If original flow rate cannot be reestablished, a new venipuncture may be necessary.

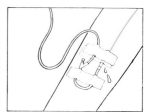

Fast flow: Patient may have manipulated tubing, or needle may have pulled out of venipuncture site unnoticed under tape or dressing. Examine site. Make new venipuncture (with new I.V. equipment) if necessary.

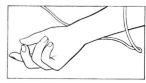

No flow: Check for kinked tubing. Patient may be lying on tubing. Or flow through tubing is completely blocked as above.

When adding medication: Remember that change in the viscosity of the I.V. fluid may affect flow rate. After adding medication, check drop count and readjust flow clamp as necessary.

I.V. FLOW RATES

Figure 21.7
Calculating and adjusting I.V. flow rate. *(Courtesy of Abbott Laboratories, Chicago, Illinois)*

person may also equate IV therapy with severity of illness. The procedure and its implications are carefully explained to the individual and the family and/or significant others. Only qualified professionals should insert IVs, and limits should be placed on the number of attempts made to start an IV. The nurse makes frequent checks on the IV and does not allow the bottle to run dry. This not only provides safety, but reassures the individual that he or she is being observed carefully. Mobility can be increased by teaching the ambulatory individual to utilize a portable IV pole.

Range of motion to the limb where the IV is inserted is carried out within the restrictions of the nee-

dle placement. The infant or child who is restrained to prevent dislodging of the IV is allowed frequent periods to move freely with the supervision of the nurse or parent. He or she is moved through ROM exercises frequently and encouraged to maintain activities appropriate to level of growth and development. Parents may be taught to hold or cuddle the child while the IV is in progress.

The individual is observed for any complications of IV therapy, such as infiltration (movement of the needle out of the vein resulting in the flow of solution into the surrounding tissues) and inflammation. Chart 21.11 outlines the complications of IV therapy,

1. Prepare secondary bottle

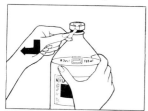

Remove Overseal. Pull the overseal tab downward and to one side (clockwise when viewed from above)—to remove in one piece.

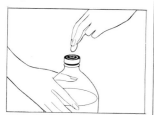

Lift Metal Disk. Expose underlying rubber stopper, exercising care not to touch stopper.

2. Prepare secondary Venoset

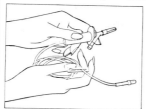

Shut Off Tubing. Remove the set from carton, but leave coiled for easy handling. Close slide clamp.

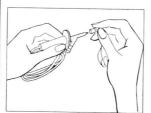

Expose Pin. Remove piercing pin cover, being careful to preserve sterility. Leave male adapter cover in place until ready to connect to primary Venoset (step 4).

3. Attach to secondary bottle

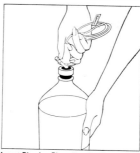

Insert Piercing Pin. Rest bottle on a firm surface. Hold with heel of hand uppermost. Thrust piercing pin straight down through bull's-eye. Do not twist or angle the pin.

Invert Immediately. Invert bottle without hesitation, and suspend. Rising filtered bubbles and a low hiss indicate vacuum. Discard any bottle without vacuum unless vacuum was previously expended in adding supplemental medications.

4. Attach to primary Venoset

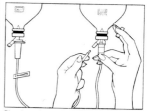

Plug into Air Inlet. Uncover secondary adapter and remove air filter from primary Venoset. Plug the Secondary Venoset firmly into primary air inlet.

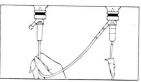

Open Slide Clamp. If adjustments to flow rate are needed use flow control device on primary Venoset.

5. Change all sets within 24 hours

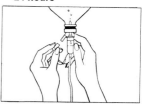

Restore Air Filter. When secondary bottle empties or is taken down primary bottle automatically restarts. If secondary is to be removed transfer its air filter to primary set. As with all I.V. sets, both secondary and primary Venoset should be changed within 24 hours.

HOW TO ATTACH THE SECONDARY VENOSET®

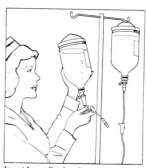

Figure 21.8

Setting up a secondary I.V. system. (*Courtesy of Abbott Laboratories, Chicago, Illinois*)

the mechanism of occurrence, and nursing responsibilities.

Fluid Loss and Nursing Measures

Any individual on gastrointestinal decompression can lose fluid and electrolytes. Figure 21.9 shows the various tubes commonly used for decompression. Figure 21.3 shows the electrolytes lost through the gastrointestinal tract. These losses occur when irrigation is done with hyper- or hypotonic solutions and when the intestine or stomach contents are removed through suction or aspiration. Other fluid and elec-

trolyte losses occur when the individual has draining wounds, fistulas, diarrhea, vomiting, diuresis, and profuse diaphoresis. Figure 21.3 also shows the electrolytes lost in these ways.

FLUID DESCRIPTION

Careful measurement of the amount, type, consistency, color, and odor of all fluid lost from the body in any of these ways helps to determine replacement needs. Indirect measurement methods such as weighing pads or linen or measuring drainage areas may have to be used when direct measurement is not possible. Comparison of electrolyte laboratory

Chart 21.11
Complications of IV Therapy

COMPLICATION	MECHANISM OF OCCURRENCE	NURSING RESPONSIBILITY

Infiltration	Needle becomes dislodged from vein and fluids flow into surrounding tissue.	Limit movement of insertion site to prevent dislodging.
		Observe site for signs and symptoms of infiltration:
		   Localized edema
		   Pallor at site
		   Coolness
		   Slowing of IV flow rate
		   Pain.
		Check for infiltration:
		   Lower bottle below the vein and observe for back flow of blood (if needle is against wall of vein or only partially infiltrated, this method will not indicate infiltration), or
		   Place tourniquet above needle insertion site. If flow continues, this indicates infiltration, or
		   Presence of edema above needle insertion indicates infiltration.
		If infiltration, remove IV, elevate arm to aid venous return, and apply warm compresses to aid absorption.

Pain at IV site	Infiltration. Too rapid infusion. Irritation of the vein by the needle or medication.	As above. Slow rate. Remove and replace at another site.

Phlebitis	Inflammation of the vein wall by needle or medication.	Check for signs and symptoms of inflammation:
		   Redness
		   Swelling
		   Tenderness or pain
		   Warmth.
		Remove IV, avoid further use of vein; apply warm moist compresses.

Thrombus	Blood clot formation at insertion site as a result of the clumping of RBCs at area of vein injury or slow flow rate.	Observe for:
		   Redness
		   Pain
		   Palpable vein
		   Slowed IV rate.
		Remove IV, apply warm, moist compresses.

(continued)

Chart 21.11 (Cont.)
Complications of IV Therapy

COMPLICATION	MECHANISM OF OCCURRENCE	NURSING RESPONSIBILITY

Thrombophlebitis	Combination of a phlebitis and thrombus.	Observe for:
		    Red streak proximal to site
		    Slowed IV rate
		    Pain at site
		    Vein hard, twisted
		    Tenderness.
		Remove IV.

Tissue necrosis	Prolonged infusion; medications.	Change sites frequently. Prevent infiltration; remove infiltrated IV immediately.
Local infection or inflammation	All of above. Poor aseptic technique. Damage to tissue during insertion.	See above. Maintain strict aseptic technique. Care on insertion.
Overhydration	Too rapid infusion; too much infusion.	Careful calculation of flow rate. Observe for signs and symptoms of overhydration.
Electrolyte imbalance	Too rapid infusion of electrolyte solution. Failure to supply electrolytes. Solution not matched to individual's needs.	Careful calculation of flow rate. Monitoring of electrolyte levels Careful checking of IV orders. Observation for signs and symptoms of electrolyte imbalance.
Air embolus	Air enters bloodstream through bubbles in tubing or solution running out.	Clear air bubbles from tubing. Prevent solution from running out.

Pyrogenic reactions	Immune reaction to foreign substances infused into blood.	Use fresh, unclouded solutions.
		Prevent contamination of solution.
		Observe for:
		    Malaise
		    Headache
		    Chills
		    Fever.
		Discontinue IV immediately; monitor vital signs; notify physician; save solution for culture.

Systemic infection	Introduction of pathogens into bloodstream.	Maintain aseptic technique; prevent contamination of solution and equipment.

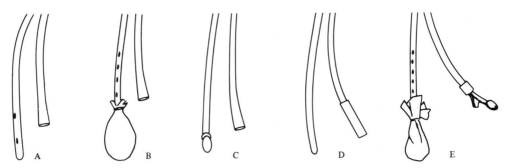

Figure 21.9

Tubing used in gastrointestinal decompression. The tube end that attaches to suction and the end that is inserted into the individual are both shown. **A.** Rubber nasogastric tube (Levin); **B.** Canto; **C.** Rehfuss, for duodenal drainage; **D.** Plastic nasogastric; and **E.** Miller-Abbott. In decompression, or deflation, of the gastrointestinal tract, fluid and/or gas is removed from the tract by means of suction. Electrolyte imbalances may result.

values helps to indicate changes in electrolyte balance as a result of drainage losses. The individual is monitored for signs and symptoms of fluid and electrolyte imbalance.

IRRIGATIONS

Gastrointestinal tubes are frequently irrigated to maintain their patency. The same principles apply to these irrigations as with any irrigation—the prescribed solution is injected into the tube and it is withdrawn by either reattaching the tube to suction or gently aspirating it with a syringe. The amount of fluid used for irrigation and the amount of fluid retrieved is charted with intake and output.

DIET

Individuals with interferences with fluid and electrolyte balance may be placed on restriction or replacement diets, depending on whether an excess or deficit exists. The nurse assists the individual in planning a diet that is either high or low in the fluid or electrolyte in question. Individual preference, lifestyle, and culture need to be considered if the plan is to be effective. Intake is scheduled throughout the day to prevent feelings of deprivation, thirst, and periodic overload. The need for restriction or replacement is thoroughly explained and options for methods of dealing with the changes are provided by the nurse.

THIRST

Thirst can be a significant concern for individuals with fluid and electrolyte imbalance, especially those on fluid restrictions. The nurse can help alleviate thirst by scheduling fluids throughout the day and by keeping the individual's mouth moist by assisting him or her in frequent mouth rinsings with water. Agents which increase the osmolarity of the mucous lining of the mouth, such as hard candy, gum, or lemon and gylcerin swabs, increase rather than decrease thirst and thus should be avoided. Lubricating the lips aids in reducing the feeling of thirst, as does a cool, well-ventilated room. Ice chips are useful in reducing thirst, since they are cold and give the feeling that the individual is receiving larger quantities of water, since ice occupies twice the space of an equal amount of water. Diversion activities and generalized comfort will assist in decreasing feelings of thirst.

CHANGES IN BEHAVIOR, SENSATION, AND COGNITION

Changes in behavior, sensation, and cognition which result from fluid, electrolyte, and acid–base imbalances require nursing interventions to insure safety, comfort, and energy conservation. If restlessness and confusion become severe, it may be necessary to restrain the individual and utilize bedrails to protect him or her from falls or other trauma. Any hallucinations the individual is experiencing is acknowledged but not validated or challenged. Sedation may be required to reduce symptoms and prevent injury to the individual. Frequent checks of the level of consciousness and orientation are necessary to assess the individual's condition (Chap. 13.)

SKIN CARE

Skin and mucous membrane changes which accompany fluid, electrolyte, and acid—base imbalance necessitate meticulous skin care. The skin is kept clean, well lubricated, and free of pressure. (Chapter 22 has a discussion of skin care.)

EVALUATION

Evaluation for maintaining fluid, electrolytes, and acid—base balance is primarily concerned with the direction of change in the individual's ability to adequately preserve or attain physiologic neutrality. Other important evaluation factors include: intake modifications that are required to prevent or counteract imbalances, the effectiveness of interventions, and the influences of fluid, electrolytes, and acid—base alteration on the body subsystems (as well as the reverse).

Specific criteria for evaluating an individual's fluid, electrolyte, and acid—base balance include:

- How do changes in fluid, electrolyte, and acid—base balance influence body functioning—physiologic? physical? psychologic?
- What is the relationship between the presenting fluid, electrolyte, and acid—base balance and the expected?
- Have the presenting fluid, electrolyte, and acid—base levels moved closer to the expected?
- What factors may account for changes in fluid, electrolyte, and acid—base levels?
- What are the changes in the degree of interference with fluid, electrolyte, and acid—base balance?
- What are the effects of fluid, electrolyte, and acid—base changes on body subsystems?
- Are there changes in knowledge (of individual, family and/or significant others) about the

influence of nutrition, elimination, other losses, subsystems, therapies (e.g., medication, diet), level of growth and development on fluid, electrolyte, and acid—base balance?
- What skills have been acquired (I & O, irrigation, weighing)?
- What changes in attitude toward fluid, electrolyte, and acid—base balance, related limitations and treatments (of the individual family and/or significant others) have occurred?

RECORDING AND TEACHING—LEARNING ACTIVITIES

Teaching—Learning Topics

- information about the relation of fluids, electrolytes, and acid—base balance to well-being, level of growth, and development
- rationale for therapeutic regimens
- care techniques for skin and thirst
- recording I & O
- restricting or increasing fluid intake
- preventive aspects
- relationship of pathologies to fluid, electrolyte, and acid—base balance
- how to modify nutrition, elimination, and subsystem patterns according to fluid, electrolyte, and acid—base interferences

Charting

Using appropriate fluid, electrolyte, and acid—base terms, objectively describe:

- objective base-line data on fluid, electrolyte, and acid—base status (e.g., tissue hydration, lab values, level of growth and development)
- objective and subjective changes that occur in the person's ability to meet fluid, electrolyte, and acid—base balance
- subjective assessment data on changes in fluid, electrolyte, and acid—base balance
- objective and subjective data on behavioral responses to fluid, electrolyte, and acid—base levels
- attitudes toward interferences and treatments
- subjective and objective reactions and responses to treatment

- schedule and methods of care
- teaching carried out
- discharge planning done
- interaction, responses, and attitudes of family and/or significant others
- degree of change in fluid, electrolyte, and acid–base balance
- update Kardex on nutritional needs

Medications to Review

- electrolyte solutions, e.g., Ky-lyte
- IV solutions, e.g., 5% dextrose/water
- diuretics, e.g., meralluride (Mercuhydrin)
- bicarbonate preparation, e.g., sodium bicarbonate
- glucocorticoids, e.g., cortisone
- mineralocorticoids, e.g., aldosterone

Diets to Review

- high fluid
- low fluid
- high and low potassium
- high and low sodium
- high and low calcium

SELECTED REFERENCES

Elbaum, Nancy. "Detecting and Correcting Magnesium Imbalance." *Nursing 77,* 7:34, August, 1977.

Hargest, Thomas S. "Start Your Count with Zero." *American Journal of Nursing,* 74:887, May, 1974.

Kemp, Ginny and Kemp, Doug. "Diuretics." *American Journal of Nursing* 78:1006, June, 1978.

Kubo, Winifred, Grant, Marcia Moeller, Walike, Barbara C., Bergstrom, Nancy, Wong, Hilda Luna, Hanson, Robert L., and Padilla, Geraldine V. "Fluid and Electrolyte Problems of Tube-Fed Patients." *American Journal of Nursing 76:*912, June, 1976.

Kurdi, William. "Refining Your I.V. Therapy Techniques." *Nursing 75,* 5:41, November, 1975.

Lambert, Martin, "Drug and Diet Interactions." *American Journal of Nursing,* 75:402, March, 1975.

Lu, Carla, Stroot, Violet, and Schaper, C. Ann. "Extracellular Volume Imbalance." *American Journal of Nursing,* 74:888, May, 1974.

Mak, Dennis, Goldman, Donald, and Rhame, Frank, "Infection Control in Intravenous Therapy." *Nursing Digest,* 3:5, May–June, 1975.

"Metabolic Acid-Base Disorders: Chemistry and Physiology" (programmed instruction, part 1). *American Journal of Nursing,* 77:1619, October, 1977.

"Metabolic Acid-Base Disorders: Physiological Abnormalities and Nursing Actions" (programmed instruction, part 2). *American Journal of Nursing,* 78:87, January, 1978.

Metheny, Norma and Snively, W. D. *Nurses Handbook of Fluid Balance,* 2nd ed. Philadelphia, Lippincott, 1974.

Michael, Sharon, "Home I.V. Therapy." *American Journal of Nursing,* 78:1223, July, 1978.

Nursing 78. *Monitoring Fluid and Electrolytes Precisely.* Horsham, Pa., Intermed Communications, 1978.

"Programmed Instruction: Metabolic Acid-Base Disorders: Clinical and Laboratory Findings." *American Journal of Nursing,* 78:44, March, 1978.

Snider, Malle, "Helpful Hints on I.V.'s." *American Journal of Nursing,* 74:1978, November, 1974.

Stroot, Violet, Lee, Carla, and Schaper, C. Ann. *Fluid and Electrolytes.* Philadelphia, Davis, 1977.

Tripp, Alice. "Hyper and Hypocalcemia." *American Journal of Nursing,* 76:1142, July, 1976.

Twombly, Marilyn. "The Shift into Third Space." *Nursing 78,* 8:38, June, 1978.

Ungvarski, Peter. "Parenteral Therapy." *American Journal of Nursing,* 76:1974, December, 1976.

UNIT VI

Security and Esteem Needs

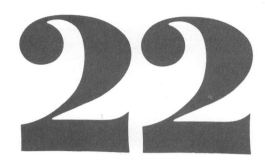

22

My body, which my dungeon is,
And yet my parks and palaces.
—Robert Louis Stevenson

BODY AESTHETICS

PRINCIPLES RELATED TO BODY AESTHETIC NEEDS

Each individual has a unique body image.

Body image is a dynamic process related to the individual's view of self and to his or her interactions with the internal and external environments.

Alterations in body image can result from actual or perceived changes.

Alterations in body image result in changes in behavioral responses and interactions.

Treating the individual with dignity and respect enhances self-esteem.

Personal care patterns are learned.

Individuals vary in their style and approach to personal care.

Individuals vary in their need for personal care.

Skin is kept lubricated by sebum.

The amount of sebum is increased during puberty and decreased in old age.

Skin irritation can result from the buildup of oily secretions.

The eccrine glands that produce sweat are located in all parts of the body.

The apocrine glands are concentrated mainly in the axillary, genital, and anal areas of the body.

Bacterial interaction with aprocine secretion results in an odoriferous smell.

Bacterial interactions with food can destroy tooth enamel and the gums.

Frequent hair brushing stimulates the production of oil and prevents drying of the scalp.

Soaps and detergents decrease the surface tension of water.

Decreased surface tension helps in fat emulsification.

The total way in which individuals view themselves and their ability to adapt these views to per-

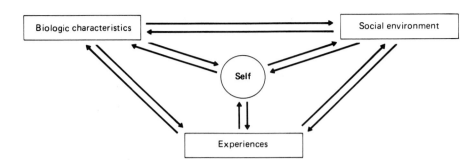

Figure 22.1
Elements that lend to the development of an individual's body image. *(Courtesy of Donovan and Pierce,* Cancer Care Nursing, *Appleton-Century-Crofts, p. 205)*

ceived or actual changes in self play an integral role in their levels of wellness. The construct of **body image** is used to describe this holistic picture of the individual. The concepts of self-esteem, self-image, and identity are intertwined with body image. The observer can never be fully aware of any individual's total body image but can indirectly piece one together from clues in the individual's behavior. Body image is a dynamic, constantly changing construct which is determined by the ever-changing stimuli the individual receives from the internal and external environments. (Fig. 22.1)

Personal appearance and maintenance of structure and form are aspects of body image. The nurse is often in a position to assist the individual in meeting these body aesthetic needs. **Body aesthetics** is the personal process of maintaining one's structure and form so that the self-image is maximized. This process involves such activities as dressing, bathing, and any personal-care measures the individual sees as important to well-being.

Body-image and body-aesthetic needs are closely tied to the individual's perception of self as a complete and functioning being. Disturbances in the individual's state of health can alter the individual's ability to meet these needs. Thus any nursing interventions which promote body integrity help the individual to maintain an optimal level of wellness.

ASSESSMENT

Body Image

COMPONENTS

Nursing assessment of the individual body image begins with an understanding of its components.

Actual, Measurable State
The first component of body image is the individual's actual, measurable traits or characteristics,

including height, weight, age, hair and eye color, muscle strength, body build, and structural components of the body.

Perception of Self
The second component is the individual's self-perception of physical, physiologic, and psychosocial characteristics. This perception is influenced by the individual's actual state, the core body image, and any changes the individual perceives as occurring in self.

The core body image is the relatively unchanging perception that each individual has about self. This core if fairly well established by the end of toddlerhood and relatively fixed by the end of adolescence. This core is manifested by feelings of good, bad, negative, positive, pretty, ugly, intelligent, stupid, big, or small, which the individual develops through his or her experiences and interactions with the environment. Toddlerhood is a critical period for this development. Chart 22.1 outlines the establishment of body image throughout the life cycle. When the body image is intact, the individual's perceptions of self are very close to what the individual's actual measurable state is. When there are distortions in body image, the individual's perceptions of self may be in extreme contrast to the actual and measurable state.

Ideal Self
The individual's view of a perfect self is the third component. Each individual has a picture of what he or she would like to look like, act like, and be. This ideal self is determined by what characteristics or traits the individual sees as important. For example, if the individual sees physical beauty as a person's most important characteristic then the ideal self will reflect this physical emphasis. In part, this ideal self is determined by what the family and/or significant others and society value. The significance of this self ideal varies greatly from individual to individual and, further, may differ in emphasis in an individual at various times of life. For example, if the self ideal is

Chart 22.1
Body Image Development through the Life Process*

STAGE	DEVELOPMENT
Infant	Perceives self as being continuous with the environment; diffuse feelings of pleasure and pain; if needs are met immediately with kindness and competency, infant will develop a positive sense of self and environment.
Toddler	First critical period for development of body image; time when child is learning many vital life skills and sense of autonomy; if child is not allowed to explore environment, try out new skills, and develop social interactions with positive reinforcement from the parenting person, will feel inadequate and negative about self. For example, during toilet training if child is repeatedly made to feel nasty, dirty, or bad without equal or greater positive reinforcements, the child will internalize these feelings as part of his core body image.
Preschooler	Time of refinement of skills and role modeling and greater exploration of environment and social interactions, especially with peers, which reinforce or negate previous image of self.
Schoolage child	Time when child enters school system and moves away from direct influence of home environment, develops feelings about self as a learner and as part of a peer social group; time of comparing physical skills and body structure with other children; if child labelled poor learner, loner, or physically inept, incorporates these feelings into core image.
Adolescent	Second critical period for development of body image and threats to it; time of body change in structure and function; tries out new skills of personality, self-governing; very susceptible to influences of peer group; social and physical abilities are paramount; rejection by peer group or having physical handicaps and differences result in feelings of worthlessness and unacceptability.
Young adult	Ability to be self-sufficient and not depend on primary family; development of long-term relationships, establishment of oneself in a career, and being "healthy" are the focuses of this period; failure to successfully meet developmental tasks negatively influences perceptions of self.
Middle-age adult	Final critical period for development of body image and threats to it; time of self-revaluation and role changes; signs of aging become apparent; menopause; if life up to this point seems wasted or inadequate or previous feelings about self-worth were negative, individual may reject self and lifestyle; particularly difficult period in American society because of emphasis on youth and youthful looks.
Older adult	Time of chronic illness, decrease in functional abilities, role losses; society rejects value of older adult in general; if dependence increases and reactions of significant others are negative, individual may lose all sense of self-worth and perceive self as insignificant.

*Chapter 25 discusses perceived and actual loss of body form and function and their relationship to growth and development.

thin and physically agile, there are times when the individual may be on diets and exercise programs to attain this. At other times, however, the individual will say it would be nice to be this way but that it takes too much effort; at those times, the individual will not try to attain this ideal.

Perception of Family's and/or
Significant Others' Views

The next component is how the individual perceives his family and/or significant others as seeing him or her, which may or may not reflect how they actually do see him or her. When the body image is intact, the views of the family and/or significant others are closely aligned with the individual's perceptions. The significance of these perceptions depends on the importance of the family and/or significant others to the person and how closely related their views are to the other components of body image. For example, if the individual does not value the opinions of the family and if these opinions contradict the individual's own perceptions of self, he or she may disregard the family's views or perceive them as similar to his or her own.

Perception of Society's View

The final component of body image is the individual's perception of how the culture and/or society views the person. This interaction is similar to the process which occurs with significant others. Again, if the individual holds the same values as the society, society's expectations are important to that individual and play a great part in how the person sees him- or herself.

INTERDEPENDENCE OF COMPONENTS

All of these five components are interdependent and each takes on more or less value at different points in the person's life. It is the total interaction of these components at any given time which results in the individual's body image. A change in any one aspect, however minor it may seem to the observer, produces a change in the individual's total body image.

DISTORTIONS IN BODY IMAGE

Any perceived or actual change in the individual's physical, physiologic, or psychosocial status can produce a distortion in body image. A **distortion in body image** is any change in the self-concept which is at variance with the individual's previous one and interferes with the individual's level of functioning. The nurse is frequently involved with individuals who are undergoing body-image changes. However, there are certain situations which are more likely to result in body image distortions than others. Such experiences can be surgery, especially when there is a loss of a body part or function which is particularly important to the individual; pain, particularly when it cannot be dealt with in the way the person thinks he or

she should be able to; role loss, including threats to sexuality; increased dependence on other persons; and loss of control of functions or activities which are highly significant to the individual.

These distortions may manifest themselves in subjective statements of worthlessness, which are often veiled in humor; in withdrawal from activities and interactions; in self-deprecating or destructive behaviors such as over- or undereating or a decrease in personal hygiene; in loss of interest in self; in exaggerated reactions to seemingly minor changes in self or environment; and in crisis (Chap. 25). Some of these behaviors may be difficult to assess because the nurse may not know the individual's previous behavioral patterns. However, a carefully taken nursing history done in collaboration with the individual and the family and/or significant others may provide a base line from which judgments can be made. Listening to the individual talk about or refer to self and events in the environment can also provide much valuable data.

Many behaviors that are labeled negative, such as hostility, seductiveness, telling risqué jokes, and being demanding or total compliance may result from threats to or distortions in body image. The nurse needs to assess those situations which may threaten the individual's body image. This can be done, in part, by determining the individual's attitudes and values toward self, the views of the family and/or significant others, and the views of the society or culture.

Nursing assessment related to body image includes descriptions of:

- measurable body characteristics
- subjective statements related to self characteristics
- subjective statements about self ideal
- subjective statements about views of family and/or significant others on self characteristics
- subjective statements about cultural and societal views on self characteristics
- previous interaction styles
- changes in interaction style
- changes in comments about self
- changes in self-care activities
- changes in interactions among individual, family and/or significant others, and staff
- potential threats to body image (e.g., role loss, disfigurement, inactivity).

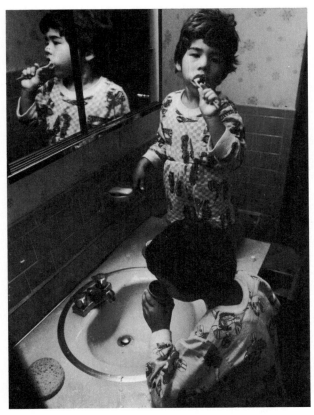

Illustration 22.1
An individual's level of growth and development influences what personal care activities are pursued and how. Here a younger sibling is refining a hygiene skill, using his brother as a role model. *(Photo by Bob Clay, from Jeroboam)*

General Body Aesthetic Needs

Each person has a unique personal-care pattern. Personal care includes maintenance of cleanliness; mouth, hair, skin, and nail care; control of odors; and use of cosmetics. Methods and degree of personal care are influenced by the individual's body image, culture, society, economics, level of wellness, level of growth and development, level of knowledge, and personal preferences. Cultural and societal expectations affect such views as what clean is, desirable body odors and characteristics, what activities are appropriate for maintaining personal appearance, and when these should be carried out and by whom. The individual's economic level influences the type and availability of facilities for personal appearance activities and the products that will be used.

The individual's state of health will determine the ability to carry out usual personal-care patterns.

The ill person may require assistance in carrying out these activities and/or may not have the energy to maintain an interest in them. In addition, the societal and cultural expectations of the ill person may not include maintenance of personal appearance.

Level of growth and development greatly influences the degree of assistance required for personal appearance activities and the attitude toward these activities. For example, the school-age child, while capable of carrying out personal-care activities, may actually value being dirty. The adolescent, on the other hand, may be preoccupied with maintaining the personal appearance standards of the peer group. The individual's level of knowledge about the implications of personal appearance and habits on health, the methods of maintaining personal appearance, and alternate methods of care are other factors in how the individual views and carries out personal-care activities. (Illustration 22.1)

Personal preferences also affect the rituals, scheduling, mode of performance, and basic level of interest in personal care activities.

ASSESSING PATTERNS OF PERSONAL CARE

When the nurse assesses the individual's patterns of personal care, the following factors should be considered: the degree of influence that these habits have, the nurse's own biases about what is clean and acceptable, and what behaviors are actually a threat to well-being rather than a variation on the expected. Many behaviors, although personally disagreeable to the nurse, do not actually interfere with the individual's ability to meet physical, physiologic, and psychosocial needs. For example, the individual may take a bath only once a week; the nurse, on the other hand, feels that bathing should be a daily activity. While this difference indicates a conflict of values, neither pattern interferes with the individual's health unless special circumstances arise. The individual in this case may recognize that his or her skin is dry and easily irritated or is in a situation where there is not enough hot water available for more frequent bathing.

On the other hand, there may be personal care habits that do threaten the individual's well-being and that the nurse may want to work on and modify with the individual. Mouth and tooth care are examples of this. The nurse knows that if the individual does not regularly brush his or her teeth, dental caries and gum pathology will result.

In some situations, the individual may have more exacting standards for personal care than the nurse has. Thus the nurse must assess each situation individually and not make value judgments based on what the nurse considers should be done.

ASSESSING NEED FOR ASSISTANCE

The nurse also assesses the personal care needs of the individual in terms of the degree of assistance the individual requires and the priority of that care in relation to other health care needs. Individuals whose level of wellness is decreased may require more assistance with personal-care activities. Their capabilities and limitations are assessed to determine which activities or parts of activities they can carry out themselves. Often, if the individual can do even a small part of his or her own care, self-esteem and feelings of control are increased. In addition, the activity benefits the individual by increasing muscle strength and activity tolerance, providing sensory stimulation, and generally increasing the activity of all body subsystems.

At times it may appear quicker and easier for the nurse to carry out personal-care activities for individuals than to assist them to do for themselves. However, if the nurse realizes the contribution the activity makes in meeting physical, physiologic, and psychosocial needs, the nurse plans to allow time for the individual to carry out those activities the individual is capable of.

CORRELATION WITH HEALTH CARE NEEDS

Personal-care activities are considered within the context of the individual's health care needs. These activities may help to meet a multiplicity of health care needs but are not health care needs in and of themselves. The individual's needs for comfort, rest, activity, self-esteem, and touch are considered along with the needs to prevent skin irritation and breakdown, dental pathologies, and infection.

The specific assessment findings of the skin, hair, nails, and mouth, which are discussed in Chapters 7, 15, 17, and 18, are now correlated with the body aesthetic needs of the individual. Since personal care activities contribute greatly to the integrity and function of the skin, hair, nails, and mouth, the nurse's assessment of their characteristics assists in determining

the particular personal-care activities to be carried out and in establishing priorities of care.

Alterations in the levels of wellness, such as fever, immobility, fluid and electrolyte imbalance, nutritional deficiencies, and respiratory interferences, produce changes in the skin and mucous membranes and in the individual's ability to prevent these changes. These health alterations can result in a buildup of skin secretions, pressure on the skin and underlying tissues, skin irritation and breakdown, the collection of secretions in the mouth, eyes, and nose, and/or drying of both the skin and mucous membranes. The nurse assesses the degree to which these interferences are present along with the factors which contribute to their occurrence.

Nursing assessment of general body aesthetic needs includes descriptions of:

- presenting care pattern
- usual care pattern
- relationship between usual care pattern and presenting pattern
- factors influencing care patterns (e.g., societal and cultural expectations, level of growth and development, and personal preferences)
- interferences in meeting body aesthetic needs
- degree of assistance required
- health care need being interfered with (e.g., comfort, safety, activity)
- personal-care activities which help to meet these needs
- skin, mouth, nails, hair, and mucous membrane characteristics
- interferences with skin, mouth, nails, and membrane form and function
- personal-care factors which contribute to interferences

NURSING DIAGNOSIS

A 16-year-old male, Tim Brown, comes to the school nurse for his annual school physical examination. The nurse notes that while all physical findings are within expected limits, he has a severe case of acne vulgaris on his face, neck, and shoulders. An assessment of the presenting behaviors is given on the facing page.

ASSESSMENT FACTOR	EXPECTED BEHAVIOR	PRESENTING BEHAVIOR
Actual measurable characteristics	—	Pustules, blackheads densely scattered on cheeks, forehead, chin, neck, and shoulders (diagram is usually drawn to show pattern); many scabbed areas; skin area red, irritated.
Perceived characteristics	—	"My zits are so disgusting I can't stand to look in the mirror."
Perception of view of family and/or significant others	—	"My mother says if I wouldn't eat all that junk and take better care of my skin I wouldn't have this problem. My girl friend has the same as I do."
Societal and cultural expectations	—	"I can't stand all those TV commercials with all those kids with clear faces selling some more junk to put on my face."
Relationship of body image to growth and development	See Chart 22.1	Same
Changes in comments about self	—	"I used to be a pretty good-looking guy, but lately, I don't know anymore."
Personal care pattern	—	Showers daily with soap Washes face once in morning and once at night with commercial antiacne soap. Uses commercial antiacne coverup cream heavily. Shaves daily with safety razor, although growth is very light. Squeezes pimples and blackheads whenever they appear.

Resulting nursing diagnoses include:

- threat to body image related to acne
- skin irritation related to lack of knowledge concerning proper skin care

PLANNING

Planning for body aesthetic needs considers the individual's personal preferences, abilities and limitations, and the time, equipment, and personnel available. The degree to which the individual can carry out activities is balanced with available resources and the actual needs of the individual. Many times individuals do not require the degree of assistance and the number of activities that routines or traditions dictate. Thus the plan is individualized and personalized rather than routinized.

The plan for one of the nursing diagnoses listed above in the situation of Tim Brown might look like that on page 612.

INTERVENTION

Body image

Measures which support the individual's feelings of self-worth and self-esteem help to promote and maintain a positive body image. By treating the individual with dignity, collaborating with the individual, providing privacy, giving the individual safe competent care, and individualizing and personalizing care, the nurse can help the individual to feel more significant and valued. Individuals who feel that they are the focus of attention and that someone is interested in

NURSING DIAGNOSIS	GOAL	PLAN
Skin irritation related to lack of knowledge proper skin care.	1. Increased level of knowledge about skin care within 2 weeks as evidenced by change in personal habits.	1. Describe relationship between shaving with safety razor and skin irritation. 2. Explain relationship between squeezing blackheads and pimples and the spread of infection. 3. Explain relationship between use of skin cover creams and clogged pores. 4. Review face-washing technique. 5. Schedule revisits for once weekly for 1 month.
	2. Decreased skin irritation within 1 month as evidenced by reduction in number of inflamed areas.	1. As above 2. Refer Tim to dermatology clinic. 3. Review nutritional habits and supplement areas of information gaps. 4. Check with dermatology clinic for diagnosis and treatment, and review with individual.

meeting their needs feel more positive about themselves.

The nurse can create an environment in which the individual has the opportunity to work through negative or ambivalent feelings about self. Recognition of these feelings by the nurse legitimizes them and lets the person know that these feelings are worthy of discussion. In this way the individual is not made to feel "crazy" or "silly" for having such feelings. Once the communication lines have been opened, the nurse can assist the individual to explore his or her attitudes and values. By clarifying what the individual values, the nurse can then find methods to support them in ways different from those used in the past. For example, if an individual values mobility and becomes paralyzed, the nurse helps the individual to find alternative ways of maintaining mobility.

DEALING WITH CHANGES

If the individual is to deal meaningfully with changes in physical, physiologic, or psychosocial status, the individual will need to recognize the reality of his or her limitations and abilities. By creating situations which present reality to the grieving individual at appropriate times, the nurse assists the individual to align the actual state with perceptions of self. For instance, when changing a dressing the nurse informs the individual of the appearance of the wound and gives the individual an opportunity to look at it. Calling changes by their appropriate names rather than using euphemisms or nicknames also helps to present reality to the individual. Providing the individual with opportunities to interact with others not only meets socialization needs but also provides another form of reality orientation. The individual needs opportunities to see the reactions of others to him or her and to test out new behaviors. Other forms of sensory stimulation further help the individual with reality orientation.

SUPPORTING THE POSITIVE

Helping the individual to improve overall appearance or replace lost body parts with prosthetic devices accentuates the positive aspects of the individual's present state. Cosmetics, clothing, wigs, hair care, shaving, and other personal appearance activities often make individuals feel more attractive and thus more positive about themselves. In addition, an improved appearance makes individuals more socially acceptable and therefore enhances interactions with others.

The effective coping behaviors that the individual uses are reinforced and new, useful ones developed. If, on the other hand, the person is in crisis, interventions appropriate to the phase of crisis are instituted (Chap. 25). By anticipating situations that may pose threats to the individual's body image, the nurse can either help the individual to avoid the situations or prepare him or her for the events that will follow.

AVOIDING NEGATIVE TERMINOLOGY

The nurse avoids the use of value terms when describing the individual's conditions, characteristics, or body forms or structures. It is not uncommon to hear nurses refer to a broken or paralyzed leg as "the bad leg." This subtly suggests and reinforces negative feelings that the individual has about self. The nurse is careful not to be drawn into situations where he or she reinforces the individual's self-deprecating remarks. Often, when the individual's statements are veiled in humor, it is easy to do so.

ASSISTING SIGNIFICANT OTHERS

The individual's interactions with the attitudes and reactions of family and/or significant others play a major role in the person's responses to perceived or actual changes in self. The nurse therefore needs to help family and/or significant others to clarify their views and attitudes and work through the grieving and loss process. The nurse includes them in the care of the individual and prepares them for changes that have occurred or will occur. Many of the same interventions are used with the family and/or significant others as are used with the individual.

Body Aesthetics

Interventions for body aesthetics include care of the skin, nails, hair, and mouth. Skin care involves keeping it clean, dry, lubricated, intact, and well supplied with nutrients. Assisting the individual with bathing helps not only to clean the skin, but to provide comfort by increasing circulation, removing odors and secretions from the skin, and providing movement, exercise, and sensory stimulation. During this time the nurse can assess the state of the individual's skin, mobility, endurance, and reactions to care. In addition, the nurse uses this time to develop rapport with the individual and to teach skills for maintaining personal care. Bathing the individual is a task frequently delegated to auxilliary personnel without evaluating

the opportunities it may give the nurse to accomplishing therapeutic goals. Therefore, the nurse needs to look at the appropriateness of bathing the individual or of delegating the task to others.

Personal Care Activities

BATHING

Bathing is often a routing procedure that is done without careful consideration or judgment. The nurse needs to weigh the benefits of complete daily bathing with its hazards. Complete daily baths often dry the skin, fatigue the individual unnecessarily, and frequently do not follow the individual's usual pattern. A partial bath, focusing only on the areas of the body which need to be bathed, often meets the individual's needs. This is especially true for infants and the elderly, who have fragile skin, and for very weak or debilitated individuals, whose energy can be used in more meaningful ways.

A variety of approaches can be used to bathe the individual. The specific approach used will depend on the individual's level of growth and development, activity orders, mobility, energy level, preferences, and the presence of casts, sutures, drains, and open wounds. Showers, tub baths, sponge baths at the sink, and bed baths are some of the most common bathing methods. Immobilized or debilitated persons can often receive showers or tub baths when special equipment is used to assist in their transfer and positioning. Illustration 22.2 A & B shows some of the equipment commonly used for these purposes.

Shower and Tub Safety

When assisting individuals with showers or tub baths, safety precautions are maintained to prevent accidents. Handrails, nonskid floors or surfaces, footstools, and some type of device to call for assistance (hand bells in the home, call bells in the institutional setting) are necessary safety measures. Bath objects and towels are placed in easy reach to prevent the necessity for the person to get up and reach. The nurse evaluates the type and degree of privacy the individual can safely have. Infants and children are not left alone while they are in the bathtub. Unless doors can be unlocked from the outside, individuals are requested not to lock them. In some cases the nurse may stay with the individual during the shower or bath; at other times, the nurse may stay within easy reach outside the bathing area. When not otherwise contraindicated, individuals with casts, catheters, and

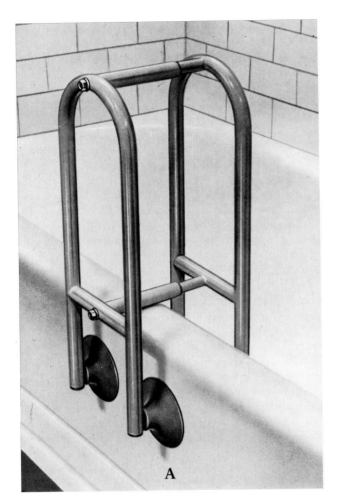

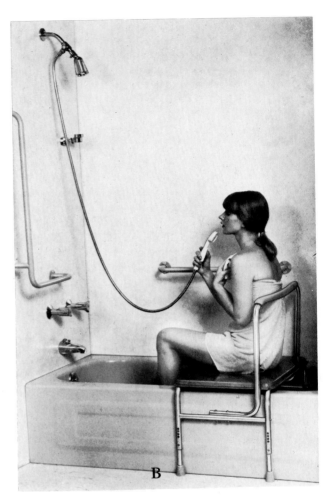

Illustration 22.2
A variety bathtub devices are available to increase the ease and safety of care activities: bathtub safety rail (A); transferable tub seat and shower hose (B). *(Courtesy of Lumex)*

other similar care devices can, when properly protected, also take advantage of showers and tub baths.

Sink Baths

When the full shower or bath is not required or desired or when treatment modalities interfere, the individual can bathe at the sink. Chairs can be placed by the sink and individuals can carry out their own baths or be assisted. As with any other type of bath, privacy and safety are maintained.

Bed Baths

The individual who is unable to utilize other bathing methods can be bathed in bed. The nurse explains the procedure to the individual and collects the necessary equipment. This includes a basin, towels, bath blankets where available, washcloth, soap, lotion, and clean clothing. If the nurse will be assisting with mouth care at this time, the nurse will also obtain a glass, a kidney-shaped basin, toothbrush, toothpaste, mouthwash, and water. If nail care is also to be included, orange sticks, a nail file, and any other necessaries such as nail clipper are obtained. Personal toiletry articles such as powders, deodorant, cosmetics, and shaving equipment are also placed within easy reach.

Once all equipment is assembled, the person is positioned comfortably. Unnecessary bedclothes are removed, and the bed is adjusted to a good working height. The person is screened to maintain privacy.

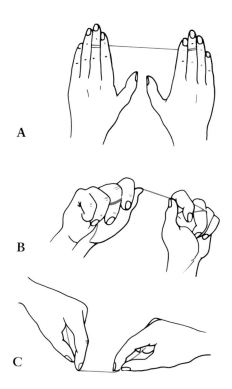

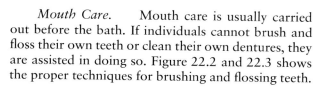

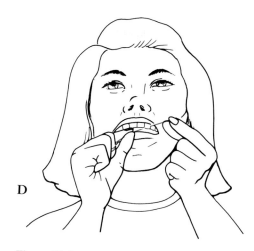

Figure 22.2

Teeth-flossing technique. **A.** First, wrap floss securely around third finger of each hand. **B.** To floss upper teeth, thumbs are used to stretch floss upward. **C.** Lower teeth are flossed with second finger stretching floss downward. **D.** Gentle back and forth movement of the floss between the teeth cleans difficult to reach surfaces.

Mouth Care. Mouth care is usually carried out before the bath. If individuals cannot brush and floss their own teeth or clean their own dentures, they are assisted in doing so. Figure 22.2 and 22.3 shows the proper techniques for brushing and flossing teeth.

If the individual cannot carry out the procedures but is able to cooperate, the nurse brushes the teeth for the individual. Dentures can be cleaned by soaking them in commercially prepared cleansers or by brushing them with toothpaste or denture cream. When

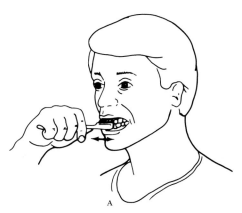

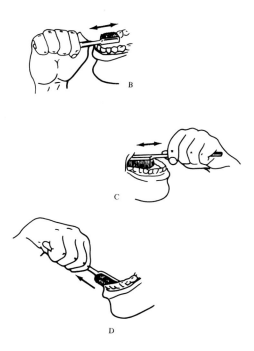

Figure 22.3

Teeth brushing technique. **A.** The outer surfaces of teeth are cleaned with short back-and-forth strokes of the brush. **B.** Inside upper and lower teeth are brushed gently back and forth, while gum tissue is brushed too. **C.** Biting surfaces are cleaned by back and forth horizontal brush movements. **D.** For inner front surfaces of teeth, the brush is moved vertically from gum line to top of crown.

handling dentures the nurse prevents their breakage by avoiding the use of very hot water and holding them with gauze to increase a grip on their usually slippery surface. If they are cleaned over a sink, the sink is filled with water to lessen the possibility of their breaking if they drop into the sink.

If the individual is unable to cooperate with mouth care, the nurse takes responsibility for cleaning. Gauze pads wrapped around a tongue blade and dipped into water or mouthwash can be used for this purpose. If the mouth is particularly crusted with ▶ **sordes** (accumulations of saliva, mucus, food, organisms, and epithelieal cells), the mouth can be cleaned with a half hydrogen peroxide, half water solution, and care is taken to prevent the individual from swallowing it. This special mouth care may be necessary several times a day with the very ill or debilitated individual, particularly if the individual is a mouth breather. Using commercially prepared mouth cleaning swabs (e.g., lemon and glycerine swabs) does not replace this cleaning process. Special mouth care serves not only to meet the aesthetic needs of the individual but also to prevent breakdown of the mucous membrane and infection.

Washing. As in any other situation where side rails are required, when the nurse gets the bath water, side rails that have been lowered are raised. The bath water should be at a comfortable temperature and changed whenever it gets dirty or cools off. The individual carries out any parts of the bath that he or she can. In washing the person, the nurse works from cleaner areas to dirtier areas. For example, the nurse begins with the face before the axilla. As water evaporates from the skin, chilling can occur. Therefore, the nurse keeps only the parts that are being washed uncovered, dries the skin thoroughly, and prevents drafts. All soap is carefully and completely rinsed off to prevent drying of the skin.

During the bath, special attention is paid to **in-** ▶ **tertrigous** areas (areas where two skin surfaces touch each other) such as under the breasts, fat folds, the perineal area, and the eyes. These areas are prone to chafing and skin breakdown as a result of friction and built-up secretions. Frequently, a light dusting of powder may help to reduce friction. However, all powder is removed each time a person is bathed. Powder and lotion are not used on the same area at the same time.

The eyes are the first part of the body to be cleaned with the clean washcloth. Soap is not used. The eyelid is cleaned from the inner aspect to the outer. A different part of the washcloth is used for each eye to prevent cross-contamination. If the secretions are so thick or tenacious that they seal the eye, gauze pads soaked in sterile water are placed over the eyelids to loosen the secretions before cleansing.

GENITAL CARE

Cleansing of the genital areas is part of the usual bath routine. However, it may be necessary at other times, particularly when the individual is incontinent. In cleaning the penis of an uncircumcised male, it is necessary to pull back the foreskin and gently wash the shaft of the penis. Particular attention is paid to thorough rinsing. The foreskin must be replaced to prevent ischemia. The tip of the penis is cleansed in a circular motion from the meatus outward and then washed toward the anus. In females, the labia are separated and gentle cleansing is done from front to back to prevent contamination of the urethra.

NAIL CARE

When the bath is completed, nail care can be carried out for individuals who cannot do it for themselves. If the nails require particular attention, the dirt can be loosened by soaking the hands or feet in warm water for 15 minutes. An orange stick is used to clean underneath the nails and around the cuticles. Care is taken to avoid breaking the skin or digging too deeply beneath the nail. A nail file is used to file down rough edges which may scratch the individual or catch on clothes or bedding. If the nails need to be cut, they are cut straight across. Individuals who have diabetes or any other peripheral vascular pathology should have their nails cut by a podiatrist, since improper technique can lead to infection and possible loss of the extremity. Lanolin may be rubbed into the skin of the feet after washing to prevent dryness and cracking. In addition, tufts of lambswool may be placed between the toes to prevent rubbing. These latter measures are usually a part of diabetic foot care.

HAIR CARE

Other personal-care activities which the nurse can assist with or perform for the individual are shaving and hair care. These activities add greatly to the individual's comfort and self-esteem.

Shaving

Using an electric razor is much easier for the nurse and more comfortable for the individual. If the individual's own electric razor is to be used, hospital policy is followed regarding grounding and other electrical safety factors. However, this type of razor may not always be available and may not be the individual's preference.

If a safety razor is to be used, the individual's face is thoroughly wet with hot water to soften the beard. Then the face is heavily lathered with soap or a commercial shaving cream. The face is shaved using short firm downward strokes. Hair and soap are rinsed off the blade frequently. The nurse uses the hand that is not holding the razor to hold the skin taut. If possible, the nurse hyperextends the individual's neck to shave this area. After the shave, the face is thoroughly rinsed and dried. When women have facial hair which is disturbing them, it is removed in the manner which they customarily use. This may be by plucking the hairs, shaving, or using facial depilatories.

Combing and Brushing

Daily hair care for the individual includes combing and brushing. If the hair is matted or tangled, it is combed in small sections. The nurse holds the lock of hair above the point of matting and combs downward, attempting to disentangle the hair. Care is taken not to pull on the scalp. If the individual desires and the hair is long enough, braids can be made. Braiding may also be done for unconscious individuals with long hair to prevent tangling and pulling on the hair during positioning and moving.

For individuals, particularly many black people, who have thick, coarse, and curly hair, daily oiling of the scalp is often necessary to prevent drying of the scalp and breaking of the hair. Commercially prepared hair oil or the individual's own preferred oil is massaged into the scalp and combed through. A wide-toothed natural comb prevents hair pulling and breakage. This type of hair usually requires no more than weekly shampooing because of the dry characteristics of the scalp and hair.

SKIN CARE

If the individual wishes it or if the skin is dry, lubricating lotions are applied after the bath and at any time in between. Alcohol or alcohol-based products are not used, since they dry out the skin and increase the possibility of skin breakdown, besides causing itchiness. A thorough back rub and massage of other bony prominences frequently accompany the bath. When giving a back rub, the nurse uses a lubricating lotion. If possible, the individual is placed in a front-lying position with the neck, shoulders, and back exposed. A back rub serves to increase circulation and to relax tense muscles. The nurse can use smooth, long, circular strokes (effleurage) up and down the back, kneading motions that concentrate on specific muscle groups (pétrissage), and alternately striking the individual's back with the ulnar surface of the hands (tapotement). Firm but gentle movements are used. The shoulder and neck muscles are included in the back rub. A back rub can be given whenever the individual is turned, to promote sleep, and anytime the individual desires. Any other bony prominences such as the elbows, ankles, and heels are concurrently massaged to reduce the effects of pressure and increase circulation. The calves are never massaged to prevent dislodging of blood clots.

SPECIAL SKIN CARE

Individuals who are prone to skin breakdown because of poor nutritional state, unrelieved pressure, immobility, fragile skin, and pathologic processes require special skin care. Special skin care helps to prevent and treat decubitus ulcer formation. A **decubitus ulcer** is an area of tissue necrosis caused by decreased blood supply to an area as a result of pressure. Figure 22.4 shows the sites where decubitus ulcers commonly occur when an individual is in a back-, side-, front-lying, or sitting position. Ulcers occur in these areas because of bony prominences under the skin that have little tissue around them to cushion the vasculature. In addition, these points present a smaller surface for diffusion of pressure and thus the pressure is concentrated at one point. As a result, blood supply to these areas is decreased when the blood vessels are compressed between the bone and the surface on which the individual is positioned.

Preventing Decubiti

Special skin care focuses on relieving pressure, increasing blood supply, preventing skin irritation, and supplying nutrients.

Relieving Pressure. Pressure is relieved by turning the individual at least every 2 hours with fre-

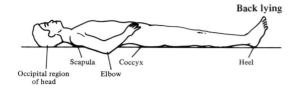

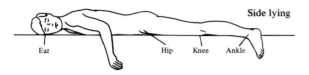

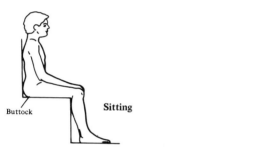

Figure 22.4

Points on the body that are susceptible to decubiti formation when an individual is in back-lying, side-lying, or sitting positions for prolonged periods with no relief to these pressure points.

quent shifting of body weight in between. Individuals who are in any type of chair for prolonged periods are also repositioned, made to stand up, or returned to bed periodically to prevent decubiti. If capable of voluntary movement, the individual is taught to consciously shift his or her weight as often as possible. Whenever the individual is moved, care is taken to avoid shearing force (Chap. 14).

Special devices such as alternating air mattresses, sheepskins, flotation pads, mattresses, and heel and elbow protector pads are often used to help relieve pressure. These items do not replace other nursing skin care measures but are used as an adjunct to them. And whenever these items are used, other pads and extra linen are not placed over them, which would decrease their beneficial effects.

Increasing Circulation. Massaging bony prominences and areas surrounding them increases circulation to the area. Any reddened area, which may indicate the beginning of a decubitus ulcer, is also massaged. Massaging is done whenever the individual is turned or repositioned and any other time circumstances warrant. Exercise and ambulation also help to increase circulation. Schedules are set up to ensure frequent and consistent exercise to help circulation, as well as to increase mobility. If the skin is starting to show signs of skin breakdown, as evidenced by a break in the skin and the leaking of tissue fluids, heat lamp treatments may be ordered. Heat causes vasodilation, thus increasing the blood supply to the area. Heat is usually applied for 15–20 minutes three to four times a day. As with any type of heat application, safety measures are instituted to prevent burns.

Preventing Irritation. Urine, feces, perspiration, drainage, water, soap, crumbs, and wrinkled bedsheets, when in prolonged contact with the skin, result in skin irritation and eventually skin breakdown. Any irritant is washed off the skin with soap and water. Thorough rinsing and drying with a patting motion are important to remove any traces of soap and moisture. Keeping the skin well lubricated also helps to prevent skin breakdown, since dry skin is more prone to loss of skin integrity. Bed linens, clothing, underpads, and dressings are kept free from wrinkles.

Supplying Nutrients. The individual's overall state of nutrition affects his or her skin integrity and the skin's ability to heal when breakdown does occur. Proper amounts of fluid, protein, vitamins, and minerals are particularly important in skin maintenance and repair. Individuals who are obese or thin are particularly prone to decubitus ulcers. Obesity not only increases the amount of pressure on a given area but, because of the avascular adipose tissue, also decreases the amount of blood circulating to any one area. The thin individual, on the other hand, has less protective padding.

Treating Skin Breakdown

Once skin breakdown has occurred, all the preventive measures mentioned above are continued, along with measures to promote healing. Irrigations with hydrogen peroxide and water, or Betadine, are frequently used to clean the area. Substances such as karaya and Maalox are often applied to the wound to help dry it. Gelfoam may also be used to promote granulation. If necrotic tissue is present, debriding ointments such as Elase, Travase, and Varidase may be used. The skin may have to be surgically debrided if the necrotic tissue is interfering with healing.

TEACHING CARE ACTIVITIES

The nurse has the opportunity to teach individuals and their families and/or significant others many personal-care activities in the home, school, community, or institutional settings. The nurse can teach ways to care for the skin; to protect it from drying, irritation, and pressure; and to promote its integrity. Also, the nurse can teach proper brushing and flossing techniques for the teeth and nail care. Safety measures which can be used in the home setting such as nonskid strips in the bathtub, installation of safety rails in the tub or shower, and arrangement of bath items within easy reach are another teaching area related to personal care. In addition, the nurse can help individuals to identify ways to match their capabilities with limitations in performing personal care activities within the individuals' usual settings.

EVALUATION

Evaluating how body anesthetic needs are being met focuses on the direction of change in the person's ability to meet these needs and the effectiveness of intervention.

Specific criteria for evaluating how body aesthetic needs are being met include:

- How do physiologic changes relate to changes in body image? Psychologic changes? Environmental changes?
- How do physiologic changes relate to changes in ability to meet personal-care needs? Psychologic changes? Environmental changes?
- Has presenting body image become more positive?
- Has presenting personal care pattern moved closer to the expected?

- What are the changes in the body image?
- What are the changes in personal-care activities?
- Are there changes in knowledge about body aesthetic needs (of individual, of family and/or significant others)?
- Are there modifications in personal habits?
- What are the changes in level of anxiety concerning meeting body aesthetic needs (of individual, of family and/or significant others)?
- What skills have been acquired in carrying out personal-care activities?
- What factors may account for changes in body aesthetic patterns?
- What are the changes in the degree of interference with meeting body aesthetic needs?
- What are the effects of changes in body aesthetic patterns on body subsystems?

RECORDING AND TEACHING–LEARNING ACTIVITIES

Teaching –Learning Topics

- rationale for therapeutic regimen
- methods of matching capabilities with limitations
- ways of structuring environment to facilitate meeting personal care needs
- safety factors related to personal care needs
- methods of decreasing anxiety related to meeting body aesthetic needs

Charting

Using appropriate terminology related to body aesthetic needs, objectively describe such factors as:

- objective base-line data on body image, skin integrity, and condition of mouth, mucous membranes, nails, and hair
- objective and subjective data on behavioral responses related to body aesthetic needs
- attitudes toward interferences and treatments
- objective and subjective reactions and responses to treatment

- schedule and methods of care
- teaching carried out
- discharge planning done
- interaction, responses, and attitudes of family and/or significant others
- degree of change in ability to meet body aesthetic needs
- update Kardex on body aesthetic needs.

Medications to Review

- chemical debriders, e.g., Varidase
- oxidizing agents, e.g., hydrogen peroxide

Diets to Review

- high protein
- high fluid
- high vitamin and mineral

SELECTED REFERENCES

"Black Skin Care Problems." *American Journal of Nursing,* 79:1092, June, 1979.

Cameron, Geraldine. "Pressure Sores: What to Do When Prevention Fails." *Nursing 79,* 9:42, January, 1979.

Di Mascio, Suzanne. "Debrisan for Decubitus Ulcers." *American Journal of Nursing,* 79:684, April, 1979.

Grier, Marian. "Hair Care for the Black Patient." *American Journal of Nursing,* 76:1781, November, 1976.

Gruendemann, Barbara J. "The Impact of Surgery on Body Image." *Nursing Clinics of North America,* 10:635, December, 1975.

Gruis, Marcia, and Innes, Barbara. "Assessment: Essential to Prevent Pressure Sores." *American Journal of Nursing,* 76:1762, November, 1976.

Kavchik-Keys, Mary Anne. "Four Proven Steps in Preventing Decubitus Ulcers." *Nursing 77,* 7:58, September, 1977.

————. "Treating Decubitus Ulcers Using Four Proven Steps." *Nursing 77,* 7:44, October, 1977.

Lang, Christine and McGrath, Anne. "Gelfoam for Decubitus Ulcers." *American Journal of Nursing,* 74:460, March, 1974.

McClosky, Joane, "How to Make the Most of Body Image Theory in Nursing Practice." *Nursing 76,* 6:68, May, 1976.

Michelsen, Dana. "How to Give a Good Backrub." *American Journal of Nursing,* 78:1197, July, 1978.

Norris, Catherine. "Body Image: Its Relevance to Professional Nursing." In *Behavioral Concepts and Nursing Intervention,* 2nd ed., Carolyn Carlson and Betty Blackwell, eds. Philadelphia, Lippincott, 1978, pp. 5–36.

"Programmed Instruction: Skin Rashes in Infants and Children." *American Journal of Nursing,* 78:1041, June, 1978.

Smith, Elaine, Liviskie, Sharon L., Nelson, Katherine A. and McNemar, Ann. "Reestablishing Body Image," *American Journal of Nursing,* 77:446, March, 1977.

Tierney, Elizabeth Ann. "Accepting Disfigurement When Death Is the Alternative." *American Journal of Nursing,* 75:2149, December, 1975.

Uhler, Elana. "Common Skin Changes in the Elderly." *American Journal of Nursing,* 78:1342, August, 1978.

Zelechowski, Gina. "Helping Your Patient Sleep—Planning Instead of Pills." *Nursing 77,* 7:62, May, 1977.

Zuchnick, Martha. "Care of an Artificial Eye." *American Journal of Nursing,* 75:835, May, 1975.

. . .—the innocent sleep;
Sleep that knits up the ravell'd sleave of care,
The death of each day's life, sore labour's bath,
Balm of hurt minds, great nature's second course,
Chief nourisher in life's feast
　　　　—William Shakespeare, Macbeth

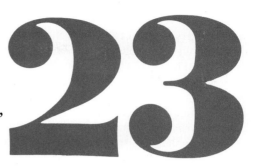

23
SLEEP AND COMFORT NEEDS

PRINCIPLES RELATED TO SLEEP AND COMFORT NEEDS

Sleep patterns vary with level of growth and development and with individual biorhythms.

Amount of sleep needed at a given time is influenced by activity level, state of health, and degree of anxiety.

Sleep habits are learned.

Sleep is necessary for wellness and survival.

Sleep is divided into five stages: stage 1 characterized by alpha waves: stage 2, characterized by spindle waves: stage 3, characterized by a mixture of spindle and delta waves: stage 4, characterized by delta waves: stage 5, REM sleep characterized by rapid eye movements and brain activity—dreaming occurs at this stage.

Usual sleep patterns can be interrupted by environmental distractions, medications, anxiety, and pain.

Sleep occurs during periods of minimum body temperature.

Sleep alterations can lead to behavioral and somatic disturbances.

Pain is a unique and subjective experience.

The pain experience is whatever the individual says it is.

Pain is increased by fatigue, anxiety, and boredom.

The sensation of pain is partially under voluntary control.

There are wide variations in individual's reactions to pain.

Pain threshholds are fairly consistent among all individuals.

Pain reactions are influenced by cultural and societal expectations, personality style, level of growth and development, meaning of pain, and past experiences with and expectations of pain.

Each individual's biorhythms can be identified as having a definite and predictable pattern.

　　Each individual has a unique internal rhythm which guides the pattern of life processes. These rhythms are known as **biologic rhythms** (biorhythms). The pattern of hormonal production, temperature regulation, cardiac output, blood pressure, urinary output, cell division, food intake, muscular activity, and sleep are just a few of the vital functions that follow these rhythmic cycles. Many biorhythms are **circadian** in nature, which means they run a full cycle within a 24-hour period (*circa*; around; *die*; day). Chart 23.1 describes some of these circadian rhythms for a person who naturally sleeps during the night and is awake during the day. Other rhythms the body follows are **ultradian,** which are shorter than circadian rhythms, for example, smooth muscle contraction; and **infradian,** which are longer than circadian rhythms, as in menstrual cycles. Infradian rhythms can extend for a long period of time, up to several months, and include seasonal variations, as seen with instances of pathophysiologic processes such as peptic ulcer.

A notable circadian rhythm is the sleep—wake cycle. During life the individual establishes a pattern of activity, rest, and sleep. This pattern is influenced by external environmental factors as well as internal biorhythms. These external factors include light—dark cycles, cultural and societal expectations, habits, and work—leisure routines. Internal biorhythms are affected by level of growth and development, state of health, drugs, and biochemical interactions. Alterations in any of these internal or external factors result in alterations in all biorhythms, including the sleep—wake cycle.

A disruption in the individual's biorhythms and interferences with physical, physiologic, and psychosocial processes affects the individual's level of comfort.

Comfort is a relative and subjective state of well-being which cannot be directly measured by anyone except the individual. Comfort is on a continuum which ranges from high-level well-being to excruciating pain, with many gradations in between. High-level comfort is usually associated with increased levels of energy and feelings of well-being, safety, and security and with the satisfaction of basic physiologic needs. When the meeting of basic needs is interfered with, when anxiety levels increase, when environmental conditions are extreme, or when pathophysiologic processes are present, discomfort occurs.

Discomfort is the feeling of unease, tension, irritation, low energy levels, or dissatisfaction experienced when needs are not met. *Pain* is an extreme form of discomfort and is most often associated with physiologic dysfunction. However, persons describe severe states of stress as painful. Exact definitions for these terms are difficult because of their

---

Chart 23.1
Circadian Rhythms of Selected Physiologic Mechanisms

PHYSIOLOGIC MECHANISM	RHYTHM
Temperature	High: late afternoon, approximately 4:00—5:00 PM Low: early morning, approximately 4:00—5:00 AM Expected variation can be up to 2°F.
Blood pressure	High: evening Low: early morning
Minute volume of the heart	High: evening, approximately 6:00 PM—12:00 AM Low: early morning, approximately 4:00—6:00 AM
Vital capacity and tidal volume	High: afternoon Low: very early morning, approximately 2:00 AM
Hemoglobin, hematocrit, and total plasma protein	Low: late evening, approximately 10:00—11:00 PM
Granulocytes	High: midnight and middle of afternoon
Skin mitosis	High: noon to midnight
Urinary secretion of water, potassium, chlorides, and urea	High: early afternoon
Growth hormone secretion	High: at night Low: during day
Adrenocorticotropic hormone secretion	High: 4:00—6:00 PM Low: midnight
Adrenalin secretion	High: morning Low: late evening
Sex hormone secretion	High: early morning

highly subjective nature. Everyone has his or her own definition for each state and the parameters within which pain and discomfort exist. Since biorhythms, sleep patterns, and comfort are frequently disrupted by changes in the physical, physiologic, and psychosocial status of the individual, the nurse needs to assess these patterns and any interferences with them. This assessment allows the nurse to plan and intervene to best meet the comfort needs of the individual and to structure care so that the biorhythms of the person are considered.

ASSESSMENT

Biorhythms

The nurse assesses the individual's biorhythms in conjunction with other health care needs. The nursing history identifies the individual's usual times of hunger, defecation, urination, sexual activity, sleep, activity, and rest. The nurse also ascertains the individual's highest and lowest energy points in the day by asking the individual to identify them. By asking the person about any recurring weekly, monthly, or seasonal variations such as menstruation, mood swings, and repeated pathophysiology, the nurse can determine a profile of infradian cycles. Any recurring pattern of behavior is part of the person's biorhythms, and since the individual may not recognize them, careful questioning by the nurse may bring these rhythms to light.

ACTUAL AND NATURAL PATTERNS

There is often a marked difference in the actual daily pattern the individual follows and the individual's naturally occurring patterns. Job and family responsibilities or societal expectations may force the individual to adopt a routine that counters the individual's natural rhythms. By differentiating between the two, the nurse can often assist the individual to a higher level of wellness by adjusting higher priority rhythms to fit within his or her daily life.

BIOCHEMICAL PROFILES

Although not commonly used at this time, biochemical profiles give much information as to the individual's physical rhythms. These profiles could assist in determining the optimum time for an individual to receive medications and treatments, to have surgery, and to participate in activities. For example, studies have shown that medications given at various times in a person's daily cycle have different effects. At some periods the action of the medication is potentiated; during others the action is notably decreased.

INTERFERENCES

The nurse also attempts to identify factors which are actual or potential interferences with the individual's biorhythms. An individual's biorhythms are altered by such factors as forced changes in usual routine, as seen with hospitalization or changes in shift rotation; medications that change biochemical interactions, activity patterns, or sensory input; surgery; changes in light–dark cycle; and travel through different time zones. An example of interference with biorhythms is seen in the person who is accustomed to sleeping during the night and working during the day who suddenly must adapt to the reverse schedule. The person may manifest behaviors indicative of a disturbance in biorhythm. These behaviors include lethargy, irritability, anorexia, disturbances in cognitive abilities, and illness. Until the individual either returns to the previous pattern or adjusts to the change (which may require several months), the individual is in a state of desynchronization.

Nursing assessment related to biorhythms includes descriptions of:

- usual patterns of daily living, e.g., eating, sleeping
- time of highest energy level, of lowest energy level
- ultradian cycles
- infradian cycles
- history of interferences with biorhythms
- behaviors manifested by interferences with biorhythms
- any available biochemical profiles
- evidence of differing treatment reactions related to the time of day

Sleep Patterns

One of the major determinants of sleep patterns is the individual's level of growth and development. Each level has a distinctive pattern, although individual variations occur at every level. As the individual matures, the proportionate amount of time spent in sleep decreases. Chart 23.2 outlines the sleep patterns and characteristics of different levels of growth and development.

ACTIVITY–REST–SLEEP PATTERN

The waking hours are not spent in constant activity but interspersed with periods of rest. **Rest** occurs when the individual is relaxed but not actually in a state of sleep. Adequate rest periods are as necessary to well-being as is sleep. As activity increases, so does the need for rest.

Activity–rest–sleep patterns are basic biorhythms. The nurse assesses the number of hours the individual spends in activity, rest, and sleep; the adequacy of these periods for the individual; factors which enhance or interfere with these patterns; ways the individual ensures these patterns; and reactions to interferences with these patterns. (Illustration 23.1)

ATTITUDES TOWARD SLEEP

The nurse also assesses the individual's attitude toward sleep. In part these assessments may be the result of cultural and societal expectations. Some persons view sleep as a luxury which is to be indulged in only when time and circumstances permit; others view it as just another part of daily life. The amount of sleep that a person thinks necessary is also partially determined by the attitudes of family and/or significant others and customary family habits. Activities which the individual uses to induce sleep or to stay awake may also be socially determined.

STAGES OF SLEEP

In order to assess the effects of interruptions in sleep patterns, the nurse needs to understand the basic stages of sleep. The *first stage of sleep* is the twilight phase. During this period the person may think he or she is awake, can be easily aroused, and may have an active thought pattern. If the individual stays in this stage for long periods during the sleep cycle, the individual may arise feeling as if he or she has not slept. An electroencephalogram will show high-peaked alpha waves at this time. This stage usu-

ally lasts up to 30 minutes before the person moves into stage 2.

Stage 2 is a relatively short period which is characterized by spindle-like spikes on an electroencephalogram. The individual is soundly asleep but still can be aroused with ease. As the spindle waves become intermingled with slower, lower peaked delta waves, the person goes into the *third stage of sleep*. This is a deeper level when a marked stimulus is needed to awaken the individual.

Approximately 30–40 minutes after the beginning of stage 1 the individual moves into the deepest phase of sleep, *stage 4*. During this stage, delta waves appear, and the person will be difficult to arouse. If awakened at this point, the individual appears disoriented and confused. (Illustration 23.2)

Rapid eye movement *(REM) sleep* is the final stage of the cycle. Before REM sleep, the individual moves back through the previous levels of sleep. This stage is characterized by rapid eye movements, an increase in minute muscle activity, and dreams. The person is difficult to arouse generally, but will awaken readily if personally significant stimuli appear in the environment. During the early part of sleep, stages 3 and 4 predominate, while stage 2 and REM sleep account for the greater proportion of middle and late sleep. Naptime sleep consists primarily of the REM stage. Chart 23.3 outlines behaviors commonly demonstrated at various stages of sleep. (Illustration 23.3)

When an individual has a decreased amount of sleep, the loss occurs predominantly in the stage of REM sleep. When the person is deprived of REM sleep, the body will attempt to compensate by increasing the amount of REM sleep during the next sleep period. When there is an increase in stage 4 sleep, there is a proportional loss in REM sleep, resulting in REM deprivation. General sleep deprivation results in lethargy, irritability, poor judgment, and a decrease in attention, coordination, and perceptual acuity, and exaggeration of somatic symptoms. A loss of REM sleep results in dream deprivation and behavioral disturbances which can last long after the REM sleep has been made up.

SLEEP INTERFERENCES

Sleep interferences can be caused by a variety of factors. Anything altering the usual sleep environment such as change in sound level or location, loss of sleep partner, drugs, illness and pain, anxiety, and change in activity level can affect the sleep pattern.

Chart 23.2
Sleep Patterns at Various Levels of Growth and Development

LEVEL	PATTERN	LEVEL	PATTERN
Neonate	Sleeps 16–20 hours per day in 3–4-hour uninterrupted blocks. Percentage of REM sleep: 50%. Respiration quiet and activity minimal during deep sleep.	Schoolage child (Cont.)	Percentage of REM sleep: 18.5%. May be afraid of the dark, may have vivid dreams and nightmares.
Infant	Sleeps 12–16 hours per day. Total amount of sleep decreases as infant gets older. Percentage of REM sleep: 30–40%. May begin to sleep through the night at around 2 months, although wide variation. May fight sleeptime in later infancy.	Adolescent	Sleeps 8–10 hours per day. Percentage of REM sleep: 20%. Often has irregular sleep patterns because of high activity level.
Toddler	Sleeps 12–14 hours per day. Majority of sleep is at night, with naps accounting for rest of sleeptime. Percentage of REM sleep: 25%. Becomes ritualistic about bedtime, e.g., must have favorite pajamas, toy; follows same procedure each night.	Young adult	Sleeps about 8 hours per day. Percentage of REM sleep: 22%. Insomnia may be present. Sleeps patterns may be interrupted by infants or small children in household.
Preschooler	Sleeps 10–12 hours, may still have nap once a day. Percentage of REM sleep: 20%. May have vivid dreams and nightmares.	Middle-age adult	Sleeps 6–8 hours per day. Percentage of REM sleep: approximately 19%. Follows sleep patterns of previous levels. Insomnia may be present.
Schoolage child	Sleeps about 10 hours a day.	Older adult	Sleeps 5–7 hours per day. Percentage of REM sleep: 20–23%. Decreased need for sleep may be upsetting to individual. Sleep may be divided between night sleep and naps. Most overlooked level for sleep patterns, especially in institutional setting, where individual may be expected to retire at 9 p.m. and not get up before 6 a.m.

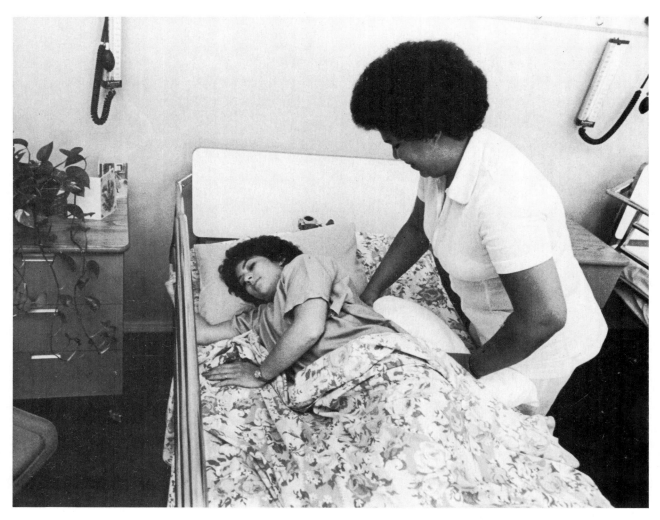

Illustration 23.1

To promote comfort, the nurse recognizes the individual's sleep needs and biorhythms when scheduling care and sees that the basic needs of the individual are met. *(Photo © Leonard Speier)*

Drugs are often prescribed to aid sleep, but actually interfere with it. For example, barbiturates decrease the amounts of REM and stage 2 sleep, resulting in REM deprivation. Alcohol is another REM inhibitor.

Within the institutional setting, nurses often do not recognize how carrying out their usual activities can disrupt an individual's sleep patterns. Activities such as talking with one another, cleaning or moving equipment, keeping lights on, giving treatments, and frequent entry into an individual's room are just a few examples of disruptive nursing behaviors. Nurses should carefully assess the necessity of their nighttime actions in relation to the individual's sleep needs. Activities which may go unnoticed during the daytime hours are frequently accentuated at night, when other environmental stimuli are decreased.

Nursing assessment related to an individual's sleep patterns includes descriptions of:

- presenting activity–rest–sleep patterns
- adequacy of these periods
- relationship between sleep patterns and level of growth and development
- usual sleep environment
- sleep-inducing techniques
- attitudes toward sleep

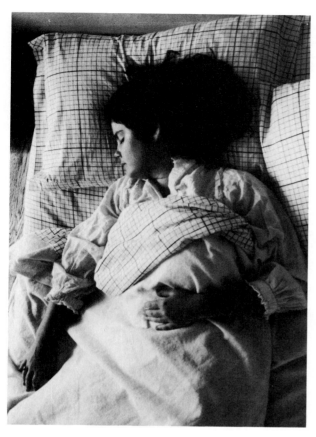

Illustration 23.2
About one-half hour after sleep begins, the fourth stage of sleep occurs. The individual demonstrates little physical activity and is difficult to arouse. *(Photo by Camilla Smith)*

Chart 23.3
Behaviors Commonly Found at Various Stages of Sleep

SLEEP PHASE	BEHAVIOR
Stage 1	Decrease in blood pressure and pulse; decrease in muscle tone; double vision; sensation of floating; sudden muscle contractions which temporarily bring individual back to waking state.
Stage 2	Eyes roll; pupils constricted; further loss in muscle tone; sensory perception decreased.
Stage 3	Muscles relaxed further; skin is flushed; sweating occurs; metabolism decreases 10–20%; further decrease in blood pressure and pulse (blood pressure reaches lowest point by end of this stage); respirations even.
Stage 4	Lowest point of physical activity; sleepwalking and enuresis may occur; positive Babinski reflex.
REM	Rapid eye movements; increase in brain temperature and activity; muscle twitching; respirations irregular; dreaming/nightmares; penile erections; talking in sleep.

- cultural and/or societal influences on sleep
- behaviors manifested by sleep loss
- factors interfering with sleep
- enuresis, sleepwalking

Comfort

The individual's level of comfort may be difficult for the nurse to assess because of its highly subjective nature. However, by ascertaining the degree to which the individual's basic physiologic needs are met and environmental conditions controlled, ensuring competent treatment, asking the individual to describe subjective feelings of well-being, and observing the individual's overt behavior, the nurse can assess the individual's level of comfort. When hunger is assuaged, the bladder emptied, muscles relaxed, and sleep needs met; when vital functions are meeting body requirements; and when other basic needs are fulfilled, the individual will feel a relatively higher level of comfort. Any time a basic physiologic need goes unmet, the individual experiences a state of physiologic tension and diffuse anxiety that is discomforting.

Discomfort may result not only from intereference with a need but also from the manner in which it is met. Therefore, the nurse assesses both the sufficiency of need fulfillment and the quality with which needs are fulfilled. For example, the person who is hungry but has to be fed may receive a sufficient amount of food to meet that physiologic need but may not enjoy the food that is given, may be dis-

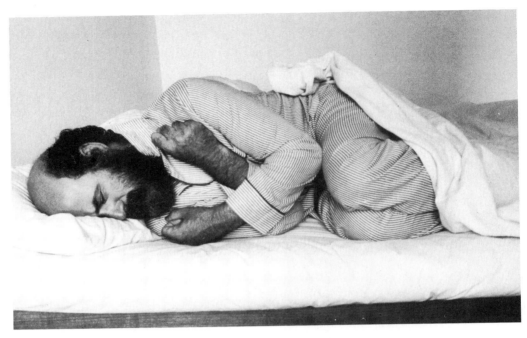

Illustration 23.3
The final stage of sleep, REM, is characterized by rapid eye movements, increased minute muscle activity, and dreams. *(Photo by Camilla Smith)*

stressed at having to be fed, or may dislike the way the food is presented. Thus a state of discomfort results.

ENVIRONMENTAL INFLUENCES

Environmental factors such as temperature, humidity, noise level, ventilation, and degree of crowding contribute to the individual's level of comfort. The types of odors and sights in the environment can also influence comfort. Each individual has a personal range of environmental conditions within which he or she is most comfortable. As a rule, people are uncomfortable when in environmental extremes. However, conditions are influenced by the individual's state of health, level of need satisfaction, cultural and societal expectations, state of mind, habits, and clothing. The nurse ascertains the individual's preferences and observes his responses to environmental changes in order to plan for any necessary modifications.

TREATMENTS

Treatments that are performed in an efficient, competent manner not only reduce the amount of physical discomfort experienced by the individual but also give the individual a sense of well-being and security. Clear, appropriate explanations of what will occur, the individual's role in procedures, and the expected outcomes reduce the fear of the unknown and increase the degree of predictability in the situation. Thus anxiety is relieved and muscle tension reduced so that treatments may actually be carried out in a more comfortable manner. Assessing the individual's level of knowledge, attitudes, and fears allows the nurse to prepare the individual appropriately and enhance his level of comfort.

OBSERVING THE INDIVIDUAL

Observation of the individual's overt behavior gives the nurse many clues as to the individual's level of comfort. Facial expressions, degree of muscle tension, body movements and posture, sounds the individual makes, skin color and tone, and quality of voice are observations the nurse can make to obtain information. Validating these observations by interviewing the individual further completes the picture.

There may often be a discrepancy between the observations the nurse makes and the statements the individual gives. This discrepancy may be the result of many different factors. The individual's cultural background, usual pattern of reactions, degree of trust, and expectations of the situation all influence the way the individual is able to express needs. For example, the child who is observed rocking back and forth, clutching a teddy bear, and on the brink of tears may respond in the negative when asked if anything is wrong. The child may indeed be in severe pain, but a lack of familiarity with the environment, fear of injections, and a feeling of desertion by mother or father may interfere with the child's ability to express discomfort.

The nurse needs to develop skill in determining when to take situations at face value and when to find alternate ways of assessing the individual's true status. Familiarity with the individual's interaction style is one way the nurse can decide what course to take. The nurse can also ask family and/or significant others for help in interpreting the individual's behavior.

Pain

The presence or absence of pain is often a major determinant in the individual's level of comfort. Pain and its intensity are totally subjective phenomena which exist whenever and however the person perceives them. The process of pain is not fully understood. However, it is currently thought that pain is mediated by the stimulation or inhibition of gating mechanisms located in the spinal cord, the central control system of the cortical and limbic areas of the brain, and a central biasing system located in the brain stem. This theory is called the gate control theory of pain and was developed by Melzack and Wall.[1] Although this is not a completely validated theory, it does provide a comprehensive view of what we presently know about pain.

GATE CONTROL THEORY

According to the gate control theory, a stimulus is picked up by large and small peripheral nerve fibers and carried to the dorsal horn cells of the spinal cord. Impulses of the small nerve fibers pass through the substantia gelatinosa (a dense network of cells along the spinal cord), where they are carried by the transmission cells to the brain unless inhibited by an equal or greater amount of larger-fiber impulses. This is the spinal gating mechanism. (Fig. 23.1)

Once the impulse reaches the cortical and limbic structures, further interpretation of the pain impulse takes place. The impulse is identified as to its type, intensity, location, and meaning, and an appropriate

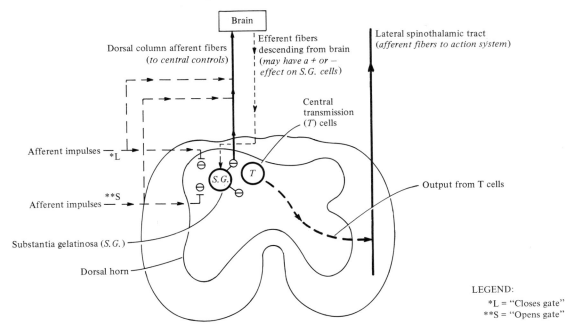

Figure 23.1
Schematic cross section of spinal cord depicting mechanism of gate control theory of pain. (*Courtesy of Donovan and Pierce,* Cancer Care Nursing, *Appleton-Century-Crofts, New York, 1976, p. 56.*

response to its presence is made accordingly. The response to the interpretation process can result in the impulse continuing along afferent pathways to the central biasing system, or the impulse can descend along efferent pathways in the spinal cord to gate cells where it can be further modified or continued to effector sites where a behavior response occurs.

It is at this point that the central control system can also independently generate impulses which travel down the spinal cord to the spinal gating mechanism for inhibition or activation of pain sensation. This type of impulse is related to psychogenic pain. **Psychogenic pain** is a sensation of pain with little or no recognized physiologic stimulation.

If the pain impulse is transmitted to the central biasing system, further inhibition may occur. The central biasing system acts as a regulator for the amount of sensory input that is sent to the rest of the brain.

OCCURRENCE OF PAIN

Pain is a protective mechanism of the body which can occur whenever there are interferences with physical, physiologic, or psychosocial processes. Pain warns the individual that some type of damage is occurring and gives the individual an opportunity to avoid its source or take some action to reduce it. Without pain the body could be damaged irreparably without the individual's awareness.

Pain occurs when there is physical and chemical damage externally; tissue death frequently related to loss of oxygen to the tissues; intrusion of one organ upon another; invasive processes that erode nerve endings; obstruction of any passageway or lumen; overstretching tissues, particularly muscles; and the filling of any body cavity with extra fluid. In addition, noxious smells or sights and anything the individual perceives as a threat to well-being can result in the individual's experiencing pain. The nurse needs to identify the source of pain whenever possible, in order to intervene appropriately. Pain from different sources requires different interventions to lessen or alleviate it. (Illustration 23.4)

CHARACTERISTICS OF PAIN

The nurse assesses the characteristics of the pain.

Location
Pinpointing the location of the pain may give some indication of its cause or treatment. The pain

can be **localized,** circumscribed within an identified area; or **diffuse,** generalized throughout the whole body or a large body area. The pain may also be described as either superficial or deep. **Superficial pain** occurs in the cutaneous tissues or supporting structures while **deep pain** is in the deep viscera or tissues. **Referred pain** originates in one organ or area of the body but is perceived in another organ or area. For example, when myocardial ischemia occurs, the pain may be felt radiating down the left arm.

Intensity and Quality
Pain is also described in terms of its intensity and quality. *Aching, dull,* and *gnawing* usually refer to persistent but not acute pain, while *sharp, knifelike, stabbing* and *crushing* refer to intermittent, higher-intensity pain. The nurse asks the individual to describe the pain in his or her own words and to liken it to other types of pain felt in the past or other experiences which are descriptive. For example, the individual might say that he or she has a sharp, crushing pain in the chest as if someone were hugging the individual with a viselike grip. Pain which is not reduced by use of traditional techniques is called **intractable pain.**

Timing
The duration of the pain is another characteristic ascertained. Pain may be **intermittent,** which implies that it comes and goes or varies in intensity over a period of time. On the other hand, it may be persistent or chronic with little change in intensity. The pain may have characteristic times of occurrence; for example, it may be more intense in the evening and less in the morning.

Precipitating Factors
Pain may be precipitated by certain events or activities. For example, the pain may occur after meals or after ambulation. Identifying the precipitating factors may help to diagnose the cause of pain as well as provide methods for preventing its occurrence.

Assessment of Characteristics
The individual may have identified methods which decrease or eliminate pain. Assessment of these methods, circumstances, or conditions allows the nurse to integrate them into the plan for pain relief and to identify the source of the pain. Written records of the characteristics of the pain experience give objective base-line data for comparison. The exact point on the body where the pain is located, the diameters of this location, along with any movement or exten-

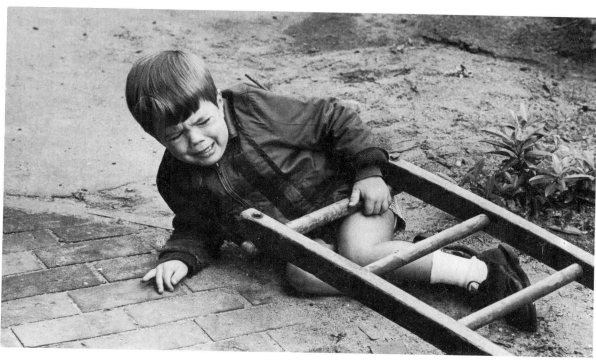

Illustration 23.4

Pain impulses are interpreted at various points along the central nervous system; their type, intensity, location, and meaning are distinguished. Here, a youngster's fall has been interpreted, or felt, as painful, and his tears are an appropriate response. *(Photo © Lynn McLaren, from Rapho/Photo Researchers)*

sion or change in intensity, quality, or duration is noted, as well as the precipitating factors and methods to alleviate it.

INFLUENCES ON PAIN RESPONSE

Studies have shown that the majority of individuals have similar threshholds for pain but vary in their reactions to the pain experience. **Pain threshhold** is that point where the person first has the sensation of pain. **Pain tolerance,** however, refers to the manner in which the individual deals with the pain. Each individual reacts uniquely to pain, and this reaction is based on how a variety of factors is integrated within the individual to produce the pain experience.

Growth and Development

The individual's level of growth and development influences that person's way of responding to pain. This in itself is related to several factors, such as the physiologic maturity of the neurohormonal system, the individual's communication skills, past ex-

periences, cultural and societal expectations as to how one should act at a certain age or as male or female, the meaning the individual is able to attach to the pain, and the amount of control the individual has over it. For example, the infant experiences pain as a diffuse sensation, can communicate discomfort only by crying, and has little or no personal control over it.

Culture

Societal and cultural expectations and attitudes toward pain also help to determine the individual's response to it. Cultures and societies have different values as to how males and females should react to pain, what pain reactions are appropriate for different age groups, how people should generally react to pain, and what actions people should take to alleviate it. Zaborowski[2] compared and contrasted the reactions to pain of four different cultural groups. Chart 23.4 summarizes these findings. While culture can play a great part in the individual's response to pain, it cannot be used as the sole determinant, and must be

Chart 23.4
Cultural Responses to Pain

CULTURAL GROUP	RESPONSE
Old American (Caucasian, Protestant, predominantly born in the United States, little ethnic identification)	Describes pain in specific terms but attempts to control verbal and behavioral responses to the pain; attempts to isolate self when in severe pain; expects medical treatment to relieve pain but usually waits to see if pain will disappear by itself before seeking attention; certain events are expected to be painful; concerned with implications of pain.
Irish (Irish-born or strong identification with Irish ethnic group)	Reacts in a similar way to Older American; not good at describing pain; will admit to having pain but chooses to handle it alone; pain itself not as great a consequence as what it may lead to; reactions may be of two types—either "grin and bear it" or "relax and let the pain take care of itself."
Jewish	Less pain tolerance than Irish or Old American; uses superlatives to describe pain experience and readily shares the experience with others; feels that the attentions of others will help in dealing with the pain; believes pain to be caused by "the worst"; seeks out medical attention for pain but may be hesitant to be treated with any measures considered addictive; like the Old American, concerned with implications of pain.
Italian	Also has less pain tolerance than Irish or Old American; very dramatic in presentation of symptoms to health care workers but stoical with friends and family; attention is centered directly on pain, not on its causes or implications; believes treatment will relieve pain and thus accepts most treatments readily.

taken within the context of the individual's total life experience.

The individual's personality style has a great bearing on the pain response. Individuals who typically react to events in a certain way will most likely react similarly to pain. The reactions depend upon the individual's usual coping mechanisms, cognitive style, and perceptions. The experiences that the individual and the family and/or significant others have had with pain and its outcomes, the meaning the individual attaches to the pain, self-concept, the importance of the affected body part, and the degree of control over the pain and its circumstances also contribute to pain responses. If, for example, the individual associates pain with death or severe disability, the individual may react more than the person who assumes that the pain can be easily treated and alleviated.

Other Influences

The individual's state of health, level of anxiety, and distractibility also influence pain responses. Fatigue and anxiety usually decrease the individual's tolerance for pain. The more the individual can concentrate on the events in the environment and not on the pain experience, the greater will be the individual's ability to deal with the pain. The individual's state of health may also give the nurse indications as to the type of pain that can be expected, its sources, and the possible alleviating and precipitating factors.

Nursing assessment of comfort and pain includes descriptions of:

- degree to which basic needs are being satisfied
- satisfaction with the way needs are met
- environmental conditions which enhance or decrease comfort
- reactions to treatments
- level of knowledge of treatments, including fears, etc.
- overt behaviors suggestive of comfort or discomfort

- subjective statements
- factors which may account for discrepancies between overt behavior and statements
- reactions to pain
- pain source
- pain characteristics
- factors which precipitate pain
- factors which decrease pain
- relationship of culture to pain reaction
- relationship of level of growth and development to pain reaction
- relationship of personality style to pain reaction
- meaning of pain
- past experiences
- level of anxiety
- state of health
- level of distractibility
- measures being used for pain relief
- effectiveness of pain relief measures

Except for testing superficial and deep pain responses (Chap. 13), there are no specific physical as-sessment measures or diagnostic tests related to sleep and comfort needs.

NURSING DIAGNOSIS

A 26-year-old woman, Ms. Collins, delivered her first baby 12 hours ago. Delivery was uncomplicated and required no anesthesia. It is now 1 A.M., and the nurse finds the new mother awake and complaining of inability to sleep.

The nurse assesses Ms. Collins' presenting (actual) behaviors to determine possible disruptions in her biorhythms and interferences with her physical, physiologic, and psychosocial processes. The following are descriptions of Ms. Collins' presenting behaviors and the behavior which the nurse would expect to find in a woman at a similar level of growth and development who has no interference with sleep and comfort.

ASSESSMENT FACTOR	EXPECTED BEHAVIOR	PRESENTING BEHAVIOR
Energy high/low	—	Usually gets up at 7 A.M. Wakes up on her own before alarm goes off. Mornings are her "best time of day." Usually experiences feelings of fatigue, lack of energy at 4 P.M. Characterizes herself as a "day person." Goes to bed between 11 and 11:30, reading for about a half-hour before falling asleep.
Actual or potential interferences with biorhythms	—	Actual: medicated with narcotics during delivery; slept for 4 hours after delivery. Potential: accustomed to stable routine, will now have new baby in home.
Sleep patterns	Young adult: 8 hours/night	Usually sleeps 7½–8 hours per night. States this is a good amount for her. Does not take naps; states she usually relaxes after dinner; does not take sleeping medication; rarely has insomnia except when she's "particularly worried or excited about something."
Sleep environment	—	Sleeps in queen-size bed with husband; is not used to sleeping alone.

(continued)

ASSESSMENT FACTOR	EXPECTED BEHAVIOR	PRESENTING BEHAVIOR
		Likes room very dark; likes soft noise of radio, especially talk shows, when falling asleep; likes cool temperature—always has window open.
Attitude toward sleep	—	"If I don't get a full night's sleep, I'm worthless the next day."
Sleep behaviors	—	Has no recall of nightmares, except for last few months of pregnancy, when she woke up during night worrying about health of baby. No sleepwalking.
Interferences related to institutional setting	—	States, "I keep thinking I hear my baby crying." Asked to have lights in hall near room turned out. States, "People keep walking past the door. I wish I had remembered to bring my radio. This bed seems so small compared to mine at home. I don't feel like I have enough room to turn over."
Comfort level physiologic	—	No hunger or thirst present; no difficulty voiding. States, "I feel tired after all the excitement." Vital signs as expected.
Environmental factors	—	See above. States room is "stuffy."
Reactions to treatment	—	"The nurses are just wonderful. Everyone seems to know what they're doing."
Overt behavior	—	Shifts weight off perineal area, grimaces when doing so. Frequently adjusts bedcovers, readjusts pillows, checks bedside clock frequently.
Subjective statements	—	"I'm a little sore all over, especially where my stitches are and my lower back. I wish I could get to sleep because I'll need all I can get for when I go home."
Pain Location		Perineal area around site of episiotomy (surgical incision made to accommodate delivery of baby); lower back at lumbar sacral area; occasional uterine cramp. Fundus firm one finger breadth below umbilicus, lochia scanty, dark red.

(continued)

ASSESSMENT FACTOR	EXPECTED BEHAVIOR	PRESENTING BEHAVIOR
Type	—	Perineal, localized, and superficial; back—radiates across buttocks and between waistline and coccyx; uterine—deep, localized.
Intensity	—	Perineal—throbbing and sharp; back—dull ache; abdomen—"crampy."
Duration	—	Perineal—constant; since delivery; back has had it "on and off" for the last 3 months but more acute since delivery. Abdominal—"every so often since delivery."
Attitudes toward pain		"It's not as bad as I expected; my mother told me it would be miserable for weeks."
Relationship of culture to pain		Italian descent; states, "I don't see any use in crying or screaming over a perfectly natural process."
Personality style		States, "I'm usually a big baby, but I'm really surprised at how well I'm able to handle it so far."
Previous experience with pain and its outcomes		First experience with childbirth; has had no major illnesses or surgery. "I figure that if the pain really gets bad you'll be able to give me something to relieve it."
Meaning attached to pain		"It's all been worthwhile. I have a beautiful, healthy baby."
State of health		No unexpected sequelae from delivery; in state of high-level wellness otherwise.
Level of anxiety		"I really worry sometime if I'll be a good mother, what'll I do if my baby chokes or something. My husband and I can't wait to take the baby home, but we know it'll really change our style of living."
Medical Orders		Acetaminophen gr X p.o. Q3-4h p.r.n. for pain. Dalmane 30 mg p.o./h.s./p.r.n. Sitz Bath b.i.d. and p.r.n. OOB ad lib. Full diet.

Resulting nursing diagnoses in the situation of Ms. Collins might include the following:

- perineal pain related to inflammation
- lower back pain related to muscle strain
- uterine cramp related to post delivery uterine muscle contraction
- inability to sleep related to change in sleep environment
- inability to sleep related to anxiety about care of baby
- inability to sleep related to physical discomfort

PLANNING

Planning to meet sleep and comfort needs requires the consideration of a full scope of nursing measures, not merely the administration of medications. The individual's biorhythms, personal preferences, and needs must be considered as real components of the care situation. This often requires a great deal of creativity and flexibility on the part of the nurse to help manipulate the environment to meet the individual's sleep and comfort needs.

The plan for one of the nursing diagnoses listed above, in the situation of Ms. Collins, might look as follows:

NURSING DIAGNOSIS	GOAL	PLAN
Inability to sleep related to physical discomfort.	1. Decreased perineal pain within 1 hour.	1. Assist individual with Sitz bath. 2. Lower head of bed so that pressure of body is not on perineal area.
	2. Relief of back pain within 1 hour.	1. Administer Acetaminophen 2. Give back rub 3. Assist into comfortable side-lying position. Place soft pillow at small of back.
	3. Maintenance of firm fundus	1. Check fundus before going to sleep and upon awakening. 2. Massage if boggy. 3. Check perineum for amount, type, and color of drainage (lochia).
	4. Sleep 7 hours without awakening	1. Decrease environmental distractions by closing door to room, window blinds; opening window; putting up side rail; straightening bed. 2. Ask day staff to have husband bring in radio. 3. Administer sleeping medication if individual desires or if still awake after 1 hour. 4. Arrange with day staff to have A.M. care and breakfast delayed until 8:30 A.M. 5. After treatments are administered, talk quietly with individual on distracting subject.

INTERVENTION

Biorhythms

The nurse uses the base-line data collected on the individual's biorhythms to schedule care. While this is sometimes difficult to carry out within institutional settings, careful scrutiny of some of the routines may show areas which can be adjusted to the individual's biorhythms. All too often the routines serve the purposes of the system rather than the individual. As more recognition is given to the effects of disturbances of biorhythms on the individual's health, greater attention will be paid to tailoring care routines to fit the individual's pattern more closely.

Until that time, however, the nurse can look at the biorhythm profiles of groups of individuals and plan each person's care within the time available according to the biorhythms. Within the nurse's work time and with recognition of priorities, the nurse can give basic care and treatments first to the early risers before doing so for later-sleeping individuals. If all other things are equal, the nurse can suggest to the late riser a breakfast that does not need to be kept warm, thus the person need not be disturbed for the meal and can sleep later. Or if an individual is used to bathing in the evening, the nurse can arrange for a bath at that time. Similarly, if a person is awake during the night and likes to sleep during the day, ambulation activities can be done during the individual's waking hours. In addition, attempts can be made to schedule tiring procedures at the individual's point of high energy, when the individual is best able to withstand them. Scheduling activities in this manner requires cooperation among all staff members and a redistribution of responsibilities to even the work load.

The nurse can assist the individual to recognize naturally occurring biorhythms and make adjustments wherever possible to follow them. For example, if a person travels between time zones frequently, the individual may be able to plan for extra time within the travel schedule to allow for readjustment of biorhythms in order to prevent fatigue and other sequelae of desynchronized biorhythms. From a safety standpoint, the nurse can help the individual not to undertake activities that require coordination, precision, and endurance at times of the day when the individual has energy lows.

Sleep

Nursing activities that can assist the individual to meet sleep needs are wide ranging. Modifying the environment to reduce distractions and to simulate the individual's usual sleep environment is one such activity. A few of the other methods available to the nurse are reducing lighting to a minimum, carrying out necessary activities as quickly as possible, adjusting the temperature by thermostat control if it is available or by adding or removing blankets, eliminating sources of odors, and providing the number of pillows or other sleep aids the individual desires. The specific actions taken will depend on the individual's preferences. Helping roommates to negotiate the environmental factors so that all participants are at least minimally satisfied is a frequently overlooked nursing intervention.

In addition to creating a conducive sleep environment, the nurse can promote relaxation by reducing pain, discomfort, and muscle tension and by allaying anxiety. There are times when the individual will require medications to help induce sleep. However, as was previously mentioned, many so-called sleep medications can actually interfere with getting the proper proportion of stages of sleep and can produce disorientation and confusion. Sleep medications that are p.r.n. should not be administered routinely, but given after careful evaluation of the individual's needs at that time. Sleep medications are not to be confused with pain medications, as both often serve different purposes. Frequently, other nursing actions can reduce the need for medications for sleep. In addition, the action of sleep medications may be enhanced by these other techniques.

The individual's bedtime ritual or routine is followed as closely as possible. Many persons enjoy a warm drink, reading to relax, a warm bath, or a snack before going to sleep. Activities which stimulate the individual should be avoided. However, what is stimulating or relaxing to one person may have the opposite effect on another. Individuals usually recognize what relaxes or stimulates them.

Scheduling procedures and activities to allow the longest possible intervals for sleep is another important aspect of meeting sleep needs. Treatments are looked at in terms of balancing their necessity with the individual's need for sleep. Physician's orders that are written in terms of time intervals (e.g., b.i.d.) rather than for specific hours can often be arranged according to the needs of the individual. Collaboration with the physician about the times that treatments and medications are scheduled results in an arrangement that benefits the individual.

The nurse assists the individual to balance activity, rest, and sleep needs. Alternating activity periods with rest periods based on the individual's endurance, limitations, and capabilities ensures conservation of energy while providing needed exercise. Many times individuals have difficulty falling asleep or sleeping through the night because of unnecessary naps taken during the day. Providing meaningful activities and stimuli during the day can prevent the individual from falling asleep out of boredom. However, if this is the usual pattern or if the individual is making up for sleep deficits, the individual should not be prevented from napping.

Comfort

Providing comfort begins with meeting basic needs. Fulfilling basic needs in a manner that is satisfying to the individual results in increased levels of comfort. Symptomatic treatment of interferences when they arise, as well as anticipation of potential interferences, serves not only to meet comfort needs but also to reduce anxiety which could potentiate feelings of discomfort by increasing feelings of safety and security (specific interventions are explained in the appropriate chapters).

Since the family and/or significant others often know the best way to comfort the individual, collaborating with them and including them in the care process is an effective way of decreasing the individual's discomfort and anxiety. Family and/or significant others should receive explanations about the care of the individual and instructions concerning it. They are not, however, forced or intimidated into carrying out care if they are unable or unwilling to do so.

As with maintenance of biorhythms, an environment conducive to relaxation and rest is important. Often when individuals are uncomfortable or in pain, environmental considerations take on greater importance. Cluttered, confined environments frequently exacerbate feelings of discomfort. Often when individuals are uncomfortable, muscle tension and perspiration increase, resulting in further discomfort. The nurse can help promote relaxation in the individual by the use of massage, body positioning, change of linen, and body aesthetic measures.

BEDMAKING

Bedmaking is usually performed in conjunction with personal-care activities; however, it is also car-

ried out any time it will add to the individual's comfort or when the bed becomes soiled. There are several types of bedmaking techniques: the occupied bed, the unoccupied bed, and the postoperative recovery bed. The occupied bed is made with the individual remaining in bed. The postoperative recovery bed is used to facilitate the transfer of an individual from a stretcher to the bed when the person's assistance is minimal. Regardless of the type of technique used, the sheets are wrinkle free, movement in bed is not impeded by the linen, and the sheets are secured so that they do not come off the mattress. The individual's preference for the number of blankets and pillows, as well as the way it is made, are followed.

Supplies needed for making a bed include a top and bottom sheet, pillowcase, spread, blanket, and a turn sheet if necessary. A turn sheet is a shorter sheet placed under the shoulders and trunk to facilitate turning and moving the individual in bed.

Charts 23.5 and 23.6 and Figure 23.2 describe the bedmaking procedure.

A postoperative bed is made in a manner similar to an unoccupied bed; however, the top sheet and spread are not tucked in but are fanfolded to one side. This allows the individual to be transferred from a stretcher to the bed without catching the individual's legs and feet in the bed linen. The top linen is then pulled over the person and tucked and mitered. Regardless of the type of technique used, the bottom sheet is pulled as tightly as possible to avoid wrinkles and to promote comfort. If underpads are used, they are placed over the bottom sheet. Underpads are not placed in multiple layers. These layers do not protect the bed better than an overlapped single layer and, additionally, bunch up and cause skin discomfort.

ANXIETY REDUCTION

Anxiety can be lessened through the use of therapeutic communication. Carefully explaining procedures, providing opportunities for the individual and family and/or significant others to ventilate their fears and anxieties, honestly answering questions, supporting the person's coping mechanisms, collaborating with the individual, spending time with the individual, and following his or her preferences whenever possible are some of the ways the nurse can use communication skills to meet the individual's comfort needs.

Chart 23.5
Making the Unoccupied Bed

TECHNIQUE	RATIONALE	TECHNIQUE	RATIONALE
Gather supplies and put in order of use.	Readily available equipment saves time and helps ensure organized carrying out of procedure.	Tuck bottom sheet securely under foot of bed.	Secures sheet.
Raise bed to proper working height and lower head of bed to horizontal.	Prevents back strain.	Repeat with spread.	
		Miter corner of sheet and spread.	Prevents slipping of sheet and spread.
Remove dirty linen and dispose of it in laundry bag, hamper, or cart.	Clears work space. Reduces opportunity for contamination of environment by linen.	Move to other side of bed and repeat procedure.	Working first on one side then the other saves time and energy.
		Fold top of sheet and spread over to make a border.	Prevents separation of sheet and spread.
Fold any linen which is to be reused.	Prepares it for use.	Pull sheet and spread out several inches at bottom.	Gives room for individual's toes and helps prevent foot drop.
Starting at head, unfold bottom sheet lengthwise. Then unfold widthwise to cover proximal side of bed.	Prevents spread of pathogens. Places sheet in position for tucking.	Fanfold sheet and spread to foot of bed.	Opens bed for easy entry by individual. If bed is not to be used for a period of time this is not done.
Tuck top of sheet under head of mattress. Make mitered corner (Fig. 23.2).	Secures sheet so it will not come loose when individual lies on it.	Put case on pillow and position pillow at head of bed.	Places pillow in position for use.
Tuck side of sheet under side of mattress. (If sheet is long enough, tuck bottom under foot of mattress and miter corner.)	Secures sheet.	Move bed to lowest position.	Safe height for individual's use.
Starting at foot of bed, unfold topsheet lengthwise. Then unfold widthwise to cover proximal side of bed.	Prevents spread of pathogens. Places sheet in position for tucking.	**Note:** If mattress is not waterproof, protective covering (e.g., rubber sheet) is placed over it before making.	Protects mattress from damage.

Chart 23.6
Making the Occupied Bed

TECHNIQUE	RATIONALE	TECHNIQUE	RATIONALE
Gather supplies and place in order of use.	Same as for unoccupied bed.	More individual to finished side of bed.	Frees other side of bed for making.
Explain procedure to individual.	Decreases anxiety and increases cooperation.	Move to other side of bed, lower side rail and proceed as with unoccupied bed.	Same as for unoccupied bed.
Raise bed to proper working height and lower head of bed to horizontal (if individual's condition allows).	Same as for unoccupied bed.	Place clean top sheet and spread over individual and remove dirty sheet and spread.	Does not uncover individual. Individual can hold clean sheet and spread to prevent them from slipping while dirty linen is removed.
Raise one side rail.	Helps prevent individual from rolling out of bed.		
Move individual to that side of bed (logrolling is used if individual cannot move spine).	Frees one side of bed for making (keep pillow under head for comfort).	Tuck and miter sheet and spread.	Same as for unoccupied bed.
		Make linen border.	As above.
Loosen bed linen on free side of bed.	Removes linen from working side of bed.	Pull out sheet and spread at feet.	As above.
Tuck or fanfold bottom linen under individual.	Tell individual that linen is being tucked under him or her.	Put case on pillow and position under individual's head.	As above. (Do not allow individual's head to drop while removing pillow.)
Proceed as with unoccupied bed until first side is made.	Same as for unoccupied bed.	Position individual as desired and in proper alignment.	Promotes comfort and safety.
Raise side rail on finished side.	Helps prevent individual from rolling out of bed.	Move bed to lowest position and raise head to desired level.	Promotes safety and comfort.

PAIN RELIEF

Any intervention that increases comfort also aids in the relief of pain.

Application of Gate Control Theory

Utilizing the gate theory of pain as a model for intervention, the nurse can take actions which decrease the pain experience at each level of the process. First, through treatment of underlying pathologies and removal of noxious stimuli, the nurse can help to stop the source of the pain. Stimulating the large afferent nerve fibers through massage, vibration, and position change helps to increase the inhibition of the smaller fibers which conduct pain impulses.

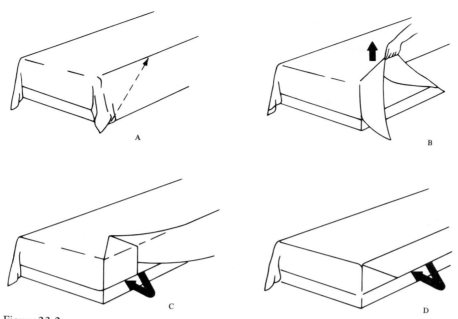

Figure 23.2
To make a mitered corner; after sheet has been tucked under at the top or bottom edge of bed, lift the sheet at the point indicated on illustrations **A** and **B**; folding sheet back on mattress, tuck loose edge (**C**) under mattress; next bring down edge of sheet that has been folded back on mattress, and tuck it under mattress, too (**D**).

Analgesics

The judicious use of medication can depress both the afferent and efferent conduction of impulses and thus interfere with pain impulse transmission. In addition, medications can decrease the individual's perceptual and cognitive abilities, altering the interpretation of the pain stimulus.

Delaying administration of analgesics in an attempt to allay pain through other nursing interventions can sometimes inhibit the effect of the medication. If analgesics are administered after the nerve pathways have been stimulated, alternate routes of administration, dosages, and even type of medication may be necessary to bring about pain relief. The reverse is also true. Overmedicating the individual can interfere with the individual's vital functions, safety, and other therapies. Therefore, a thorough assessment of the individual's pain experience and the analgesics prescribed is necessary in using pain medication to greatest therapeutic advantage.

Distraction

The central control system can be influenced to block the sensation of pain through distraction of the individual. Diversionary techniques such as recre-

ational therapy, conversation, exercise, and use of favorite leisure-time activities can divert the individual's attention away from the pain. In addition, by increasing environmental input, the central biasing system is stimulated, resulting in an inhibition of the pain sensation. Perhaps this phenomenon accounts for the increased incidence of pain reported at night when the environmental input is greatly reduced.

Exploring the Meaning of Pain

How the individual interprets pain can play a major role in the increase or reduction of the pain sensation, so helping the individual to explore the meaning and significance of the pain may also help in its relief. The manner in which pain interventions are carried out also influences the individual's interpretation. Interventions which are approached by the nurse in a positive, "this will help" manner are much more effective than those which are tentatively offered.

Individualized Relief Measures

Bringing together a combination of these methods for an integrated, coordinated approach to pain relief is more effective than employing isolated actions. Whatever interventions are used, the nurse needs to follow and check with the individual frequently to evaluate the intervention as well as to reassure the individual of continued interest. Not every measure will meet with success each time; therefore, the nurse will want to develop a wide repertoire of approaches to prevent frustration on the part of both the individual and the nurse. The nurse may want to explore newly recognized techniques of biofeedback, meditation, relaxation through exercises, yoga, and acupuncture. Successful and unsuccessful interventions are recorded to increase the use of successful ones and to prevent the repetition of unsuccessful methods.

EVALUATION

Evaluating how sleep and comfort needs are being met focuses on the direction of change in the person's ability to rest and relax. How interferences within body subsystems affect the individual's comfort and sleep patterns and vice versa is also evaluated.

Specific criteria for evaluating whether sleep and comfort needs are being met include:

- How do physiologic changes influence comfort, sleep, and biorhythms? Psychologic changes? Environmental changes?
- What is the relationship between presenting patterns and needs?
- Have the presenting comfort, sleep, and biorhythm patterns moved closer to the expected?
- What factors may account for the changes in comfort, sleep, and biorhythms?
- What are the changes in degree of interference with comfort, sleep, and biorhythms?
- What are the effects of changes in comfort, sleep, and biorhythms on body subsystems?
- Are there changes in knowledge (individual, family and/or significant others) about sleep, comfort, and biorhythms?
- Are there modifications in personal habits which relate to sleep, comfort, and biorhythms?

- What skills have been acquired to assist the individual, family and/or significant others in meeting sleep and comfort needs?
- Are there changes in attitudes toward these needs?

RECORDING AND TEACHING–LEARNING ACTIVITIES

Teaching–Learning Topics

- relationship of comfort, sleep, and biorhythms to well-being and level of growth and development
- sleep patterns at various levels of growth and development
- rationale for therapeutic regimens
- relaxation techniques for comfort, pain, and sleep
- ways to promote, maintain, and restore comfort, sleep, and biorhythms
- ways to modify personal habits which affect comfort, sleep, and biorhythms
- proper use of sleep and pain medications
- preventative aspects of discomfort, pain, and sleep deprivation
- ways to balance sleep activity and rest needs

Charting

Using appropriate terminology related to sleep and comfort needs, describe such factors as:

- objective base-line data on biorhythms, sleep patterns, sleep and comfort enhancers and interferences, precipitating factors, level of growth and development, cultural influences
- objective and subjective data on changes in the individual's ability to meet sleep and comfort needs
- subjective data on pain, sleep, comfort, biorhythms
- attitudes toward pain, sleep, comfort
- responses to treatments
- schedule and methods of care
- teaching carried out
- discharge planning done

- interactions and responses of family and/or significant others
- update Kardex on changes in goals and plans for meeting sleep and comfort needs

Medications to Review

Central Nervous System Depressants
- nonnarcotic analgesics, e.g., acetaminophen
- narcotic analgesics, e.g., codeine sulfate
- hypnotics, e.g., chloral hydrate
- sedative, e.g., secobarbital (Seconal)
- alcohol
- tranquilizers, e.g., diazepam (Valium)

NOTES

1. Ronald Melzack and P. D. Wall. "Pain Mechanisms: A New Theory." *Science*, 154:971, November, 1965.
2. M. Zaborowski. "Cultural Components in Responses to Pain." *Journal of Social Issues*, 8:16, 1952. See also, *People in Pain*, San Francisco, Jossy-Bass, 1969, by the same author.

REFERENCES

Breeden, Sue and Kondo, Charles. "Using Biofeedback to Reduce Tension." *American Journal of Nursing*, 75:2010, November, 1975.

Cady, Jane W. "Dear Pain. . ." *American Journal of Nursing*, 76:962, June, 1976.

Davitz, Lois, Davitz, Joel, and Sameshima, Yasuko. "Suffering as Viewed in Six Different Cultures," *American Journal of Nursing*, 76:1296, August, 1976.

DeBlas, Marie and Washburn, Carolyn. "Using Analgesics Effectively." *American Journal of Nursing*, 79:74, January, 1979.

Jacox, Ada "Assessing Pain." *American Journal of Nursing*, 79:895, May, 1979.

McCaffery, Margo and Hart, Linda. "Undertreatment of Acute Pain with Narcotics." *American Journal of Nursing*, 76:1586, October, 1976.

McMahon, Margaret and Sister Patricia Miller. "Pain Responses: The Influence of Psycho-Social Cultural Factors." *Nursing Forum*, 17(1):58–71, 1978.

Natalini, John. "The Human Body as a Biological Clock." *American Journal of Nursing*, 77:1130, July, 1977.

O'Dell, Margaret. "Human Biorhythmology." *Nursing Forum*, 14(1):43, 1975.

Pace, J. Blair. "Helping Patients Overcome the Disabling Effects of Chronic Pain." *Nursing 77*, 7:38, July, 1977.

"Pain and Suffering—A Special Supplement." *American Journal of Nursing*, 74:489, March, 1974.

Putt, Arlene. "A Biofeedback Service by Nurses." *American Journal of Nursing*, 79:88, January, 1979.

Ryan, Betty Jane. "Biofeedback Training: The Voluntary Control of Mind Over Body and Mind." *Nursing Forum*, 14(1):48–55, 1975.

Silman, Judith. "The Management of Pain: Reference Guide to Analgesics." *American Journal of Nursing*, 79:74, January, 1979.

Sterman, Lorraine Taylor. "A Review of Clinical Biofeedback." *American Journal of Nursing*, 75:2006, November, 1975.

Stewart, Elizabeth. "To Lessen Pain—Relaxation and Rhythmic Breathing," *American Journal of Nursing*, 76:958, June, 1976.

Storlie, Frances. "Pointers for Assessing Pain." *Nursing 78*, 8:37, May, 1978.

"Symposium: Biological Rhythms." *Nursing Clinics of North America*, 11:569–638, December, 1976.

"Symposium: Pain." *Nursing Clinics of North America*, 12:609–668, December, 1977.

Wilson, Robin. "An Introduction to Yoga." *American Journal of Nursing*, 76:261, February, 1976.

The omnipresent process of sex,
as it is woven into the whole texture
of our man's or woman's body,
is the pattern of all the process
of our life.
　　—Havelock Ellis, "The New Spirit"

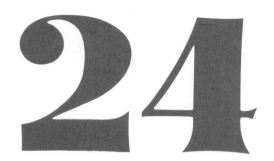

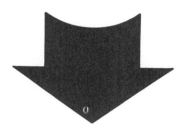

SEXUALITY NEEDS

PRINCIPLES RELATED TO SEXUALITY NEEDS

Sexuality is a basic human need.

Sexuality is a component of all aspects of human life.

Sexual identity is related to physical, psychologic, social, cultural, and religious influences.

Sexuality needs and sexual behavior are manifested throughout the entire growth and development process.

Patterns of expected sexuality fall within a wide range of behaviors.

Many disease processes and medications interfere with expression of sexuality and sexual behavior.

Environmental changes such as hospitalization can interfere with an individual's usual expression of sexuality and sexual behavior.

Sexuality is a general manifestation of human beings and is reflected in all aspects of our lives. Leif has theorized that "sexuality may be described in terms of a system analogous to the circulatory or respira-

tory system."[1] He categorizes the sexual system according to **biologic sex,** which includes actual physical sex characteristics and the chromosomal and hormonal makeup of the individual; **sexual identity,** which comprises the individual's feeling of being of the male or female sex; **gender identity,** which is the sense of being a masculine or feminine person; and **sexual role behavior,** which is the way the individual manifests his or her biologic sex and sexual and gender identities.[2] In accordance with this outline, most theorists today view sexuality as a broad concept. They define the individual's sexuality as pervading all of his or her behavior and not just those activities involved in the sex act itself.

Controversy arises when the concept of sexual normality is considered, and two distinct schools of thought have evolved. One is best demonstrated by Leif's definition that sexual "normality is a process, a dynamic, shifting, changing interplay among discovery, invention, dissemination of information, and behavioral and attitudinal changes."[3] Within this framework many expressions of sexual behaviors (e.g., homosexual and extramarital relationships) are considered variations and not deviations, as they are within the framework of the second school of thought.

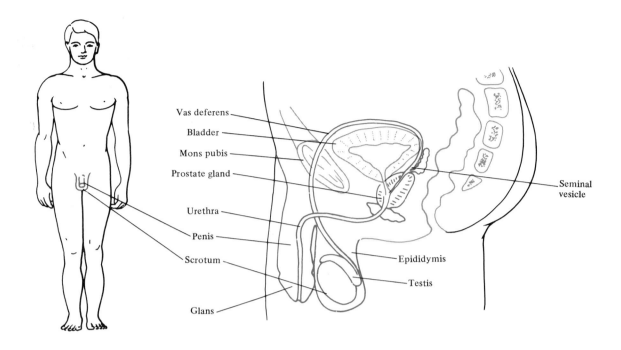

Vas deferens

Bladder

Mons pubis

Prostate gland

Urethra

Penis

Scrotum

Glans

Seminal vesicle

Epididymis

Testis

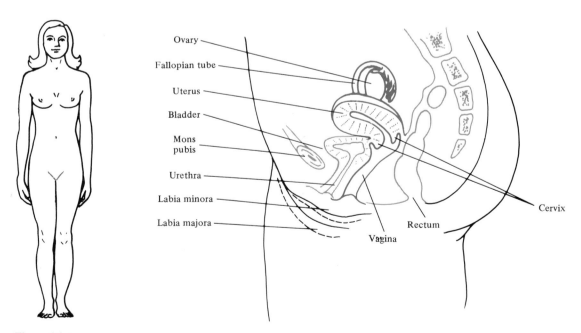

Ovary

Fallopian tube

Uterus

Bladder

Mons pubis

Urethra

Labia minora

Labia majora

Cervix

Rectum

Vagina

Figure 24.1
Male and female reproductive systems.

For the other school of thought, normality is "that which best serves survival of the species" and is "functioning in harmonious accord with design [biological function]."[4] In this definition, normality is not seen as a reflection of the social and cultural mores of the times, but as an inherent pattern of human behavior.

Sexuality, therefore, is a basic human need that must be considered along with any other basic need in assessing, planning, and implementing nursing care.

ASSESSMENT

Nursing assessment of sexuality needs is important not only in the individual who has an interference with sexuality needs because of his or her health state, but also for any individual whom the nurse encounters in the health care system.

Interferences may be a result of genital subsystem pathology such as **vaginitis** (inflammation of the mucosal lining of the vagina), hormonal imbalances such as decreased testosterone levels in males, impairment of the nervous system as with spinal cord injuries, psychologic conditions such as depression, or interferences with other body subsystems such as myocardial infarction (heart attack) or arthritis.

Nursing assessment of sexuality needs for an individual with no direct interference is necessary because factors such as stress, lack of information, or misinformation may alter the expression of sexuality. The individual's level of growth and development, manner of expressing sexuality needs, attitudes, culture, level of knowledge, and interferences with sexuality are major areas in the nursing assessment of sexuality needs.

Growth and Development

INTRAUTERENE LIFE

It has long been known that genetic sex is determined at conception. However, only recently has it been demonstrated that uterine life plays an important role in the sexual development of the individual. While genetic sex is determined at conception, all embryos will develop female characteristics unless the male embryo (bearing the XY chromosome) secretes sufficient testosterone to offset the mother's estrogen.

The embryonic hormonal environment is believed to have significance in the later development of sexual identity.

INFANCY

The infant derives a general feeling of well-being from stroking and cuddling. While not specifically sexual in nature, these pleasurable sensations have implications for the individual's developing sense of sexuality and feelings about the self. Sexual role behavior begins to develop at this stage through the attitudes of the parents toward the infant. For example, if a parent provides typically female clothing and toys for the girl baby, she will soon begin to identify those things as feminine. Studies have shown that the way in which adults handle and talk to boy and girl infants are stereotypic of perceived male and female behavior: the boy gets "rough-housed," while the girl gets cuddles and kisses.

Infants at this stage exhibit oral behavior, which has been identified by some psychoanalytic schools of thought as being a precursor to sexual behavior.

As infancy progresses the child begins to explore his or her body and finds that certain body parts such as the clitoris or penis provide more pleasure when stroked or manipulated than other body parts—the hands or feet, for example. Again, there is no specific sexual connotation to the activity of **masturbation;** the infant is only attempting to explore those parts that "feel good." Negative sexual feelings can begin to develop at this time when significant people attach a sexual overtone to masturbation and attempt to stop it through use of physical or verbal discipline. Even at this early age, the baby learns to carry out this perceived "bad" behavior when adults are not around.

TODDLERHOOD

Toddlerhood is a very significant stage in psychosexual development. By the age of three the child learns gender identity and can accurately verbalize his or her sex. Toilet training, a major life event, usually occurs during this stage. Since excretory function and sexual function are strongly associated in the American culture, toilet training can become a critical point for the toddler's identification of the feelings of "dirty" or "bad" with the sexual organs and self.

Masturbation is a frequent behavior of the toddler. Not only does the toddler engage in it routinely, but it also provides a sense of security in times of stress, anxiety, or isolation. Again, adult reaction to the behavior is an important factor in the toddler's emotional association of his or her own behavior. At this level parents can effectively teach the child to masturbate in private rather than in public situations, which would cause embarrassment.

At this time there is a strong attraction to the parent of the opposite sex, with little girls wanting to marry their fathers and little boys their mothers. This may be viewed as the oedipal stage.

THE PRESCHOOLER

The preschooler is now able to identify accurately not only his or her gender but also that of others. This may result in exploration of other children's bodies, particularly those of the opposite sex. This is a usual pattern of behavior, not a deviant one. However, the way in which significant others react to the situation can markedly affect the child's feelings of self and sexuality.

This is a period of marked sexual identification through engaging in stereotypic masculine and feminine activities. The girl becomes "mother's little helper" and the boy "daddy's little worker." Behavior is very imitative of the same sex and may even be exaggerated. For example, the little girl will always want to wear dresses and feminine accessories. Deviations from the perceived stereotype is distressing for the child. This type of behavior may be viewed as an attempt to resolve the oedipal conflict. (Illustrations 24.1 and 24.2)

Questions the preschooler may have about sexuality should be answered in relation to what the child really wants to know. Adults often think that children of this age want more information than they really do. A familiar story which exemplifies this is the parent, who, in response to being asked by the child "Where do I come from?" gives a long involved discussion of human reproduction, only to have the child say, "No, I mean where do I come from; my friend Johnny comes from Detroit."

THE SCHOOLAGE CHILD

The schoolage child is in the so-called stage of sexual latency. This term reflects the fact that the child's behavior does not seem to be directly related

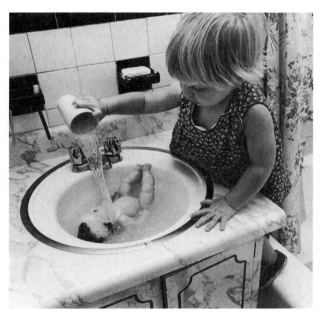

Illustration 24.1

In the preschool period of marked sexual identification, this child, typically, is learning to engage in activities that are stereotypic of her sex. *(Photo © Abigail Heyman, from Magnum)*

to sexuality. In actuality, the child is consolidating previously learned sexual behaviors and attitudes and is testing out these sexual role behaviors with members of the same sex. Generally, the child "hates" members of the opposite sex, although sneaking looks and peeking at them is a common behavior. (Illustration 24.3)

At this age the child chooses some adult of the same sex, usually famous, who epitomizes the ideal of masculinity or femininity. They not only imitate these people, but also constantly compare their parents with him or her. Dress at this age is usually asexual. Worries about the body center on mutilation and castration. Since schoolage children are interested in the working aspects of the world around them, this is an excellent time to teach them the functional aspects of sex.

PREADOLESCENCE

Children once again become interested in and occupied with the opposite sex during preadolescence. Signs of puberty may be evident, such as developing breasts and changing body shapes through the redistribution of adipose tissue. Preadolescence is a transition stage.

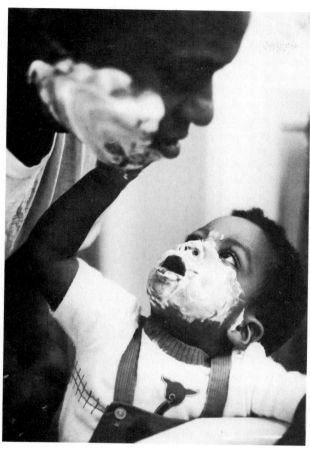

Illustration 24.2
Imitating the behavior of persons of their own sex is one way that preschoolers develop their sexual identity. *(Photo by Burk Uzzle, from Magnum)*

ADOLESCENCE

During adolescence the sexual system matures. Therefore, the adolescent must deal with a multiplicity of feelings related to changes in body form and function, peer group pressures, and the attitudes and mores of society. Hormonal changes produce the secondary sex characteristics, growth spurts, redistribution of adipose tissue, menarche in females, and spermatogenesis in males. Hormone production, particularly early in adolescence, is not regulated and accounts, at least in part, for mood swings and emotional lability.

These physiologic and physical changes result in body image changes. The individual seems to be changing on a daily basis and often has difficulty stabilizing the self-concept of who or what he or she is. The adolescent is occupied with the appearance and function of the body. Thus any situation which threatens physical form or function is very frightening and overwhelming.

Psychosocially, adolescence is a time of attempting to establish oneself as a sexual being. One "tries on for size" new ways of behaving as a sexual being. Sexual experimentation is very common at this time. However, a great deal of ambivalence is felt toward sexual behavior. Their peer group, society, and the adolescents' changing physical form and function place great pressure on them to be sexually oriented, but many mixed messages are interspersed with these factors. The family usually discourages sexual experimentation, although encouraging popularity and keeping up with the peer group. The society says sexy is beautiful but does not sanction the adolescent to follow through with sexual behavior. Sexual activity is usually seen as a pure expression of love.

The male adolescent is often very concerned with "machismo" and being "macho." Thus he may take on extremes of what he considers to be masculine. He fears the idea of homosexuality and often severely ridicules any behavior which does not fit his idea of masculinity. On the other hand, adolescence is a time when some males and females come to realize they are homosexuals. However, by the end of adolescence, young women commonly need to prove their feminity and sexual desirability. Clothing, makeup, and general appearance often reflect this need. They often compare their peers in terms of sexual ideals. Some adolescents deal with their sexual ambivalence by directing their sexual energies in other ways—into sports, academic achievement, and school activities.

Adolescents may appear to be very knowledgeable about sex and sexuality. They may fear appearing unsophisticated or naive and thus will not directly express their need for information. In addition, adolescents often feel that sexual desires and needs are unique to them. Thus adults may be seen as having no real understanding of what they are going through. A fear of recrimination from older people can also limit their ability to ask for information and to use adults to clarify their feelings about sex.

Major health concerns related to sexuality during this period include venereal disease and birth control. In many states the dissemination of information concerning birth control and prescriptions of birth control to minors is forbidden without parental consent. This also applies to treatment of venereal disease. Therefore, adolescents may be reluctant to seek help in these areas and may not be aware of services available to them.

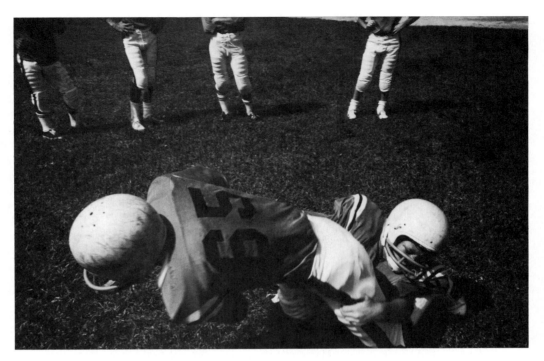

Illustration 24.3
The schoolage child's behaviors most often seem unrelated to sexuality; however, during this
period he tests what he has already learned about his six role with members of his own sex.
(Photo by Charles Harbutt, © Magnum)

THE YOUNG ADULT

By the end of adolescence, extreme sexual role behaviors are usually modified. The young adult can now begin to establish relatively permanent intimate relationships. This is the peak period for first marriages and childbearing. Marriage, childbearing, and child rearing may alter feelings of sexuality and sexual expression. These alterations may be either negative or positive, depending on how these roles fit into the individual's perception of masculinity or femininity.

Today, however, many people feel that marriage is not the only option for establishing intimate ties. It is not uncommon to find both heterosexual and homosexual couples living together, single-parent families, and individual's living by themselves. Since this is the traditional time of pairing, people who are involved in nontraditional situations may feel many stresses from society and family. In addition, the single person may feel out of the mainstream and pressured into unwanted sexual activity. (Illustration 24.4)

Birth control and venereal disease continue to be major health concerns. Because of career and education concerns, many people are now delaying childbearing until later in young adulthood. Still others are deciding not to have children at all. Sterility may also be a concern for individuals who wish to have children but are unable to conceive. Difficulties related to sexual performance and satisfaction, such as impotence and frigidity, may require health counseling and intervention. Knowledge about sexuality may be limited and myths widespread. Embarrassment may hinder the individual's ability to seek information and treatment.

MIDDLE AGE

As the person enters middle age there is again a period of ambivalent feelings about sexuality. Middle age is a time of maximum career productivity and many of the preoccupations of earlier years, such as finishing educations and starting careers, are resolved. The person may have a feeling of "coming into one's own." However, he or she may be receiving mixed messages from peers, family, and society. Since youth is often equated with sexuality in American culture, the middle-aged person may feel a loss of desirability and sexual ability.

Menopause in women creates definitive physical

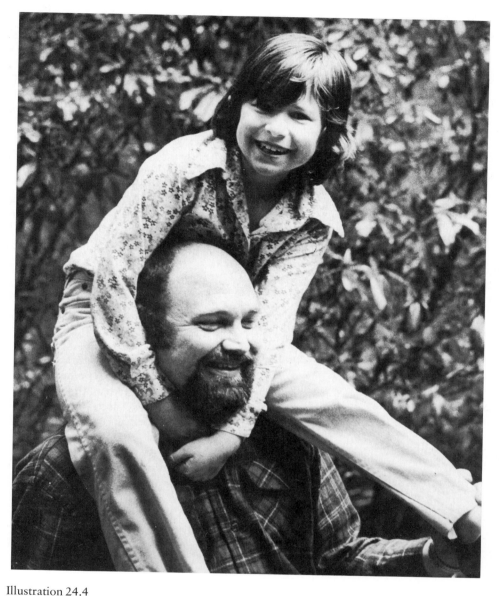

Illustration 24.4
Single parent families are not uncommon in today's American culture. *(Reprinted with permission from* The Single Parent, © *1978, Parents Without Partners, Inc.)*

changes and may result in feelings of loss of feminity. On the other hand, many women may look on this change more positively, since they no longer need fear pregnancy. The loss of parental roles as children grow up and leave home may affect both males and females. If much of the sexual identity is invested in the role of mother or father, this change can further increase feelings of sexuality loss.

The increase in extramarital sexual relationships and divorce seen in this group may, in part, result from these feelings of loss. Both people may feel guilt and a sense of inadequacy during this developmental stage.

The individual who has remained single may look back and wonder what he or she has missed. Labels such as "old maid" or "perennial bachelor" may threaten the person's sense of sexuality. The availability of partners may be limited, and the social acceptability of seeking them out may be decreased.

Chronic illnesses such as arthritis and heart conditions may alter expressions of sexuality. Sexual performance and satisfaction difficulties may again cause concern. Knowledge of alternate sexual options and the implications of the pathology on sexuality may be incomplete and inaccurate. Myths about sexuality in middle age abound.

OLD AGE

Old age is often thought to be a period of asexuality. This is not the case. However, older adults do have many assaults made on their feelings of sexuality. Physical and physiologic changes which affect appearance, function, and strength alter their ability to meet their sexuality needs. Society's view that old age is "not sexy" or that expressions of sexuality typify the "dirty old man" make any expression of sexuality difficult. Loss of partners through death or disease further attacks the older adult's ability to meet sexuality needs. As in middle age, the availability of partners, especially males, makes companionship and sexual expression difficult. Those older adults who do find partners often must resort to subterfuge or a negation of lifelong beliefs because of family disapproval, societal attitudes, or economics. (Illustration 24.5)

In old age, as with any other age, people who have had positive views toward their sexuality and their expressions of it find that this continues in this period until death. The older adult may, however, have to modify intercourse positions as a result of chronic illness. Often sexual intercourse is possible if the partners recognize that the arousal period lengthens while the ejaculatory period shortens. Alternative sexual activity such as masturbation and mutual manual manipulation may replace or supplement sexual intercourse.

Older adults may be stereotyped as senile and without inhibitions as to sexual behaviors, constantly grabbing others or exposing themselves. Again, this is not a true picture of most of the elderly. However, those older persons who, because of cognitive or psychologic impairments, do sexually act out are punished, humiliated, and isolated, which serves only to increase the cognitive or psychologic impairment.

Nursing assessment of growth and development related to sexuality needs includes descriptions of:

- expected sexuality pattern
- presenting sexuality pattern
- relationship between the expected and presenting sexuality patterns
- attitude toward sexuality pattern (individual? family and/or significant others?)
- knowledge of growth and development (individual? family and/or significant others?)
- manner of dealing with variations from the expected
- ways of expressing sexuality
- outlets for expression of sexuality
- restrictions on expressions of sexuality.

Expression of Sexual Role Behaviors

Sexuality is expressed in every aspect of life. Individuals have their own unique way of expressing themselves as sexual beings. The style of dress, use of makeup and cosmetics, and hairstyle are some of the physical ways that people manifest their femininity or masculinity.

IN OCCUPATIONS

The occupations people choose, their hobbies, fields of interest, and recreational activities often reflect the feelings of what is appropriate for their

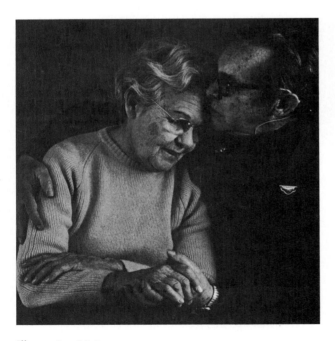

Illustration 24.5
Positive expressions of sexuality may continue throughout old age. *(Photo © Joel Gordon)*

sexual identification. For example, until recently men would not do traditionally female activities such as needlepoint or sewing. Certain occupations were once considered the strict domain of either men or women. Nursing and medicine are examples of this.

WITHIN THE FAMILY AND SOCIETY

Roles within the family and society also are based on one's attitudes and beliefs about what is masculine or feminine. Roles such as child rearing and care of the home are often perceived to be feminine, while economic support of the family is often seen as the masculine responsibility. Economics and changes in societal attitudes have brought more women into the work force. In some ways this has caused a blurring of strictly defined masculine and feminine roles.

INTERACTION STYLE

The interaction style of the individual is another reflection of sexuality. How one person interacts with another person of the same or opposite sex is defined according to the way one identifies oneself sexually. The way one is allowed to greet someone, rules of etiquette, spatial distancing, and touch are some of the modes of interaction that demonstrate sexual feelings. The perception of the appropriateness of being dependent is also linked to attitudes of sexuality.

NURSING ASSESSMENT

The nurse needs to identify the definitions individuals have of themselves as sexual beings in order to plan and implement care that will best support positive self-concept. Care that is offered based on the nurse's belief system rather than the individual's may not be effective or even accepted. Thus an assessment of the person's pattern of expressing sexuality is necessary in order to avoid basing care on assumptions or stereotypes.

Nursing assessment of the individual's pattern of sexual role behaviors includes descriptions of:

- ways sexuality is expressed
    physical appearance
    social roles

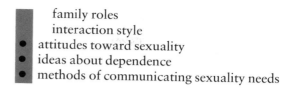

- family roles
    interaction style
- attitudes toward sexuality
- ideas about dependence
- methods of communicating sexuality needs

Attitudes Toward Sexuality

Attitudes and values toward sexuality are based on such factors as the individual's life experience, culture, religious beliefs, and sexual orientation. Attitudes about acceptable masculine and feminine behaviors, acceptable sexual practices, and acceptable sexual outlets are all based on these factors.

SEXUAL ATTITUDES IN ILLNESS

The individual's reaction to illness or disability may, in part, depend on the degree to which the illness or disability threatens his or her sense of sexuality. The belief that becoming ill or dependent is not an acceptable aspect of sexual identity may result in an individual's denial and/or rejection of illness or treatment.

Attitudes of what is acceptable sexual practices may influence one's ability to adjust to limitations imposed by illness. For example, a man who is paralyzed from the neck down (**quadriplegia**) may not be able voluntarily have or maintain an erection, thus preventing him from having vaginal–penile intercourse. His sexual beliefs may hinder him in exploring other methods of sexual expression such as oral–genital sex.

Attitudes will also affect one's ability to accept birth control information or comply with health regimens. Treatments ordered as douches or as applications of medication to the genital area may create anxiety or an inability to comply because of sexual beliefs and attitudes. An inability to carry out one's definition of one's sexual role because of illness may cause an individual to fear a loss of sexuality. A man who cannot work, for example, may feel that he is no longer a "real man" because he cannot support his family.

Nursing assessment of sexual attitudes includes descriptions of:

- attitudes toward sexuality
- ways of expressing attitudes

- influence of attitudes on sexuality pattern
- sexual expectations based on attitudes
- religious beliefs
- cultural beliefs
- degree to which religious and cultural beliefs about sexuality influence health care

Knowledge About Sexuality

Knowledge of sexuality, sexual practice, and sexual outlets often influences an individual's attitude about sexuality. Conversely, the individual's attitudes and beliefs may influence his ability to seek and accept information about sexuality. Due to their sensitivity about sexuality, many people have not been exposed to full and accurate information, and myths and misconceptions have developed in place of accurate information. Such myths suggest that masturbation causes mental illness, that all homosexuals molest children, that one cannot engage in physical activity while menstruating, that nurses are promiscuous, and that elderly persons interested in sex are perverted. Chart 24.1 lists other common myths and misconceptions.

Many fears develop as a result of a lack of knowledge. Individuals who have recovered from an illness or who are chronically ill may be afraid to engage in sexual activity for fear of being injured. Lack of knowledge may also prevent an individual from seeking health advice, obtaining treatment, or carrying out sexual role behaviors. Lack of knowledge about the influence of pathology, health state, medications, or diet on sexuality may also interfere with the individual's ability to meet sexuality needs. These influences may cause the individual to have unrealistic expectations. A woman who is a diabetic may feel that her inability to have an orgasm is due to her failure as a woman, but in fact it is a result of longstanding diabetes.

Many people who have an interference with their sexual pattern of sexual expression may be unaware of the alternate options available to them. They may see their sexuality only in terms of their ability to carry out the sexual act and not in terms of their whole pattern of interactions. Options which are available to the individual for sexual gratification may include such activities as being physically close to someone, stroking, oral-genital sex, or masturbation.

Nursing assessment of an individual's knowledge about sexuality includes descriptions of:

- accuracy of sexual information
- effect of knowledge on sexuality patterns
- availability of information and resources
- knowledge of options available to them
- attitude toward seeking information
- myths and misconceptions
- relationship about knowledge of sexuality to health care
- knowledge of effects of health state and care regimen on sexuality

Sexual Pattern

Part of the individual's sexuality is manifested in his or her pattern of sexual activities. This pattern includes such considerations as sexual preferences, variations, frequency of sexual activities, and the degree of satisfaction that results from sexual activities.

PREFERENCES

Sexual preferences are the types of sexual activities in which the person regularly engages. Some of the activities frequently utilized are penile–vaginal intercourse, anal intercourse, oral–genital sex, and masturbation. An individual may primarily use one of these methods for sexual satisfaction or regularly engage in a variety of these. Chart 24.2 presents a glossary of sexual activity terms. These activities are frequently preceded or followed by various methods of touching, stroking, hugging, or kissing. Sexual preference information becomes an important part of nursing assessment when some interference in sexual function occurs. The nurse can utilize this base-line data in providing information to the individual about alternative methods which are acceptable.

VARIATIONS

Variations in sexual activity include homosexuality, bisexuality, sadomasochism, fetishism, and transvestism. These variations become nursing considerations when an individual whose sexual pattern is a variation enters the health care system and whose health care is directly or indirectly affected by this

Chart 24.1
Sexual Myths

MYTHS OR COMMON MISCONCEPTIONS	FACTS (BASED ON RESULTS OF CURRENT RESEARCH)
The sex drive or "libido" is of primary importance in early development and behavior in infancy.	The bases for one's developing sexuality are established during the first five years of life as a result of learning, mainly through nonverbal channels. The self-gratifying behavior and pleasure-seeking activities of the infant are not "sexual" in the adult sense of the word, for sex, as such, is rarely a human need prior to adolescence.
Each person is endowed with a finite amount of sexual drive which if overdrawn in youth or in young adult life leaves little reserve for the later years.	Actually the correlation between sexual activity and length of time it persists throughout life is just the opposite. The more sexually active a person is, the longer it continues into the later years of life.
The need for expressing one's sexuality becomes less important in the latter half of one's life.	Physiologically, sexual desire and ability do not decrease markedly after middle age. The expression of one's sexuality, as an integral part of development, follows the overall pattern of health and physical performance.
Sexual abstinence is necessary in training for the development of optimum physical performance in sports, dance, or other strenuous activities.	While there is great variation in sexual activity, physiologically the achievement of orgasm is rarely more demanding than most activities encountered in daily life. The desire for sleep which often follows is most commonly due to factors other than physical exhaustion from sexual activities. Orgasm may bring a relief of sexual tension with a feeling of relaxation and a readiness for sleep. A sense of weariness is more likely due to related activities resulting in improper eating, sleeping, drinking, or feelings of guilt.
Excessive sexual activity can lead to mental breakdown.	The biological significance of man's sexuality is of no greater impact on his total development than any other necessary biological function. Most behavioral scientists do not regard sex as *the* prevailing instinct in man so that his sex life must be paramount in his emotional development. There is no scientific basis for believing that one will develop a mental or physical illness unless one's sex needs are satisfied.
Nocturnal emissions (wet dreams) are indicators of sexual disorders.	Erotic dreams that culminate in orgasms are common physiological phenomena in at least 85% of all men. They occur at any age, beginning in the teens when the maturing sex organs exert a new primacy in masculine development. The phenomena is also common among females, who report in clinical studies that their sexual dreams culminated in orgasm. In women, this practice is believed to increase with advancing age.
Because of the antomical nature of the sex organs, the female is inherently passive and the male inherently aggressive.	Physiologic studies disprove this myth by showing the woman to be far from passive. Maximum gratification requires each partner to be *both* passive and aggressive in participating mutually and cooperatively.
It is "unnatural" for a woman to have as strong a desire for sex as a man—for women normally do not enjoy sex as much as men.	These myths have been reinforced by a society which has traditionally taught women that they are to suppress sexual desires to gain love, security, and society's respect—based on the assumption that it is the "basic nature" of women to be submissive, dependent, and subordinate. Physiologic studies indicate that, in some respects, the woman's sex drive is not only as strong but may be even stronger than that of the male.

(continued)

Chart 24.1 (Cont.)
Sexual Myths

MYTHS OR COMMON MISCONCEPTIONS	FACTS (BASED ON RESULTS OF CURRENT RESEARCH)
Women who have multiple orgasms or who readily come to climax are actually nymphomaniacs.	Physiologic studies at this time suggest that we do not know women's sexual potential—but indicate that there is a wide range of intensity and duration of orgastic experience—and the potential for multiple (or frequent orgasms within a brief period of time) is not at all uncommon. Therefore, women have greater orgastic capacity than men with regard to duration and frequency of orgasm.
There is a difference between vaginal and clitoral orgasm. The former being the more "mature" according to Freudian theory; the latter indicating signs of narcissism or inadequacy.	Physiologic misunderstanding has produced the myth of separate clitoral and vaginal orgasms rather than their interrelationships. Female orgasm is normally initiated by clitoral stimulation, but since it is a total body response there are marked variations in intensity and timing. There is no reason to believe that the quantitative differences in the female response to the sex act are due to vaginal rather than a clitoral orgasm.
A mature sexual relationship requires the male and female to achieve simultaneous orgasm.	While simultaneous orgasm may be desirable, it is an unrealistic goal in view of the complexity of human sexuality. Often it is possible only under the most ideal circumstances and is not a determinant of sexual achievement or of satisfaction (except to someone who accepts this as dogma).
It is dangerous to have intercourse during menstruation.	Since the source of the menstrual flow is from the uterus rather than the vagina, there is no basis for concern about tissue damage to the vagina nor is there any reason for the woman's sexual drive to diminish during the menstrual period. There is no physiologic basis for abstinence during the menses.
The larger penis has greater possibilities for pleasurable stimulation or for producing orgasm in the female.	Physiologically, there is practically no relationship between the size of the penis and a man's ability to satisfy a woman sexually. Furthermore, there is very little correlation between penile size and body size and their relationship to sexual potency.
The face-to-face coital position is the proper, moral, and healthy one for it is this position that distinguishes the sexual activity of man from the remainder of the animal kingdom.	Recent knowledge of human sexual practices dispel this myth with the recognition that there is no *normal* or *single most acceptable* sexual position. Whatever position offers the most pleasure and is acceptable to both partners is correct for them. Any variation is normal, healthy, and proper if it satisfies both partners.
The ability to achieve orgasm is an indicator of an individual's sexual responsiveness.	Achievement of a satisfactory sexual response is the result of the successful interaction of numerous physical, psychologic, and cultural influences. Too often the physical fact of orgasm (or lack of orgasm) is taken to be symbolic of sexual responsiveness and seen out of context of the entire relationship between man and woman. Such distortions add to the tension and anxiety of those who strive to attain this singular goal—contributing to conditions of impotence and frigidity.

From: Doris Sutterley and Gloria Donnelly. Perspectives in Human Development. *Philadelphia, Lippincott, 1973, pp. 132–134.*

Chart 24.2
Sexuality Terms

Bisexual—individual who maintains characteristics of both sexes; individual who engages in sexual activity with members of both sexes.

Fetishism—sexual arousal by certain objects or body parts.

Frigidity—inability of an individual (usually used in reference to women) to attain sexual satisfaction or to reach orgasm.

Gay—commonly used term for homosexual.

Heterosexual—individual who engages in sexual activity and whose sexual identification is centered on persons of the opposite sex.

Homosexual—individual who engages in sexual activity and whose sexual identification is centered on persons of the same sex.

Impotence—inability of a man to engage in sexual intercourse because of inability to have a penile erection.

Lesbian—female homosexual.

Sadomasochism—use of and reception of hurting activities to attain sexual satisfaction.

Sterility—inability to conceive children.

Transsexual—individual who changes physical sex through hormonal and surgical treatment; individual who identifies completely with the opposite sex.

Transvestite—person who receives sexual satisfaction from dressing in clothes of opposite sex; individual may be heterosexual or homosexual in basic orientation.

Orgasm—the height of sexual excitement (climax).

sexual pattern. Societal attitudes toward sexual variations may result in the individual's receiving a biased type of health care or being denied an opportunity to have significant others near in time of physical or psychologic stress. For example, a homosexual in an intensive care unit may be allowed to have only relatives or a spouse visit. This may result in the individual's being deprived of the support and love of the most significant person at that time—a homosexual partner.

The nurse may have to assess his or her own feelings toward these variations to see if they influence the ability to accept the individual and give effective nursing care. Caring for individuals with sexual variations may cause anxiety, as may any unfamiliar situation or one that is counter to the nurse's belief sys-

tem. Nurses need to explore their own sexuality needs to come to terms with their actions.

The frequency of sexual activities may become a nursing assessment factor when the individual's pattern is interrupted by a health interference or hospitalization. Hospital routine rarely allows individuals the privacy in which intimacy needs can be met. Too often, individuals who are hospitalized are thought to be asexual or "too sick" to be concerned with sexual activities. Thus any sexual behavior is thought to be inappropriate, and the individual and partner are made to feel as if they have done something wrong.

COUNSELING

Nurses often encounter situations in which the individual seeks guidance concerning satisfaction of sexual activities. The actual pattern of the individual's sexual activities is not as important as the gratification the individual receives from these activities. Frigidity, impotence, failure to reach orgasm, and boredom are commonly manifested dissatisfactions. Although the nurse who has not had special preparation is not a sexual therapist, she can provide information and guidance and act as a resource person to the individual who has indicated difficulties in attaining sexual gratification.

Nursing assessment related to sexual patterns includes descriptions of:

- sexual actvities utilized
- interferences with usual sexual activities
- attitudes toward activities and interferences (individual, family and/or significant others)
- intimacy patterns (e.g. stroking, touching)
- sexual variations
- relationship of sexual variations to health care
- attitude of nurse/health care team toward variations
- frequency of sexual activities
- interferences in frequency resulting from health interference or hospitalization
- attitude toward interferences in frequency (individual, family and/or significant others, health team)
- degree of sexual satisfaction
- interferences with sexual satisfaction
- resources available

Interferences with Sexuality

Sexuality patterns may be interfered with by pathology (either directly related to the genital subsystem or not), therapeutic regimen (e.g., medications, surgery), hospitalization, fear, anxiety, lack of knowledge, or anything the individual considers to be an interference. Interferences may be manifested in a wide variety of behaviors. Self-denigration as shown by such statements as, "I'm only half a woman," "I'm no good to my wife anymore," "I used to be so beautiful," or "What kind of a man am I when I can't even support my family," may be an expression of interference with sexuality. Flirting, use of obscene language, telling sexual jokes, relating stories of sexual prowess, genital exposure or public masturbation may also be ways that the individual may express interferences. Often these behaviors are misinterpreted by the health care team because no relationship is seen between the individual's illness and sexuality or threats to it. These behaviors may be seen as perversion, as sexual advances, or as inappropriate. The health care team may not realize that these are expressions of a threat to the individual's sexuality.

> **Nursing assessment related to interferences with sexuality includes descriptions of:**

- the relationship between the individual's health state and expressions of sexuality, hospitalization, stress, anxiety, lack of knowledge, therapeutic regimen
- ways interferences are communicated
- ways interferences are interpreted
- attitudes toward interferences (individual, family and/or significant others)
- ways individual, family and/or significant others deal with interference

Physical Assessment

Although sexuality is a total body response and not measured by any one body subsystem, the examination of the male and female genitalia is covered here because of the close association with sexuality. Assessment of the genitalia involves inspection and palpation only.

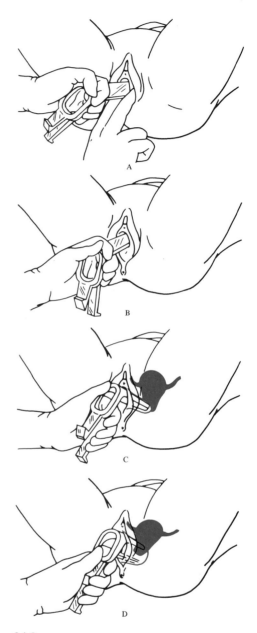

Figure 24.2
Insertion of vaginal speculum. **A.** Opening the entrance introitus) to the vagina. **B.** Oblique entrance of speculum into vagina. **C.** Completed insertion of speculum. **D.** Opening speculum blades.

INSPECTION

Body Hair
The distribution of body hair is the first area of inspection. After puberty the hair distribution takes

Chart 24.3
Insertion of a Vaginal Speculum

TECHNIQUE	POINTS TO NOTE	TECHNIQUE	POINTS TO NOTE
Explain procedure to individual.	Increases cooperation, decreases anxiety	Tell individual to bear down.	Relaxes perineal muscles and opens vaginal opening
Place woman in lithotomy position.	Optimum position for insertion and observation of the cervix	With other hand insert speculum with blades oblique in downward motion following the vaginal canal.	Follows vaginal canal
Warm and lubricate speculum.	Makes insertion easier and more comfortable	When the speculum is well inserted into the vagina, remove fingers from opening.	Avoids trauma
	Warm only to body temperature as vagina is sensitive to heat		
	If Pap smear is to be done, the speculum should be lubricated only with water	Rotate blades of speculum horizontally.	Positions speculum for observation
Place 2 fingers of one hand an inch or two into the vaginal canal and apply moderate downward pressure with fingers.	Accommodates insertion and avoids pressure on and trauma to internal structures	Insert speculum full length of vagina.	Opens entire vagina
		Open blades and observe cervix (at this time a Pap smear can be taken).	A Pap smear is the collection of cells for cytology.

on a characteristic pattern in males and females. Men usually have concentrated hair growth on the face, chest, axillae, back, abdomen, pubic area, and extremities. The pubic hair distribution is diamond shaped, with one point beginning below the umbilicus. Women have hair concentrations on the axillae, lower abdomen, pubic area, and extremities. The pubic hair distribution is triangular in shape, with the base over the mons. Changes in these characteristic distributions result from hormonal imbalance, pathology, and drug reactions.

Genitals

In males, the inguinal area, penis, the testes are observed for rashes, masses, scars, and inflammation. The penis is inspected for discharge. (If the foreskin is present, it is retracted for observation.) The position of the urinary meatus is noted for any varia-

tion (e.g., **hypospadias**—the opening of the meatus is on the undersurface of the penis; **epispadias**—the opening of the meatus is on the top surface of the penis). In addition, the testes are observed for symmetry (the right testis is usually higher than the left) and descension. **Undescended testicles** are located in the abdominal or inguinal canal rather than externally.

Inspection of the female genitals includes observation of the labia majora and minora, clitoris, vaginal opening and the canal, and cervix. Inspection of the vaginal canal and the cervix requires inserting a vaginal speculum. Chart 24.3 outlines the procedure. Figure 24.2 illustrates insertion of speculum.

The cervix is inspected for color, signs of erosion, lesions, position, discharge, and shape of the os. Chart 24.4 shows the expected cervical characteristics.

Chart 24.4
Expected Cervical Characteristics

FACTOR	FINDING
Color	Pink
	Cyanotic in pregnancy
	Light pink after menopause
Shape	Cervix: round or oval
	Os: round or lateral
Surface	Smooth, glossy
Discharge	Mucus is expected—can be clear
	or cloudy, thick or thin
	Odorless

PALPATION

Of Males

The inguinal and femoral areas in males are palpated for **hernias.** A hernia is an outpouching of tissue through the supporting structures. To palpate for inguinal hernias, the index finger of the examiner gently pushes the scrotal skin upward following the spermatic cord to the inguinal ring, while the man coughs. The inguinal ring feels fibrous and firm. Any bulges or masses are noted. Figure 24.3 illustrates the method of palpating inguinal hernias. Femoral hernias are palpated by feeling the anterior superior spine of the ilium for masses or tenderness.

The scrotum is palpated for masses or tender-

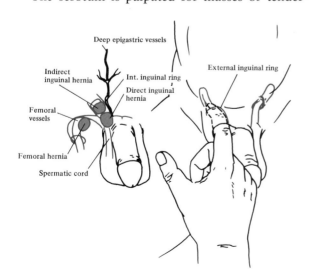

Deep epigastric vessels

Indirect inguinal hernia

Int. inguinal ring

Direct inguinal hernia

External inguinal ring

Femoral vessels

Femoral hernia

Spermatic cord

Figure 24.3
Sites of hernias in the inguinal area and technique used to palpate for protuberance.

ness. Each testis and the epididymis should be palpated individually. Young adult males are taught to do testicular self-examination periodically.

Of Females

In females, the vagina, cervix, uterus, and pelvic organs are palpated by the bimanual technique (Figure 24.4). The examiner inserts one or two gloved fingers of one hand into the full length of the vagina and places the other hand on the abdomen just below the umbilicus. By pressing the hand on the abdomen toward the fingers in the vagina, the uterus is identified as to size, shape, consistency, and mobility (Chart 24.5). Any masses or tenderness are noted. The ovaries are palpated, and other pelvic organs are similarly palpated.

NURSE'S INTERVIEW

In assessing any of these sexuality factors, the nurse must consider the relevance of the information collected. Due to the personal nature of this information and prevailing societal attitudes toward discussing sexuality, the individual may not readily understand the need for sexuality assessment. Any information obtained is for the direct purpose of helping plan the individual's care and is not done only for the sake of gathering information. Most people are approachable concerning sexuality information if the interviewing technique is nonthreatening and nonjudgmental. The beginning nurse usually finds herself or himself more ill at ease than the person being interviewed.

NURSING DIAGNOSIS

A 43-year-old, widowed Puerto Rican male, Mr. Rivera, has been hospitalized for hypertension which has been treated by a low-sodium, 1800-calorie diet; aldomet (an antihypertensive), 250 mg, p.o., b.i.d.; a diuretic, Lasix (furosemide), 20 mg, p.o., o.d.; and a potassium supplement, KCl, 20 cc, p.o., o.d. He enters the hospital this time for evaluation studies. Mr. Rivera is 6 feet tall, weights 240 pounds, and works as a longshoreman. His weight fluctuates between 220 and 240 pounds.

The admitting history states that Mr. Rivera does not consistantly take his medications or follow

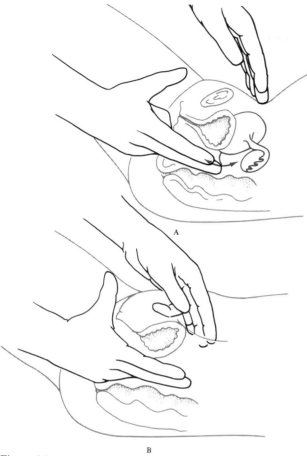

Figure 24.4
Bimanual palpation of the uterus (top) and adnexa (bottom).

Chart 24.5
Expected Characteristics of the Uterus and Ovaries

CHARACTERISTIC	FINDING
Uterus	
Size	In women who have never been pregnant: 5.5–8 cm long 3.5–4 cm wide 2.0–2.5 cm anterior-posterior diameter. Each dimension enlarges 2–3 cm in women who have been pregnant.
Consistency	Firm; cervix feels like tip of nose.
Shape	Elongated, pear shaped
Position	Cervix, midplane Body of uterus may be displaced forward, back, or upward.
Surface	Smooth
Mobility	Cervix can move 2–3 cm in any direction. Uterus can be moved forward and upward.
Tenderness	None
Ovary	
Location	Right and left side of midline (deep pressure is necessary to palpate).
Size	3–4 cm
Shape	Almond
Consistency	Soft
Tenderness	Sensitive to pressure

his prescribed diet. The expected weight for an individual of Mr. Rivera's height and body build is 185 pounds.

While the nurse is talking with Mr. Rivera, he states "that diet is not enough to keep a man strong." Further assessment reveals that according to Mr. Rivera, "a skinny man is no man at all." He also indicates that losing weight will cause him to "lose my abilities as a man." Mr. Rivera also states that "I don't feel sick, so why should I junk myself up with medicine."

Some of the resulting nursing diagnoses for this situation include:

- threatened masculinity related to personal and cultural beliefs
- poor nutritional habits related to threatened masculinity
- poor nutritional habits related to lack of knowledge of effects of diet on pathologic process
- irregular medication patterns related to lack of knowledge of medication actions
- irregular medication patterns related to lack of knowledge of pathologic process.

PLANNING

Planning for sexuality needs focuses on the influence of health state, knowledge, hospitalization, pathologic process, and therapeutic regimen on the individual's ability to satisfactorily meet these needs. The plan should be centered on the individual's needs as he or she sees them, and not on the needs of the health team.

In the situation of Mr. Rivera, the plan for one of the nursing diagnoses listed above might look as follows:

NURSING DIAGNOSIS	GOAL	PLAN

Poor nutritional habits related to threatened masculinity	*Short term:*
	1. Increased knowledge of diet's effects on hypertension within 1 week
	2. Decreased sodium intake within 1 day
	3. Maintains steady weight at 220 lb during hospital stay
	4. Reinforced positive feelings of masculinity during hospital stay
		1. Explain low-calorie, low-sodium diet
		    Benefits
		    Rationale
		    Effects
		2. Explain methods of weight reduction in relationship to cultural preferences
		    Buying food
		    Preparing meals
		    Eating out
		3. Explain weighing schedule
		    Methods
		    Frequency
		    Benefits
		4. Explain options for maintanence of weight and weight loss
		    Increase exercise
		    Low-sodium diet
		    Usual pattern
		    Combination of dieting with usual patterns
		5. Sincere compliments on appearance
		6. Explore feelings about masculinity
		7. Encourage planning of own care
		8. Active involvement in decision making
		9. Support choices made
		10. Encourage usual life-style

	Long term: 1. Decreased body weight 2. Sustained improvement of **feelings of masculinity**	1. Refer to neighborhood dietary clinic 2. As above

INTERVENTION

Nursing intervention for sexuality needs centers on therapeutic communication and information and option giving. The nurse also acts as a resource and referral person.

Therapeutic Communication

Therapeutic communication enables the nurse to help the individual recognize and explore available options in meeting sexuality needs or coping with interferences. Available options help the individual to participate in his or her own care and to choose those behaviors which are consistent with his or her beliefs, attitudes, and cultural mores.

The nurse uses both verbal and nonverbal skills to communicate acceptance of the individual's choice and mode of sexuality expression. Often, the nurse's recognition of the individual's sexuality needs is a means of "giving permission" to the individual to discuss patterns of sexual expression. Since the topic of sexuality is one that is frequently avoided or discussed only with intimates, it is necessary to indicate that sexuality is an acceptable topic. Thus the nurse "gives permission" to open the discussion.

Providing Information

Information on sexuality can be given to the individual and family and/or significant others within the context of other information related to a health interference. For example, when the nurse is giving information about the resumption of activities after colostomy surgery, one of the activities that the nurse includes—along with diet, exercise, and stoma care—is sexual expression.

By supporting the individual's masculine or feminine behaviors, the nurse is helping the individual to meet sexuality needs. For instance, by assisting with body aesthetic needs, whether shaving an individual or helping to apply makeup, the nurse validates the individual's sense of self-worth and value as a sexual being.

Many times the nurse is not prepared to handle the interferences with sexuality which the individual may present. In those instances the nurse acts as a resource person and may make referrals to other health professionals and provide information on available agencies and services.

Option Giving

Facilitating the individual's choice of sexuality expression does not imply that all sexuality behaviors are acceptable at all times and in all places. Inappropriate behavior includes actions which embarrass or compromise other people or place the individual in a situation that is unsafe or threatening to his or her self-esteem. For example, masturbating in the hospital corridor not only infringes on the rights of others, but also places the individual in the position of being humiliated and rejected. The nurse can intervene effectively by providing a private place such as the bed with the curtains drawn, where the person can continue without interruption or embarrassment.

The beginning nurse may be unfamiliar with situations such as an individual who displays seductive behavior or the man who has an erection while care is being administered. Such behaviors as telling sexual reference jokes, propositioning the nurse, referring to sexual prowess, or touching the nurse in an intimate manner may be classified as seductive. The nurse can intervene with the individuals who demonstrate these behaviors by setting limits as to which behaviors are acceptable and exploring the underlying motivation for those that are unacceptable. Often, the seductive behaviors are indications of a threat to the individual's basic feelings of sexuality.

The man who experiences an erection while being given care may be offered the choice of continuing with the care or having the nurse leave the bedside for a short time until the erection subsides. This gives recognition to the fact that the erection has occurred and that the man can choose the method of dealing with the situation. Spontaneous erections take place without the conscious intent of the individual when the bladder is full or neurologic damage is present, or in response to tactile stimulation. Ignoring the erection may only serve further to embarrass the individual.

Sex Education

Sex education is an important aspect of nursing intervention. Family members, particularly parents, are given information as to the expected sexuality behaviors at various levels of growth and development and the roles family attitudes play in the sexual development of the child. The nurse also directly provides sexuality information to various age groups in many settings—schools, clinics, and community meetings.

EVALUATION

Evaluation of sexuality needs is directed toward the changes that have taken place in the person's ability to express, explore, and meet these needs to the satisfaction of the individual and the family and/or significant others. In addition, evaluation is made of the changes resulting from the individual's health state and/or therapeutic regimen which affect the meeting of sexuality needs.

Specific criteria for evaluating how sexuality needs are being met include:

- How do physiologic changes relate to changes in meeting sexuality needs? Psychologic?
- What are the changes in the degree of sexuality need satisfaction?
- What changes have occurred in knowledge (individual, family and/or significant others)?
- What changes have occurred in attitude (individual, family and/or significant others)?
- What changes have occurred in expression of sexuality behavior (individual, family and/or significant others)? Exploration?

RECORDING AND TEACHING–LEARNING ACTIVITIES

Teaching–Learning Topics

- What are the alternative options for sexuality expression?
- What are the available resources and how are they used?
- What are expected sexual behaviors according to the level of growth and development?
- Basic sex information (e.g., anatomy, physiology, contraception)
- What are the common health concerns related to sexuality?
- Influence of therapeutic regimen on sexuality
- Factors which support sexuality.

Charting

Using appropriate sexuality terms, objectively describe:

- level of sexuality growth and development
- expression of sexuality needs, roles assumed, manifestations of masculinity and femininity, interaction styles
- attitudes toward sexuality

- fears related to sexuality
- level of knowledge
- teaching carried out
- results of physical assessment
- interferences with sexuality
- family and/or significant others' interactions and responses
- variations from the expected in relationship to health care needs
- influences of therapeutic regimen on meeting sexuality needs
- influences of pathology on meeting sexuality needs
- update Kardex on changes in goals and plans for meeting sexuality needs.

Medications to Review

- hormones, e.g., estrogen, testosterone
- antihypertensives, e.g., guanethidine (Ismelin)
- CNS depressants, e.g., alcohol
- oral contraceptives, e.g., norethynodrel-mestranol (Enovid-E)

NOTES

1. Harold I. Leif. In *The Sexual Experience,* edited by Benjamin Sadock, Harold Kaplan, and Alfred M. Freeman. Baltimore, Williams & Wilkins, 1976, p. 4.
2. *Ibid.*
3. *Ibid.*
4. Warren J. Gadpaille. *The Cycles of Sex.* New York, Scribner's, 1975, p. 5.

SELECTED REFERENCES

"All about Sex . . . After a Coronary, Despite Dialysis, After Middle Age, Education for Students." *American Journal of Nursing,* 77:602, April, 1977.

Allen, Andra J. "All-American Sexual Myths." *American Journal of Nursing,* 75:1770, October, 1975.

Bates, Barbara. *A Guide to Physical Examination.* Philadelphia, Lippincott, 1974.

Comarr, A. Estin and Gunderson, Bernice. "Sexual Function in Traumatic Paraplegia and Quadriplegia." *American Journal of Nursing,* 75:250, February, 1975.

Conklin, Margaret, Klint, Karen, Morway, Ann, Shepherd,

Roberta and Sawyer, Janet. "Should Health Teaching Include Self-Examination of the Testes?" *American Journal of Nursing,* 78:2074, December, 1978.

Diecklemann, Nancy, Galloway, Karen, Dresen, Sheila E., Johnson, Linda, Owen, Bernice Doyle, Prock, Valencia N., and Granquist, Joanne F. "The Middle Years—A Symposium." *American Jounral of Nursing,* 75:993, June, 1975.

Feely, Ellen and Pyne, Helen. "The Menopause: Facts and Misconceptions." *Nursing Forum,* 14(1):74, 1975.

Fontaine, Karen Lee. "Human Sexuality: Faculty Knowledge and Attitudes." *Nursing Outlook,* 24:174, March, 1976.

Griggs, Winona. "Sex and the Elderly." *American Journal of Nursing,* 78:1352, August, 1978.

Krozy, Ronna. "Becoming Comfortable with Sexual Assessment." *American Journal of Nursing,* 78:1036, June, 1978.

Lanahan, Colleen. "Homosexuality: A Different Sexual Orientation." *Nursing Forum,* 15(3):314, 1976.

Laurence, John C. "Homosexuals, Hospitalization and the Nurse." *Nursing Forum,* 14(13):305, 1975.

Lief, Harold and Payne, Tyana. "Sexuality—Knowledge and Attitudes." *American Journal of Nursing,* 75:2026, November, 1975.

Malasanos, Lois, Barkauskas, Violet, Moss, Muriel, and Stoltenberg-Allen, Kathryn. *Health Assessment.* St. Louis, Mosby, 1977.

McCoy, Norma L. "Innate Factors in Sex Differences." *Nursing Forum,* 15(3):277, 1976.

Meers, Linda B. "An Approach to Concerns of the Professional Dealing with Sexuality." *Health Values: Achieving High Level Wellness,* 1:114, May-June, 1977.

Mindler, Laurie. "Sex Education on a Psychiatric Unit." *American Journal of Nursing,* 74:1859, October, 1974.

Mims, Fern H., ed. "Symposium on Human Sexuality." *Nursing Clinics of North America,* Vol. 10, September, 1975.

Moore, Karen, Lighty, Marie, and Nolen, Mary. "The Joy of Sex After a Heart Attack." *Nursing 77,* 7:52, June, 1977.

Murray, Barbara and Wilcox, Linda J. "Testicular Self-Examination." *American Journal of Nursing,* 78:2075, December, 1978.

"Patient Assessment: Examination of the Female Pelvis. Part 1" (Programmed Instruction). *American Journal of Nursing* (Suppl.), 78:1717, October, 1978.

"Patient Assessment: Examination of the Female Pelvis. Part 2" (Programmed Instruction), *American Journal of Nursing* (Suppl.) 78:1913, November, 1978.

"Patient Assessment: Examination of the Male Genitalia" (Programmed Instruction). *American Journal of Nursing* (Suppl.), 79:689, April, 1979.

Sana, Josephine and Judge, Richard D. *Physical Appraisal Methods in Nursing Practise.* Boston, Little, Brown, 1975.

Sheey, Gail. "The Sexual Diamond: Facing the Facts of the Human Sexual Life Cycles." *New York* January 26, 1976.

Smith, Jim and Bullough, Bonnie. "Sexuality and the Severely Disabled Person." *American Journal of Nursing,* 75:2194, December, 1975.

Stephen, Gwen J. "The Creative Contrariness: A Theory of Sexuality." *American Journal of Nursing,* 78:76, January, 1978.

Stoller, Robert J., et al. "A Symposium—Should Homosexuality Be a Diagnosis." *Nursing Digest,* 3:55, March-April, 1975.

VanBree, Nancee S. "Sexuality, Nursing Practise and the Person with Cardiac Disease." *Nursing Forum,* 14(4):396, 1975.

Watts, Rosalyn J. "The Physiological Interrelationships Between Depression, Drugs, and Sexuality." *Nursing Forum,* 17(2):168, 1978.

"When the Patient Is Gay." *Nursing Digest,* 3:60, March-April, 1975.

Woods, Nancy F. and Mandetta, Anne P. "Sexuality in the Baccalaureate Nursing Curriculum." *Nursing Forum,* 15(3):294, 1976.

Zalar, Marianne. "Human Sexuality—A Component of Total Patient Care." *Nursing Digest,* 3:40, November-December, 1975.

Our joys as winged dreams do fly;
Why then should sorrow last?
Since grief but aggravates thy loss,
Grieve not for what is past.
Anonymous, The Friar of Orders Gray

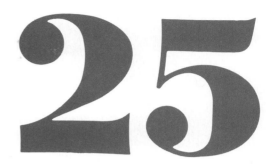

25

GRIEVING AND LOSS

PRINCIPLES RELATED TO GRIEVING AND LOSS

Maturational crises are a series of stressful life events which arise out of the growth and developmental process and for which the individual's coping mechanisms are inadequate.

Situational crises are those unexpected stressful events for which the individual's coping mechanisms are inadequate.

Grieving is the wholistic process experienced by an individual in response to or in anticipation of an actual or perceived loss.

Loss is the absence, actual or perceived, of a significant person, object, body part, function, or emotion which was formerly present.

A young child grieves in three stages: protest, despair, and denial

Dying is a physiologic, physical, psychologic, and sociologic crisis process which ends with death.

Death is the termination of the physical existence of an individual.

The medical, legal, and moral definitions of death are controversial.

Biologic death is the cessation of cellular function.

Brain death is used in some states as the legal criterion for death. It is the spontaneous cessation of brain activity.

Subjective reactions to dying, death, grieving, and loss are based on the individual's culture, philosophy of life, past experience, level of growth and development, values, and attitudes.

Each culture has a set of rituals concerned with death, dying, and grieving.

Physiologically, death may be manifested as a gradual decline in vital function.

The sense of hearing is thought to be the last sensation present in the individual.

The cells and functions of different organs die at different rates.

The impact of a loss depends, in part, on the visibility of the change, the duration of the loss process, the suddenness of the occurrence, recovery time, degree of lifestyle disruption, financial

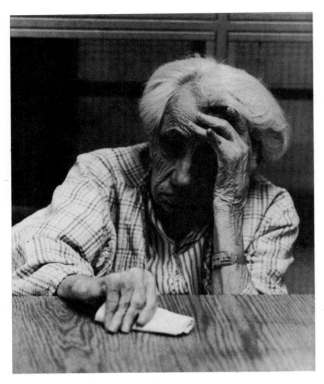

Illustration 25.1
When any individual loses security, love, self-esteem, or self-respect, grief is experienced. *(Photo © Sepp Seitz, from Woodfin Camp & Assoc.)*

demands, interaction patterns, and the available support systems.

Loss and the resulting grief are phenomena common to all people. The degree of grief experienced is proportional to the significance of the loss to the individual. Although a sense of grief is associated with death and dying, it also accompanies the loss of a body function or part, an object, or an emotional satisfaction. Emotional satisfaction includes such areas as security, love, relationships, self-esteem, self-respect, and self-realization.

Losses can be either actual or perceived. Actual losses are those visible and obvious to people other than the individual who is suffering the loss. Actual losses may include loss of a body part, physiologic function, significant object or person, or role or position. Actual losses in the psychosocial realm may not be immediately obvious to the observer but can be determined through careful assessment.

Perceived losses are those which the individual feels have occurred but which are not directly veri-fiable by another. Perceived losses can be directly related to actual loss. For example, the individual who retires does lose the role of worker and income earner. However, that person may also perceive that he or she has lost the role of independent person or decision maker. Whether a loss is actual or perceived, it can result in the grieving process. (Illustration 25.1)

Our American culture discourages recognition of loss, grief, death, and dying. Thus many individuals are unprepared for these crises when they occur. These crises, both situational and maturational, are intricate parts of the life process. Most individuals with the appropriate support can personally learn and grow from these experiences.

In an attempt to explore and deal with the feelings, attitudes, and implications aroused by the concepts of grieving, loss, death, and dying, many controversial issues have arisen which greatly influence nursing practice. The ethical, legal, and sociologic questions of what constitutes death, of organ transplantation, the right to die, the right to live, informed diagnosis, prognosis and treatment, options available for treatment, and life after death represent a few issues facing the health professional.

Part of the process for the nurse who is assisting the individual confronted with loss, grief, death, and dying is a realization of the nurse's own feelings, attitudes, values, and responses. Self-assessment is a necessary prerequisite for the therapeutic use of self in caring for individuals involved in resolution of these crises. An awareness of how his or her own feelings influence the nurse's behavior makes the assessment of the individual's needs and their effects on that person's behavior more effective.

ASSESSMENT

Level of Growth and Development

The level of growth and development of individuals plays a major role in their recognition of and reaction to loss. Gaining experience with loss, deepening their understanding of and exposure to philosophical and religious concepts, and increasing their interaction patterns and responses help to crystallize a conceptualization of and reaction to death, dying, and loss. Chart 25.1 summarizes typical concepts of death and dying at varying levels of growth and development.

SIGNIFICANCE OF THE LOSS

As the individual develops an awareness of his or her body and attaches personal significance to it and its function both as a whole and in its separate parts, the importance of the loss of a body part or function will change. The meaning and importance of a body part is influenced by a person's body image, interaction patterns, lifestyle, and basic beliefs and values. The significance of each body part and its function and of the body as a whole will vary from person to person. Consequently, the reaction to the loss will be different for each individual. Chart 25.2 summarizes concepts of loss of body part or function at different levels of growth and development. (Illustration 25.2)

The meaning of and reaction to the loss of an object, possession, significant person (including the self), or emotional satisfaction will also partly depend on the individual's level of growth and development. The losses that result in the grief of the young child are centered more around objects, possessions, and people in the immediate, here-and-now environment; the adult, on the other hand, focuses not only on the immediate environment, but also on the past and future significance of the loss.

BLURRING OF LEVELS

The major consideration for the nurse in assessing the relationship of the level of growth and development to grieving is not how the individual should be reacting, but how he or she is actually reacting. This is true since there is no clear-cut delineation of any aspect of growth and development, and the beliefs and values of one level may carry through the entire life process. For example, the magical thinking of the toddler by which he or she believes that the death of an individual resulted from his or her wishes may carry through into adulthood. As an adult he or she may intellectually realize that wishing does not cause another's death; emotionally, however, the individual may feel a personal responsibility in the death for having wished it.

Chart 25.1
Concepts of Death and Dying Throughout the Life Process
At Differing Levels of Growth and Development

Infant (up to 5 years)	Not believed to understand the concept.
	Fears separation (separation anxiety) from significant caretaker; may believe death is not permanent; may see death in terms of going away and not coming back; cannot separate wishes from causality, therefore if a person "wished away" dies, feels guilty.
Child (5–10 years)	Growing awareness of death, particularly if he or she has had a family experience with it; death is personified as someone permanently taking you away; often feels that death is avoidable and magical, has morbid thoughts about the destruction of the body after death; fears pain and mutilation accompanying death.
Preadolescent (10–12 years)	Has a concept that death happens to all people, including himself, and that it is irreversible; beliefs about afterlife and philosophy of death greatly influenced by the belief of significant adults in his or her life.
Adolescent (12–18 years)	Has developed a philosophy of death; rarely thinks about death unless confronted by it and then may not be able to express accompanying feelings; may see self as immortal or challenged by death; often willingly takes risks with own safety.
Young adult (18–45 years)	Although has a philosophy of death and a realization of it for self, does not often consider it until faced with the situation.
Middle age (45–65 years)	Sees parents and some peers dying; often becomes preoccupied with death as old age approaches; may make many plans for own death (e.g., insurance policies, purchasing burial plots, making wills).
Older adult (65+ years)	Fears lingering, incapacitating illness; realizes imminence of death (although usually not in the immediate future); fears loss of peers and significant others.

Chart 25.2
Concepts of Loss of Body Part or Function at Differing Levels
Of Growth and Development

Infant (1–15 months)	Loss of body part or function seen in the context of overall somatic comfort; adjusts well to body part loss.
Toddler (15 months–3 years)	Awareness and significance of body parts and functions produce grief over loss of part or function; fears mutilation (particularly of genital parts); still adjusts well to body part loss; body function and mastery are important, so loss of function is significant.
Preschool and school age (3–12 years)	As awareness and dependence on physical body increases, the sense of grief over loss of body part or function increases; since children at this age are aware of differences or abnormalities in others and themselves, deformities are undesirable.
Adolescent (12–18 years)	Physical attractiveness and prowess very important; loss of body part and function particularly traumatic; fears rejection by peers; sees body loss as thwarting all life plans.
Young adult (18–45 years)	Depends on significance of body part or functions for lifestyle and roles; the presence or absence of long-term intimate relationship may influence degree of threat to ego.
Middle age (45–65 years)	Another peak period of physical awareness; may see body loss as a sign of loss of youth, attractiveness, ability, and a movement closer to death.
Older adult (65+ years)	May have some expectation of loss of body function and roles; fears loss of independence and self-care abilities.

Nursing assessment related to level of growth and development and conceptualization of grieving, loss, death, and dying includes descriptions of:

- comparison of present conceptualization with what is expected at that level of growth and development
- comparison of presenting responses to loss with what is expected at that level of growth and development
- significance of body parts and function
- previous experiences with loss and ways of dealing with it
- reactions to loss
- effects of loss on lifestyle and interactions
- how grief is communicated

Influence of Culture

Culture is another aspect of assessment which helps determine how the individual views and responds to loss. Attitudes and values the person holds are influenced by cultural background and religious beliefs. How the individual expresses grief is often derived from cultural expectations. For example, the Nordic or Anglo-Saxon person may adopt a stoic, calm behavior pattern when faced with loss; the Jewish, Italian, or Greek person, on the other hand, may openly express feelings by crying or moaning. When assessing the cultural influence on the reaction to loss, the nurse recognizes that the outward manifestations of grief may in no way reflect the degree of emotion felt by the individual but instead be a fullfillment of cultural expectations. In the United States today, grief reactions of individuals are usually a combination of traditional customs of the cultural group and of the larger American culture.

Nursing assessment of the cultural influence on loss, grief, death, and dying includes descriptions of:

- cultural beliefs about loss, grief, death, and dying (including religious beliefs)
- cultural significance of body parts or functions

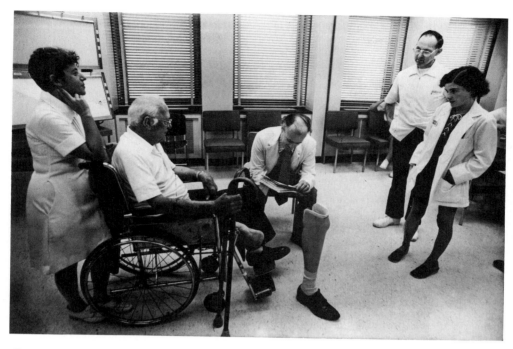

Illustration 25.2

The extent and pattern of grieving that occurs in an individual at the loss of a body part depends on the significance of that part to the individual. Using a prosthesis, a step taken here toward rehabilitation, is part of resolving grief. *(Photo by Chris Maynard, from Magnum)*

- cultural rites and rituals directed toward loss, grief, death, and dying
- adherence to and variation from cultural pattern
- ways of expressing grief in cultural context
- relationship of cultural patterns to nursing intervention

Other Factors Influencing Grief

Attitudes and values toward loss are also affected by the individual's level of knowledge, sex, socioeconomic level, age, role in the family and society, life satisfaction, and lifelong interaction patterns.

KNOWLEDGE

The individual's knowledge about the process of loss and his or her prognosis and diagnosis, care options, types of recovery available after the loss of body parts or function, resources available, and problem-solving ability all contribute to the ways he or she reacts to, thinks about, and responds to loss. However, it is not the possession of knowledge alone which determines the individual's values and at-

titudes, but the way in which he or she chooses to use this knowledge. Informed people don't always follow through on their knowledge, but may react in ways which do not appear to be logical in light of the facts.

SEX ROLES

The social expectations of the male and female roles in the United States play a part in how the individual reacts to loss. Men may have more difficulty in openly expressing their grief, whereas it is socially acceptable for women to do so. Men tend to reestablish relationships after the loss of a significant other sooner than women do, since women often have a longer-lasting sense of loyalty. In addition, men and women attach different significance to body parts, functions, and objects (see Chap. 22). (Illustration 25.3)

SOCIOECONOMIC SUPPORT

Although socioeconomic status does not influence the degree of emotion experienced, the support systems available to channel the emotion are affected. Financial resources—including insurance policies,

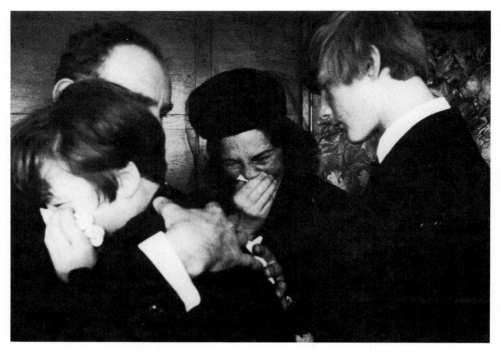

Illustration 25.3
Among several factors influencing expressions of grief are an individual's sex, age, and his or her role within the family. In the American culture when someone dies, it is generally acceptable for the female to openly grieve and less acceptable for the older male. *(Photo from Magnum)*

pensions, and savings—may provide the individual with more options to deal with the loss. For example, the financially secure individual with a disabling handicap may be able to obtain an education, sophisticated devices, and trained personnel for care, all of which may help him or her to better cope with the changes brought about by loss.

Life Expectations and Goals

Individuals who feel they have reached their goals and enjoyed their life may feel less frustrated by the prospect of loss than individuals who have not. When the loss interferes with the achievement of life goals, it is often viewed as more devastating by the individual and those around him or her. Phrases commonly heard when an individual suffers a significant loss directly reflect this view. For example, "It is so unfair. He just got married." Or, "She was just starting the new project which she had been planning for years and this had to happen."

The values and attitudes the individual holds about the quality of life and the expectations he or she has about life also enter into the picture. If life is seen as a series of frustrations the individual may consider a loss just another frustration; however, the individual who considers life to be a series of victories may feel loss to be a personal failure.

CRISIS

The individual's usual pattern of coping will be carried through to his or her reaction to loss. Individuals suffer losses throughout life and learn ways of dealing with them. Thus the individual who has relied on others to handle difficult situations will continue to do so, while the individual who feels self-reliant and does not depend on the help of others will continue with that approach. When lifelong methods are not adequate to deal with a loss, the individual is in ▶ **crisis.** (Illustration 25.4)

Shock Phase

The *shock phase* is characterized by a high level of anxiety, loss of control, failure to realize the implications of the situation, and a generalized inadequacy in dealing with the event. The person feels overwhelmed and disorganized. He or she attempts to

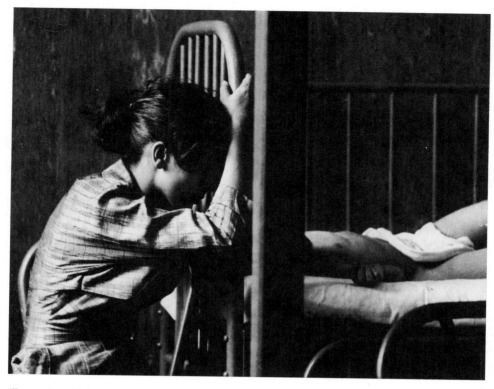

Illustration 25.4

The threat of losing a child may provide a crisis reaction within parents. Their fear and guilt may be overwhelming. *(Photo by Charles Harbutt, from © Magnum)*

move in several problem-solving directions at one time; his social interactions are often inappropriate and unfulfilling. This phase usually lasts a relatively short time (a few hours to a couple of days). However, it may seem like a very long period of time to the individual.

General Realization

The second phase of crisis, when the reality of the situation begins to hit home, is known as general *realization*. The individual realizes the facts of the situation but still cannot cope with or understand their implications.

Defensive Retreat

In defensive retreat, the third phase, the individual utilizes avoidance techniques to protect him- or herself from the reality of the situation. The individual may deny the situation, rationalize it away, project on others, or completely withdraw from the environment. He or she resists attempts by others to resolve the situation. The individual may feel in con-

trol of the situation and feel physically and psychologically well; however, the situation still exists.

Acknowledgment

Acknowledgment, the fourth phase of crisis, occurs when the individual faces the situation and recognizes the implications. Grieving usually begins at this point. The individual attempts to problem solve with increasing effectiveness. However, he or she may be depressed, have low self-esteem and decreased feelings of self-actualization, and recognize the effects of his or her previous behaviors on others.

Resolution

The final stage of crisis is *resolution*. In successful resolution the individual has learned new coping mechanisms and gained new attitudes and behaviors which allow dealing effectively with the situation. He or she has accepted the situation and adjusted to the changes necessary in lifestyle and behaviors.

With ineffective resolution the individual may

acquire a variety of negative behaviors. These may take the form of psychosomatic disorders, apathy, withdrawal, antisocial behavior, or suicide. With maladaption, similar events can trigger another crisis.

Nursing assessment of influences on attitudes and values toward grieving includes descriptions of:

- level of knowledge
- ways knowledge is used
- feelings about appropriateness of grief reaction for age and sex
- influence of socioeconomic status on grieving
- attitudes about quality of life and influence of these attitudes on grieving
- usual coping patterns
- previous experience with loss and methods of coping with it
- effectiveness of coping mechanisms in dealing with present loss
- perception of the significance of loss
- presence of crisis
- phase of crisis
- how stage of crisis is expressed
- type of resolution of crisis

Family and/or Significant Others' Reactions to Loss

The individual undergoing a loss must be considered in the context of the family and/or significant other system. While the individual is suffering the primary loss, the family and/or significant other must deal not only with the individual's reactions, but also with their concurrent loss. The family and/or significant others can provide a support system for the individual in which the individual may deal with the loss or they can hinder him or her in working through the loss. In providing a support system, the family and/or significant others may assist the individual to explore options and help him or her to follow through on the choices the individual has made. They may join in collaborative problem solving and willingly take on responsibilities and actions delegated to them by the individual. They may mutually share feelings and openly communicate both negative and positive emotions related to the loss.

In contrast, the family and/or significant others may feel in some way responsible for the loss and thus guilty. They may be angry at the individual for

having sustained the loss or feel abandoned or deserted; they may feel shame; they may tend to overprotect the individual (or the reverse); they may withdraw from the situation or may be hostile toward the individual; they may identify with the loss; or they may feel helpless and hopeless. They, too, may react to the loss as a crisis and go through the same stages of grieving and loss, although not at the same time as the individual, resulting in conflict and misunderstanding.

The reactions of family and/or significant others to grief are influenced by the same factors as those of the individual. However, their attitudes, beliefs, and responses may not be congruent with the individual's, causing further conflict and crisis.

In assessing the reactions of the individual and the family and/or significant others, the nurse should identify the prior interaction style of the system. Although this system may be acting in a "socially unacceptable" manner, the method may work for them. The nurse may have expectations that a family should act in a certain way during periods of crisis (e.g., be supporting and loving). However, a crisis may only serve to perpetuate previous interaction styles.

Nursing assessment related to the reactions of the individual and family and/or significant others to grief includes descriptions of:

- meaning of loss to family and/or significant others
- reactions of family and/or significant others to loss
- ways family and/or significant others express grief
- attitudes of family and/or significant others, their values and beliefs toward loss
- comparison of the attitudes, values, and beliefs of the individual and those of the family and/or significant others
- areas of congruence and incongruence concerning loss between individual, family and/or significant others
- interaction pattern between individual, family and/or significant others (preexisting, present)
- differences between preexisting and present pattern
- family's and/or significant others' usual coping style
- family's and/or significant others' previous experience with loss and ways of dealing with it

- presence of crisis in family and/or significant others
- phase of crisis, how manifesting
- resolution of crisis
- comparison of crisis phase of individual with that of family and/or significant others
- the effects on the individual of the responses of family and/or significant others to loss

Physiologic Responses to Loss and Dying

The stress produced by actual or potential loss results in activation of the stress response, causing physiologic changes (Chap. 3). The nurse assesses for signs and symptoms of the stress response and the influence it has on the overall ability of the individual to cope. Grieving over a loss may also manifest itself in psychosomatic symptoms.

The physiologic changes the individual who is dying experiences will depend on the specific nature of the pathologic process he or she is suffering from. Some pathologic processes advance mainly by attack on one organ or subsystem, while others may spread throughout the body. The dying process may occur within a very short time or extend for many years. Treatment often results in periods of remission (absence or decrease of symptoms) during which the individual feels, and is, relatively well. Some people remain well until just before death and others have gradual deterioration of body form and function.

The individual who is dying as a result of one pathologic process is not immune from others. In fact, resistance to disease may be decreased as a result of the pathology itself or its treatment. Thus the individual needs not only to be assessed for signs and symptoms of other disease processes, but also protected from their occurrence.

The individual whose death is imminent experiences physiologic changes. Vital signs may become irregular and depressed. Breathing may be periodic (as in Cheyne-Stokes respiration) and difficult. Diaphoresis occurs as the peripheral circulation fails and mottling results in dependent areas of the body. The skin is pale and cold. However, the person may subjectively feel warm and thus be restless. Feelings of great thirst are common. As muscles relax, there is a loss of muscle tone and sphincter control. The reflexes are diminished, but pressure sensation remains. Hearing is thought to be the last sensation to remain. Speech is difficult and slurred, and the swallow reflex becomes diminished. The level of con-

sciousness may range from complete consciousness to a comatose state.

After death the cells of different organs die at varying rates. Several processes occur: **algor mortis,** the loss of body heat; **livor mortis,** mottling of dependent areas of the body; and **rigor mortis,** the stiffening of muscles.

Nursing assessment of the physiologic changes that result from loss and dying includes descriptions of:

- signs and symptoms of stress response
- somatic manifestations
- physiologic changes resulting from pathologic process
- potential or actual superimposed pathologies
- attitudes toward physiologic changes (individual, family and/or significant others)
- effect of physiologic change on family and/or significant others
- therapeutic regimen
- effectiveness of therapeutic regimen
- physiologic interferences with lifestyle
- nursing implications

Psychosocial Responses to Loss

No person grieves according to schedule or plan. However, certain patterns of the grieving process have been identified by various researchers. The dying person grieves for himself and the resulting losses to him. The family and/or significant others grieve for the loss to themselves, as well as for the loss to the individual. Grieving patterns are seen with the loss of body parts and functions, objects, and emotional satisfaction, as well as the loss of life.

GRIEVING PROCESS (KÜBLER/ROSS)

Kübler-Ross has identified five stages in the grieving process—denial, anger, bargaining, depression, and acceptance.

Denial
Denial is the phase when the individual rejects the existence of the loss and continues to act as if nothing were wrong. The individual will often not seek treatment or assistance during this phase.

Anger

The second stage, anger, occurs with the beginning of recognition of the loss. The individual may be angry at self, family and/or significant others, the health care team, God, or the world in general. He or she is often hostile, abusive, and hypercritical at this time. However, the anger reaction signifies the beginning realization of the loss. The family and/or significant others and the health team may respond in a like manner and accept the responsibility for the anger and the loss, giving rise to guilt feelings.

Bargaining

Bargaining, the third stage, is the attempt by the individual to make a deal with someone or something to recoup or to prevent the loss. These deals may be very subtle or overt. If these bargains appear to be effective, the person may continue to make them. The individual who adopts "model behavior" while hospitalized may be covertly making a deal with the staff. In other words, the individual may be saying, "If I'm good and do everything you say, you will make me better."

Depression

The fourth stage, depression, occurs when the full impact of the loss hits the individual. He may isolate himself from social interactions and try to cut himself off from ties with the external environment. The depression stage gives the individual an opportunity to work through the situation and begin to problem solve.

Acceptance

Acceptance occurs when the individual recognizes the situation and its implications and begins to interact in new ways based on the situation. Kübler-Ross points out that this is not necessarily resignation or hopelessness, but a coming to terms with oneself.

GRIEVING PROCESS (ENGEL)

While the scheme of Kübler-Ross is behavior oriented, that of Engel is process oriented. Kübler-Ross identifies the predominant behaviors which individuals manifest when faced with the loss, while Engel recognizes the processes which occur throughout grieving. Engel identifies three steps in the grieving process— *shock and disbelief, developing awareness,* and *restitution and recovery.*

Shock and Disbelief

The shock and disbelief stages are similar to the shock phase of crisis and the denial stage in Kübler-Ross's model. This is the phase in which the individual attempts to protect himself from the reality of the loss.

Developing Awareness

In the second step of developing awareness, the individual acknowledges the loss and experiences an acute feeling of desperation. He may simultaneously experience anger, guilt, depression, frustration, and emptiness. Engel states that "crying, with tears, is typical of this phase. . . . In general, crying seems to involve both an acknowledgement of the loss and the regression to a more helpless and childlike status."[1]

Restitution and Recovery

The third and final phase is restitution and recovery, when the inevitability of the situation becomes clear to the individual and the loss situation can be handled in proper perspective.

IDENTIFYING GRIEVING METHODS

The individual and the family and/or significant others may react according to one of the above patterns or in their own totally unique way. Changes in interaction patterns, lifestyles, feelings of dehumanization, pride about the ability to handle the situation, reintegration of body image, and adoption of new coping mechanisms are just a few of the ways reaction to grief may be evidenced. Labeling the individual's and the family's and/or significant others' stage of grief is not important in nursing assessment, but the identification of the methods which work for them is. Whatever behavior is manifested, it is not negative until it interferes with the process of living.

Nursing assessment of the psychosocial responses to grief includes descriptions of;

- behavior manifested (individual, family and/or significant others)
- effect of behavior on lifestyle, interaction patterns, and the ability to live

The Individual's Plans

When faced with a loss or the threat of a loss, many individuals make future plans for themselves and their family and/or significant others. Writing a will, arranging to donate organs, investigating types of funerals and burials, and making financial arrangements are examples of such planning. Knowledge of the plans made by the individual helps the nurse to comply with the individual's wishes, to make special arrangements, and to support the choice of options available. Assisting him or her to plan for the future helps the individual to gain a measure of control over the situation and may help relieve anxiety about the future of the family and/or significant others, as well as of the self.

THE LIVING WILL

One example of a therapeutic care option for the individual is the Living Will. This document states the type of care the individual is to receive, if and when he or she is incurably ill. Although not legally binding in many states, the Living Will helps the nurse to intervene in a manner that is most compatible with the individual's wishes. Figure 25.1 illustrates the Living Will.

To My Family, My Physician, My Lawyer and All Others Whom It May Concern

Death is as much a reality as birth, growth, maturity and old age—it is the one certainty of life. If the time comes when I can no longer take part in decisions for my own future, let this statement stand as an expression of my wishes and directions, while I am still of sound mind.

If at such a time the situation should arise in which there is no reasonable expectation of my recovery from extreme physical or mental disability, I direct that I be allowed to die and not be kept alive by medications, artificial means or "heroic measures". I do, however, ask that medication be mercifully administered to me to alleviate suffering even though this may shorten my remaining life.

This statement is made after careful consideration and is in accordance with my strong convictions and beliefs. I want the wishes and directions here expressed carried out to the extent permitted by law. Insofar as they are not legally enforceable, I hope that those to whom this Will is addressed will regard themselves as morally bound by these provisions.

Signed_____

Date _____

Witness_____

Witness_____

Copies of this request have been given to _____

_____

_____

_____

Figure 25.1
A living will. (Reprinted with permission of Concern for Dying, 250 West 57th Street, New York, New York, 10019)

UNIFORM DONOR CARD

of _____ Dawn F. Kilts
Print or type the name of donor

In the hope that I may help others, I hereby make
this anatomical gift, if medically acceptable, to take
effect upon my death. The words and marks below
indicate my desires. I give:

(a) ☒ any needed organs or parts
(b) ☐ only the following organs or parts

_____
Specify the organ(s) or part(s)

for the purpose of transplantation, therapy, medical
research or education.

(c) ☒ my body for anatomical study if needed.

Limitations or
special wishes, if any: _____

KEEP THIS CARD WITH YOUR DRIVER LICENSE

RTN-11609B

FRONT

Figure 25.2
Example of a donor card used in New York State. *(Courtesy of the New York State Department of Motor Vehicles)*

ORGAN OR BODY DONATION

If an individual has specified disposition of his or her organs for transplant or body for research, the body will be cared for after death and the appropriate agencies notified. Figure 25.2 gives an example of an organ and body transplant donation card currently used by the New York State Department of Motor Vehicles.

Having a knowledge of plans and knowing that they will be carried out may comfort the family and/or significant others at the time the death occurs.

Nursing assessment related to plans made in anticipation of loss includes descriptions of:

● plans made
● nursing implications

Nursing Self-Assessment Related to Grieving and Loss

The nurse's personal attitudes, beliefs, values, and responses to loss, grief, death, and dying influence the effectiveness of the care the nurse gives to the individuals undergoing loss. Studies have shown that nurses frequently spend less interaction time with dying individuals, foster inappropriate coping mechanisms, and focus on their own needs rather than on those of the individual and family and/or significant others. In assessing personal behaviors, the nurse needs to look at the impact of these behaviors on the individual and the family and/or significant others, as well as the derivation of the behavior. The nurse's responses to loss are determined by the same factors as anyone else's.

The level of development and growth, cultural background, age, sex, socioeconomic background, level of knowledge, experience with loss, and interaction style are just some of the factors which contribute to the formation of the nurse's responses to grieving and loss. In addition, a sense of professional failure may color the nurse's reactions to the individual who is dying or encountering a loss of body part or function. Chart 25.3 shows a questionnaire which the nurse can use to explore personal attitudes and feelings toward death, loss, and other issues related to the practice of nursing.

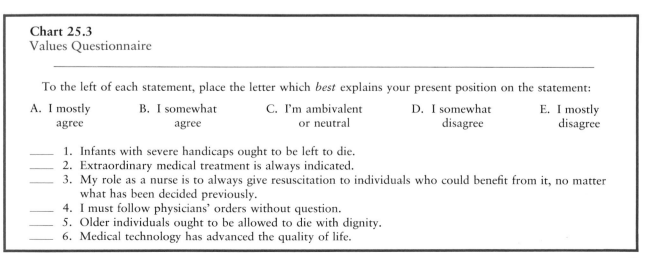

Chart 25.3
Values Questionnaire

To the left of each statement, place the letter which *best* explains your present position on the statement:

A. I mostly   B. I somewhat   C. I'm ambivalent   D. I somewhat   E. I mostly
   agree   agree   or neutral   disagree   disagree

_____ 1. Infants with severe handicaps ought to be left to die.
_____ 2. Extraordinary medical treatment is always indicated.
_____ 3. My role as a nurse is to always give resuscitation to individuals who could benefit from it, no matter what has been decided previously.
_____ 4. I must follow physicians' orders without question.
_____ 5. Older individuals ought to be allowed to die with dignity.
_____ 6. Medical technology has advanced the quality of life.

(continued)

Chart 25.3 (Cont.)

Values Questionnaire

_____ 7. Children ought not to be involved in giving consent for treatments.

_____ 8. Families or significant others ought to make the decisions about life or death situations without involving the client.

_____ 9. Children ought to participate in human experimentation that is not harmful, even if it has no benefit to them.

_____ 10. Prisoners ought to participate in scientific experiments to repay society for their wrongdoings.

_____ 11. Vasectomy is the safest and best type of sterilization.

_____ 12. Adults with developmental lag ought to be sterilized.

_____ 13. Women ought to seek medical supervision from female physicians to avoid potential discriminatory practices.

_____ 14. Children whose parents refuse to have them receive medical care ought to be removed from their families through court action.

_____ 15. Research using fetuses ought to be vigorously pursued.

_____ 16. Abortion is the right of the woman which she should exercise in collaboration with her physician.

_____ 17. Life support systems ought to be discontinued after several days of a flat electroencephalogram.

_____ 18. Health professionals are a scarce resource in many parts of the country.

_____ 19. Nursing is a subservient profession, especially to the medical profession.

_____ 20. As a nurse, I must relinquish my personal philosophy to support the philosophies of others.

_____ 21. All individuals, regardless of differences, ought to be treated in a humanistic way.

_____ 22. I ought to give mouth to mouth resuscitation to a derelict if he needs it.

_____ 23. A child who is disabled has value.

_____ 24. All forms of human life have value.

_____ 25. I ought to be involved in decision-making regarding ethical issues in practice.

_____ 26. Committees should decide who receives scarce resources, such as kidneys.

_____ 27. Individual rights ought to be more important than the rights of society-at-large.

_____ 28. A person has the right to make a Living Will.

_____ 29. Women of childbearing age ought to be sterilized after two pregnancies to maintain zero population growth.

_____ 30. Underdeveloped countries ought to be given health and financial support from developed countries.

_____ 31. I should support all the positions on ethical questions taken by my professional organizations.

_____ 32. I should aggressively support my own values when they conflict with values of others.

_____ 33. Consideration of the cultural values of individuals under care is a waste of time.

_____ 34. The _care_ component of nursing practice is not as important as the _cure_ component of medical practice.

_____ 35. The nurse's primary role in decision-making on ethical issues is to implement the selected alternative.

_____ 36. I feel afraid when caring for an individual who is dying.

_____ 37. Children who have disabilities ought to be institutionalized.

_____ 38. Individuals in mental health institutions and prisons ought to be given behavior modification therapy to make them conform to society.

_____ 39. Personal possessions ought to be removed to guarantee safekeeping during hospitalization.

_____ 40. Persons under care ought to have access to their own health information.

_____ 41. Withholding health information fosters recovery.

_____ 42. A person with kidney failure is always able to get kidney dialysis when needed.

_____ 43. Society ought to bear the cost of extraordinary medical interventions.

_____ 44. Confidentiality is an important part of the nurse's role.

_____ 45. As a nurse, I ought to value responsibility.

_____ 46. Homosexuality ought to be discouraged.

_____ 47. Nurses have a right to withhold information to facilitate nursing research on human subjects.

_____ 48. An individual who refuses treatment ought to be dropped from the health supervision of an agency or professional.

_____ 49. Sexually active adolescents ought to be encouraged to use contraceptives.

_____ 50. Transplantations ought to be done whenever needed.

(continued)

Chart 25.3 (Cont.)

Values Questionnaire

After completing all the statements, add up the number of As, Bs, Cs, Ds, and Es that you have. How many statements do you have the clear ideas about? _____

	Yes	No
Do these outweigh the number of ambivalent or neutral statements you have?	___	___
Do the statements you agree with (include "mostly" and "somewhat") outweigh the statements you disagree with (include "mostly" and "somewhat")?	___	___
Look at the questions you *mostly disagree* with. Do you see any relationship between the statements which influenced your responses (e.g., age of client, severity of condition, etc.)?	___	___
Look at the questions you mostly agree with. Do you see any relationship between these statements which influenced your responses?	___	___
Now go back and look at the way you rated the particular clusters of statements identified below. Do you see any consistency in the way you rated these statements due to such variables as age, sex, etc.? Try to think why you might be consistent or inconsistent in the way you rate the statements.	___	___
Statements 5, 8, 16, 17, 28, and 36 relate to issues pertaining to *death*. Do you see any consistency in the way you rated these statements? What variable(s) influenced your decision?	___	___
Statements 11, 12, 16, 29, 46, and 49 relate to *human sexuality and reproductive issues*. Do you see any consistency in the way you rated these statements? What variable(s) influenced your decision?	___	___
Statements 3, 4, 19, 20, 25, 31, 34, 35, 44, and 45 relate to *nurses and the profession of nursing*. Do you see any consistency in the way you rated these statements? What variable(s) influenced your decision?	___	___
Statements 2, 6, 15, 17, 24, 42, 43, and 50 relate to the issues raised by *advanced medical technology*. Do you see any consistency in the way you rated these statements? What variable(s) influenced your decision?	___	___
Statements 1, 7, 9, 14, 23, 37, and 49 relate to *children*. Do you see any consistency in the way you rated these statements? What variable(s) influenced your decision?	___	___
Statements 9, 10, 15, and 47 relate to *human experimentation*. Do you see any consistency in the way you rated these statements? What variable(s) influenced your decision?	___	___
Statements 3, 7, 8, 13, 14, 21, 22, 27, 28, 33, 39, 40, 41, 44, and 48 relate to *rights of clients*. Do you see any consistency in the way you rated these statements? What variable(s) influenced your decision?	___	___
Statements 9, 10, 27, 29, 30, 32, and 43 relate to the *rights of society*. Do you see any consistency in the way you rated these statements? What variable(s) influenced your decision?	___	___
Statements 18, 26, 40, and 42 relate to the issues of *scarce resources*. Do you see any consistency in the way you rated these statements? What variable(s) influenced your decision?	___	___
Statements 3, 4, 20, 21, 22, 25, 26, 31, 32, 35, 39, and 45 relate to your perception of what you feel are *obligations* in certain circumstances. Do you see any consistency in the way you rated these statements? What variable(s) influenced your decision?	___	___

What have you learned about yourself from completing this exercise? Was it easy to stick to your decision after discussing the choices with others?

From: Shirley M. Steele, Vera M. Harmon. Values Clarification in Nursing. *New York, Appleton-Century-Crofts, 1979, pp. 70–74.*

NURSING DIAGNOSIS

Mr. Zee, a 19-year-old male college sophomore, is referred to the nurse liaison in mental health for the outpatient *oncology* (study of cancer and its treatment) unit. At the time of his first visit Mr. Zee has been under treatment for *metastatic* testicular cancer for 2 years. (Metastatic refers to the spread of cancer cells from the original site to other parts of the body.) At the time of referral he is in the terminal stage of illness. He is enrolled at a local college which is 2,500 miles from his hometown. He moved to the Southwest from the Northeast because of the climate. He currently lives with his 68-year-old widowed father in a small off-campus apartment. Mr. Zee is informed about his diagnosis and prognosis.

ASSESSMENT FACTOR	EXPECTED BEHAVIOR	PRESENTING BEHAVIOR
Concept of death and dying at level of growth and development	Late adolescent: developed philosophy of death; rarely thinks about death unless confronted by it; may not be able to express accompanying feelings; may see self as immortal or challenged by death.	Makes frequent out-of-context references to death by relating stories of other people's death and injury; in discussing a friend's serious accident, states, "It kinds shakes you when someone whom you've known quite well gets racked up. Not only do you feel sorry for him, but it makes you realize that disaster is never very far from yourself."
Previous experience with loss	—	Mother died of cancer when he was age 7; recently moved to area—separated from longstanding friends.
Reactions to loss	—	Rarely refers to mother; talks about high school friends frequently: "My friends back home and I were really close. I see many of the times we had together very vividly but reminiscing about the past isn't for me." "I'd like to find another version of those high school years but so far no luck. Things are different as are the friends, but I can't explain it."
Effects of loss on lifestyle	—	"Unfortunately the last four weeks have been hell. I've been sick and I've missed a lot of classes. I feel like saying the hell with everything and just going. As it is, I dropped most of my courses, and I'm trying to hold on in the others. God, I sometimes think I'm really going crazy now. I'm completely fed up with the world and utterly confused. I'd like to quit altogether, but then I'd most likely go bananas. With luck everything will be okay with me in two or three weeks. Now I don't know what to do. I'd like to quit school for the rest of the year. I want to go out and live and the hell with everything. If you've gotten the impression that I'm feeling very sorry for myself and very bitter, you're right."

(continued)

ASSESSMENT FACTOR	EXPECTED BEHAVIOR	PRESENTING BEHAVIOR
Cultural beliefs	Individual, depending on cultural background and assimilation into general American culture.	Very religious Roman Catholic but makes no references to religious aspects of death and dying. Scottish-English, Polish background; believes person should be stoic. States, "I'm somewhat of a stoic and that helps. Descartes mentioned that we can never be happy until we fully realize that we can't control the external world. I really think that this is a great secret of happiness to be able to accept what fate brings. I'm not a complete stoic—you've got to fight, too, but you can understand what I mean in general. Actually, it's hard to say what I really mean, but I hope you have a glimmer of what I mean." "I used to dislike emotions in others, but now I see that they can be very useful—no use holding your real feelings back."
Attitudes	—	"No matter how black things may seen, I can tell you there is a silver lining in those clouds." "I'm from a group of fighters and that's what really counts." "Most likely I will begin a full schedule again next semester. I won't be in the best possible condition, but I'm more than well enough to make it. Yet, the strange thing is I can't understand why I'm so damned determined to get back. Frankly, it seems senseless and purposeless to work at an education for a future I might never have and can't really envision right now. All I can do is live each day as it comes. Yet I feel going back to school is something I *have* to do. It would be much better if I could be back home with my friends, but I won't allow myself. You're so good at analyzing people. Help me and tell me why I'm so crazy to feel I have to spend the next precious months here at school. I'm certainly no martyr, but why this?" "I'm going for a full medical checkup tomorrow, so you'll have to suffer through a lengthy account of my condition and all future plans and ideas. I'd sincerely like you to sorta hope with me that all the news would be good. OK? The story is that the doctors, and believe me I have many of them, want to try a new experimental drug on me which has a good chance of clearing up most of the trouble. Actually, the whole situation is just making the best of a bad situation, but there really isn't much choice. After all, there is a chance that I'll be helped a lot, and I certainly don't have anything to lose. So wish me luck, and when I get back I hope I'll be able to surprise you."

(continued)

ASSESSMENT FACTOR	EXPECTED BEHAVIOR	PRESENTING BEHAVIOR
Presence of crisis	—	At this time coping mechanisms appear to be working as evidenced by ability to accept treatment and function within physiologic limits.
Reaction of family and/or significant others to loss	—	Father totally denies any possibility of impending death of son. States, "He's so much better everyday," despite weight loss of 50 lb and beginning neuromuscular and renal deterioration.
Individual's reaction to responses of family and/or significant others	—	"I can't talk to anyone, especially my father."
Physiologic responses	Gradual decrease in bodily functions.	Same.
Life goals	—	Originally had been an anthropology major; last term changed to premed major; talks about life as surgeon. "The only problem is I can't stand to see anybody get stuck with a needle, especially a biopsy or bone marrow test. I don't really give a damn about the person getting stuck, but I always see myself in his place and that's what bothers me.." "With my innate talents, I'll probably find cures for cancer, heart disease, and chapped lips while I'm an intern."
Attitudes toward staff	—	"Maybe most of my troubles are only hypochondriacal now; I hope so; but I can't help but have visions of the poor patients resignedly given up to fate by their doctors. God! That really scares me."
Psychologic reactions	—	See above. "I read in today's paper where the volunteer bureau needs people to visit lonely people of all ages. If I could work it out I'd like to do a little of that. I certainly have the time and I'm sure if I could visit a shut-in of about my own age we would have a lot to offer each other. Of course, this might be a way to meet more interesting people, so it's far from a personal sacrifice. So tomorrow I'll give the bureau a call and get some more information." Never uses the words cancer or death in reference to himself; uses euphemisms, e.g., situation, trouble, condition. Constantly refers to "how great the Southwest is" while conversely wishing he were back home.
Plans	—	States, "Whatever happens, I'll go back East to home."

Resulting nursing diagnoses in order of priority might include:

- ambivalence about dying related to lack of resolution of loss
- fear of abandonment by health team related to perception of the health team's attitude toward dying process
- loneliness related to separation from significant others
- inability to discuss dying process with father related to father's denial of son's impending death

PLANNING

Helping the individual to live at the highest possible level is the major focus of planning for loss. Supporting the coping mechanisms that work for him or her while helping to develop new ones when necessary are important aspects of the nurse's plan. Rehabilitation, physical comfort, prevention of further dysfunctions and deformities, maintaining present functions, and acting as a resource person for the individual are nursing interventions which are planned to assist the individual in living at his or her optimum level.

Planning for the family and/or significant others as part of the individual's support system and as individuals who are simultaneously going through a loss themselves is a significant component of the nursing care plan. Working with the individual and the family and/or significant others as a system provides the context for the plan.

In the situation of Mr. Zee, the plan for one of the nursing diagnoses listed above could be as follows:

NURSING DIAGNOSIS	GOAL	NURSING PLAN

Ambivalence about dying related to lack of resolution of loss	*Short term:*
	1. Clarification of perception of expected sequelae of dying process within 2 weeks as evidenced by decreased number of conflicting statements about future plans
		1. Explore level of knowledge of dying process by asking individual to tell what he knows about his illness and the succession of events.
		
		2. Identify areas of incongruity.
		
		3. Evaluate purpose that incongruities serve for the individual.
		
		4. Discuss areas of incongruity by:
		  a. Validating accurate perceptions
		  b. Correcting misinformation
		  c. Supporting useful coping mechanisms of incongruity by accepting them.
		5. Provide any additional information requested by the individual.
		6. Share plans with physician.

	2. Increased verbalization of feelings of loss within 1 week	1. Continue existing interaction pattern. 2. Accept statements of individual. 3. Allow time for individual's verbalization. 4. Maintain confidentiality. *(continued)*

NURSING DIAGNOSIS	GOAL	NURSING PLAN
		5. Provide information about 24-hour counseling service.
		6. Set up schedule of availability to individual.
	3. Increased feelings of control over daily events within 1 week	1. Provide options such as time of appointments, use of resources.
		2. Devise plan with individual for scheduling of daily activities which take into account physical, emotional, and monetary resources.
		3. Support choice of options.
	Long term:	
	4. Maintenance of supportive coping mechanisms until death	1. As above.
		2. Observe for signs of crisis.
		3. Intervene immediately if crisis situation appears.
	5. Maintenance of open relationship with therapeutic others until death	1. As above.
		2. Devise contingency plan if nurse is not available.
		3. Explore ways of increasing communication between father and son.
		4. Explore ways of increasing communication with friends.
		5. Explore ways of maintaining communication with health team.
	6. Maintenance of realistic hope until death	1. As above.
		2. Discuss pros and cons of therapeutic regimen.
		3. Accept future plans.
		4. Assist with formulation of realistic future plans.
	7. Maintenance of participation in life activities until death	1. As above.
		2. Identify resources needed to maintain life activities as condition deteriorates.
		3. Explore ways of obtaining resources.
		4. Explore ways of manipulating physical environment to enhance functioning.

INTERVENTION

Promotion, maintenance, or restoration of dignity, self-esteem, comfort, function, and interaction patterns underlie the nursing intervention with an individual and his or her family and/or significant others who are experiencing a loss.

Fostering Dignity

The dignity of an individual is, to a large extent, a reflection of the respect he or she is given by the people in the environment. By maintaining the individual's privacy and confidentiality, listening and responding to statements and requests, accepting the person as he or she is, and providing the highest level of care possible, the nurse can support and help restore the individual's sense of dignity. Since self-esteem is allied to a sense of dignity, actions which enhance one will enhance the other.

Both the quality and quantity of time spent with the individual are important factors in supporting these needs. When the nurse can honestly and openly project a feeling of wanting to spend time with the individual, discuss the person's feelings, and help him or her in meeting needs, then the individual's feelings of worth are increased and reinforced.

Regardless of the individual's level of knowledge, the isolation of the individual from the staff and his or her family and/or significant others will provide a loss of self-esteem and fears about the severity of the loss. The individual may wonder if he or she is so insignificant, deformed, or hopeless as to be abandoned, rejected, given up, or ignored.

The isolation of the individual who is experiencing a loss often reflects the inability of the health care team and family and/or significant others to face and deal with the loss. A common reaction by the nurse and other health team members is assuming an attitude of being too busy to spend time with the individual. This not only rationalizes the nurse's decreased interaction time, but may also result in the individual's decreasing the number of demands for interaction. Another reaction is to treat the individual as if he or she were an inanimate object or already dead. This particularly occurs with the comatose individual. Conversations carried out in the presence of the individual should be directed toward and not about him or her.

Still another reaction is a failure of the nurse to recognize the impact of the loss on the individual, or even to be aware that a loss has occurred. The latter situation occurs predominantly when the individual undergoes nonphysical actual losses or perceived losses.

Providing Comfort Measures

Specific comfort measures for the individual experiencing loss will depend on the underlying pathology. In the case of an individual who has lost a specific body part or function, assistive devices, medications, exercises, and treatments are part of the therapeutic regimen aimed at increasing his or her level of comfort and function. In the case of the dying individual, there may be these same types of interventions or the nurse may gear comfort measures toward

the support of deteriorating systems. Alleviating thirst, providing oral hygiene and skin care, decreasing pain, supporting temperature regulation, maintaining safety measures, and decreasing anxiety and stress are just some of the supportive measures the nurse utilizes.

The maintenance of body function through exercise and the scheduling of activities, treatments, and medications are necessary to assist the individual to function at an optimal level. The nurse supplements loss of function without demeaning the individual or treating him or her like a child.

Establishing Trust

By establishing a trust relationship with the individual and the family and/or significant others, the nurse can do much to facilitate positive interaction patterns. When the nurse is available to and accepting of the reactions of the individual and the family and/or significant others to loss and expressions of grief, the nurse helps create an environment conducive to the expression of grief and resolution of loss. Thus the nurse can help prevent withdrawal of the individual and his or her family and/or significant others, their use of unsuccessful coping mechanisms, and the experience of crisis. By providing truthful information, the nurse can assist the individual and the family and/or significant others in anticipating events, establishing a trust relationship, and planning for the future.

Individuals and families and/or significant others who have had the opportunity to express grief are often better able to cope with the loss and maintain interaction patterns that are in keeping with abilities, lifestyles, roles, developmental tasks, and life goals. For example, the young adult who has a leg amputated can be assisted to modify preexisting life plans so that he or she can then learn how to maintain roles, facilitate career choices, carry on social interactions, and follow through on life goals.

Crisis Intervention

When the individual is in crisis, the nurse must rapidly assess the individual for his or her inability to utilize the coping mechanisms to resolve the stress-producing situation through identification of the negative behaviors that the individual is presenting. The nurse then immediately devises a plan specific to the situation and intervenes.

► **Crisis intervention** is a process of mutual problem solving between the individual and the nurse. The nurse may also be called on to intervene with the family and/or significant others in crisis. During the stage of crisis, the individual is more open to the suggestions of others than at other times of his or her life. This provides the nurse with the opportunity to support and direct the individual in purposeful problem solving until he or she is able to do so alone. This vulnerability of the individual places a great responsibility on the nurse to be decisive, accurate, and trustworthy.

The nurse presents the individual with facts—not theories, suppositions, or opinions—and helps the individual to explore the cause-and-effect relationship of the crisis and the events which helped precipitate it. In effective intervention the nurse accepts the individual's behavior so as to provide a structure from which to work and to prevent the person from hurting him- or herself or others.

The nurse and the individual may role play problem-solving methods to help prepare the individual to use these methods in actual situations. The nurse also helps the individual to build a support network from community resources and significant others which will help him or her with the crisis, as well as assisting in avoiding future crises.

Throughout the crisis intervention process, the nurse should help the individual to take ultimate responsibility for his or her actions. Once resolution of the crisis has taken place, the situation is reviewed, the successful problem-solving methods reinforced, and realistic plans for the future formulated. The person is provided with a crisis referral system which would be available to him or her should the need arise. Crisis intervention may occur in a short time period—a few minutes, as in an emergency room—or it may extend for several weeks in therapy sessions.

Introducing Options

The individual and the family and/or significant others undergoing loss often need the expertise of other health care and related professionals. In these situations the nurse recognizes his or her own limitations and refers the individual to the appropriate individual or agency.

In assisting the individual and family and/or significant others to cope with loss, the nurse provides opportunities for them to be together as often as they desire in a private environment. The family and/or

significant others can be taught to provide as much of the individual's care as they wish and are capable of. Techniques such as feeding, bathing, assisting in ambulation or suctioning are just some examples of the activities which family and/or significant others can carry out, whether in the home or institutional setting. However, these responsibilities should not be demanded or expected of those who are unable to cope.

CARE SETTING

Care-setting options are available for the individual who is in the terminal stages of illness.

The Home
One such setting is the home. Many individuals and their families and/or significant others do not realize, however, the feasibility of this option because of the American trend toward hospitalizing the terminally ill. The alternative can be explored with the interested individual and family and/or significant others. A combination of home care and hospital care may be a viable approach for individuals who require technologic support during periods of the dying process.

The Hospice
Another alternative which is becoming more available to the dying is the hospice. The hospice provides a therapeutic environment for the terminally ill. The personnel are specially prepared to work with the dying, and while physical care is readily available, the emphasis is on productive living. The individual participates in all care decisions, and the family and/or significant others are free to participate in the entire care environment. (Illustration 25.5)

Respecting the Individual

Once the available care setting options have been fully explored, the choice made by the individual and family and/or significant others should be supported. They should not fear recrimination.

All too often, the beginning nurse fears saying something that may hurt the individual. However, in any interaction with the grieving individual and his or her family and/or significant others, concern for the individual's dignity and worth is the deciding factor in providing effective care.

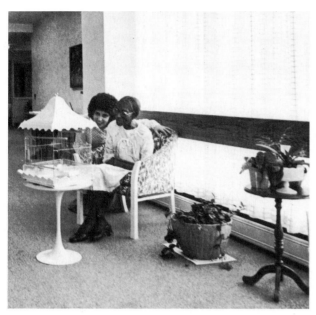

Illustration 25.5
Hospice provides a supportive therapeutic environment for the terminally ill person. *(Photo by Don Selchan, from the Audio-Visual Department of the Forbes Health System)*

EVALUATION

Evaluation of the nursing care of the grieving individual centers on the direction of change in the individual's ability to cope successfully with the loss.

Specific criteria for evaluating change in the individual experiencing loss include:

- Has the individual's ability to cope with loss increased or decreased?
- Has the interaction with family and/or significant others changed?
- Has crisis been resolved? In what way?
- Have expressions of grief been facilitated?
- Have effects on lifestyle changed?
- Have attitudes and values toward loss changed?
- How do physiologic changes relate to changes in the ability to cope with loss?
- What are the changes in knowledge?
- What skills have been acquired in coping with loss? With crisis?
- What are the changes in body image resulting from dealing with the loss?

RECORDING AND TEACHING–LEARNING ACTIVITIES

Teaching–Learning Topics

- rationale for therapeutic regimens
- methods of matching capabilities with limitations
- problem-solving techniques
- ways to structure environment to facilitate coping with loss
- how to perform care activities
- possible reactions to grief
- acceptability of grieving behaviors
- available resources and how to use them
- expected sequelae of events
- care options

Charting

Using appropriate terms, objectively describe such factors as:

- objective base-line data on level of growth and development, coping mechanisms used, phase of crisis, physiologic changes, factors influencing grieving
- subjective and objective changes that occur in the individual's ability to cope with the loss
- subjective assessment data on responses to therapeutic regimen, interaction patterns
- objective and subjective data on behavioral responses to loss, attitudes toward loss, therapeutic regimen, and interaction patterns
- family's and/or significant others' interactions and responses
- schedule and methods of care
- teaching carried out
- discharge planning done
- update Kardex on changes in goals and plans for assisting individual to cope with loss.

NOTES

1. George L. Engel. "Grief and Grieving." *American Journal of Nursing*, 64:95, September, 1964.

SELECTED REFERENCES

Aquilera, Donna and Messick, Janice. *Crisis Intervention,* 3rd ed. St. Louis, Mosby, 1978.

Armstrong, Margaret. "Dying and Death—and Life Experiences of Loss and Gain: A Proposed Theory." *Nursing Forum,* 14(1):95, 1975.

———. *Dealing with Death and Dying.* Jenkintown, Pa., Intermed Communications, 1976.

Benton, Richard. *Death and Dying.* New York, Van Nostrand, 1978.

Burgess, Karen. "The Influence of Will on Life and Death." *Nursing Forum,* 15(3): 238, 1976.

Carlson, Carolyn and Blackwell, Betty, eds. *Behavioral Concepts and Nursing Intervention,* 2nd ed. Philadelphia, Lippincott, 1978.

Cohen, Florence S. "Removal of the Dead: From Room to Morgue." *Journal of Nursing Education,* 17:36, March, 1978.

———. "Encounters with Grief—A Special Supplement." *American Journal of Nursing,* 78:414, March, 1978.

Engel, George. "Grief and Grieving." *American Journal of Nursing,* 64:95, September, 1964.

Fulton, Robert, ed. *Death and Identity.* Bowie, Md., Charles Press, 1976.

Garfield, Charles. *Psychosocial Care of the Dying Patient.* New York, McGraw-Hill, 1978.

Jackson, Patricia Ludder. "The Child's Developing Concept of Death: Implications for Nursing Care of the Terminally Ill Child." *Nursing Forum,* 14(2): 204, 1975.

Kastenbaum, Robert and Aisenberg, Ruth. *The Psychology of Death.* New York, Springer, 1972.

Kübler-Ross, Elisabeth. *Death: the Final Stage of Growth.* Englewood Cliffs, N.J., Prentice-Hall, 1975.

———. *On Death and Dying.* New York, Macmillan, 1969.

Pennington, Elisabeth. "Postmortem Care: More than Ritual." *American Journal of Nursing,* 78:846, May, 1978.

Rosenthal, Ted. *How Could I Not Be Among You.* New York, George Braziller, 1973.

Sharer, Patricia. "Helping Survivors Cope with the Shock of Sudden Death." *Nursing 79,* 9:20, January, 1979.

Stanford, Gene and Perry, Deborah. *Death Out of the Closet.* New York, Bantam, 1976.

The International Work Group in Death, Dying and Bereavement. "Assumptions and Principles Underlying Standards for Terminal Care." *American Journal of Nursing,* 79:296, February, 1979.

Waechter, Eugenia. "Bonding Problems of Infants with Congenital Anomalies." *Nursing Forum,* 16(314):298, 1977.

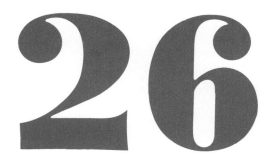

*This was the most unkindest
cut of all . . .*
—*William Shakespeare,* Julius Caesar

THE SURGICAL EXPERIENCE

The surgical process threatens the individual's ability to meet basic needs. The nurse, through understanding the process and appropriate interventions, can do much to promote, restore, and maintain the individual's high-level wellness in the face of these threats. *Surgery* is the deliberate invasion of the body tissues which creates a change in the structure and/or function of the body. Surgery is performed to diagnose and cure pathologies by removing abnormal tissues or secretions, repairing damaged structures or inborn defects, slowing the progress of pathophysiologic processes, and relieving undesirable symptoms.

▶ The surgical process consists of three components. The **preoperative phase** starts when the individual is apprised of the need for surgery and ends
▶ when anesthesia is induced. The **intraoperative phase** begins with the induction of anesthesia and finishes when the surgical procedure is completed. The final phase of the surgical process covers the time from when the surgery ends and continues until the healing process is completed. This phase includes the immediate postoperative phase, the intermediate post-
▶ operative phase, and the later **postoperative phase.**
▶ **Surgery,** as an invasive process, results in the holistic response of the individual. All body systems are affected and all needs, physical, physiologic, and

psychosocial, are compromised. Chart 26.1 outlines these general interferences and responses to the surgical process. A wide variety of factors influence the individual's responses to the surgical process. These influences include the individual's state of health prior to surgery, level of growth and development, cognitive abilities, level of knowledge, level of anxiety, cultural and societal expectations, the meaning of the lost body part, and previous experiences with hospitalization and surgery. (Illustration 26.1)

THE PREOPERATIVE PHASE

The aim of surgery is to produce the desired effects with the fewest risks and complications and to return the individual to an optimum state of health in the shortest possible time. Since surgery entails a total body response and carries the risk of many complications, the individual needs to be in the best physical, physiologic, and psychosocial state possible. The nurse plays a major role in assisting the individual to

---

Chart 26.1
General Interferences Produced by Surgery

SYSTEM OR NEED	INTERFERENCE	POSSIBLE NEGATIVE RESPONSE
Skin	The protective barrier is disrupted and open to invasion from microorganisms.	Localized or systemic infection. Evisceration Dehiscence
Oxygen uptake	Depression of the central nervous system by anesthesia/analgesics. Buildup of secretions or decreased diffusion of gases.	Respiratory arrest Pneumonia
Oxygen transport and utilization	Circulation disrupted—blood loss.	Shock, anemia, increased cardiac workload, cardiac arrest, cardiac arrhythmias.
Energy input	Gastrointestinal tract slowed. Food and fluids withheld. Protein catabolism. Increased energy needs (increased BMR).	Protein, vitamin, and mineral depletion. Nausea and vomiting. Malnutrition
Energy output— elimination	Gastrointestinal tract slowed and innervation decreased. Decreased renal blood flow. Loss of sphincter control. Decrease in smooth muscle tone.	Intestinal obstruction, paralytic ileus. Renal shutdown. Incontinence or retention. Atonic bladder.
Fluid and electrolyte, acid–base balance	Fluid withheld, retention of fluids, fluid and electrolyte loss during surgery. Carbon dioxide buildup.	Dehydration Edema Fluid and electrolyte imbalance. Acidosis or alkalosis.
Body kinetics	Decrease in muscle activity and tone resulting from central nervous system depression. Forced immobility. Pain Weakness and debilitation.	Muscle atrophy, contractures; poor muscle tone; all hazards of immobility.

(continued)

enter surgery at the individual's highest level of functioning.

Types of Surgery

The degree to which the individual can achieve the highest level of functioning depends, in part, on the amount of time available for preparation. If the surgery is of an emergency nature, the preparation time is minimal because the individual requires immediate surgical intervention. **Emergency surgery** is usually performed in life-threatening situations, such as to stop hemorrhaging after trauma or to repair se-

vere damage to a vital organ. Other situations may require **urgent surgery** within a day or two after diagnosis. Although surgery of this type is still done for life-threatening conditions, the time delay occurs because either the risks of immediate surgery may outweigh its possible benefits and the individual's condition is allowed to stabilize or alternative methods of treatment are being attempted to eliminate the need for surgery.

Other surgeries are *required* interventions, but the nature of the condition allows for a period of weeks or months to elapse before they are performed. The actual time frame will depend on the condition being treated, the stage of the pathologic process, and

Chart 26.1 (Cont.)

General Interferences Produced by Surgery

SYSTEM OR NEED	INTERFERENCE	POSSIBLE NEGATIVE RESPONSE
Sensory	Sensory input altered. Central nervous system depression. Decreased oxygenation	Sensory deprivation. Cerebral anoxia.
Body image	Invasion of body space. Mutilation Loss of body part or function. Loss of independence	Distortions of body image. Anxiety
Sleep and comfort	Alteration in biorhythms. Pain receptors stimulated. Central nervous system depression.	Sleep disturbances, behavioral alterations. Pain
Communication	Communication disrupted.	Anxiety, fear, behavioral changes.
Neurohormonal	Increased physical, physiologic, and psychosocial interferences resulting from initiation of stress response.	Increased blood pressure, pulse. Pupillary dilation. Increased blood glucose levels. Increased BMR. Increased secretion of adrenalin. Decreased gastric and intestinal activity. Increased muscle tone. Decreased urinary excretion. Fluid and sodium retention. Exhaustion
Sexuality	Interference with sexual activity. Interference with role performance.	Sexual frustration. Threat to self-image.
Grieving and loss	Loss of body part or function. Threat of death.	Distortion of body image. Crisis Death

▶ the individual's state of health. **Elective surgery** needs to be performed to prevent the possible sequelae of a condition but does not require immediate treatment and can be performed at the convenience of the individual and the surgeon. This surgery may be performed within a matter of weeks, months, or even years.

General Preoperative Interventions

Promotion of highest level of functioning for the individual is accomplished by carefully assessing all body systems for actual or potential interferences and intervening where they exist. Major nursing interventions during the preoperative period are teaching, helping to reduce the individual's anxiety and fears concerning the surgery, establishing base-line data for intraoperative and postoperative comparison, and creating an atmosphere of trust and open communication for the individual and the family and/or significant others.

COLLECTING DATA

The individual undergoes a series of diagnostic tests and physical examinations to ascertain his or her

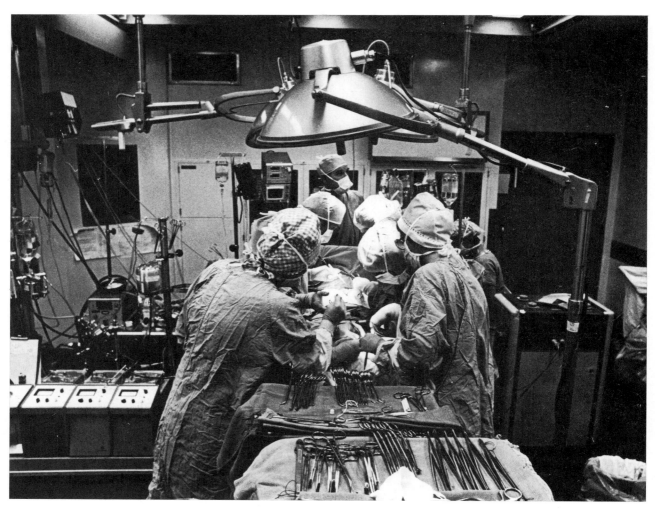

Illustration 26.1
Surgery: a deliberate invasion of the body tissue to diagnose pathology, remove or repair body parts, or to relieve undesirable symptoms. *(Photo © Will McIntyre, from Photo Researchers)*

present state of health. Chart 26.2 lists the diagnostic tests routinely carried out prior to surgery. In addition to the routine tests, diagnostic tests specific to the existing pathology are carried out to assist the surgeon to focus on the surgical area. Any underlying conditions which are identified are further investigated and treated.

The physician interviews the individual to obtain a medical, surgical, and family history. The nurse obtains a nursing history to determine the individual's nursing care needs and to identify actual and potential negative health behaviors.

Once the nursing history has been obtained and negative health behaviors identified, the nurse can plan to intervene.

ESTABLISHING AN ATMOSPHERE OF TRUST

Through the establishment of a trusting and open environment, the nurse can assist the individual and family and/or significant others to cope with the surgical process in the most effective manner. Many individuals when presented with the necessity for surgery fear the outcomes of the surgery, pain, the effects of surgery on their lifestyle, loss of control, and the unknown. Often they are unable or afraid to seek out information and clarification from the physician or other members of the health team. The nurse not only can explain the course of the surgery, but also can act as a liaison between the individual

Chart 26.2
Routine Diagnostic Tests
In Preparation for Surgery

TEST	RATIONALE
Chest x-ray	To identify any signs of respiratory pathology or compromise in respiratory status.
ECG	To identify any cardiac abnormalities.
Urinalysis and C/S	To identify urinary tract infections, indirect assessment of metabolic and renal function.
CBC with differential	To identify the blood's ability to carry oxygen, the presence of anemia, the blood-forming capabilities of the body, and the presence of infection, and to assess indirectly the clotting ability of the blood.
Serum electrolytes	To identify electrolyte imbalances.
FBS	To identify metabolic disorders, particularly diabetes mellitus.
BUN	To indirectly assess renal function.

and the health team. Through the use of all the nurse's therapeutic communication skills, the person can be helped to explore fears, understand the meaning of the surgery, and choose the course of action which is most appropriate. The family and/or significant others often share the same anxieties and fears as the individual and may be reluctant to discuss the prospect of surgery with the individual and the members of the health team. The nurse can be as effective in intervening with the family and/or significant others as with the individual.

TEACHING

Preoperative teaching serves to help allay the fears and anxieties of the individual as well as to pro-

vide the individual with the basic skills needed during the postoperative period. In this way, the individual can have an increased feeling of control over the situation and events. Preoperative teaching also reduces the fear of the unknown, thus facilitating the postoperative course. Fear is lessened because the individual is faimilar with the procedures and equipment to be used and with the rationale for the care to be received. The individual's level of anxiety and stage of grieving may interfere with acceptance or comprehension of the preoperative teaching. Thus repetition and reinforcement are necessary during the postoperative period.

General areas of preoperative teaching include methods and rationale for coughing, deep breathing, incision splinting, turning, ambulating, and exercising. The individual is familiarized with the equipment which will be in the postoperative environment, as well as any ongoing treatments such as intravenous therapy, oxygen therapy, and cardiac monitoring. Since many individuals are concerned about the pain they might experience after surgery, information as to the availability of analgesics is also given. For example, telling the person that medication may be requested prior to coughing and deep breathing (if this is the case) may increase the individual's willingness to participate in the procedure and decrease anticipatory fears. If it is known that the individual is going to a specialty unit after surgery, the individual should be informed of it and the rationale for placement there, and should be familiarized with the environment.

Immediate Preoperative Interventions

INFORMATION SHARING

The events that immediately precede surgery, such as administration of preoperative medications, skin preparations, transfer to the surgical suite, and the activities following this transfer are discussed with the individual.

The family and/or significant others should be informed as to the sequence of events, where they may wait while the individual is in surgery, whom they can contact for information, and what the individual will look like and what equipment will be surrounding the individual when returning from surgery. Family and/or significant others are often needlessly frightened by the general appearance of their loved one and all the paraphernalia that seem to be present. They frequently assume that the individual's appearance and equipment signify a more severe situation than actually exists.

CONTINUITY OF CARE

The nurse often has to carry out these essential interventions in a relatively short span of time. Frequently the individual is not admitted to the hospital until a day or two prior to surgery. Therefore, a general protocol for preoperative interventions which can be adapted to the individual's special needs is developed. The clinic or community-health nurse who works with the individual prior to admission to the hospital begins the preparation process as soon as the need for surgery has been ascertained. Notations of the assessment and interventions that have taken place outside the hospital setting should be placed in the individual's record so that continuity of care can occur.

Although the type of surgery and the preferences of the individual and the surgeon determine the actual preoperative procedures that are carried out prior to surgery, certain activities are carried out the night before and the day of surgery.

DIET MODIFICATION

► Individuals who are undergoing **general anesthesia** have food and fluid withheld 8–12 hours prior to surgery (n.p.o.). This helps prevent aspiration of stomach contents during surgery and nausea and vomiting after surgery. If surgery is to be performed on the stomach or bowel, the individual may have been placed on a liquid or low-residue diet for several days prior to surgery. If the withholding of food and fluids will in any way compromise the individual's nutrition and fluid and electrolyte balance, intravenous therapy is instituted to supply some of these needs.

ENEMA OR LAXATIVE ADMINISTRATION

Since anesthetic agents reduce peristalsis and relax the anal sphincter, the intestines are frequently evacuated prior to surgery. This is always performed prior to gastric and intestinal surgery to prevent contamination of the peritoneal cavity. Evacuation is accomplished through cleansing enemas, laxatives, or a

combination of both. Usually the enemas are given until results are clear. Attempts are made to schedule these preparations so that the individual's sleep is interrupted as little as possible. The procedures may further weaken the already debilitated individual, and thus careful evaluation of the individual during the preparation is made and any adverse reactions reported.

SKIN PREPARATION

The skin may be specially prepared by shaves and/or bathing with disinfectant solutions. The exact areas prepared depend on the type of surgery, hospital policy, the preferences of the individual and the surgeon, and the amount of body hair. The frequency of skin shaves before surgery is decreasing because of recent evidence of its lack of effectiveness and potential hazards. Some skin shaves are done in the operating area just prior to surgery. If a shave is done, care is taken to remove all hair from the designated area and to prevent any nicks or cuts. Skin shaves are done under bright, oblique lighting, shaving against the grain of the hair to ensure a close, clean shave. The individual may be instructed to bathe in disinfectant solution several days prior to surgery. These solutions should remain on the skin for several minutes before rinsing.

FACILITATING SLEEP AND COMFORT

Sleeping medications are usually ordered the night before surgery to help promote sleep. Their administration should be timed with other preparations to aid their effectiveness.

The night before surgery is often especially stressful for the individual. The nurse can help relieve anxiety and increase comfort by the therapeutic use of self, creating a restful environment and being available to the individual. Having the family and/or significant others present may provide additional reassurance and support.

PROVIDING FOR SAFETY

Final safety and preparatory measures are carried out on the day of surgery. Special preoperative checklists are usually available to have a written record of the preparations which are needed and the times they are done. Figure 26.1 shows an example of a preoperative checklist. All jewelry is removed to prevent it from getting lost during surgery and interfering with the surgical process. If the individual desires, the wedding ring may be left on and taped securely around the finger. Jewelry and other valuables may be taken home by the family and/or significant others or locked in the hospital safe. Nail polish and other cosmetics are removed to allow for careful assessment of the skin and nailbeds and to prevent any possibility of fire from these highly flammable substances. Any prostheses that the individual wears—including dentures, wig, eyelashes, artificial eyes or limbs—are removed and safely stored to prevent their loss or interference with surgery. Many times the nurse may not be aware that the individual uses any of these devices and should specifically ask about them by name. The individual may be reluctant to go without these articles, but careful explanation of the rationale behind removing them for surgery will help to increase cooperation. The individual should have an accurate nameband securely attached to the wrist to insure proper identification during the time the individual is unconscious.

Current laboratory reports are attached to the chart to provide a last-minute update on the individual's condition. Any evidence of colds, fever, decreased hemoglobin and hematocrit, and overwhelming anxiety may necessitate the cancellation of surgery and must be reported to the surgeon. Vital signs are checked and recorded to provide base-line data and to assess for any change in the person's status. The individual empties the bladder just prior to receiving preoperative medication (if an indwelling catheter is not in place) to prevent incontinence during surgery, which contaminates the sterile field, and to promote the comfort of the individual.

OBTAINING INFORMED CONSENT

All individuals must sign an informed consent before any surgical process. (Figure 26.2 shows a sample consent form.) If the individual is under 18 years of age or incapable of signing the form, the closest relative does so. This consent not only gives the surgeon permission to perform surgery, but also states that the individual has been informed of exactly what procedure is being done, its outcomes, and the possible complications. The nurse checks that this form is present on the individual's chart before sending the individual to surgery.

THE BROOKLYN HOSPITAL

PRE-OPERATIVE CHECK LIST

NURSE CHECKING IS TO INITIAL EACH ITEM CHECKED

Check the following before 11P.M. on eve of elective surgery:

	Initials
1. Height and weight on chart	
2. Operative consent signed, witnessed, dated (If minor, legal consent)	
3. Transfusion consent signed, witnessed, dated (If minor, legal consent)	
4. Identification band on patient's wrist	
5. History and physical written	
6. Shave prep done	
7. Recent (48 hr.) CBC & urine report on chart	
8. Blood available in blood bank	
9. Seen by clergy	

Nurse preparing patient for O.R. check the following:

1. Pre-op orders & medications given & recorded	
2. T.P.R. & B.P. taken & charted on T.P.R. sheet	
3. Dentures, contact lens, hearing aids, prosthesis, wigs, etc. removed	
4. All clothing removed except for hospital gown	
5. All jewelry removed	
6. Patient voided	
7. All make-up removed — lipstick, nail polish, etc	

Figure 26.1
A preoperative checklist helps assure that necessary measures have been carried out for the individual prior to surgery. (*Courtesy of The Brooklyn Hospital*)

ADMINISTERING MEDICATIONS

Preoperative medications are given approximately 30 minutes before the scheduled time of surgery. This allows the medications to reach their

THE BROOKLYN HOSPITAL

CONSENT FORM

Only consent of a competent patient over 18 years of age (or emancipated, if under 19 years) is valid.
Otherwise, signature of spouse or parent or nearest legally responsible relative or guardian is required.

CONSENT FOR TREATMENT (Patient, parent, nearest relative or guardian)

Knowing that _____ is suffering from a condition requiring diagnosis and/or medical or surgical treatment, I hereby voluntarily consent to such diagnostic procedures, hospital care and/or medical or surgical treatment as may be deemed necessary in the judgment of the staff physicians of THE BROOKLYN HOSPITAL concerned in the patient's case.

Witness: _____   Signature: _____
                                                     (Patient, parent, nearest relative or guardian)

Date: _____   Relationship to patient _____

CONSENT FOR OPERATION and/or SPECIAL PROCEDURE (Patient, parent, nearest relative or guardian)

I, the undersigned, hereby consent to and authorize the performance of _____
_____ and/or surgical or other procedures upon _____
as may be deemed necessary to treat my/his/her condition or conditions; said procedures to be performed by
Dr. _____ and/or such other physicians or surgeons under his direction as he may
designate or as may be designated, all of whom are in attendance at THE BROOKLYN HOSPITAL. Consent is hereby given
to administer whatever anesthetic agent or agents as may be deemed necessary or appropriate by said physicians or surgeons.
Any tissues surgically removed may be disposed of by the hospital in accordance with established practice. I hereby certify
that I fully understand the nature of the above consent which has been explained to me.

Witness: _____   Signature: _____
                                                     (Patient, parent, nearest relative or guardian)

Date: _____   Relationship to patient: _____

CONSENT FOR DELIVERY

I authorize Dr. _____, and whomever he may designate as his assistant(s) to perform
upon _____ any operation which he deems advisable in the course of (my) (her)
obstetrical care and delivery. I consent to the administration of such anesthetics as may be considered necessary or advisable by the
physician responsible for this service, with the exception of _____
                                                                           (State "None" or specify)

I certify that I understand the nature of the above consent which has been explained to me.

Witness: _____   Signature: _____

Date: _____ Time: _____ A.M. P.M.   Relationship to patient: _____

FRONT

Figure 26.2

Consent forms for various health care procedures. *(Courtesy of The Brooklyn Hospital)*

RELEASE (For patient signing out against advice)

_____, a patient in THE BROOKLYN HOSPITAL, wishes to leave the hospital contrary to the advice of the attending physicians. They have advised that the patient's condition is such that to do so may result in injury and/or aggravation of his/her present condition. Despite this advice, the patient wishes to leave and therefore releases the hospital, its physicians, and its personnel from all responsibility for the possible consequences of his/her actions.

Witness: _____   Signature: _____
                                                          (Patient)

Date: _____   Signature: _____
                                                          (Parent, nearest relative or guardian)

                                          Relationship to patient: _____

RELEASE OF RESPONSIBILITY FOR LEAVE OF ABSENCE

I hereby absolve THE BROOKLYN HOSPITAL from all responsibility and liability for myself during my leave of absence from the hospital of not more than six (6) hours. I understand that the party/parties that pay for any part of my hospitalization may not pay for the time I am on Leave of Absence; therefore, I assume responsibility for such payments.

Witness: _____   Patient's Signature: _____

Date: _____ Time: _____ A.M. Approved By: _____ M.D.
                                          P.M.

Reason for Leave of Absence: _____

CONSULTATION FOR STERILIZATION

We, the undersigned physicians, have examined _____ and find that sterilization is an urgent medical necessity for this patient. The detailed reasons for this opinion have been incorporated in the progress notes of the patient's hospital chart.

Witness: _____   Signature: _____ M.D.

Date: _____ Time: _____ A.M. Signature: _____ M.D.
                                          P.M.

STERILIZATION PERMIT

I, the undersigned, hereby authorize and direct Dr. _____ and assistants of his/her choice to perform the following operation _____ upon _____ at THE BROOKLYN HOSPITAL and to do any other procedure that his/her/their judgment may dictate during the above operation. It has been explained to me that this operation is intended to result in sterility although this result has not been guaranteed. I voluntarily request the operation and understand that if it proves successful, the results will be permanent and it will therefore be physically impossible fo the patient to inseminate or to conceive or bear children.

Witness: _____   Signature: _____
                                                          (Patient)

Date: _____ Time: _____ A.M. Signature: _____
                                          P.M.

BACK

Figure 26.2 (Cont.)

peak level of action by the time anesthesia is induced. Most individuals receive one medication to reduce respiratory tree secretions and others to promote relaxation. These drugs reduce the chance of aspiration of secretions during and immediately after surgery and enhance the induction of the desired level of anesthesia. Chart 26.3 outlines the medications commonly used preoperatively and their actions. Once the preoperative medications are given, the individual is placed in bed with the side rails up to prevent falls or other accidents. The individual may relax more if a family member and/or significant other or health team member quietly sits beside the bed during this time.

The individual is now transported to the surgical suite.

THE INTRAOPERATIVE PHASE

The intraoperative phase begins when the individual enters the surgical suite. Most individuals are temporarily held in a waiting area while final preparations are made in the operating room. Many surgical suites have separate anesthesia rooms where the anesthesia is induced. The individual is then transferred to the operating room and moved to the operating table. The individual is positioned on the table according to the type of surgery being done. Additional skin preparation may be carried out at this time and anesthesia induced if it has not already been done. The surgical site is then draped with sterile sheets and the actual surgery begins. Throughout the surgery the anesthesiologist (or anesthetist) monitors the individual's vital signs and level of consciousness to determine anesthesia needs. Illustrations 26.2 and 26.3 show the operating room environment.

Surgical Team

The surgical team usually consists of the surgeon, the surgeon's assistants, the anesthesiologist (or anesthetist) and assistants, the surgical nurse, the scrub nurse (or technician), and the circulating nurse (or technician). In addition, the x-ray technician, pathologist, and other specialists are part of the team as needed. Chart 26.4 outlines the responsibilities of each member of the surgical team.

Chart 26.3
Common Preoperative Medications

TYPE	ACTION
Vagolytics	
1. Atropine sulfate	Decreases respiratory tree secretions.
2. Scopolamine	Decreases vagus actions.
Sedatives and tranquilizers	
1. Barbiturates (Nembutal, Seconal)	Results in muscle relaxation; lowers vital signs; allays anxiety.
2. Hydroxygene pamoate (Vistaril)	
3. Diazapam (Valium)	
4. Promethazine (Phenergan)	Phenergan also has an antiemetic effect.
Analgesics	
1. Nonnarcotic: Pentazocine (Talwin).	
2. Narcotic: Morphine sulfate, Meperidine hydrochloride (Demerol)	Given for sedative effect.

The Anesthesia Process

The anesthesia the individual receives may be local, regional, or general. The choice depends on the type of surgery, the individual's state of health, and the preferences of the surgeon and the anesthesiologist.

LOCAL ANESTHESIA

Local anesthesia is the blocking of the peripheral nerve endings within a circumscribed area to prevent transmission of stimuli during surgery. It is used for suturing wounds, dental work, examination of larynx, bronchi, and rectum, and removal of small lesions, such as polyps, warts, or external hemorrhoids.

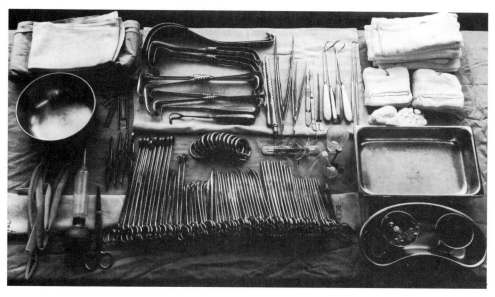

Illustration 26.2
A sterile setup of surgical instruments. *(Photo by Stan Levy, from Photo Researchers, Inc.)*

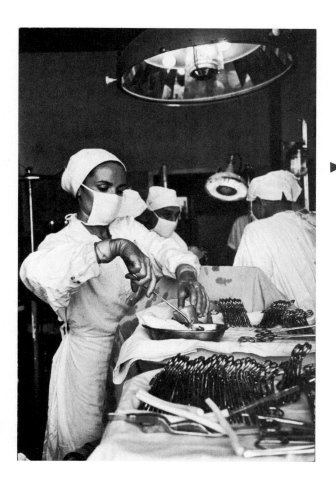

Local anesthesia may be administered topically through the use of sprays or drops or by subcutaneous or intracutaneous injection. Xylocaine, procaine, lidocaine, and cocaine are examples of local anesthetics.

REGIONAL ANESTHESIA

▶ **Regional anesthesia** is used to block the transmission of afferent impulses by anesthetizing large nerve bundles or transmission sites in or around the spinal cord. Some types of regional anesthesia are epidural block, intradural block, and deep cervical block. When the anesthesia is injected into the spinal cord, the procedure is similar to that of a lumbar puncture. Agents commonly used are xylocaine, lidocaine, and procaine. Regional anesthesia is frequently used for orthopedic procedures, childbirth, and lower abdominal and inguinal procedures. This method is often used with debilitated individuals or persons with heart or respiratory pathologies who require surgery.

Illustration 26.3
The scrub nurse, an integral part of the surgical team, passes to the surgeon instruments that she has prepared, being careful to maintain sterile technique. *(Photo by Stan Levy from Photo Researchers, Inc.)*

Chart 26.4
Responsibilities of the Members of the Surgical Team

ROLE	RESPONSIBILITY
Surgeon	Has primary responsibility for the performance of the surgical procedure; performs the complex aspects of the surgical procedure.
Assistant to surgeon	Usually surgical resident in training; assists surgeon; may incise the surgical site at the beginning of surgery and close the incision at the end; helps control bleeding and drainage, exposure of surgical site; holds instruments; may perform less complex aspects of surgery.
Anesthesiologist (Physician specializing in the anesthesia process) *or* anesthetist (Nurse specializing in the anesthesia process)	Has primary responsibility for evaluating the individual's anesthetic needs preoperatively; inducing and maintaining anesthesia during surgery; monitoring vital functions during surgery. Administers blood and medications as needed and supervises the recovery-room course.
Assistants to anesthesiologist or anesthetist	Usually anesthesia residents in training—assist with anesthesia activities.
Surgical nurse	Supervises the overall function of the operating room; coordinates activities of nurses and technicians; provides nursing care where necessary.
Scrub nurse (or technician)	Sets up instruments and equipment; assists surgeon in gowning and gloving; hands instruments to surgeon; anticipates equipment and supply needs; is responsible for the maintenance of sterile technique; carries out sponge, needle, and instrument counts.
Circulating nurse (or technician)	Supervises setup and cleanliness of the operating room; checks equipment for functioning; assists surgical team in gowning and gloving; obtains equipment and supplies as they are needed during surgery; assists in bringing individual into operating room and in nonsterile preparations; reviews preoperative checklist.

GENERAL ANESTHESIA

General anesthesia is used to depress the central nervous system and produce total body anesthesia. General anesthesia may be administered by inhalation, intravenously, or rectally. There are four stages of general anesthesia: analgesia, excitement, surgical anesthesia, and medullary paralysis. Chart 26.5 outlines the stages of general anesthesia. Commonly used inhalational anesthesias are nitrous oxide, cyclopropane, and halothane; intravenous anesthesias are sodium pentothal, propanidid, and sodium methohexitol; rectal anesthesias include pentothal. Anesthesia is frequently first induced intravenously. Once the third stage is reached, an endotracheal tube is inserted and inhalational anesthesia used. (Illustration 26.4)

Surgical Environment

STERILE FIELDS

A sterile environment is maintained throughout the surgical process. Tables, lights, and large equipment are rendered surgically clean by use of disinfectants. All drapes, instruments, dressings, and sutures used are sterile and handled using sterile technique. All surgical team members who come in contact with the individual undergoing surgery and/or the sterile field are dressed in sterile gowns, gloves, and masks. They are changed whenever there is a possibility they have been contaminated. Contamination of the surgical incision during surgery is one of the major hazards facing the individual and affecting post-

Chart 26.5
Stages of General Anesthesia

STAGE	ONSET	RESPONSE
One: Analgesia	Begins with the administration of anesthesia.	Reception of sensory input distorted, all reflexes present, blood pressure remains stable, respiratory rate may increase, euphoria present. Used for childbirth, performance of minor procedures, relief of pain.
Two: Excitement	Begins with loss of consciousness.	Reflexes present but may be hyperactive with stimulation, increased muscle and rapid eye movements, pupils dilate, blood pressure increases, pulse increases and becomes irregular (this stage is avoided whenever possible).
Three: Surgical anesthesia	After stage of excitement.	
Plane one		Respirations regular, pupils constricted, reflexes absent, relaxation of small muscles, blood pressure returns to usual.
Plane two		Vital signs stable, but expiratory phase of respiration lengthened; large muscles relax; no movements.
Plane three		Complete relaxation; respirations increase and become shallower; diminished respiratory movement; temperature drops (plane used for abdominal surgery).
Plane four		Pupils dilated; blood pressure and pulse decreased, skin pale, cold, and clammy.
Four: Medullary paralysis		Respiratory arrest, vascular collapse, impending death.

operative recovery. Thus scrupulous care must be taken by all members of the surgical team to prevent any chance of contamination during surgery. Cultures are periodically done from all standing operating-room equipment and the ventilation shafts in order to prevent spread of organisms through these routes.

FIRE PREVENTION

Since many anesthesias and the oxygen used in the operating room are either highly flammable and/or support combustion, care is taken to reduce the risk of fire and explosions. All personnel wear nonconductive shoes and underclothing. Equipment must be well grounded and in good repair to prevent the emission of sparks. No smoking or lighting of flames is allowed in surgical areas.

QUIET, NONSTIMULATING ATMOSPHERE

Maintenance of a quiet, nonstimulating environment in the operating room is conducive to the induction of anesthesia and the reduction of the individual's anxiety. Persons having local and regional anesthetics may be fully aware of all the stimuli in the environment and can be easily agitated by conversation, banging of equipment, and other distractions. Individuals in stages 1 and 2 of general anesthesia are not only aware of stimuli, but also may distort the input they receive. In addition, environmental stimuli exaggerate reactions in stage 2.

The Phase Ended

When the surgery is completed, the incision is appropriately dressed and the individual is transferred

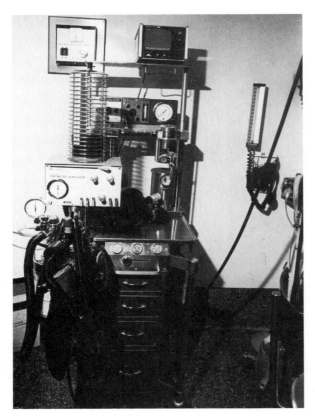

Illustration 26.4
Machinery used to administer general anesthesia. *(Photo © Leonard Speier)*

to the postoperative recovery area. Records of the individual's vital signs during the surgery, medications received, blood transfused, and any other immediately pertinent information are transferred with the individual. This provides data for comparison in the recovery room.

THE POSTOPERATIVE PHASE

Immediate Postoperative Period

The individual remains in the recovery area until he or she has completely reacted from the anesthesia and vital signs are stable. In some instances the individual may be transferred to an intensive care unit, depending on the type and severity of the surgery. The goal of the recovery room nurse is to maintain adequacy of all vital functions, to prevent the early complications of surgery, and to relieve discomfort.

MAJOR COMPLICATIONS

The major complications of the immediate postoperative period are respiratory obstruction, shock, hemorrhage, and cardiac arrest.

Respiratory Obstruction

Respiratory obstruction may be the result of the occlusion of the pharynx by the relaxed tongue, the inability of the individual to remove secretions from the airway, aspiration of secretions or vomitus, or edema of the airway. Signs of respiratory obstruction include noisy, irregular respirations; pallor or cyanosis; restlessness; anxiety; use of accessory muscles for breathing; and a rapid, irregular pulse. Respiratory obstruction can be prevented by close observation of vital signs; frequent oral and oropharyngeal suctioning; positioning the individual with the head to one side; auscultating the chest for adventitious sounds; and inserting an airway. Deep breathing and coughing are instituted as soon as the individual is alert enough and continued at least every 2 hours throughout the postoperative period.

Shock

Shock may result from massive hemorrhaging, peripheral vascular shutdown, and cardiac insufficiency. Signs of shock include cold, clammy skin, increases in pulse and respiration, decreases in blood pressure, thirst, and restlessness. This complication can be prevented by replacement of lost fluids, careful observation for signs of hemorrhage, close monitoring of vital signs (q. 15 minutes until stable, then q½h for 2 hours), and application of elastic stockings.

Hemorrhage

Hemorrhage occurs when blood vessels have not been tied off during the surgical process or when sutures tying off vessels are disturbed. The signs of hemorrhage are the same as for shock. In addition, bloody drainage on dressings or on bedclothes posterior to the wound indicates bleeding. The prevention of hemorrhage is also the same as for shock.

Cardiac Arrest

Cardiac arrest occurs as a result of hypoxia, respiratory obstruction, cardiac insufficiency, and fluid and electrolyte imbalance and as a reaction to the anesthesia. (Chapter 18 discusses signs, symptoms, and treatment.)

NURSING IMPLICATIONS

In the immediate postoperative period, the nurse assesses the patency and function of all drainage tubes and adjusts them as necessary. The individual's level of consciousness is assessed and the individual is appropriately oriented to self, place, and time. The nurse assesses the individual for pain and administers analgesics accordingly and as ordered. The individual is turned frequently and positioned as determined by the surgical site. Individuals may frequently experience nausea and vomiting because of air swallowing, the return of peristalsis, and the effects of anesthesia and/or medications. The nauseated individual is encouraged to take deep breaths, and the head is turned to one side in case of vomiting. Antiemetics may be administered to reduce the nausea and prevent vomiting. Any orders or treatments specific to the surgery are assessed and appropriately carried out. Intake and output records are kept on all individuals.

When the vital signs are stable and the individual has reacted, the individual is transferred to his or her room.

The Intermediate Postoperative Period

The intermediate postoperative period covers the first 72 hours after surgery. Upon the individual's return to his or her room, vital signs and dressings are checked and drainage tubes and equipment are connected, the individual is positioned comfortably and according to the surgery, levels of orientation and consciousness are assessed, and postoperative orders are reviewed and carried through. The individual may still be very groggy and special measures to ensure safety are taken. Side rails are raised, the bed is in lowest position, and the call bell is made readily available to the person. Any questions the individual has are answered, but the nurse should realize that the individual may not remember the answers, so reinforcement of this information may be necessary at a later time. Family and/or significant others should be allowed to see the individual, but they are first apprised of the individual's condition, appearance, and behavior. (Illustration 26.5)

DEEP BREATHING/COUGHING

Deep breathing, coughing, and positioning are carried out at least every 2 hours during this period. In the early part of this stage, the nurse may have to reinforce preoperative teaching and provide a great deal of assistance to the individual in performing these activities.

ANALGESIA

If the individual has had major surgery, analgesics should be offered prior to carrying out deep breathing and coughing. During this period the individual usually experiences pain, and analgesics should be made available approximately every 3–4 hours. By the fourth postoperative day, incisional pain should be markedly decreased, and the analgesics are evaluated for type and dosage.

VOIDING REQUIREMENTS

The person should void within 10 hours after surgery; if not, the individual is usually catheterized to prevent urinary retention. The individual is offered the bedpan regularly. Abdominal discomfort is assessed to determine whether it is the result of the surgical procedure or a full bladder. Intake and output records are kept during this period.

AMBULATION

Progressive ambulation is usually started within the first 24 hours, depending on physician's orders and the condition of the individual. Many individuals are ambulated as early as the evening of surgery. Early ambulation helps prevent many of the complications of surgery, including thrombophlebitis, gastric distension, pneumonia, and loss of muscle tone. In addition, early ambulation assists in the reactivation of body function and form and helps to counteract the effects of central nervous system depression during surgery. Elastic stockings are frequently ordered to aid in venous return.

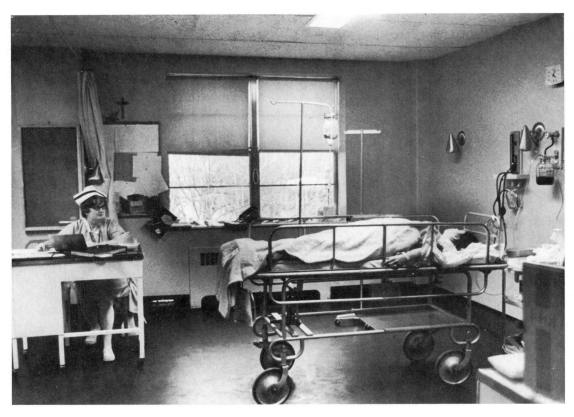

Illustration 26.5
In the recovery room during the immediate postoperative period, the nurse closely monitors
an individual's vital functions and promotes his comfort until the individual has completely
reacted from anesthesia. *(Photo by David Strickler, from Monkmeyer)*

BODY TEMPERATURE

The individual may experience a slightly lower body temperature right after surgery. This is caused by the central nervous system and hypothalamic depression, and some peripheral vasoconstriction. However, the individual's temperature usually rises to a low-grade fever within the 24 hours as a result of the inflammatory response. This response may last for up to 2 days. Temperatures that are above 100 F (37.7 C) or that remain elevated for longer periods need to be evaluated, as they may indicate pneumonia or a wound infection.

FOOD AND FLUIDS

Food and fluids are withheld until the individual's gag and swallow reflexes have returned. Depending on the type of surgery, extent of anesthesia, and individual differences, bowel sounds may be absent up to 48 hours after surgery. Food is usually withheld until bowel sounds return, although sometimes the individual will be allowed fluids before this time. Nausea, vomiting, and prolonged absence of peristalsis may indicate paralytic ileus or obstruction. It is during this time that catabolism is exceeding anabolism and a negative nitrogen balance exists. Weight is lost and fluid and electrolyte imbalance may occur if careful monitoring is not done. Hyperalimentation is used for those individuals who have marginal or deficit nutritional states, since protein is lost during this period and is not replaced by food intake.

NURSING IMPLICATIONS

The individual is assessed for signs of crisis, body image distortions, grieving and loss, and sensory deprivation. These signs may be very subtle and easily overlooked by the nurse in an attempt to meet the variety of physical needs the individual has at this time. However, the implications of these signs for the individual's recovery are great. They often impede the individual's return to the highest level of functioning and interfere with the ability to meet basic needs. The family and/or significant others may experience many of the same feelings during this time. Interaction between the individual and family and/or significant others may therefore be affected. Thus the nursing interventions are focused not only on the individual, but also on the family and/or significant others.

The Later Postoperative Period

As the initial postoperative period ends, the individual begins to meet more of his or her own health care needs. Nursing actions are those which will help to maximize the individual's recovery and assist the individual to attain the highest level of well-being within the usual life setting. This later postoperative period covers the time from the second or third postoperative day until the individual is functioning at a maximum level of wellness. The nurse continues to assess health behaviors and intervenes to meet the individual's needs.

CONTINUED PHYSICAL AND PHYSIOLOGIC CARE

Physical and physiologic care is still a focus because, during the early part of this period, the individual is still in an acute phase of recovery. This phase requires a great deal of energy as the healing process continues. Protein, vitamin, and calorie intakes are increased to meet the energy needs of the healing process. Ambulation is steadily progressed to increase muscle strength and endurance as well as to promote healing. The individual may assume poor posture in an attempt to protect injured muscles and thus needs to be reminded to stand and sit correctly. Gaseous exchange may be decreased because the individual is still reluctant to breathe deeply, cough, and move. Movement, deep breathing, and coughing may be improved if the nurse explains to the individual that they will not in any way be injurious and that some pain is initially an expected part of the process. Reinforcing information on splinting and

judicious use of analgesics will also further the movement process. The individual may have difficulty reestablishing bowel and bladder habits. The nurse can assist in this area by suggesting foods which will promote elimination, by teaching the individual the relationship between exercise and elimination, and by administering laxatives when appropriate. Fluid and electrolyte needs are also a concern, particularly after the initial fluid-retention period. The nurse needs to continue careful observation of the wound since many wound disruptions can occur at this time. Sutures are usually removed around 7–10 days after surgery, depending on the amount and type of tissues involved and the progression of healing. Chart 26.6 outlines the major complications of the acute postoperative period.

PSYCHOLOGIC ASSISTANCE

It is during this period that many individuals and their family and/or significant others come to a full realization of the implications of surgery on their lifestyles. Before this time, preoccupation with surgery, pain, disability, and activities of care limited their abilities to focus on the future and internalize the effects of the surgery. The individual's usual coping behaviors may become exaggerated at this time. If they are not sufficient to deal with the situation, the individual may enter a crisis. These behavioral changes can place extra strain on the interactions among the individual, the family and/or significant others, and staff. Passivity, depression, anger, negativism, and denial are just some of the behaviors frequently seen.

TEACHING–LEARNING

Many new health behaviors may have to be learned at this time. Although the nurse has been teaching all along, this is when the major emphasis will be placed on the teaching–learning process. Self-care skills, changes in habits, and modification of environment and lifestyle are some of the behaviors with which the individual may require help. The family and/or significant others should be included in this teaching–learning so that they too are aware of the individual's capabilities and limitations and can assist the individual in meeting health care needs. Although most persons will be able to return to their daily activities within a matter of weeks, measures to match

Chart 26.6
Major Complications of the Acute Postoperative Period and Nursing Preventions

NEED	INTERFERENCE	MECHANISM OF OCCURRENCE	NURSING PREVENTION
Biologic safety	**Wound** infection, as evidenced by increased pain, swelling, and redness in incisional area; purulent drainage, foul odor; fever, increased pulse. Usually manifests itself within 36–48 hours.	Contamination of surgical site during surgery. Untreated preoperative infection. Breaks in aseptic technique during wound care and dressing changes.	Maintenance of sterile environment during surgery. Assessing and reporting signs of infection; Proper aseptic technique during wound care and dressing Give prophylactic antibiotics as ordered, maintain nutrition, recognize predisposing factors (e.g., age, weight).
Oxygen uptake	**Atelectasis,** manifested by fever, dyspnea, cyanosis, tachycardia.	Collapse of alveoli posterior to mucous plug. Increased viscosity and amount of respiratory secretions. Depression of respiratory activity.	Positioning, complete suctioning Coughing, deep breathing, hydration.
	Pneumonia, manifested by fever; collection of fluid in lungs; thick, viscous sputum; dyspnea, lethargy. Can develop as early as the first 34 hours after surgery.	Central nervous system depression. Inadequate expansion of lungs. Immobility Aspiration	Coughing, deep breathing, positioning. Good mouth care. Ambulation as soon as allowed. Good nutrition. Increased fluid intake. Judicious use of narcotics.
Oxygen uptake, transport, and utilization; waste removal	**Pulmonary embolism,** manifested by chest pain, dyspnea, cyanosis, cardiac arrest, cor pulmonale (right-sided heart failure), hemoptysis, cough, tachycardia, wheezing.	Foreign body such as air, fat, or clot travels through bloodstream and lodges in blood vessels of the lung.	Prevention of thrombophlebitis and phlebothrombosis (see below).
	Thrombophlebitis, as evidenced in localized red area or red streak, Homan's sign present, area warm to touch, calf pain. Usually occurs 7–14 days postoperatively.	Injury to vessel wall results in buildup of clot. Venous stasis contributes to clot formation.	Elastic stocking Exercise Ambulation No pressure on ankles. Prevention of infiltration of IVs.

(continued)

Chart 26.6 (Cont.)

Major Complications of the Acute Postoperative Period and Nursing Preventions

NEED	INTERFERENCE	MECHANISM OF OCCURRENCE	NURSING PREVENTION
Elimination	Constipation (bowel movement should occur within 3–4 days postoperatively.)	Peristalsis slowed by anesthesia and/or manipulation of the bowel.	Exercise, diet with sufficient residue, fluids, laxatives, privacy.
Nutritional intake and elimination	**Gastric distention,** manifested by enlarged abdomen, sharp, stabbing abdominal pains, rectal pressure, decreased bowel sounds.	Peristalsis slowed by anesthesia, air swallowing. Gas accumulates in intestine.	Exercise, movement, rectal tube. Solid food as soon as allowed.
	Paralytic ileus, manifested by vomiting, absence of bowel sounds, gastric distention (can lead to shock), constipation.	Peristalsis stopped because of anesthesia. Manipulation of the bowel. Electrolyte imbalance. Peritonitis.	Observe for bowel sounds, gastric distention, and constipation. Maintain fluid and electrolyte balance.
Elimination	**Urinary retention,** manifested by distended bladder, decreased urinary output, residual urine.	Catheterization Manipulation of bladder. Central nervous system depression.	Privacy Offer bedpan. Help person attain usual voiding position as soon as possible. Perineal exercises
Biologic safety	**Dehiscence,** manifested by separation of wound edges; unexpected appearance of drainage; can occur 5th to 8th postoperative day.	Poor healing process. Stress on wound.	Maintain good nutrition. Wound splinting when engaged in vigorous activity or when vomiting.
	Evisceration, manifested by separation of wound edges and protrusion of internal organs and tissues. Can occur 5th to 8th postoperative day.	Poor healing process. Stress on wound.	See above. If it occurs, immobilize person. Cover area with sterile dressing soaked in sterile saline and call surgeon immediately.

capabilities with limitations will be needed, since *complete* healing and adaptation to changes may take many months. However, misconceptions often arise about what can or cannot be done. The nurse clarifies when and how the individual can resume activities of daily living. There are discussions of such things as the foods the individual can eat, exercise tolerance, and when the individual can resume sexual activities.

Many resources exist within the community to assist the individual in the latter part of the postoperative period. Apprising the individual of these resources and how to use them is an important intervention. Community health and clinic nurses reinforce the individual's learning and assist in promoting and maintaining the highest level of functioning. Communication and planning between hospital-based and community-based nurses is a prerequisite for the continuity and follow-through of nursing care for the individual who has undergone surgery.

SELECTED REFERENCES

Chouinard, Fern, Foley, Noreen, and Millar, Kathryn. "Vigilant Nursing Care After Reconstructive Microsurgery." *Nursing 79,* 9:18, June, 1979.

Croushore, Theresa. "Postoperative Assessment: The Key to Avoiding the Most Common Nursing Mistakes." *Nursing 79,* 9:46, April, 1979.

Damstregt, D. "Pastoral Roles in Pre-Surgical Visits." *American Journal of Nursing,* 75:1336, August, 1975.

"Dealing With Depression After Radical Surgery." *Nursing 79,* 9:46, February, 1979.

"Defeated Patient: Her Wories Come First." *Nursing 77* 7:28, April, 1977.

Dziurbejko, Marsha and Larkin, Judith Candib. "Including the Family in Preoperative Teaching." *American Journal of Nursing,* 78:1892, November, 1978.

Hegyvary, St. "The Hospital Setting and Patient Care Outcomes." *Journal of Nursing Administration,* 5:36, May, 1975.

Laird, Mona. "Techniques for Teaching Pre- and Postoperative Patients." *American Journal of Nursing,* 75:1338, August, 1975.

LeMaitre, George and Finnegan, Janet. *The Patient in Surgery: A Guide for Nurses.* Philadelphia, Saunders, 1975.

Marcinek, Margaret Boyle. "Stress in the Surgical Patient." *American Journal of Nursing,* 77:1809, November, 1977.

McConnell, Edwina. "After Surgery: How You Can Avert the Obvious Hazards. . . and the Not-So-Obvious Ones, Too." *Nursing 77,* 7:32, March, 1977.

Merkatz, Ruth, Smith, Dorsey, and Seitz, Pauline. "Preoperative Teaching for Gynecologic Patients." *American Journal of Nursing,* 74:1072, June, 1974.

Metheny, Norma and Snively, William. "Perioperative Fluids and Electrolytes." *American Journal of Nursing,* 78:840, May, 1978.

Parsons, Mickey Camp and Stephens, Gwen J. "Postoperative Complications: Assessment and Intervention." *American Journal of Nursing,* 74:240, February, 1974.

Roberts, Melville, Vilinskas, Juliet, and Owen, Gary. "Technicians or Nurses in the Operating Room?" *American Journal of Nursing,* 74:906, May, 1974.

Robinson, Lisa. *Psychological Aspects of the Care of Hospitalized Patients.* Philadelphia, Davis, 1976.

Ryan, Rosemary. "Thrombophlebitis: Assessment and Prevention." *American Journal of Nursing,* 76:1634, October, 1976.

Scott, Steve. "Operating Room Follies." *American Journal of Nursing,* 77:467, March, 1977.

Smith, Betty J. "Safeguarding Your Patient Against Anesthesia." *Nursing 78,* 8:52, October, 1978.

"Symposium: Perspectives in Operating Room Nursing." *Nursing Clinics of North America,* 10:613, December, 1975.

Walters, Jean. "Four Practical Questions to Ask When Organizing Preoperative Classes." *American Journal of Nursing,* 79:1090, June, 1979.

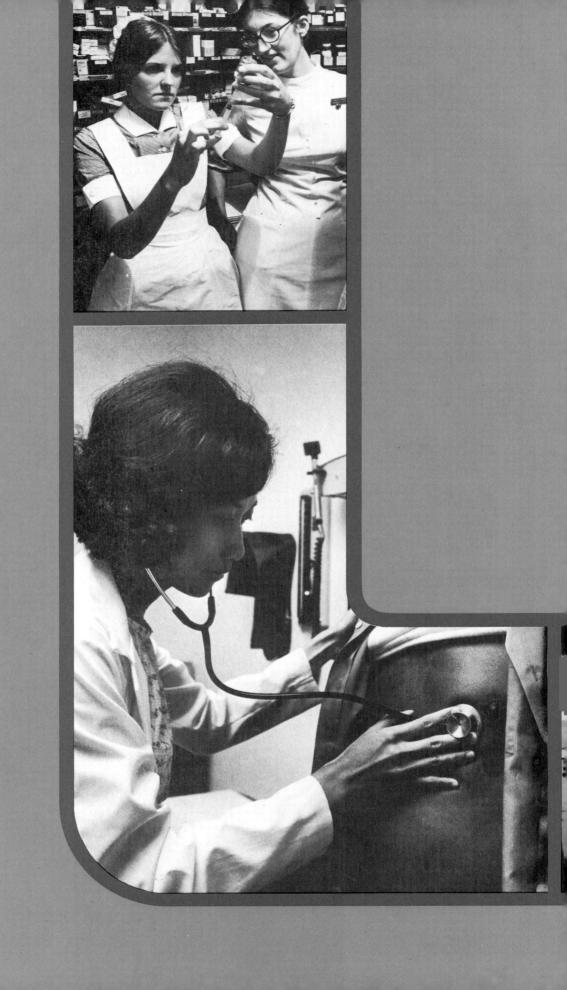

Intervention: Nursing Process in Action

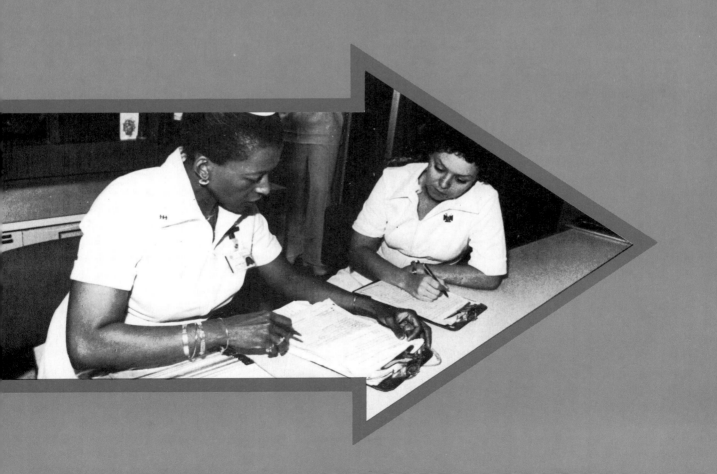

THE NURSING PROCESS IN ACTION

The following is a nursing process presentation of a real care situation adapted from a beginning nursing student's case study.*

ASSESSMENT: 7/13

General Assessment

Initials.   A. S.

Age.   33 years old.

---

*Adapted, with permission, from a case study by Nancy Newman, former nursing student, Long Island University, Department of Nursing, Brooklyn Center, Brooklyn, New York.

Sex.   Male.

Religion.   Protestant (nonpracticing).

Race.   Black.

Reason for Hospitalization.   Fifth admission within last year for sickle cell crisis.

Perception of Situation.   "My sickle cell crisis was so bad I couldn't control it."

Expectations of Hospital Stay.   "Maybe all of you can get me through this crisis even though I know you can't cure me."

Social Aspects.   Four brothers, three sisters, mother died of sickle cell anemia. Siblings do not reside near one another but are in contact by phone at least once a day. Father is alive and well. One other brother has sickle cell anemia.

A. S. is presently living with a woman. They are not legally married. They have 7-year-old twin daughters. He feels being married would "tie him down." He does not wish to remain living with the mother of his children—would like to date, "especially one of the nurses."

Level of Growth and Development.   Selected a mate, has a family, does not manage own home or actively participate in child rearing. States he is unwilling to settle down as yet and "give up" his "freedom."

A. S. involves himself more with his father, brothers, and sisters than with his children and their mother. His children call him repeatedly and ask if he is not coming home because he doesn't love them.

Occupation.   A. S. is presently unemployed because of his "medical condition." Receives unemployment insurance. Was previously a real estate salesman. His children's mother is a nurse at M. Hospital and provides the major source of income. He is also receiving social service benefits.

Education.   Finished high school; attended vocational high school and was graduated. Has one more semester left to complete college degree in accounting. Had to "discontinue for a while due to my medical condition."

Modes of Transportation.   Has own car, which he loans to his brother when hospitalized—which has been quite often of late. His children's mother doesn't drive. He is happy about this, as he states, "She would always take the car."

Habits.   Alcohol intake: denies any. Drugs: only those prescribed by his physician. Does not smoke. Personal: says he has habit of putting things off that he doesn't like to do (paperwork from his job) because he doesn't know how much longer he has to live so he'd rather do the things he enjoys. Showers daily, uses deodorant; states he likes to look nice.

Allergies.   Sensitive to Compazine, Talwin.

Hobbies.   Likes to draw; has steady hand.

Housing.   Resides with his two children and their mother in a two-bedroom apartment on the fifth floor of an elevator building in a public housing project.

Cognitive Status
State of Consciousness.   Receives Demerol, 125 mg, q2h, so at times he appears drowsy and slow to respond.

Orientation.   Well oriented to time, date, day, and people around him. Has calendar by bed and wears a wristwatch.

Level of Education.   Three-and-a-half years of college. His ability to recall events recent and past is excellent. He still recalls minute details of past events.

Attention Span.   Even when heavily sedated with pain medication, his attention span is very long, and he never appears unwilling to carry on a conversation.

Vocabulary Level.   Uses complex technical words.

Ability to Understand Ideas.   Quick to gain meanings and make relationships. Excellent insight into his health problems. Because of repeated medical explanations and own research, he is able to explain very explicitly and technically his condition. States he is presently writing a book entitled *Sickle Cell Anemia: The Killer of Many.* He has been prompted to do so by his many medical referrals. He explains all the whys and wherefores of his disease and hopes it will help others gain insight. States he hopes he lives long enough to finish it.

Emotional Status
Emotional Reactions.   Mood is usually smiling, cheerful, and talkative. However, expresses some agitation about the woman across the hall who is always in his room bothering him. States that "she takes advantage of me by using my phone all the time." Makes frequent remarks about his limited life span.

Body Image.   Expressed concern over his abdomen, as it has become distended over the past few weeks. Concerned over the possibility his clothes might not fit him and he might have to buy new ones. States that he might not be great looking but that he is no idiot. This was expressed as a concern over a conversation he had had with his doctor.

Ability to Relate to Others
Family.   Receives many phone calls from his brothers and sisters. He is always joking with them

and seems to get along well with them. Says they were a close family growing up. Says his children call him "a lot and want me to go home." Was grimacing and shook head "no" at this point. The children's mother visits him, and he says they argue from the time she comes until she leaves.

Other Patients. Interacts with most of the individuals on the unit. Walks around the floor occasionally. Even though his roommate speaks French, he interprets what he needs and helps him when he can. States, "Being hospitalized is like my second home."

Health Team Members. Well-liked by staff; jokes and flirts around with all of them. Impression: flirting reaction to threats to body image.

Physical Assessment

General Appearance
Male in early thirties, in no acute distress. Medium body build, evenly proportioned. Well nourished.

Height. 5 feet, eleven inches.

Weight. 160 pounds on admission 4 weeks ago. Now 166 pounds.

Skin. Dry, intact except for ulcerated area on left ankle; mobile, returns to place immediately.

Hair. Even distribution over body, thick, shiny curly hair on head.

Gait. Moves slowly, posture upright, movements coordinated. Ambulates with assistance; uses no supportive devices.

Equilibrium. Steady; assumes high Fowler's position when in bed.

Speech Pattern and Affect. See above.

No obvious breath or body odors.
Complains of abdominal "swelling," pain in joints and abdomen, shortness of breath on exertion, "sore" on left ankle, "swelling" of feet and legs. States, "I have sickle cell anemia."

Head and Neck
Hair. Thick, shiny, curly, evenly distributed.

Scalp. No scaliness, lumps or lesions.

Skull. No deformities, lumps, or tenderness.

Skin. Full beard pattern, chocolate colored, evenly pigmented.

Eyes. Pupils equal, reacting to light and accommodation; coordinated bilateral movements symmetrical. Sclera—jaundiced. Retina—red reflex present. Complains of "spots in front of my eyes." Can read print in newspaper unilaterally and bilaterally. Does not wear eyeglasses. Eyebrows—full hair distribution; eyelid—full eyelashes, no edema or lesions. Lacrimal gland—no swelling or signs of irritation. Cornea and lens—clear. Irises—symmetrical; even brown color.

Ears. Auricle—no deformities, tenderness, or lesions. Auditory acuity—midline lateralization; AC>BC (air conduction greater than bone conduction); hears full range of sounds.

Nose. No deformities, tenderness, lesions, or discharge.

Sinuses. No tenderness.

Buccal Mucosa. Intact, light pink in color, patchy pigmentation.

Gums. Moist, intact.

Teeth. Upper, left medial incisor missing; overbite of upper teeth.

Tongue. Symmetrical, mobile, no nodules, tenderness, or lesions.

Pharynx. Rises appropriately on testing.

Tonsils. Removed at age six.

Lymph Nodes. No tenderness or swelling.

Trachea. Midline; no difficulty swallowing.

Thyroid. Symmetrical; no swelling, nodules, or tenderness.

Neck Vessels. No distention; carotid-bilateral fullness; rate 76 at rest; no jugular distention on assuming sitting position.

Thorax and Lungs

Anterior – Posterior Diameter. Approx. 1:2.

Respiration Rate. Twenty per minute.

Rhythm. Shallow; uses neck and accessory muscles when experiencing pain.

Chest Expansion. Limited when experiencing pain and on exertion.

Respiratory Excursion. Symmetrical, even, 3 cm.

Fremitus. Present.

No deformities, bulging of interspaces or retraction, nodules, or areas of tenderness.
No adventitious sounds.
Experiences dyspnea on exertion.

Heart

Murmurs, thrills. None heard.

Rate. 76 at rest.

Rhythm. Regular.
Cardiomegaly reported on x-ray examination.

Blood Pressure. 140/80.

Breasts and Axillae
No lumps, nodules, or tenderness; symmetrical.

Abdomen
Protuberant, distended, symmetrical; umbilicus slightly protruded. No masses; old scar on RUQ from gall bladder surgery. Limited abdominal respiratory actions. Frequent gurgling sound in bowel.

Liver. Enlarged, 14 cm from midclavicular line, tender.

Abdomen. Tympanitic, tender in RUQ.

Spleen. Enlarged, slightly palpable.

Kidneys. Not palpable, no tenderness.

Genitalia
Penis. No lesions or nodules.

Scrotum. No swelling or nodules.

Testes. Symmetrical; no tenderness or nodules; no hernias noted.

Anus and Rectum. No lesions, lumps, tenderness; prostate not enlarged, smooth, movable.

Peripheral Vascular System
Arms. Symmetrical, no distended vessels, no edema. Left radial pulse, 76; right radial pulse, 76.

Nails. Smooth, clean, trimmed, very white nail beds.

Legs. 1+ bilateral edema of feet and ankles; no varicosities; crusty, red ulceration 5 cm in diameter on left malleolus. Left posterior tibial pulse—slightly diminished. Left foot has purplish undertones; left ankle mottled.

Musculoskeletal System
Equal strength in limbs: 3.5, between fair and good on Lovett scale; has full ROM in all joints but resists movements because of joint pain. Limited exercise tolerance.

Knees. Tender, swollen, slightly warm to touch.

Ankles. Tender, swollen.

Neurologic System
Mental Status and Speech Pattern. See foregoing.

Cranial Nerve Function. Intact.

Motor System. Coordinated, steady, slow movements.

Reflexes. 2+.

Sensations. Symmetrical, intact.

State of Rest and Comfort
Ability to Sleep. Character of sleep—Intermittent.

Quantity of Sleep. Six to eight hours per night; day—rarely any.

Presence of Pain. States, "It's always there in different degrees." Receives pain medication every 2 hours. States, "Sometimes you know when a crisis is coming on and sometimes you don't. Anything can precipitate it, especially stress." Often walks around holding stomach and grimacing. Requests for pain medication have increased over time. States, "Injections don't last as long as they used to." Duration of pain is variable; attempts to control it with rest, medication. When it becomes severe and uncontrollable, he has to be hospitalized. Presently has pain mostly in joints and in abdomen. Joint pain limits his motion; abdominal pain limits chest expansion.

Response to Environment. Orderly room; does not feel strange or unfamiliar in surroundings. Impression: reaction to repeated hospitalizations.

Daily Eating Habits. Time and amounts—states he hasn't a good appetite since hospitalized. Also is a "finicky" eater. He mostly enjoys sweets, dislikes all vegetables except spinach, peas, and carrots. Dislikes roast beef. Never eats breakfast at home. "Usually pick here and there." Always leaves some food on tray but takes dessert and saves it. Does not have knowledge concerning basic four or relationship between food intake and body requirements.

Eating Habits. Self-feeding, no difficulty in mastication or swallowing. Has decreased salivation. States "always thirsty." Impression: related to diuretic therapy.

Elimination
Urination. Bathroom privileges without assistance. No bedpan, urinal, indwelling catheter, or incontinence. No pain or difficulty in voiding.

States he drinks and drinks as hydration is necessary to dilute blood so it doesn't sickle and pool, yet he doesn't urinate that often.

Defecation. Normal, no incontinence.

Previous Bowel Habits. Unchanged when hospitalized. Has bowel movement every other day.

Physician's Diagnosis and Orders

Diagnosis. Sickle cell anemia.
[Although a description of pathology is not given in assessment, one is included here to assist the student. Sickle cell anemia is a genetic hemolytic anemia which results in a malformation of the hemoglobin

molecule when subjected to decreased blood oxygen levels. Lowered oxygen levels may be caused by stressors such as anxiety, physical activity, environmental temperature extremes, and infections. Sickle cell anemia is found predominantely in blacks.

The symptoms which result are secondary to the hemolysis of red blood cells and the subsequent clumping of these cells. Symptoms include anemia; jaundice, particularly in the sclera; bone enlargement (as a result of bone marrow hypertrophy); severe joint swelling and pain; tachycardia; cardiomegaly; cardiac arrhythmia; heart failure; infarctions of vital organs; and susceptibility to infections.

Treatment is geared toward relief of symptoms and includes oxygen therapy to increase oxygen levels, bed rest to decrease oxygen needs, narcotics for the relief of pain, increased fluids to decrease blood viscosity, blood transfusions, and modification of life style to decrease the risk of crises. See a medical–surgical text for detailed description of pathology and treatment.]

Diet. Regular, force fluids.

Activity. OOB, no strenuous exercise.

Medications. Demerol, 125 mg, q2h IM p.r.n.
Digoxin, 0.25 mg, p.o.q.d.
Lasix, 80 mg, p.o. q.d.
Folic acid, 1 mg, p.o. t.i.d.
Aldactone, 25 mg, p.o. b.i.d.
Tetracycline, 500 mg, p.o. b.i.d.

Special Treatments
Nasal O_2 5–8 liters p.r.n. via mask.
Wash ulcer on left ankle b.i.d. with H_2O_2 and coat with Betadine solution. Apply dry sterile dressing (DSD).
Keep legs elevated when not ambulating.
TPR, blood pressure q6h.
Force fluids.

Significant Laboratory Data
Three transfusions (0 Rh+) given previously (no adverse reactions).

Hgb. 8 g.

Hct. 28%.

Urinalysis. Many bacteria present, primarily enterococcus.

Culture of Leg Ulcer. Moderate amounts of Staphylococcus aureus.

X-ray Examination. Abdomen—Mild gaseous distention of numerous large and small bowel loops, no suggestion of obstruction. May have distended urinary bladder. Pelvic mass should not be ruled out.

Lumbosacral spine—Bones mildly demineralized.

Chest—Bone changes compatible with sickle cell anemia. Heart shows cardiomegaly, pulmonary markings prominent, minimal atelectasis.

Liver—Enlarged, changes compatible with sickle cell anemia.

NURSING DIAGNOSIS: 7/13

Actual Nursing Diagnoses

1 Pain in joints related to clumping of hemolysed cells.
2 Abdominal pain related to gaseous distention and decreased blood flow through peritoneal organs.
3 Dyspnea on exertion related to decreased oxygen tension.

4 Ulcer on left malleolus related to decreased blood flow to area.
5 Edema of lower extremities related to venous stasis.
6 Threat to positive body image related to physical changes and dependence.
7 Anxiety related to fear of limited life expectancy.
8 Unbalanced diet and fluid intake related to nutritional habits.

Foreseeable Nursing Diagnoses

9 Precipitation of sickle cell crisis related to physical and psychologic stressors.
10 Urinary tract infection related to presence of bacteria in urine and lowered hemoglobin levels.
11 Fluid and electrolye imbalance related to depletion of fluid and potassium resulting from diuretic therapy and nutritional habits.

Possible Nursing Diagnoses

12 Drug dependency related to frequent long-term administration of narcotics.

Planning 7/13
Goals*

IMMEDIATE GOALS	INTERMEDIATE GOALS	LONG RANGE GOALS
ACTUAL		
1. a. Decrease joint size within 1 week.	Maintain reduced joint size for hospital stay.	Decrease recurrence of joint swelling.
b. Decrease subjective feeling of joint pain on movement within 2 days.	Increase subjective feeling of well-being during hospital stay.	Maintain subjective feeling of well-being.
c. Decrease requests for medication for pain in joints within 2 days.	Maintain reduced pain level for hospital stay.	Decrease recurrence of pain.
2. a. Decrease abdominal girth within 1 week.	Continue decrease in abdominal girth for hospital stay.	Maintain expected abdominal girth size.
b. Decrease bowel sounds within 1 week.	Maintain expected bowel sounds.	Maintain expected bowel sounds.

*Numbers refer to the corresponding nursing diagnosis.

(continued)

IMMEDIATE GOALS	INTERMEDIATE GOALS	LONG RANGE GOALS
c. Decrease tenderness of RUQ within 1 week.	Absence of tenderness of RUQ during hospital stay.	Maintain absence of tenderness of RUQ.
d. Increase subjective feelings of well-being within 1 week.	Maintain subjective feelings of well-being during hospital stay.	Maintain subjective feelings of well-being.
e. Decrease requests for medication for abdominal pain within 1 week.	Maintain reduced abdominal pain level for hospital stay.	Decrease recurrence of abdominal pain.
3. a. Walk full length of corridor without changes in respiratory rate or rhythm or changes in heart rate within 1 week.	Walk full length of corridor 3 times a day without changes in respiratory rate or rhythm or changes in heart rate within 2 weeks.	Resume activities of daily living.
b. Decrease subjective feelings of SOB within 1 week.	Maintain decreased subjective feelings of SOB during hospital stay.	Maintain decreased subjective feelings of SOB.
c. Decrease number of requests for O_2 within 1 week.	Continue reduction of requests for O_2 during hospital stay.	Eliminate need for supplemental O_2.
4. a. Decrease size of ulcer within 5 days.	Absence of ulcer within 2 weeks.	Prevent recurrence of ulcer.
b. Prevent further skin breakdown in legs and ankles.	Prevent further skin breakdown in legs and ankles.	Prevent further skin breakdown in legs and ankles.
5. a. Decrease edema of legs within 3 days.	Absence of edema within 2 weeks.	Prevent recurrence of leg edema.
b. Decrease mottling of legs within 4 days.	Absence of mottling within 2 weeks.	Prevent recurrence of mottling of legs.
c. Decrease subjective feeling of swelling of ankles and feet within 3 days.	Continue increase in subjective feeling of swelling of ankles and feet during hospital stay.	Absence of subjective feeling of swelling in ankles and feet.
6. Decrease number of self-deprecatory remarks concerning appearance within 1 week.	Makes positive comments concerning appearance within 2 weeks.	Maintain positive attitude toward appearance.
7. Within 3 days expresses feelings about threat of death.	Increase in number of long-term life goals.	Increase in future orientation of life goals.
8. a. Decrease in subjective feelings of thirst within 3 days.	Continue decrease in subjective feelings of thirst during hospital stay.	No unexpected feelings of thirst.
b. State the basic 4 food groups within 3 days.	Plans balanced menu for 1 day of meals within 1 week.	Plans daily balanced meals.
c. Explain relationship between food intake and body needs within 1 week.	Increases intake of basic 4 foods within 1 week.	Increases daily intake of basic 4 foods.

Planning 7/13 (Cont.)
Goals

IMMEDIATE GOALS	INTERMEDIATE GOALS	LONG RANGE GOALS
FORESEEABLE GOALS		
9. State relationship between stress and sickle cell crisis within 3 days.	State modifications in daily living to reduce physical and psychologic stress within 1 week.	Devise plan balancing rest and activity in ADL within 2 weeks.
10. a. No symptoms of frequency, urgency, or dysuria.	No symptoms of frequency, urgency, or dysuria during hospital stay.	No symptoms of frequency, urgency, or dysuria.
b. Negative urine culture within 2 weeks.	Maintain negative urine culture during hospital stay.	Maintain negative urine culture.
11. a. Maintain balance between fluid intake and fluid output.	Maintain balance between fluid intake and fluid output.	Maintain balance between fluid intake and fluid output.
b. Maintain expected potassium levels.	Maintain expected potassium levels.	Maintain expected potassium levels.
POSSIBLE GOALS		
12. a. Decrease requests for narcotics consistent with increased subjective feelings of well-being within 2 weeks.	Continue decrease in requests for narcotics consistent with increased subjective feelings of well-being during hospital stay.	Freedom from narcotics.
b. Increase knowledge of implications of drug dependency within 1 week.	Continue increase in knowledge of implications of drug dependency during hospital stay.	Freedom from narcotics.
c. Increase knowledge of alternative methods of pain relief within 2 weeks.	Use of alternative methods for pain relief during hospital stay.	Freedom from narcotics.

Planning 7/13
Plan

PLAN FOR IMMEDIATE GOAL: 1C	RATIONALE FOR NURSING ACTION
Explain relationship between fluid intake and joint pain.	Increases cooperation. Gives individual options. Understanding of relationships increases change in long-term behavior.
Ascertain fluid preferences.	Matching plan with individual preferences increases compliance.

(continued)

Planning 7/13 (Cont.)
Plan

PLAN FOR IMMEDIATE GOAL: 1C	RATIONALE FOR NURSING ACTION
Offer 6 oz. of fluids of choice especially juices with potassium every hour from 7 AM to 11 PM and record.	By increasing availability of fluid, intake increases. Frequent contact with staff increases feelings of self-worth. Increased fluid intake reduces clumping of RBCs and counterbalances potassium depletion by diuretics. Written record available for comparison with output. Verifies plan carried out. Outline of times insures spacing of fluid throughout day and prevents interruption of sleep.
Encourage to drink fluids on tray.	Supplements fluid intake.
Teach to record own intake and output.	Increases feelings of independence adds to feelings of self-worth.
Ascertain meaning of rest for individual and what activities he considers restful.	Matching plan with individual preferences increases compliance. Helps individual to begin to identify restful ADL.
Explain relationship between rest and decrease in joint pain.	Increases cooperation. Increases understanding of need for long-term modification of behavior.
Devise plan with individual to rest in bed with feet elevated for 1 hour out of every 4.	Incorporates individual's preferences. Collaborative efforts increase feelings of control over situation. Increases compliance. Prevents nurse from imposing own will. Elevation of feet assists venous return.
Record results and reactions.	Provides record for comparison and modification of plan.
Measure ankle and knee joint girth 8 AM and 8 PM.	Provides basis of comparison, evaluates effectiveness of plan.
Teach purposes and procedures of leg elevation.	Increases knowledge base, increases compliance.
Determine preferences of methods for elevating legs and plan.	Increases compliance.
Suggest sitting location that has maximal stimulation.	Decreases feelings of isolation.
Teach precautions for leg elevation —pressure on popliteal and inguinal nerves and vessels —prevention of circulatory overload.	Prevents complications of therapy. Increases knowledge base.
Check q1h for follow-through when sitting up or lying in bed.	Reinforces importance of procedure. Allows for modification of method. Increased contact increases feelings of self-worth.

(continued)

Planning 7/13 (Cont.)
Plan

PLAN FOR IMMEDIATE GOAL: 1C	RATIONALE FOR NURSING ACTION
Place call bell, fluids, and desired personal items within reach.	Prevents interruption of therapy.
Determine reactions to therapy.	Provides input from individual for evaluating effectiveness of therapy. Allows for modification of therapy according to individual's needs. Recognizes importance of input.
Explain procedures, purposes, and precautions of antiembolic stockings.	Increases compliance.
Apply antiembolic stockings before rising in AM and remove at night.	Applying before rising prevents venous stasis. Removal at night prevents skin breakdown.
Check q4h for signs of circulatory embarrassment.	Prevents complications of therapy.
Explain purposes, procedures, and precautions of active ROM of extremities.	Increases compliance. Gives individual options. Understanding of relationships increases change in long-term behavior.
Devise plan with individual to carry out active ROM at least q2h when awake.	Increases compliance. Collaborative efforts increase feelings of control over situation, prevents nurse from imposing own will, incorporates individual's preferences.
Record reactions to therapy.	Written record available for comparison, verifies plan carried out.
Devise plan with individual for diversionary activities.	Increases compliance. Increases feelings of control over situation. Prevents nurse from imposing own will. Diversionary activities help take mind off pain if actively meaningful to individual. Incorporates individual's preferences.
Consult with occupational therapist.	Utilizes expertise of other professionals.
Consult with family to supply necessary equipment.	Provides needed supplies, incorporates family.
Introduce to other individuals on unit with similar interests.	Increases socialization.
Discuss meaning of pain to individual.	Allows for ventilation of feelings.
Discuss precipitating factors and means of alleviating pain.	Increases nurse's data base and helps individual to make associations between activities and pain.
Devise plan with individual to incorporate his methods of alleviating pain into plan.	Decreases pain. Increases control over situation. Increases compliance. Prevents nurse from imposing own will. Incorporates individual's preferences.

(continued)

Planning 7/13 (Cont.)
Plan

PLAN FOR IMMEDIATE GOAL: 1C	RATIONALE FOR NURSING ACTION
Discuss relaxation techniques with individual: —meditation —yoga —displacement of pain —attitude change toward pain.	Increased use of relaxation methods aids in decreasing pain.
Devise plan with individual for using alternate methods of pain relief.	Increases control over situation. Increases compliance. Prevents nurse from imposing own will. Incorporates individual's preferences.
Administer Demerol q2h when alternative methods for pain relief are not effective.	Helps prevent reliance on medication. Reduces pain.
Administer Lasix 80 mg, q.d. at 10 AM and Aldactone 25 mg at 7 AM and 7 PM.	Promotes diuresis.

INTERVENTION: 7/15

This phase is illustrated by the nurse's notes written two days after the initial assessment.

7:00 AM   Found awake lying in bed. States he slept "pretty well through the night. I only needed pain medication twice." Aldactone 25 mg, p.o., given. Skin on ankles and feet still mottled from dorsum of foot to 7.5 cm above malleolus. Decubitus ulcer remains 5 cm in diameter, scab intact, color red. Washed with H_2O_2; Betadine and dry sterile dressings applied. Antiembolic stockings applied from ankles to midcalf. Orange juice, 6 oz., taken. Assisted OOB to chair. Legs elevated on footstool. Explanation of antiembolic stockings and leg elevation reinforced. States, "It's more comfortable now that I'm using the footstool."

8:00 AM   Breakfast of 6 oz. prune juice, one slice buttered toast, and 8 oz. coffee with sugar and cream taken. Assisted to record intake sheet. States, "This is easy, just like a balance sheet in accounting." Legs not elevated at this time. States, "Who can eat with feet up in the air." No c/o joint pain. Ankle girth: 34 cm; knee girth: 47 cm.

9:00 AM   Refusing any fluids. States, "Next thing you know I'll be floating away." Rationale for forcing fluids repeated. Only shook head and smiled in response. No tingling, redness, or numbness distal to antiembolic stockings. Toes warm to touch bilaterally.

10:00 AM   Lasix, 80 mg, p.o., given. Ginger ale, 3 oz., taken. c/o "achy feeling in ankles and knees." Sat with him while he put feet, ankles, and legs through full ROM. States activity "helps some." Art supplies set out at his request.

11:00 AM   Orange juice, 6 oz., taken. States he would like to visit man next door, "but my ugly legs won't hold me." Swelling acknowledged, plan to reduce swelling discussed. Requested pain medication but decided to defer it until he tried deep breathing relaxation exercises. Assisted to bed with feet elevated. Refused to do ROM.

11:15 AM   Requesting pain medication. States, "Those stupid exercises don't work."

11:20 AM   Demerol, 125 mg, IM, given. Lights dimmed.

11:45 AM   Sleeping, as evidenced by breathing pattern.

12:00 noon   Still sleeping.

12:45 PM   Awake. Assisted out of bed to chair. Would not elevate legs until after lunch. Ate Salisbury steak, boiled potato, 8 oz. milk, 8 oz. tea, one serving ice cream. Refused vegetables. Stated, "Even though I know I should, I can't force myself to eat those things." Needed reminding to chart intake. Antiembolic stockings adjusted; no tingling, redness, or numbness distal to stockings; toes warm bilaterally. States joint pain back to "its usual dull ache."

2:00 PM   Orange juice, 8 oz., taken. Reviewed food components of basic four. He made lists of food likes and dislikes from each group. Assisted to practice breathing relaxation exercises. Legs elevated; full ROM to feet and legs.

2:30 PM   Visited by occupational therapist. Called to bring in sketching pad.

3:00 PM   Water, 6 oz., taken; c/o sharp pain in knees; requesting medication. Refuses alternate pain relief methods; assisted to bed with legs elevated.

3:05 PM   Demerol, 125 mg, IM, given. Requested radio music and to be "left alone for a couple of hours."

5:00 PM   Stated, "Why didn't anyone bring me my 4 o'clock juice?" Explored feelings concerning contradictory statements; states, "You should know me well enough by now to know I don't always mean what I say." Ambulated around room; left sitting in chair with legs elevated talking with roommate.

6:00 PM   Antiembolic stockings adjusted; no numbness, redness, or tingling noted; toes warm bilaterally. Dinner of 4 oz. orange juice, breast of chicken, french fried potatoes, strawberry shortcake, 8 oz. coffee with cream and sugar; still refusing vegetables. C/o moderate pain in knees and ankles. States, "I can stand it for a while." While reviewing plan for relief of joint pain stated, "What's the use of planning, I'm going to die anyway." Discussed feelings about dying, plan for relief of joint pain.

7:00 PM   Six oz. orange juice taken with Aldactone, 25 mg, p.o. Stated, "I spend more time in the bathroom than anyplace else." Reviewed rationale for diuretic therapy. Left writing in book.

8:00 PM   Four oz. water taken. Assisted to bed, legs elevated; requesting medication of pain in knees. Stated, "I already tried those relaxation exercises. I want my Demerol." Ankle girth: 35 cm; knee girth: 47.5 cm.

8:05 PM   Demerol, 125 mg, IM, given; back rub given; left watching TV in bed with legs elevated.

9:00 PM   Six oz. ginger ale taken. Stated, "I don't feel too badly now."

10:00 PM   Antiembolic stockings removed. Skin mottling from dorsum of foot to 5 cm above malleolus; informed of decrease in mottling; ulcer remains 5 cm in diameter. Washed with H_2O_2; Betadine and dressing applied. Six oz. orange juice taken. Left watching TV.

11:00 PM   Six oz. water taken; requesting pain medication. States, "I can't get to sleep without it."

Back rub given. Sat with him while practiced breathing exercises; still requesting pain medication.

11:05 PM   Demerol, 125 mg, IM, given. Lights turned out. Stated, "I'll try to sleep now."

3:30 AM   Awake, up to bathroom, requesting water and pain medication. Back rub given. Assisted with full ROM to feet and legs.

3:45 AM   Sleeping as evidenced by breathing pattern and relaxed body state.

EVALUATION: 7/16

This phase is illustrated by a summary note for goal 1 written on the day projected for evaluation.

No longer requesting pain medication q2h. Delaying injections without apparent severe discomfort. No medications needed from 11 AM to 7 PM. Nursing interventions of exercises effective at times. No effects seen as yet with breathing relaxation exercises. To continue with breathing relaxation exercises and explore other alternatives, e.g., pain deferrment areas. Consult with M.D. re: decrease in dosage. Continue nursing actions for relief of pain.

Appears to understand relationship between fluid intake and joint pain; can list basic principles of it. Requests fluids when schedule is not kept. Follows fluid schedule most of time. Potassium levels remain at expected values. Intake and output balanced; knows how to chart own intake and output, but still needs reminding at times. Drinking all fluids on meal tray. Complaints of thirst decreased. Plan: decrease hourly fluid to 5 ounces; ask family to bring in ginger beer.

No success in ascertaining meaning of rest for individual. Seek additional data from family, observe behavior patterns more closely to determine restful activities. Plan devised with individual for rest periods of staying up 3 hours and resting in bed 1 hour; however, resists plan at times stating, "I'm not a baby." Review plan with individual for possible modifications, reexplore feelings about rest and activity with individual.

No decrease in knee and ankle girth but mottling on ankles decreased 2.5 cm. Continue with leg elevation plan and rest and fluid plans with above modifications.

NURSING HISTORY FORM*

Name   Age

Occupation   Marital status

Religion   Sex

Address

Number of admissions/visits to agency
 Reasons

Perceptions of illness

Expectations of health care

Present concerns

Social history
 Position in family
 Family interactions/roles
 Significant others
 Significant others' interactions/roles
 Community/social interactions

Educational level

Usual transportation pattern

Housing

Habits/patterns of activities of daily living
 Nutrition
 Elimination
 Sleep
 Drugs
 Others
Preferences

Hobbies

Cognitive status
 Level of consciousness
 Orientation
 Intellectual ability
 Attention span

Vocabulary
 Words used to describe ADL
 General word usage

Ability to make relationships

Ability to learn

Emotional status
 Affect
 Level of anxiety
 Coping mechanisms

Body image

Sexuality

Level of growth and development

Ability to relate to others

Physical assessment†

Medical diagnosis

Medical plan/orders

Diagnostic tests

Understanding of medical diagnosis, orders, plan

Deficits in knowledge

---

*The following assessment was used for the basic nursing assessment of this individual.
†This format follows that of Barbara Bates in *A Guide to Physical Examination*. Philadelphia, Lippincott, 1974.

APPENDIX A: EXAMPLES OF THERAPEUTIC DIETS

BLAND ULCER DIET PLAN

For _____ Date _____

GENERAL INSTRUCTIONS

The bland diet is a flexible diet which can be adjusted to your food likes and dislikes. Its principles are:
- Eat slowly and chew well.
- Eat meals at the same hour each day.
- Eat small meals at frequent intervals, never skip meals.
- If possible, relax a few minutes before and after each meal.
- Eat protein-rich foods because they buffer stomach acid. Milk and Carnation Instant Breakfast are excellent sources, along with meats, fish, poultry, eggs, cheese and peanut butter.
- Avoid all foods with rough skins, seeds or rough fiber. Avoid fried or highly seasoned foods, black pepper, chili powder, cloves, mustard seed, nutmeg, caffeine, cocoa, coffee, tea,

and alcohol. Other spices, seasonings, and beverages may be tried in moderate amounts.
- Avoid extremely hot or cold foods.
- Include a citrus juice or fruit daily for Vitamin C, but be sure to sip juices throughout the meal so that they are well mixed with other foods.
- Choose a good source of Vitamin A every other day. These are dark green or yellow fruits and vegetables.
- If your normal activities are restricted or limited due to existing conditions, it may be desirable to lower caloric intake initially and increase intake gradually as conditions and activity improve. Body weight should be monitored on a regular basis.

Basic Meal Plan	Sample Menu	Calories	Special Instructions
BREAKFAST	**BREAKFAST**		**Adjustment to Sample Menu**
1 serving fruit	½ grapefruit	40	(use milk beverage as checked below)
1 serving eggs	1 poached egg	72	1. ☐ Use*CIB prepared with Whole Milk.
1 serving bread	1 slice white toast	63	2. ☐ Use Whole Milk only.
1 serving fat	1 tsp. margarine	34	3. ☐ Use Carnation Instant Nonfat Milk only.
1 serving sweets	½ Tbsp. jelly	24	
1 serving milk beverage	*CIB mixed with 8 oz. Nonfat milk or see special instructions	210	
Beverage (optional)	Decaffeinated coffee	2	
MID-MORNING	**MID-MORNING**		
1 small serving bread	1 (whole) graham cracker	55	
1 small serving meat or substitute	1 Tbsp. peanut butter	186	
1 serving milk beverage	1 cup Carnation Instant Nonfat Milk	80	
NOON MEAL	**NOON MEAL**		
1 serving cheese	½ cup creamed cottage cheese	111	
1 small serving fruit or vegetable	¼ cup canned cherries packed in water	32	
1 small serving bread	2 saltine crackers	24	
1 serving soup	1 cup cream of chicken soup (made with milk)	179	
½ serving milk beverage	½ cup Carnation Instant Milk	40	
MID-AFTERNOON	**MID-AFTERNOON**		
1 small serving dessert	½ cup pudding made with milk, cooked	170	
½ serving milk beverage	½ cup Carnation Instant Nonfat Milk	40	
EVENING MEAL	**EVENING MEAL**		
1 small serving meat or substitute	3 oz. broiled steak	176	
½ small serving potato, rice, or noodles	½ cup mashed potatoes (made with milk)	68	
2 servings fat	2 tsp. margarine	68	
2 small servings vegetables	¼ cup cooked carrots	11	
	¼ cup cooked green beans	8	
Beverage (optional)	Decaffeinated coffee	2	
1 small serving dessert (optional)	1 small fruited gelatin salad	80	
BEDTIME	**BEDTIME**		
1 serving milk beverage	*CIB mixed with 8 oz. nonfat milk or see special instructions	210	
1 serving cheese	1 slice cheddar cheese	96	
1 small serving bread	4 saltine crackers	48	By _____

*Carnation Instant Breakfast. You may use any flavor   Total: 2129

	FOODS PERMITTED	**FOODS TO OMIT**
MILK	Whole Milk, Carnation Instant Nonfat Milk, Carnation Evaporated Milk, Carnation Instant Malted Milk, Half and Half, Buttermilk, and Carnation Instant Breakfast.	None
EGGS	Poached, scrambled, soft or hard cooked, baked, creamed, plain omelet or souffle.	Fried
CHEESE	Plain, mild-flavored, such as American, cottage, cream.	Cheese with added spices, nuts, or relishes
MEATS	Very tender beef, veal, lamb, fresh pork, liver, poultry or fish which has been broiled, roasted, boiled or steamed. Crisp bacon.	Bologna, luncheon meat, sausage, frankfurters, ham and all pickled, salted and smoked meats. Rich gravies and sauces. Fatty meats and all fried meats, fried fowl or fried fish.
VEGETABLES	Cooked tender asparagus tips, beets, carrots, green or waxed beans, mushrooms, pumpkin, green peas, white or sweet potato, spinach, summer or winter squashes. Vegetables may be creamed, escalloped, or served in cream soups or gelatin salads. Mild-flavored vegetable juices.	All raw vegetables. Skins of potato. All other cooked vegetables not listed in "Foods Permitted." Avoid gas forming vegetables such as cabbage, broccoli, cauliflower, brussels sprouts, garlic, onion, dried beans, or peas. Pickles and olives. Pickled vegetables.
FRUITS	Canned or cooked applesauce, cherries, peeled apricots, peaches or pears. Baked apple without skin. Fresh ripe banana and avocado. All fruit juices. Other pureed fruits.	All other fruits except those listed in "Foods Permitted." Avoid figs, raisins, pineapple, berries, melon, fruits with coarse skins or seeds. Spiced or pickled fruits.
SOUPS	Cream soups made with foods permitted. Oyster stew.	Broth, bouillon, consomme, commercial creamed soups which are highly seasoned. Any soup with a meat broth base.
BREADS & CEREALS	Plain white and wheat bread. Refined cooked cereals such as cream of wheat, cream of rice, farina, oatmeal; refined dry cereals such as puffed wheat, cornflakes. Crisp waffles. Spaghetti, rice, noodles, macaroni. Saltine, graham, soda or plain crackers.	Whole grain cereals, breads and crackers. Pancakes and hot breads. Omit breads and cereals with seeds, nuts or raisins.
DESSERTS	Jello, gelatine, custard, plain pudding. Plain cake, cookies, pound cake, sponge cake, angel food cake, ice cream, sherbet.	All rich foods as pies, pastries, candies, chocolate, any with fruits not recommended, coconut or nuts.
SWEETS	Jelly, sugar, syrup, honey, marshmallows and molasses. Gum drops and fruit flavored hard candy.	Chewing gum, chocoaltes, candy made with fruit not recommended, coconut or nuts. Jam.
FATS	Butter, margarine, mayonnaise, mild salad dressings, salad oil, cream, and smooth peanut butter.	Spicy seasoned dressings, nuts, rich gravies and sauces, crunchy peanut butter.
BEVERAGES	Any noncarbonated, nonalcoholic. Coffee substitute, decaffeinated coffee, postum.	Coffee, tea, alcoholic and carbonated beverages (unless approved by physician).
SPICES	Cinnamon, salt, sugar, mace, parsley and paprika. Flavorings and extracts.	All other spices.

CHOLESTEROL CONTROL DIET PLAN for Normal Weight Patients

For _____ Date _____

GENERAL INSTRUCTIONS

Eat regularly as indicated on your sample menu. Servings of margarine and oils, breads and cereals, fruits or vegetables may be added or substracted from the diet plan to adjust the calorie intake.

Choose fish, poultry, and other protein foods in List II (on back) often. Eat less beef, lamb, pork, regular cheese, and other foods in List IV which are extremely high in cholesterol. Limit meat, fish, or poultry servings to 6 oz. per day, as indicated in your Basic Meal Plan.

Prepare foods with corn, cottonseed, soybean, or safflower oil and choose margarines which are polyunsaturated.

Choose a good source of Vitamin C daily. They are citrus fruits, strawberries, broccoli, brussels sprouts, papaya, and cantaloupe. Choose a good source of Vitamin A every other day. These are dark green or yellow fruits and vegetables.

Basic Meal Plan See substitution lists on back for other allowable foods.	Sample Menu	Calories	Chol. Mg.	Special Instructions
BREAKFAST	**BREAKFAST**			
1 serving fruit or juice	1 grapefruit half	40		
1 serving cereal with	1 cup enriched shredded oat cereal	171		
½ cup nonfat milk	½ cup Carnation Instant Nonfat Milk	40	2.5	
2 servings bread	2 slices white toast	124		
*2 servings margarine	2 tsp. margarine	68		
1 serving sweets	1 Tbsp. jam	54		
Beverage	Coffee without cream	2		
NOON MEAL	**NOON MEAL**			
1 serving cooked vegetable	1 cup vegetable soup	78		
1 serving bread or crackers	4 saltine crackers	47		
1 serving fish or poultry	3 oz. roast turkey, white meat	150	65.5	
2 servings bread	2 slices white bread	124		
*2 servings margarine	2 tsp. margarine	68		
1 serving raw vegetable	3 carrot & 3 celery sticks	19		
1 serving fruit	1 medium apple	87		
1 serving nonfat milk	1 cup Carnation Instant Nonfat Milk	80	5	
Beverage	Tea or coffee without cream	2		
EVENING MEAL	**EVENING MEAL**			
1 serving meat, fish, fowl	3 oz. broiled halibut	154	54	
1 serving starchy vegetable	1 baked potato	188		
1 serving bread	1 slice French bread	43		
*3 servings margarine	3 tsp. margarine	102		
1 serving cooked vegetable	½ cup green beans	17		
2 servings raw vegetables	Large lettuce & tomato salad	23		
2 servings salad dressing	2 Tbsp. Italian dressing	166		
1 serving dessert	½ cup orange sherbet	129		
1 serving nonfat milk	1 cup Carnation Instant Nonfat Milk	80	5	
Beverage	Tea or coffee without cream	2		
BEDTIME	**BEDTIME**			
1 serving Carnation Instant Breakfast with	8 oz. Carnation Instant Breakfast with	130		
nonfat milk	8 oz. nonfat milk	80	5	
1 serving bread or crackers	2 graham crackers	55		By _____

*Use only a polyunsaturated margarine such as Fleischmann's   Total: 2323   142 mg.

SUBSTITUTION LISTS

LIST I — Foods of plant origin contain no cholesterol. These are fruits, vegetables, cereals, grains, nuts, and vegetable oils. However, choosing liquid or unsaturated vegetable oils, rather than "hydrogenated" (solid) vegetable oil products is sometimes recommended as these oils may have a cholesterol-lowering effect. Exceptions to this rule are coconut and olive oil.

LIST II — These animal-origin foods are low in cholesterol:

	Chol. mg.		Chol. mg.		Chol. mg.
3 oz cottage cheese	8	3 oz haddock	51	1 cup nonfat milk	5
3 oz chicken, white	67	3 oz halibut	51	1 cup buttermilk	5
3 oz cod	48	3 oz salmon	40	1 cup yogurt (low fat)	17
3 oz (bass, whiting, carp, sole, pollack, pike, perch)	50-70	3 oz trout	47	Egg white	0
		3 oz tuna	55	¼ cup egg substitute (such as Fleischmann's "Egg Beaters" which contains less than 1 mg. chol. and approx. 100 calories)	
3 oz flounder	43	3 oz turkey, white	65		

LIST III — These animal-origin foods are higher in cholesterol, but may still have a cholesterol-lowering effect because of their unsaturated or low-total fat content.

	Chol. mg.		Chol. mg.		Chol. mg.
3 oz chicken, dark	77	3 oz herring	82	3 oz turkey, dark	86
3 oz crab	85	3 oz lobster	72		

LIST IV — These animal-origin foods are high in cholesterol or may have a cholesterol-raising effect. They should be limited.

	Chol. mg.		Chol. mg.		Chol. mg.
3 oz beef	80	3 oz lamb	83	3 oz cheese, cheddar	84
3 oz brains	1,700	3 oz liver	372	3 oz cheese, Swiss	85
3 oz chicken gizzards	166	3 oz pork	76	3 oz cheese, American	77
3 oz heart	233	3 oz sardines	119	*3 oz clams	43
3 oz kidneys	683	3 oz sausage	53	*3 oz oysters	43
3 oz sweetbread	396	3 oz shrimp	128	*3 oz scallops	45
		3 oz veal	86		
1 cup milk, whole	34	1 Tbl. butter	35	1 Tbl. ½ & ½	6
1 egg (50 g), whole	252	1 Tbl. chicken fat	9	1 Tbl. sour cream	8
1 egg yolk (17 g)	252	1 Tbl. cream cheese	16	1 Tbl. whipping cream, unwhipped	20
		1 Tbl. lard	13		

LIST V — Cholesterol content of products which contain animal-origin foods.

	Chol. mg.		Chol. mg.		Chol. mg.
1 piece angel cake	0	1 muffin (40 g)	21	1 popover	59
1 piece yellow cake (75 g)	33	1 corn muffin (40 g)	28	1 waffle	119
1 piece sponge cake (66 g)	162	½ cup noodles	25	**1 Tbl. mayonnaise	10
1 cream puff (130 g)	188	⅛ apple pie	120		
½ cup custard	139	⅛ lemon pie	117		
½ cup ice cream (10% fat)	27	⅛ pumpkin pie	70		
½ cup ice milk	13	½ cup potato salad	81		
½ cup pudding (mix)	15	½ cup white sauce	17		

*Cholesterol accounts for only 30% of the total sterol in scallops and only 40% in oysters and clams. The other sterols in these shellfish require further study and may have nutritional significance.

**Imitation mayonnaise and mayonnaise made with safflower oil contain less cholesterol.

DIABETES MELLITUS DIET PLAN

For _____ Date _____

GENERAL INSTRUCTIONS

The principles of a diabetic diet are as follows: *Eat regularly* —do not omit a meal. Eat foods in the portion sizes indicated on your diet plan. Use the exchange list to add variety to your diet. *Work to attain and then maintain the optimal weight for your age, frame, and physical activity.* Follow a regular exercise program.

Choose a good source of Vitamin C daily and Vitamin A every other day. Good sources of Vitamin C are marked with (**), fair sources with (*) on the exchange list. Good sources of Vitamin A are dark green or yellow fruits and vegetables.

Broiling, roasting, boiling, or baking methods of preparation are preferable. Any fat used in preparation of food must be taken from the fat allowance of your meal plan. Meats should be weighed or measured after preparation.

Avoid concentrated sweets, pies, frosted cakes, pastry, rich desserts, sugar, honey, syrups, regular soft drinks and chewing gum, and sweetened condensed milk.

Real labels. "Dietetic" differs from "diabetic" in that dietetic may refer to food restrictions other than sugar-free. Diabetic does not mean you can consume the product in unlimited quantities.

Basic Meal Plan 1500 Calories	Sample Menu	Calorie Variations			
		1000 Calories	1200 Calories	1800 Calories	2400 Calories
BREAKFAST 1 fruit exchange (List 2) 1 meat exchange (List 4) 2 starch exchanges (List 3) 1 fat exchange (List 5) 1 milk exchange (List 6) free food list	**BREAKFAST** ½ cup orange juice 1 medium poached egg 1 slice whole wheat toast 2/3 cup enriched bran flakes 1 tsp. margarine 1 cup Carnation Instant Nonfat Milk 1 cup black coffee or tea	OMIT 1 starch exc. 1 fat exc.	OMIT 1 starch exc. 1 fat exc.	ADD 1 fat exc.	ADD 1 meat exc. (List 4) 1 starch exc. 2 fat exc.
NOON MEAL 2 meat exchanges (List 4) 2 starch exchanges (List 3) 3 fat exchanges (List 5) 1 vegetable exchange (List 1) free food list 1 fruit exchange (List 2) free food list	**NOON MEAL** 2 oz. cheddar cheese 2 slices white bread, grilled with 1 tsp. margarine (subtract 1 fat exch. per ounce of cheese consumed.) 1 cup fresh spinach salad 1 Tbsp. low calorie dressing ¾ cup strawberries 1 cup black coffee or tea	2 starch exc. 2 fat exc.	1 starch exc. 2 fat exc.	1 starch exc.	2 starch exc. 1 fat exc. 1 cup Carnation Instant Nonfat Milk (List 6)
EVENING MEAL free vegetable (List 1) free food list 4 meat exchanges (List 4A) free food list 2 starch exchanges (List 3) 1 vegetable exchange (List 1) 2 fat exchanges (List 5) 1 fruit exchange (List 2) free food list	**EVENING MEAL** 1 cup tossed lettuce salad 1 Tbsp. low calorie dressing 4 oz. broiled halibut with lemon wedge ½ cup steamed rice 1 hard roll ½ cup broccoli 2 tsp. margarine 1 small orange 1 cup black coffee or tea	1 meat exc. (List 4A) 1 starch exc. 1 fat exc.	1 meat exc. (List 4A) 1 fat exc.	1 starch exc. 1 fat exc. 1 cup Carnation Instant Nonfat Milk (List 6)	1 starch exc. 1 fat exc. 1 fruit exc. 1 cup Carnation Instant Nonfat Milk (List 6)
BEDTIME 1 milk exchange (List 6) 1 starch exchange (List 3)	**BEDTIME** 1 cup Carnation Instant Nonfat Milk 2 graham cracker squares	Follow 1500 Calorie Meal Plan at Bedtime			1 meat exc. (List 4) 1 fat exc. 1 starch exc.

SPECIAL INSTRUCTIONS: Please note the fat and calorie difference between meat exchanges 4 and 4A. When substituting these meats in your diet, remember to adjust your fat exchanges accordingly.

By _____

FREE FOODS—ALLOWED AS DESIRED—Negligible carbohydrate, protein, and fat.

Coffee	Gelatin, unsweetened	Diet salad dressings	Pepper	Artificially sweetened
Tea	Rennet tablets	(less than 2 calories/Tbsp.)	Herbs	beverages furnishing
Clear Broth	Cranberries	Mustard	Spices	less than 5 calories/cup
Bouillon	Lemon, Lime	Pickle, sour	Flavorings	
		Pickle, dill-unsweetened	Vinegar	

LIST 1 VEGETABLE EXCHANGES—Approximately 5 grams carbohydrate, 2 grams protein and 25 calories per cooked serving—½ cup, raw—1 cup.

Artichokes	Carrots	*Spinach, *Turnip	*Tomatoes
Asparagus	Cauliflower	Mushrooms	*Tomato or vegetable Juice (½ cup)
Bean sprouts	Celery	Okra	**FREE VEGETABLES**—The following raw vegetables
Beans (green or wax)	Cucumbers	Onions	may be eaten as desired.
**Broccoli	Eggplant	*Peppers (red or green)	
Beets	Greens (Beet, Chard)	Rutabaga	Chicory Lettuce (all kinds)
**Brussels sprouts	*Collard, Dandelion,	Sauerkraut	Chinese cabbage Radishes
*Cabbage (all kinds)	*Kale, *Mustard,	Summer Squash	Endive Watercress
			Escarole Parsley

LIST 2 FRUIT EXCHANGES—Approximately 10 grams carbohydrate, 40 calories per serving. Fruits and juices may be fresh, cooked, dried, frozen or canned WITHOUT SUGAR OR SYRUP.

Fruits

Apple—½ medium	Cherries—10 large	Mango—½ small	Peach—1 medium	**Juices**
Applesauce—½ cup	Dates—2	Melon, **Cantaloupe—	Pear—1 small	Apple, Pineapple—1/3 cup
Apricots, fresh—2 medium	Figs, fresh—1 large	¼ med. (6″ dia.)	Persimmon—1 medium	**Grapefruit, orange—½ cup
Apricots, dried—4 halves	Figs, dried—1 small	*Honeydew—⅛ (7″ dia.)	Pineapple—½ cup	Grape, prune—¼ cup
Bananas—½ small	Fruit cocktail,	*Watermelon—1 cup cubed	Prunes, dried—2	
Berries (**straw., boysen.,	canned—½ cup	Nectarine—1 small	Raisins, dried—2 Tbsp.	
*rasp., black)—¾ cup	**Grapefruit—½ small	**Orange—1 small	**Strawberries—¾ cup	
Blueberries—½ cup	Grapes—12	**Papaya—1/3 medium	*Tangerine—1 large	

LIST 3 STARCH EXCHANGES—Approximately 15 grams carbohydrate, 2 grams protein, 68 calories per serving.

Bread: (1 slice)	Cornbread (2″x2″x1″)—1	**Other**—Omit 2 fat exchanges:	**Vegetables:**
White, wholewheat, rye,	Pancake, waffle (5″x½″)—1	Chips, corn or potato—15	Beans or Peas, dry cooked
raisin, pumpernickel,	Potatoes, French fried (3″)—8	**Cereals:**	(lima, navy, kidney, blackeyed,
French or Italian	Sherbet—¼ cup	Hot cereal—½ cup	split pea, etc.)—½ cup
Bagel—½	**Crackers:**	Dry flakes—2/3 cup	Beans, baked (no pork)—¼ cup
Dinner roll—1 (2″ dia.)	Graham (2½″ sq.)—2	Dry puffed—1½ cups	Corn—1/3 cup or ½ med. ear
English muffin—½	Matzoth (4″x6″)—½	Rice or grits, cooked—½ cup	Hominy—½ cup
Bun, Hamb. or hot dog—½	Melba Toast—4	Spaghetti, macaroni, noodles,	Parsnips—2/3 cup
(8 to the pound)	Oyster (½ cup)—20	other pastas, cooked—½ cup	Peas, green (canned or froz.)—½ cup
Cornbread (1½″)—1 cube	Pretzels (3⅛″)—25		*Potatoes, white (1 small)—½ cup
Tortilla (6″ dia.)—1	Round, thin—6		Potatoes, sweet or yams—¼ cup
Other—Omit 1 fat exchange:	Ry-Krisp—3		Pumpkin—¾ cup
Biscuit, muffin (2″ dia.)—1	Saltine—5		Winter squash—½ cup

LIST 4 MEAT EXCHANGES—Approximately 7 grams protein, 5 grams fat, 73 calories per exchange.

Medium Fat Meat	Egg, whole—1	**Other**—omit 1 fat exchange:
(Poultry with skin, beef, lamb,	Salmon, red, canned or	Cheese, brick, cheddar, roquefort, Swiss,
pork, veal, ham, etc.)	smoked—¼ cup	& processed—1 oz.
cooked—1 oz.	Sardines—3 medium	Frankfurters—1 (8-9 per pound)
Cold cuts—1 oz. slice	Tuna, canned in oil—¼ cup	**Other**—omit 2 fat exchanges:
Vienna sausages—2		Peanut butter—2 Tbsp.

LIST 4A MEAT EXCHANGES—Approximately 7 grams protein, 3 grams fat, 55 calories per exchange. CHOOSE ONLY LEAN, UNMARBLED CUTS OF MEAT: TRIM OFF ALL VISIBLE FAT; DO NOT ADD FAT IN COOKING.

Beef, Dried chipped—1 oz.	Poultry without skin—1 oz.	Lobster—1 small tail
Beef, lamb, pork, ham, veal	(Cooked)	Oysters, clams, shrimp—5 medium
LEAN ONLY cooked—1 oz.	Fish, any except those in	Tuna, packed in water—¼ cup
Cottage cheese—¼ cup	List 5—1 oz.	Salmon, pink, canned—¼ cup

LIST 5 FAT EXCHANGES—Approximately 5 grams fat, 45 calories per exchange.

Avocado (4″ dia.)—⅛	Cream, sour—2 Tbsp.	Roquefort—2 tsp.	**Nuts:** Almonds—
Bacon, crisp—1 slice	Cream cheese—1 Tbsp.	1000 Island—2 tsp.	10 whole, peanuts
Butter, margarine—1 tsp.	Dressing, French—1 Tbsp.	Oil—1 tsp.	10 whole, pecans
Cream, light (20%)—2 Tbsp.	Mayonnaise—1 tsp.	Olives—5 small	2 large, walnuts
			6 small

LIST 6 MILK EXCHANGES—Approximately 12 grams carbohydrate, 8 grams protein, trace fat, 80 calories per serving.

Carnation Instant Nonfat	**Other**—omit 1 fat exchange:	**Other**—omit 2 fat exchanges:
Milk (Liquid)—1 cup; (Dry)—1/3 cup	Lowfat milk—1 cup	Whole milk—1 cup
Buttermilk, fat free—1 cup	Yogurt made with lowfat milk—1 cup	Carnation Evaporated Milk—½ cup
Yogurt, plain, made with nonfat milk—1 cup		Buttermilk made from whole milk—1 cup

DIET PLAN DURING PREGNANCY AND LACTATION

Date _____For _____

GENERAL INSTRUCTIONS

The principles of the pregnancy and lactation diet plan are as follows:

- Eat regularly—do not omit a meal.
- Choose a minimum of four servings per day from List A, three servings per day from List B, and four servings per day from Lists C & D.
- Choose one good source, or two fair sources of Vitamin C per day (see List C).

- Choose a good source of Vitamin A every other day (see List C).
- Follow a regular exercise program as directed by your physician.
- Increased nutrient intake is recommended during lactation—add 1 serving from List A per day. Drink two to three quarts fluids per day. The sample menu provides about 1.5 quarts of fluid.

Basic Meal Plan	Sample Menu	Special Instructions
See substitution list on back for other allowable foods		Do Not follow the instructions for Sodium Weight Control without your physician's knowledge.

BREAKFAST
1 serving fruit—List C
1 serving meat—List B
1 serving bread—List D
1 serving—List E
1 serving cereal—List D
1 serving—List E
1 serving milk—List A
1 serving—List E

NOON MEAL
1 serving vegetable—List C
1 serving cheese—List B
2 servings bread—List D
2 servings—List E
1 serving vegetable—List C
1 serving fruit—List C
1 serving milk—List A

AFTERNOON SNACK
1 serving milk—List A

1 serving—List E

EVENING MEAL
1 serving vegetable—List C
1 serving—List E
2 servings meat—List B

1 serving cereal—List D
1 serving vegetable—List C
1 serving bread/cereal—List D
1 serving—List E
1 serving fruit—List C

1 serving—List E

BEDTIME
1 serving milk—List A

BREAKFAST
½ cup orange juice
2 poached eggs
1 slice whole wheat toast with
1 tsp. margarine
¾ cup 40% Bran Flakes with
2 tsp. sugar
1 cup Carnation Instant Nonfat Milk
Coffee

NOON MEAL
7 oz. tomato soup prepared w/water
2 oz. Cheddar Cheese on
2 slices white bread, grilled with
2 tsp. margarine
2/3 cup coleslaw
1 medium apple
1 cup Carnation Instant Nonfat Milk

AFTERNOON SNACK
1 package Carnation Instant Breakfast made with Carnation Instant Nonfat Milk
2 Vanilla Wafers

EVENING MEAL
1 cup fresh spinach salad with
1 Tbsp. French dressing
4 oz. broiled halibut garnished with chopped parsley and lemon slices
½ cup steamed rice
4 oz. broccoli spears
1 hard roll with
1 tsp. margarine
½ cup sweetened rhubarb w/1 Tbsp. whipped cream
Hot tea with lemon

BEDTIME
1 package Carnation Instant Breakfast made with Carnation Instant Nonfat Milk

---

☐ **For Sodium Control**
1. Use salt free margarine and salad dressings.
2. Use salt free bread & cereals only. (Dry cereals contain added salt except for puffed wheat, rice & shredded wheat)
3. Prepare all foods without salt
4. Avoid salted or cured meats such as: bacon, sausage, luncheon meats, ham, chipped beef & cheeses.
5. Avoid canned vegetables, canned meats and meat substitutes unless they are labeled salt-free.
6. Check with your local water supplier as water may contain a lot of sodium. Distilled water may be neecssary.

☐ *For Controlled Weight Gain
Follow the special instructions given in the boxes at the bottom of each of the 5 food groups listed on the back of the diet.

By _____

SUBSTITUTION LISTS

LIST A: MILK GROUP Foods included:

Milk—fluid whole, Carnation evaporated, fluid skim, Carnation instant nonfat milk, buttermilk, low fat milk

Cheese—cottage (1 cup = 1 cup milk); cheddar-type, natural or processed (1 oz. = ¾ cup milk)

Ice cream

Carnation Instant Breakfast

Carnation Slender

Yogurt

Amount recommended: At least 4 eight oz. cups per day

Milk is a leading source of calcium which is needed for bones and teeth. It also provides high quality protein, riboflavin, vitamins A, D, E, B_6, B_{12}, phosphorus, magnesium, and zinc.

> *If controlled weight gain is desirable, use skim milk, Carnation instant nonfat milk, low fat yogurt, cottage cheese, and Carnation Slender to fulfill the requirements of this group.

LIST B: MEAT GROUP Foods included:

Beef; veal; lamb; pork; variety meats, such as liver, heart, kidney

Poultry and eggs

Fish and shellfish

As alternates—dry beans, dry peas, lentils, nuts, peanuts, peanut butter.

Amounts Recommended: The equivalent of at least 3 servings daily. Count as a serving: 2 to 3 ounces of lean cooked meat, poultry, or fish—all without bone.

2 eggs

1 cup dry beans, dry peas, or lentils

4 tablespoons peanut butter

Foods in this group are valued for their protein, which is needed for growth and repair of body tissues — muscles, organs, blood, skin, and hair. These foods also provide iron, thiamin, riboflavin, vitamins B_6, B_{12}, phosphorus, zinc, and iodine. Vegetable protein foods provide protein, iron, thiamin, folacin, vitamins B_6, and E, phosphorus, magnesium, and zinc.

> *If controlled weight gain is desirable, select lean cuts of meats and choose poultry and fish often. Use broiling, roasting, steaming, boiling or baking methods of cooking and avoid the use of fats and oils in food preparation.

LIST C: VEGETABLE-FRUIT GROUP Foods included:

All vegetables and fruits

Valuable sources of vitamin C and vitamin A are listed below:

Sources of Vitamin A: Dark green leafy and deep yellow vegetables and a few fruits, namely: Apricots, broccoli, cantaloupe, carrots, chard, collards, cress, kale, turnip greens, pumpkin, spinach, sweet potatoes, winter squash (Hubbard, acorn, etc.)

Sources of vitamin C: Good sources: Grapefruit or grapefruit juice, cantaloupe, raw strawberries, broccoli, brussels sprouts

Fair sources: Honeydew melon, tangerine or tangerine juice, watermelon, raw cabbage, greens—collards, kale, mustard, turnip, green pepper, potatoes and sweet potatoes cooked in the jacket, spinach, tomatoes or tomato juice, fresh or frozen raspberries.

Amounts recommended: Choose 4 or more servings daily including: 1 serving of a good source of vitamin C or 2 servings of a fair source. 1 serving, at least every other day, of a good source of vitamin A.

Count as 1 serving:

½ cup vegetable or fruit

a portion as ordinarily served such as 1 medium apple, orange, banana, or potato; ½ a medium grapefruit or cantaloupe.

Fruits and vegetables are valuable chiefly because of the vitamins and minerals they contain. In this plan, the group is counted on to supply nearly all the vitamin C needed and over half of the vitamin A.

> *If controlled weight gain is desirable limit consumption of corn, potatoes, or sweet potatoes to 1 serving per day. Use fresh or water pack fruits and avoid those canned with sugar.

LIST D: BREAD-CEREAL GROUP Foods included:

All breads and cereals that are whole grain, enriched or restored. (Brown rice & converted rice are in this group)

Cereals, cooked or ready-to eat, cornmeal, grits

Enriched or whole grain flour

Macaroni, spaghetti, noodles made from enriched flour

Quick breads and other baked goods if made with whole grain or enriched flour.

Amounts recommended: Choose 4 servings or more daily. Count as 1 serving: 1 slice of bread, 1 ounce of ready-to eat cereal, ½ to ¾ cup cooked cereal, cornmeal, grits, macaroni, noodles, rice, or spaghetti.

Foods in this group furnish worthwhile amounts of protein, iron, several of the B vitamins, phosphorus, zinc, and food energy.

> *If controlled weight gain is desirable, avoid the use of quick breads and other baked goods which contain large amounts of sugar, honey or fat. Limit total number of servings in this group to 5 per day.

LIST E: OTHER FOODS

Foods other than those listed in Lists A, B, C & D can usually be included to meet daily energy requirements and to add variety to meals. Refined breads, cereals, flours; sugars; butter; margarine, and other fats are examples. It is recommended that some vegetable oil be included among the fats used.

The use of the following is also recommended:

Iodized salt

Pasteurized milk fortified with 400 International Units of vitamin D.

Foods not specifically mentioned in the food groups supply additional food energy (calories) and may add to the total nutrients in meals.

> *If controlled weight gain is desirable avoid sugar, honey, concentrated sweets, pies, cakes, pastry, rich desserts, regular soft drinks and alcoholic beverages. Limit the use of fats and oils to 2 Tbsp. per day.

HIGH PROTEIN DIET PLAN

For _____ Date _____

GENERAL INSTRUCTIONS

The protein content of the Sample Menu has been adjusted to approximately 150 grams per day. Daily protein requirements normally range from 44 to 78 grams.

The principles of the High Protein Diet are as follows:

Eat regularly—do not omit a meal.

Exercise regularly and monitor your weight.

Vary the sample menu by choosing different foods as offered in the indicated substitution lists on the back of the diet.

Choose a good source of Vitamin C daily. They are citrus fruits, strawberries, broccoli, brussels sprouts, papaya, and cantaloupe.

Choose a good source of Vitamin A every other day. These are dark green or yellow fruits and vegetables.

Patients on a high protein diet should pay special attention to maintaining a high level of calcium and magnesium in their diet. Good sources of calcium include dairy products, green leafy vegetables, legumes and nuts. Good sources of magnesium include nuts, soybeans, cocoa, seafood, whole grains, dried beans and peas.

Basic Meal Plan	Sample Menu	Calories	Choles-terol mg.	Special Instructions
BREAKFAST	**BREAKFAST**			☐ Calories may be reduced by following the suggestions on the reverse side.
Fruits	½ cup orange juice	56		
Meat/eggs/cheese	1 med. poached egg	72	222	
Fats	2 strips bacon	91	13	
Breads and cereals	1 cup bran flakes	106		☐ Cholesterol may be lowered by following the suggestions on the revere side.
Milk beverage	1 cup Carnation Nonfat Milk	80	5	
Sweets (optional)	1 tsp. sugar	15		
Beverage	Coffee or tea	2		
MID-MORNING	**MID-MORNING**			
Milk beverage	1 cup CIB* with nonfat milk	210	10	
NOON	**NOON**			
Meat/eggs/cheese	2 oz. cheddar cheese	223	56	
Meat/eggs/cheese	3 oz. grilled hamburger patty (lean)	243	80	
Breads and cereals	1 hamburger bun	81		
Vegetable/fruit	3 slices tomato on a lettuce leaf	11		
Fats	2 tsp. mayonnaise	67	6	
Vegetable/fruit	French fries (10)	137		
Beverage	Coffee or tea	2		
MID-AFTERNOON	**MID-AFTERNOON**			
Milk beverage	1 cup CIB* with nonfat milk	210	10	
DINNER	**DINNER**			
Salad—vegetable/fruit	Fresh salad made with ½ cup lettuce, ½ cup spinach	9		
Fats	1 Tbsp. Italian dressing	83		
Meats/eggs/cheese	5 oz. broiled halibut garnished with lemon wedge	244		
Starchy vegetable	½ cup steamed rice	112	90	
Vegetable/fruit	½ cup broccoli	33		
Fats	2 tsp. margarine	68		
Breads/cereals	1 hard roll	78		
Fats	1 tsp. margarine	34		
Dessert	½ cup sweetened rhubarb	190		
Beverage	Coffee or tea	2		
BED-TIME	**BED-TIME**			
Milk beverage	1 cup CIB* with nonfat milk	210	10	

CIB*—Carnation Instant Breakfast (any flavor)   total: 2669   502 mg.

By _____

General Instructions: Eat regularly as indicated on your sample menu. The protein in this diet has been adjusted to approximately 150 grams (daily protein requirement is normally 44-78 grams per day). Foods which increase protein are meat, milk, fish, poultry, cheese, eggs, and CIB. Plan to consume these foods in the quantities indicated in your sample menu so that the total food intake contains at least 3 cups Carnation Instant Breakfast, 1 cup nonfat milk, and 9 oz. of cooked meat, fish, fowl, or cheese each day. Breads, cereals, fruits, vegetables, fats and sweets may be added to provide extra calories and balance meals. Noon and evening basic meal plans may be interchanged when desired.

SUBSTITUTION LISTS

Milk group: Approximately 8 grams protein per 8 oz.*
Nonfat, lowfat, or whole milk
Carnation Instant Nonfat milk, reconstituted

Buttermilk
Yogurt, plain

*CIB with 8 oz. milk provides 15 grams protein.

Meat/Eggs/Cheese group: Approximately 7 grams protein per measure listed.
Beef, lamb, pork, veal, poultry, fish—1 oz.
Canned salmon, tuna, mackerel, crab, lobster—¼ cup
Clams, oysters, scallops, shrimp—1 oz.
Dried beans and peas, lentils—½ cup

Sardines, drained—3
Egg—1
Cheese, aged & processed—1 oz.
Cottage cheese—¼ cup
Peanut butter—2 Tbsp.

Breads, Cereals, & Starchy Vegetables Group: Approximately 2 grams protein per measure listed.

Bread:
White, wheat, rye, raisin, pumpernickel, French, Italian—1 slice
Bagel, English muffin—½
Bun, hamburger, hotdog—½
Hard roll (2″)—1
Muffin, biscuit (2″)—1
Pancake, waffle (4″)—1

Crackers:
Graham (2½ sq.)—2
Matzoh (4″ x 6″)—½
Melba toast—4
Oyster—½ cup
Pretzels (3⅛″)—25
Round, thin—6
Ry-Krisp—3
Saltines—6
Soda (2½″)—4

Cereals:
Hot cereal—½ cup
Dry flakes—2/3 cup
Dry puffed—1½ cup
Rice or grits, cooked—½ cup
Pasta, cooked—½ cup
Popcorn, popped—3 cups
Wheat germ—¼ cup

Starchy Vegetables:
Corn—1/3 cup or ½ med. ear
Hominy—½ cup
Parsnips—2/3 cup
Peas, green—½ cup
Potatoes, white—½ cup
Potatoes, sweet—¼ cup
Pumpkin—¾ cup
Winter squash—½ cup

Vegetable group:
Approximately 2 grams protein per ½ cup cooked or 1 cup raw. All vegetables are included in this group except those listed under Starchy Vegetables. Leafy green vegetables may contain less than 2 grams protein per above serving.

Fruit group: Contains less than 1 gram protein per average serving.

Fat group: The following foods are included in the fat group due to their high fat content. They contain varying amounts of protein.
Butter, margarine, oil, fats—zero protein
Salad dressings—negligible protein
Bacon (1 slice, 20/lb.)—2 grams
Cream, sour or light (2 Tbsp.)—1 gram
Cream, heavy (2 Tbsp.)—less than 1 gram
Cream cheese (1 Tbsp.)—1 gram

Nuts:
Peanuts (1 oz.)—7 grams
Pecans (1 oz.)—3 grams
Walnuts, almonds, cashews (1 oz.)—5 grams

Special Instructions:

Calories may be adjusted with the following foods:
sugar—1 Tbsp. - 45 calories
bread—1 slice - 65 calories
butter, margarine, mayonnaise—1 tsp. - 34 calories

Cholesterol may be lowered by the reduction or elimination of the following foods:
1 med. egg yolk - 222 mg. cholesterol
3 oz. heart - 233 mg.
3 oz. liver - 372 mg.
3 oz. shrimp - 128 mg.
3 oz. sardines - 119 mg.
3 oz. lamb - 83 mg.
Also brains, chicken gizzards, kidneys, and sweetbreads.

LOW FAT DIET PLAN

For_____ Date _____

GENERAL INSTRUCTIONS

The principles of the Low Fat Diet are as follows:

- Foods should be used in the amounts specified and only as tolerated.
- Prepare all foods without the addition of butter or other fats.
- Trim all visible fat from meat before eating.
- Include at least 4 or more servings of breads and cereals and 4 or more servings of fruits and vegetables per day.

- Choose a good source of vitamin C per day. They include citrus fruits, strawberries, broccoli, brussels sprouts, papaya and cabbage.
- Choose a good source of vitamin A every other day. They include dark green or yellow fruits and vegetables.
- CIB* prepared with nonfat milk adds protein, vitamins, minerals, and needed calories to a diet restricted in fat.

Basic Meal Plan	Sample Menu	Calories	Special Instructions
BREAKFAST	**BREAKFAST**		☐ **FOR WEIGHT CONTROL**
Fruits	1 small banana	119	1. Follow a regular exercise program as directed by your physician.
Breads and cereals	1 cup bran flakes	106	
Sweets (optional)	1 tsp. sugar	15	2. Limit breads and cereals to 4 servings per day.
Eggs	1 medium poached egg	72	
Breads and Cereals	2 slices whole wheat toast	133	3. Use Carnation Slender with nonfat milk in place of CIB.
Fats	1 tsp. margarine	34	
Sweets	2 tsp. jelly	33	4. Use only unsweetened or fresh fruits for dessert. Avoid sugar, concentrated sweets and regular soft drinks. Artificial sweeteners may be used.
Milk Beverage	1 cup Carnation Instant Nonfat Milk	80	
Beverage	Coffee or tea without cream	2	
MID-MORNING	**MID-MORNING**		
Milk Beverage	1 cup CIB* with nonfat milk	210	5. Avoid the use of potatoes or other starchy vegetables (including corn, lima beans, sweet potatoes, dried peas and beans).
NOON	**NOON**		
Soups	1 cup vegetable soup, prepared with water	78	
Breads or cereals	4 saltine crackers	48	
Vegetables	3 celery sticks	7	
Meats	3-oz. roast turkey, white meat	150	
Breads or Cereals	2 slices white bread	124	
Fats	1 tsp. mayonnaise	33	
Fruits	1 medium apple	87	
Milk Beverage	1 cup Carnation Instant Nonfat Milk	80	
Beverage	Coffee or tea without cream	2	
DINNER	**DINNER**		
Salad	1 cup fresh spinach with	14	
	½ medium tomato and	11	
	1 Tbsp. diet salad dressing	15	
Meat	3 oz. broiled halibut with	154	
	lemon wedge	6	
Starchy vegetable	½ cup steamed rice	112	
Vegetable	½ cup green beans	17	
Fats	1 tsp. margarine	34	
Breads or cereals	1 hard roll	78	
Fruits	½ cup sweetened rhubarb	190	
Beverages	Coffee or tea without cream	2	
BEDTIME	**BEDTIME**		
Milk Beverage	1 cup CIB* with nonfat milk	210	

By _____

*CIB — Carnation Instant Breakfast (any flavor)   Total   2256

GENERAL INSTRUCTIONS

Eat regularly as indicated on your sample menu. The fat content of your diet has been decreased to approximately 15% of the total calories. The average American diet contains approximately 40% fat. Limit fat servings in your diet to 3 teaspoons of fats, 6 oz. meats, and one egg per day. If no egg is desired, 7 oz. meat may be used per day. Breads, cereals, fruits, vegetables and sweets may be added to provide extra calories and balance meals.

	FOODS PERMITTED	FOODS TO OMIT
MILK	Nonfat milk, buttermilk, CIB prepared with nonfat milk or instant dry nonfat milk (Carnation Instant Nonfat Dry Milk can be prepared double strength as a substitute for cream or half & half.).	Whole milk, low fat milk, whipped cream, ice cream, ice milk, half and half, chocolate milk, evaporated milk, yogurt, non-dairy creamer.
EGGS	1 daily, cooked without fat. Egg whites permitted.	More than 1 daily; eggs fried in fat.
CHEESE	Cottage cheese or whey cheeses. Especially made low fat yellow cheeses clearly labeled as such.	All other cheeses.
MEATS	All lean meats, fish, fowl, vegetable meat substitutes (if fowl is breaded and fried, remove skin and breading before eating), water-packed canned fish. Choose poultry and fish often.	Fried meats, fish and poultry, fish canned in oil, fatty cuts of meat such as brisket, short ribs, pork chops, bacon, sausage, luncheon meats, frankfurters, duck, goose, peanut butter.
VEGETABLES	All vegetables permitted.	Creamed vegetables, vegetables in cheese sauce, hollandaise sauce or other rich sauces, fried vegetables, buttered vegetables unless buttered with fat allowance.
FRUITS	All fruits and fruit juices permitted.	Avocado and coconut.
SOUPS	Broths, bouillon, canned broth-based soups prepared with water or nonfat milk.	Creamed soups or canned soups prepared with whole milk.
BREADS AND CEREALS	Bread, cereals, pastas, crackers, popcorn (unbuttered).	Biscuits, waffles, rich rolls, pancakes, sweet rolls, doughnuts, popovers, other rich breads.
DESSERTS	Gelatin, puddings prepared with nonfat milk, angel food cake, sherbet, ices, meringues, vanilla wafers.	Custards and puddings prepared with whole milk or egg yolks, cakes (except angel), cookies, ice cream, pie crusts, pastries, any dessert made with chocolate or nuts.
SWEETS	Jelly, jam, sugar, syrup, honey, molasses, plain hard candy, gumdrops.	Chocolate and any candy containing chocolate, cream, or fat. (Cocoa may be used.)
FATS	Diet salad dressing, LIMIT OF ONE TEASPOON oil, mayonnaise, salad dressing, or margarine per meal.	Butter, shortening, lard. Oil, mayonnaise, salad dressing, or margarine in amounts GREATER than 1 TEASPOON PER MEAL.
BEVERAGES	Coffee, tea, coffee substitute, carbonated beverages.	None.
MISC.	Salt, spices, herbs, condiments, cocoa, vinegar, pickles, catsup, mustard, steak sauce, etc.	Olives, nuts, gravy, rich sauces such as cream sauce.

SODIUM-RESTRICTED DIET PLAN

For _____ Date _____

GENERAL INSTRUCTIONS

Your diet plan primarily uses foods which are prepared without salt and stresses the use of foods that are low in natural sodium.

Eat regularly as shown in your basic meal plan.

Select a variety of foods and do not add salt.

Carefully read the labels of all prepared foods. Look not only for salt, but also for bicarbonate of soda (baking soda), baking powder, MSG, and sodium compounds such as sodium benzoate, sodium citrate, etc. Most frozen dinners, instant dinner mixes, sauces, canned foods (except fruits and fruit juices) and prepared foods contain salt unless they are especially prepared for sodium-restricted diets and labeled as such.

Eat only the amount of List II foods (on back) specified in your basic meal plan. These foods are moderately high in sodium.

Choose a good source of Vitamin C daily. They are citrus fruits, strawberries, broccoli, brussels sprouts, papaya, and cantaloupes.

Choose a good source of Vitamin A every other day. These are dark green or yellow fruits and vegetables.

Water varies in sodium content from one area to another. Check with your local water supplier and if the water in your area contains more than 20 mg. sodium per quart, bottled water should be used. The use of water-softeners may add significant amounts of sodium to the water supply.

Avoid medicines, laxatives, and salt substitutes unless prescribed by physician.

Basic Meal Plan	Sample Menu	Calories	Sodium mg.	Cholesterol mg.	Special Instructions
BREAKFAST	**BREAKFAST**				FOR WEIGHT CONTROL
1 serving fruit or juice—List I	½ grapefruit	40	1		
1 serving cereal—List I	1 cup Puffed rice cereal (enriched) with	60	tr.		1. Follow a regular exercise program as directed by your physician.
1 serving nonfat milk—List II	1 cup Carnation Instant Nonfat Milk	80	115.8	5	2. Avoid the use of wine, beer, or other alcoholic beverages.
1 serving fruit—List I	1 small banana	120	1		3. Use only unsweetened or fresh fruits for desserts; avoid sugar, concentrated sweets, regular jelly and jams, regular soft drinks, etc. Artificial sweetener may be used.
1 serving salt-free bread—List I	1 slice salt-free whole wheat toast	61	5		
1 serving fat—List I	1 tsp. unsalted margarine	34	—		
1 serving sweets—List I	1 tsp. jam	18	0.8		
Beverage	Coffee or tea	2	2		
NOON MEAL	**NOON MEAL**				4. Limit breads and cereals to 4 servings per day.
2 oz. cooked fresh meat—List II	2 oz. unsalted roasted chicken (light meat)	95	36	68	5. Limit margarine and other fats to 4 servings per day.
2 servings salt-free bread—List I	2 slices salt-free white bread and	124	5		6. Avoid the use of potatoes or other starchy vegetables (including corn, lima beans, sweet potatoes, dried peas and beans).
1 serving fat—List I	1 tsp. salt-free mayonnaise with	33	—	3	
1 serving vegetable—List I	lettuce (3 small leaves)	2	1		
1 serving fruit—List I	1 box (1½ oz.) raisins	124	12		
1 serving fruit—List I	½ medium apple	40	1		
1 serving nonfat milk—List I	1 cup Carnation Instant Nonfat Milk	80	115.8	5	
EVENING MEAL	**EVENING MEAL**				
1 serving vegetables—List I	1 cup chopped fresh spinach	14	39		
1 serving vegetables—List I	½ medium tomato	11	1.5		
2 servings fat—List I	2 Tbsp. oil and vinegar dressing	166	1		
1 serving salt-free bread—List I	1 slice salt-free whole wheat bread	61	5		
1 serving fat—List I	1 tsp. unsalted margarine	34	—		
1 serving wine—List I (optional)	7 oz. wine	173	10.2		
4 oz. cooked fresh meat—List II	4 oz. broiled lean steak	234	67.8	103	
1 serving vegetable—List I	1 baked potato	188	6		
2 servings fat—List I	2 Tbsp. sour cream	57	12	16	
1 serving vegetable—List I	6 asparagus spears	18	1		
1 serving vegetable—List I	½ cup cooked rhubarb with sugar	191	2.5		
1 serving dessert—List II	½ cup ice cream	129	42	26	
Beverage	Coffee or Tea	2	2		
BEDTIME	**BEDTIME**				By _____
1 serving fruit—List I	1 medium orange	64	1		
	Total:	2255	487	226	

LIST I: FOODS WITH LOW SODIUM CONTENT—These foods may be used as desired unless calories are also restricted.

All fruit and fruit juices

All fresh or frozen vegetables except those in LIST II or LIST III

BREAD & CEREALS:	Puffed wheat/rice or shredded wheat Most hot, unsalted cereals Salt-free breads Pearl barley, rice, noodles, macaroni, spaghetti Popcorn, unsalted

FATS:	Sweet butter Unsalted margarine Vegetable oils	Salt-free mayonnaise Sour cream Nuts, unsalted
MISC:	Vinegar Wines Jams or jellies	Honey & syrup Sugar

Herbs and spices which do not contain salt or MSG (monosodium glutamate)

Special salt-free foods (read the label to determine milligram level per serving—under 15 mg. per serving foods may be used as desired)

LIST II: FOODS WITH MODERATE SODIUM CONTENT—These foods must be limited in amounts as specified.

MILK:	(Whole, Carnation Instant Nonfat, diluted evaporated, skim, low fat)—Limit to 2 cups Daily.
EGGS:	Limit to 1 per day.
DESSERTS:	Limit to one choice per day—serving portion as indicated. Cake—1½ oz. Cookies, assorted—1 oz. Gelatin—½ cup Ice Cream—½ cup Regular cooked puddings such as tapioca, rice, etc.—½ cup Sherbet—½ cup

*Meat/fish/fowl (other than those in List III)—Limit to 6 oz. cooked weight daily.

VEGETABLES: Limit to one choice per day—½ cup serving only (fresh, frozen or salt-free canned)

Beets	Frozen Lima Beans
Beet greens	Frozen peas
Carrots	Kale
Chard	Mustard greens
Dandelion greens	Turnips, white
Celery	

*Fresh crab, lobster, shrimp, scallops, brains, kidneys, and frozen fish which have been flumed in brine contain higher amounts of sodium than other fresh meats. These foods should be chosen infrequently.

LIST III: FOODS WITH HIGH SODIUM CONTENT—These foods should be avoided.

MILK:	Buttermilk
CHEESE:	All excepting special low sodium cheese or low sodium cottage cheese.
MEATS/FISH/FOWL:	Bacon, ham, frankfurters, sausages, bologna, luncheon meats; canned, salted, dried, smoked or pickled meat, fish or poultry. Herring, caviar, regular canned tuna & salmon, anchovies, sardines and salted cod. Canned crab, shrimp, lobster and oysters. Salt pork, chipped or corned beef, brain, kidney, meats koshered by salting. Regular peanut butter.
VEGETABLES:	Sauerkraut, olives, pickles, regular canned vegetables and canned vegetable juices. Any vegetable prepared in brine.
FATS:	Salted butter or margarine, commercial salad dressings and regular mayonnaise, bacon fat, salted nuts, canned gravies.

BREADS & CEREALS:	Regular and yeast breads and rolls prepared with salt, dry cereals other than those listed in List I, regular pancakes, muffins, biscuits, cornbread, crackers and mixes. Potato chips, corn chips, pretzels, salted popcorn, etc. Quick cooking cereals if a sodium compound has been added in processing. Cornmeal and self-rising flour.
SOUPS:	All regular canned soups, soup mixes, broth, bouillon, consomme, commercial bouillon cubes, powders or liquids.
DESSERTS:	Instant puddings, pie crust unless prepared without salt, desserts in excess of the amount allowed in List II.
BEVERAGES:	Dutch process cocoa, soft drinks or beer which have been bottled in areas with high sodium content in their water supplies.
CONDIMENTS:	Salt, seasonings which contain salt or monosodium glutamate, worcestershire sauce, soy sauce, meat tenderizers, regular catsup, chili sauce, barbecue sauce, horseradish sauce, etc. Pickles, relishes and olives.

REDUCING DIET PLAN

For _____ Date _____

GENERAL INSTRUCTIONS

Effective and sustained weight reduction can best be achieved through a regular plan of diet and exercise. The principles of the Reducing Diet Plan are as follows:

Eat regularly—do not omit a meal.

Follow a regular exercise program as directed by your physician. Between meal snacks should be chosen from the free list.

Vary the sample menu by choosing different foods as offered in the indicated substitution lists on the back of the diet. Eat those foods in the measured amounts indicated. Noon and evening basic meal plans may be interchanged when desired.

Choose a good source of Vitamin C daily. They are citrus fruits, strawberries, broccoli, brussels sprouts, papaya, and cantaloupe.

Choose a good source of Vitamin A every other day. These are dark green or yellow fruits and vegetables.

Broiling, roasting, steaming, boiling, or baking methods of food preparation are preferable. Avoid the use of fats and oils except in the amounts allowed. Avoid sugar, honey, concentrated sweets, pies, cakes, pastry, rich desserts, regular soft drinks and alcoholic beverages.

Basic Meal Plan 1200 Calories   **Sample Menu**   **Calories**   **Special Instructions**

See substitution list on back for other allowable foods.

BREAKFAST	**BREAKFAST**		**Special Instructions**
1 serving fruit—List 3	1 grapefruit half	40	☐ **1000 Calories:** Omit 1 serving non-fat milk, 1 serving starch and 1 serving fat per day from basic meal plan.
1 serving starch—List 4	1 oz. enriched concentrate cereal	107	
1 serving nonfat milk	1 cup Carnation Instant Nonfat Milk	80	
Miscellaneous—List 1	Sugar substitute	—	
Miscellaneous—List 1	Black Coffee	2	
NOON MEAL	**NOON MEAL**		☐ **1500 Calories:** Add 2 measures meat, 1 serving starch, 1 serving fat, and 1 serving fruit per day to basic meal plan.
2 measures meat/fish/fowl/cheese—List 5	2 oz. Cheddar cheese	223	
1 serving starch—List 4	5 small whole wheat crackers	57	
2 servings fruit—List 3	1 medium apple	86	(OR)
½ serving nonfat milk	½ cup Carnation Instant Nonfat Milk	40	
EVENING MEAL	**EVENING MEAL**		☐ **1500 Calories:** Add 1 package Carnation Slender with 6 ounces nonfat milk. Add 1 measure meat and 1 serving starch.
1 serving vegetable—List 1	1 cup fresh spinach salad	14	
Miscellaneous—List 1	1 Tbsp. low calorie French dressing	15	
4 measures meat/fish/fowl/cheese—List 5	4 oz. Broiled Halibut garnished with	205	
Miscellaneous—List 1	1 lemon wedge	4	
1 serving starch—List 4	½ cup steamed rice with	112	
1 serving fat—List 6	1 tsp. margarine	34	
1 serving vegetable—List 1	6 asparagus spears	18	
Dessert—List 1	½ cup dietetic gelatin	8	
Miscellaneous—List 1	Hot Tea	2	
BEDTIME	**BEDTIME**		
1 serving Slender w/nonfat milk	1 package Carnation Slender	110	
	with 6 oz. nonfat milk	60	
	total	1217	

By _____

*Choose a multivitamin and iron supplemented cereal

SUBSTITUTION LISTS

LIST 1 FREE FOOD LIST—These foods may be used as often as desired provided cream, sugar or honey, or fat is NOT added to them.

Miscellaneous
Coffee
Tea
Clear broth
Bouillon
Beverages, artificially sweetened containing less than 5 calories per 8 ounces
Jelly, artificially sweetened
Sugar substitute

Parsley
Herbs
Spices
Seasonings
Flavorings
Vinegar
Mustard
Horseradish
Salad dressing (dietetic)

Desserts & fruits
Cranberries
Lemons
Gelatin, unsweetened
Rennet tablets

Juices
Lemon juice
Tomato Juice
Vegetable juice

Vegetables
Asparagus
Bean sprouts
Beet greens
Broccoli
Brussels sprouts
Cabbage (all kinds)
Cauliflower
Celery
Chard
Chicory

Collard greens
Cucumbers
Dandelion greens
Escarole
Eggplant
Green beans
Kale
Lettuce (all kinds)
Mushrooms
Mustard greens

Okra
Peppers (green or red)
Radishes
Sauerkraut
Spinach
Squash, summer
Tomatoes
Turnip greens
Watercress
Wax beans

LIST 2 OTHER VEGETABLES—Limit these vegetables to one ½ cup serving per day (approximately 36 calories per serving)

Artichokes
Beets

Carrots
Onions

Peas, green
Pumpkin

Rutabaga
Squash, winter

Turnips

LIST 3 FRUITS AND FRUIT JUICES May be fresh, cooked, dried, frozen or canned—NO SUGAR OR SYRUP (approximately 40 calories per serving or amounts indicated)

Fruits
Apple, medium — ½
Applesauce — ½ cup
Apricots, medium, fresh — 2
Apricots, dried halves — 4
Banana, small — ½
Blackberries — 1 cup
Blueberries — ⅔ cup
Boysenberries — 1 cup
Cantaloupe, medium — ¼

Cherries, large — 10
Dates — 2
Figs, fresh, large — 1
Figs, dried — 1
Fruit cocktail, canned — ½ cup
Grapefruit, small — ½
Grapes — 12
Honeydew melon — ⅛
Mango, small — ½

Nectarine, small — 1
Orange, small — 1
Papaya, medium — ⅓
Peach, medium, fresh — 1
Peach, canned — ½ cup
Peach, dried halves — 2
Pear, small, fresh — 1
Pear, canned — ½ cup
Pear, dried halves — 2

Pineapple — ½ cup
Plums, medium, fresh — 2
Prunes, dried — 2
Raisins, dried, Tbsp. — 2
Raspberries — 1 cup
Strawberries — 1 cup
Tangerine, large — 1
Watermelon, cubed — 1 cup

Juices
Apple — ⅓ cup
Grape — ¼ cup
Grapefruit — ½ cup
Orange — ½ cup
Pineapple — ⅓ cup
Prune — ¼ cup

LIST 4 STARCHES (approximately 70 calories per serving of amounts indicated)

Breads:
White, whole wheat or rye — 1 slice
Bagel — ½
Biscuit or muffin — 1 (2″ diameter)
Bun, hamb. or hot dog — ½ (8 to the pound)
Cornbread (1½″ cube) — 1
English muffin — ½

Crackers
Graham (2½″ sq.) — 2
Melba toast — 4
Oyster (½ cup) — 20
Saltine — 5
Round, thin — 6
Ry-Krisp — 3
Tortilla (6″ dia.) — 1
Wheat crackers — 5

Cereals
Hot cereal — ½ cup
Dry flakes — ⅔ cup
Dry puffed — 1½ cups
Rice or grits, cooked — ½ cup
Spaghetti, macaroni, noodles or other pastas, cooked — ½ cup

Vegetables
Beans or peas, dry cooked (lima, navy, kidney, black-eyed split, etc.) — ½ cup
Beans, baked (no pork) — ¼ cup
Corn — ⅓ cup or ½ med ear
Potatoes, white (1 small) — ½ cup
Potatoes, sweet or yams — ¼ cup
Popcorn, popped (no butter) — 1 cup

LIST 5 MEATS, FISH, FOWL The following meats and meat substitutes are lowest in calories (approximately 50 calories per amount indicated). Select them as often as possible. Choose lean, unmarbled cuts; trim off all visible fat; do not add fat in cooking.

Beef, dried chipped — 1 oz.
Beef, lamb, pork, ham, veal LEAN ONLY, cooked — 1 oz.
Liver — 1 oz.

Poultry without skin, cooked — 1 oz.
Fish, any except those listed below — 1 oz.
Crab — ¼ cup
Clams, shrimp, or oysters — 5 medium

Scallops (12/lb.) — 1 large
Tuna, packed in water — ¼ cup
Salmon, pink canned — ¼ cup
Cottage cheese — ¼ cup

The following meats and meat substitutes are higher in calories (approximately 73 calories per amount indicated). Select them sparingly.

Medium-fat meat (beef, lamb, pork, veal), cooked — 1 oz.
Duck — 1 oz.
Goose — 1 oz.
Poultry with skin — 1 oz.

Cold Cuts — 1 oz.
Frankfurters (8-9/lb.) — 1
Vienna sausages — 2
Cheese (brick, cheddar, roquefort, swiss, processed etc.) — 1 oz.

Egg, whole — 1
Salmon, red canned or smoked — ¼ cup
Sardines — 3 medium
Tuna, packed in oil — ¼ cup
Peanut butter — 2 Tsp.

LIST 6 FATS (approximately 45 calories per amount indicated)

Avocado (4″ diam.) — ⅛
Bacon, crisp — 1 slice
Butter, margarine — 1 tsp.

Cream, sour — 2 Tbsp.
Cream cheese — 1 Tbsp.
Nuts — 6 small

Dressing, french — 1 Tbsp.
Mayonnaise — 1 tsp.
Roquefort dressing — 2 tsp.

1000 Island dres — 2 tsp.
Oil — 1 tsp.
Olives — 5 small

RESIDUE CONTROLLED DIET PLAN

For_____Date_____

GENERAL INSTRUCTIONS

The Low Residue diet is a flexible diet which can be adjusted to your food likes and dislikes.

Its principles are:

Eat regularly as indicated on sample menu.

Avoid all rich gravies, desserts and fried foods.

Use all fats in moderation.

Chew all foods well.

Plan to include one citrus juice or fruit daily for Vitamin C.

Include one dark green or yellow fruit, vegetable, or juice every other day for Vitamin A.

Basic Meal Plan	Sample Menu	Special Instructions
BREAKFAST	**BREAKFAST**	Calories may be adjusted with the following foods:
Fruit	½ cup Orange juice	sugar—1 tsp.=18 calories
Egg	1 poached egg	honey—1 tsp.=22 calories
Bread	1 slice white toast	bread—1 slice=65 calories
Sweets	2 tsp. jelly	butter or margarine—
Cereal	½ cup Instant Cream of Wheat	1 tsp.=34 calories
Sweets (optional)	1 tsp. honey	
Beverage	Coffee	
10 AM SNACK	**10 AM SNACK**	
Milk beverage or substitute	1 cup CIB* made with Carnation Nonfat Milk	
Fruit	1 small banana	
NOON MEAL	**NOON MEAL**	
Lean meat or substitute	2 oz. Cheddar cheese, grilled with	
Bread	2 slices white bread	
Fat	1 tsp. margarine	
Vegetable	6 oz. tomato juice	
Fruit	½ cup canned pears	
2 PM SNACK	**2 PM SNACK**	
Milk beverage or substitute	1 cup CIB* made with Carnation Nonfat Milk	
Sweets	2 sugar cookies	
EVENING MEAL	**EVENING MEAL**	
Fruit or vegetable	1 cup fruit cocktail packed in water	
Lean meat or substitute	4 oz. roast turkey	
Potato or substitute	½ cup white, enriched rice	
Vegetable	½ cup pureed asparagus	
Bread	1 hard roll	
Fat	2 tsp. margarine	
Dessert	1 slice angel food cake topped with	
Fruit	¼ cup canned cherries	
Beverage	Coffee	By _____

*CIB—Carnation Instant Breakfast (any flavor)

	FOODS PERMITTED	FOODS NOT ALLOWED
EGGS	Prepared in any manner, except fried.	Fried eggs.
MEAT & MEAT SUBSTITUTES	Roasted, baked, or broiled beef, chicken, turkey, bacon, ham, lamb, veal, or fish. Cottage, cream, and mild American cheese.	Highly-seasoned or highly-salted meats and fish. Fatty meats, luncheon meats or frankfurters. (Crisp bacon is allowed in moderate amounts.) Fried meats or shellfish with tough connective tissues. Highly flavored cheeses.
VEGETABLES	Canned or cooked pureed vegetables such as asparagus, beets, carrots, peas, pumpkin, squash, spinach and young string beans. Cooked potato without skin. Mild flavored vegetable juices.	All raw vegetables. Fried potato, potato chips, and brown rice.
FRUITS	Cooked or canned apples, apricots, cherries, peaches, and pears. Fruit juices. Ripe banana or avocado without skins or seeds.	All fresh fruits.
SOUP	Bouillon, broth, strained cream soups made from the foods allowed.	Any others.
FATS	Butter, margarine, and oils.	Highly spiced salad dressings.
BREADS & CEREALS	Refined bread, toast, rolls, and crackers. Cooked cereal such as Cream of Wheat. Cornmeal, corn-flakes, puffed rice, and puffed wheat.	Any with whole grain or graham flour, bran, seeds or nuts; hot breads and quick breads. Whole grain or bran cereals. Whole grain rice, dried legumes, popcorn.
DESSERTS	Gelatin desserts, tapioca, angel food or sponge cake, plain custard, ice cream without fruit or nuts, cookies, and pudding.	Any made with coconut, nuts, or fruits.
SWEETS	Sugar, honey, jelly, syrups, hard candy, and milk chocolate.	Jam, marmalade, candy with coconut, nuts or whole fruits.
BEVERAGES	Milk as directed by your physician or dietitian. Coffee, tea, and carbonated beverages.	Alcohol.
MISCELLANEOUS	Salt, plain gravy, and cream-style peanut butter.	Garlic, seed spices, pickles, olives, nuts, pepper, chili powder, popcorn, rich gravies, and vinegar.

APPENDIX B: VITAMINS AND MINERALS

Table 1.
Summary of Information on Vitamins

NAME	DAILY RECOMMENDED ALLOWANCES FOR ADULTS	RICH FOOD SOURCES	PHARMACEUTICAL SOURCES	STABILITY	BIOLOGICAL ROLE
FAT-SOLUBLE VITAMINS					
Vitamin A (retinol; pro-vitamin A; α, β, γ carotene)	5000 I.U.	Liver, kidney, milk fat, fortified margarine, egg yolk, yellow and dark green leafy vegetables, apricots, cantaloupe, peaches	Fish liver oils	Stable to light, heat, and usual cooking methods. Destroyed by oxidation, drying, very high temperature, ultraviolet light.	Essential for normal growth, development and maintenance of epithelial tissue. Essential to the integrity of night vision. Essential for health of the eyes. Helps provide for normal bone development and influences normal tooth formation. Toxic in large quantities.
Vitamin D (calciferol)	Sunlight and normal diet are adequate. (400 I.U. in children, pregnancy, and lactation)	Vitamin D milk, irradiated foods, some in milk fat, liver, egg yolk, salmon, tuna fish, sardines	Fish liver oils, concentrates.	Stable to heat and oxidation.	Essential for normal growth and development; important for formation of normal bones and teeth. Influences absorption and metabolism of

	RDA / Daily Requirement	Sources	Synthetic Source	Stability	Functions
					phosphorus and calcium. Prevents and cures rickets and osteomalacia.
Vitamin E (tocopherols)	25–30 mg	Wheat germ, vegetable oils, green leafy vegetables, milk fat, egg yolk, nuts. (Synthesized in intestinal tract)	Wheat germ oil, synthetic	Stable to heat and acids. Destroyed by rancid fats, alkali, oxygen, lead, and iron salts, and ultraviolet irradiation.	Is a strong antioxidant. As such may help prevent oxidation of unsaturated fatty acids and vitamin A in intestinal tract and body tissues. Protects red blood cells from hemolysis. Reproduction (in animals).
Vitamin K (menadione)	Not established. Oral dose of 1–2 mg considered adequate for prophylaxis. Normal diet adequate for healthy persons.	Liver, soybean oil, other vegetable oils, green leafy vegetables, tomatoes, cauliflower, wheat bran. (Synthesized in intestinal tract.)	Synthetic	Resistant to heat, oxygen, and moisture. Destroyed by alkali and ultraviolet light.	Aids in production of prothrombin, a compound required for normal clotting of blood. Toxic in large amounts.
WATER-SOLUBLE VITAMINS					
Thiamin (vitamin B_1)	0.4 mg per 1000 kcalories; older person 1.0 mg per day.	Pork, liver, organs, meats, legumes, whole grain and enriched cereals and breads, wheat germ, potatoes. (Synthesized in intestinal tract.)	Yeast, wheat germ, synthetic.	Unstable in presence of heat or alkali or oxygen. Heat stable in acid solution.	Prevents beriberi. As part of cocarboxylase, aids in removal of CO_2 from alpha keto acids during oxidation of carbohydrates. Essential for growth, normal appetite, digestion and healthy nerves.

(continued)

Table 1. (Cont.)
Summary of Information on Vitamins

NAME	DAILY RECOMMENDED ALLOWANCES FOR ADULTS	RICH FOOD SOURCES	PHARMACEUTICAL SOURCES	STABILITY	BIOLOGICAL ROLE
WATER-SOLUBLE VITAMINS (Cont.)					
Riboflavin (vitamin B_2)	0.6 mg per 1000 kcalories.	Milk and dairy foods, organ meats, green leafy veg., enriched cereals and breads, eggs.	Yeast, liver concentrates, synthetic.	Stable to heat, oxygen, and acid. Unstable to light (especially ultraviolet) or alkali.	Essential for growth. Essential for health of the eyes. Plays enzymatic role in tissue reproduction, and acts as a transporter of hydrogen ions. Coenzyme forms FMN and FAD. Prevents fissures at corners of mouth, around nose and ears, eye irritation, photophobia.
Niacin (nicotinic acid)	13 – 18 mg niacin equivalent or 6.6 mg per 1000 kcalories.	Fish, liver, meat, poultry, many grains, eggs, peanuts, milk, legumes, enriched grains.	Yeast, liver concentrates, synthetic.	Stable to heat, light, oxidation, acid and alkali.	As part of enzyme system, aids in transfer of hydrogen, acts in metabolism of carbohydrates and amino acids. Prevents pellagra, nervous depression, neuritis.
Vitamin B_6 (pyridoxine, pyridoxal and pyridoxamine)	2.0 mg	Pork, glandular meats, cereal bran and germ, milk, egg yolk, oatmeal, legumes.	Yeast, wheat germ, liver concentrates.	Stable to heat, light and oxidation.	As a coenzyme, aids in the synthesis and breakdown of amino acids and in the synthesis of unsaturated fatty

	Functions	Stability	Sources	Requirement
	acids from essential fatty acids. Essential for conversion of tryptophan to niacin. Prevents hypochromic anemia, seborrheic dermatitis, mucous membrane lesions and peripheral neuritis. Essential for normal growth.			
Pantothenic acid	As part of coenzyme. A, functions in the synthesis and breakdown of many vital body compounds. Essential in the intermediary metabolism of carbohydrate, fat, and protein.	Unstable to acid, alkali, heat and certain salts.	Present in all plant and animal foods. Eggs, kidney, liver salmon and yeast are best sources. Yeast, wheat germ, liver concentrates.	Level not yet determined but believe 10 mg adequate. Supplied in normal diet.
Biotin	Probably an essential component of a coenzyme. Appears to be involved in synthesis and breakdown of fatty acids and amino acids through aiding the addition and removal of CO_2 to or from active compounds, and the removal of NH_2 from amino acids. It is closely related metabolically to folic acid and pantothenic acid.	Stable.	Liver, mushrooms, peanuts, yeast, milk, meat, egg yolk, most vegetables, banana, grapefruit, tomato, watermelon, and strawberries. (Synthesized in intestinal tract.) Yeast, liver concentrates.	Not known but 150 to 300 mcg will provide daily needs.

(continued)

Table 1. (Cont.)
Summary of Information on Vitamins

NAME	DAILY RECOMMENDED ALLOWANCES FOR ADULTS	RICH FOOD SOURCES	PHARMACEUTICAL SOURCES	STABILITY	BIOLOGICAL ROLE
WATER-SOLUBLE VITAMINS (Cont.)					
Folacin (folic acid)	Not yet determined but probably 0.1 to 0.2 mg is adequate.	Green leafy vegetables, organ meats (liver), lean beef, wheat, eggs, fish, dry beans, lentils, cowpeas, asparagus, broccoli, collards, yeast. (Synthesized in intestines.)	Yeast, concentrates.	Stable to sunlight when in solution; unstable to heat in acid media.	Appears essential for biosynthesis of nucleic acids and probably for normal fat metabolism. Appears essential for normal maturation of red blood cells. Functions as a coenzyme, tetrahydrofolic acid.
Vitamin B_{12} (cyanocobalamin)	5 μg	Liver, kidney, milk and dairy foods, meat, eggs.	Concentrates, synthetic.	Slowly destroyed by acid, alkali, light and oxidation.	Involved in the metabolism of single-carbon fragments. Essential for biosynthesis of nucleic acids and nucleoproteins, and thereby in normal red blood cell formation, role in metabolism of nervous tissue; probably essential for normal fat metabolism. Related to certain anemias, especially pernicious anemia. Related to growth.

| Ascorbic acid (vitamin C) | 70 mg | | Puerto Rican cherry, citrus fruits, tomatoes, melons, peppers, greens, raw cabbage, guava, strawberries, pineapple, potatoes. | Synthetic. | Unstable to heat, alkali, and oxidation, except in acids. Destroyed by storage. | Essential for growth. Possibly functions as coenzymes in the metabolism of amino acids, particularly phenylalamine and tyrosine; facilitates conversion of folic acid to folinic acid and is essential for many hydroxylation reactions. Role in tooth and bone formation. Maintains intracellular cement substance with preservation of capillary integrity. Promotes healing of wounds and fractures; and reduces liability to infections. Enhances absorption of iron. Essential for production of collagen, the basic substance of connective tissue. Related in some way to biosynthesis of steroid hormones. Prevents scurvy. |

From: Marie V. Krause and Martha A. Hunscher, Food, Nutrition and Diet Therapy, 5th ed. Philadelphia, Saunders, 1972, pp. 111–113.

Table 2.
Mineral Elements in Human Nutrition (Known or Believed to be Essential)

MINERAL	LOCATION IN BODY AND SOME BIOLOGICAL FUNCTIONS	ESTIMATED DAILY REQUIREMENT FOR ADULT	FOOD SOURCES	COMMENTS ON LIKELIHOOD OF A DEFICIENCY
MACROMINERALS				
Calcium	99% in bones and teeth. Ionic calcium in body fluids essential for ion transport across cell membranes. Calcium is also bound to protein, citrate or inorganic acids.	Recommended Dietary Allowance: 800 mg.	Milk and milk products; sardines, clams, oysters, kale, turnip greens, mustard greens, broccoli.	Dietary surveys indicate that many diets do not meet Recommended Dietary Allowances for calcium. Since bone serves as a homeostatic mechanism to maintain calcium level in blood, many essential functions are maintained, regardless of diet. Long term dietary deficiency is probably one of the factors responsible for making osteoporosis (bone-thinning) a significant clinical problem.
Phosphorus	About 80% in inorganic phase of bones and teeth. Phosphorus is a component of every cell and of highly important metabolites including DNA, RNA, ATP (high energy compound), phospholipids. Important to pH regulation.	In ordinary diets, phosphorus intake of adults is approx. 1½ times that of calcium. On an intake of 800 mg calcium, phosphorus intake is approx. 1200 mg.	Cheese, egg yolk, milk, meat, fish, poultry, whole grain cereals, legumes, nuts.	Dietary inadequacy not likely to occur if protein and calcium intake is adequate. However, increased need for phosphorus is postulated with diet leading to acid urine and during prolonged therapy with certain antacids.
Magnesium	About 50% in bone. Remaining 50% is almost entirely inside body cells with only about 1% in extracellular fluid. Ionic Mg functions as an activator of many enzymes and must influence almost all processes.	120 mg/1000 kcal in average diets (200 to 300/mg day)	Whole-grain cereals, nuts, meat, milk, green vegetables, legumes.	Dietary inadequacy considered unlikely, but conditioned deficiency is often seen in clinical medicine, associated with surgery, malabsorption, loss of body fluids, certain hormone and renal diseases, etc.

Magnesium deficiency has a profound effect on other minerals.

	Function	Intake	Food Sources	Remarks
Sodium	30 to 45% in bone. Major cation of extracellular fluid and only a small amount is inside cell. Regulates body fluid osmolarity, pH and body fluid volume.	About 10 g NaCl/day usual intake in U.S. Average diet 2 to 6 g.	Common table salt, seafoods, animal foods, milk, eggs. Abundant in most foods except fruit.	Dietary inadequacy probably never occurs, although low blood sodium requires treatment in certain clinical disorders. Evidence is accumulating that requirements increase during pregnancy. Sodium restriction is practiced in certain cardiovascular disorders.
Chlorine	Major anion of extracellular fluid, functioning in combination with sodium; serves as a buffer, enzyme activator; component of gastric hydrochloric acid. Mostly present in extracellular fluid; less than 15% inside cells.	(Included under sodium).	Common table salt, seafoods, milk, meat, eggs.	In most cases, dietary intake is of little significance except in presence of vomiting, diarrhea or profuse sweating.
Potassium	Major cation of intracellular fluid, with only small amounts in extracellular fluid. Functions in regulating pH and osmolarity, cell membrane transfer. Ion is necessary for carbohydrate and protein metabolism.	Usual diet in U.S. contains from 0.8–1.5 g potassium, 1000 kcal. Average diet 2–4 g	Fruits, milk, meat, cereals, vegetables, legumes.	Dietary inadequacy unlikely, but conditioned deficiency may be found in kidney disease, diabetic acidosis, excessive vomiting or diarrhea, hyperfunction of adrenal cortex, etc. Potassium excess may be a problem in renal failure and severe acidosis.
Sulfur	Bulk of dietary sulfur is present in sulfur-containing amino acids needed for synthesis of essential metabolites; functions in oxidation-reduction reactions. Sulfur also functions in thiamin, biotin, and as inorganic sulfur.	Need for sulfur is satisfied by estimated daily requirements for essential sulfur-containing amino acids and vitamins.	Protein foods (meat, fish, poultry, eggs, milk, cheese, legumes, nuts).	Dietary intake is chiefly from sulfur-containing amino acids and adequacy is related to protein intake.

(continued)

Table 2. (Cont.)
Mineral Elements in Human Nutrition (Known or Believed to be Essential)

MINERAL	LOCATION IN BODY AND SOME BIOLOGICAL FUNCTIONS	ESTIMATED DAILY REQUIREMENT FOR ADULT	FOOD SOURCES	COMMENTS ON LIKELIHOOD OF A DEFICIENCY
MACROMINERALS (Cont.)				
Iron	About 70% is in hemoglobin; about 20% stored in liver, spleen and bone. Iron is component of hemoglobin and myoglobin, important in oxygen transfer; also present in serum transferrin and certain enzymes. Almost none in ionic form.	Recommended Dietary Allowance: 10 mg for adult man; 18 mg for women during child-bearing years.	Liver, meat, egg yolk, legumes, whole or enriched grains, dark green vegetables, dark molasses, shrimp, oysters.	Iron deficiency anemia occurs in women in reproductive years and in infants and preschool children. May be associated in some cases with unusual blood loss, parasites, malabsorption.
MICROMINERALS				
Zinc	Present in most tissues, with higher amounts in liver, voluntary muscle, and bone. Constituent of essential enzymes and insulin. May be of importance in nucleic acid metabolism.	Daily intake estimated as 10–15 mg. Possibility of higher requirements in adolescent boys.	Milk, liver, shellfish, herring, wheat bran (widely distributed).	Zinc deficiency has been demonstrated in Iran and Egypt in certain patients whose diet is also inadequate in protein and iron. Possibility of dietary inadequacy in this country considered remote, but conditioned deficiency may be seen in systemic childhood illnesses; and in patients who are nutritionally depleted or have been subjected to severe stress such as surgery.

Copper	Found in all body tissues; larger amounts in liver, brain, heart and kidney. Constituent of enzymes; of ceruloplasm and erythrocuprein in blood. May be integral part of DNA or RNA molecule.	Daily intake of 2 mg appears to maintain balance; ordinary diets provide 2–5 mg/day.	Liver, shellfish, whole grains, cherries, legumes, kidney, poultry, oysters, chocolate, nuts.	No evidence that specific deficiencies of copper occur in the human.
Iodine	Constituent of thyroxine and related compounds synthesized by thyroid gland. Thyroxine functions in control of reactions involving cellular energy.	100–150 μg.	Iodized table salt, seafoods, water and vegetables in non-goitrous regions.	Iodization of table salt is recommended especially in areas where food is low in iodine. Certain foods contain goitrogens which may accentuate effect of low dietary iodine.
Manganese	Highest concentration is in bone, also relatively high concentrations in pituitary, liver, pancreas and gastrointestinal tissue. Constituent of essential enzyme systems; rich in mitochondria of liver cells.	3–9 mg. For children: 0.2 mg/kg.	Beet greens, blueberries, whole grains, nuts, legumes, fruit, tea.	Unlikely that deficiency occurs in humans.
Fluorine	Present in bone. In optimal amounts in water and diet, reduces dental caries and may minimize bone loss. This effect appears to be due to its combination with bone crystal to form a more stable compound.	Essentiality not established, but appears to be necessary for optimal health of bones and teeth.	Drinking water (1 ppm Fl), tea, coffee, rice, soybeans, spinach, gelatin, onions, lettuce.	In areas where fluorine content of water is low, fluoridation of water (1 ppm) has been found beneficial in reducing incidence of dental caries. (Excess may be toxic.)

(continued)

Table 2. (Cont.)

Mineral Elements in Human Nutrition (Known or Believed to be Essential)

MINERAL	LOCATION IN BODY AND SOME BIOLOGICAL FUNCTIONS	ESTIMATED DAILY REQUIREMENT FOR ADULT	FOOD SOURCES	COMMENTS ON LIKELIHOOD OF A DEFICIENCY
MICROMINERALS (Cont.)				
Molybdenum	Constituent of essential enzyme (xanthine oxidase) and of flavoproteins.	Little quantitative evidence of requirement.	Legumes, cereal grains, dark green leafy vegetables, organs.	No information.
Cobalt	Constituent of cyanocobalamin (vitamin B_{12}), occurring bound to protein in foods of animal origin. Essential to normal function of all cells, particularly cells of bone marrow, nervous system and gastrointestinal system.	3–5 µg vitamin B_{12}.	Liver, kidney, oysters, clams, poultry, milk, variable in vegetables and grains– depends upon cobalt content of soil.	Primary dietary inadequacy is rare except when no animal products are consumed. Deficiency may be found in such conditions as lack of gastric intrinsic factor, gastrectomy, and malabsorption syndromes.
Selenium	Associated with fat metabolism, component of "Factor 3" with vitamin F to prevent fatty liver.	Minute amounts.	Grains, onions, meats, milk, vegetables: variable–depends upon selenium content of soil.	No known deficiency disease seen in man.
Chromium	Associated with glucose metabolism.	Ordinary intake 80–100 µg; approx. 2–5 µg absorbed.	Corn oil, clams, whole-grain cereals, meats, drinking water: variable.	Deficiency found in severe malnutrition, diabetes and cardiovascular diseases.

From: Marie V. Krause and Martha A. Hunscher. Food, Nutrition and Diet Therapy, 5th ed. Philadelphia, Saunders, 1972, pp. 146–147.

Table 3.
Potassium Content of Fruits

Amounts listed are for ¹/₂ cup servings. Foods are listed in order of increasing potassium content.

GROUP I (0.0–1.3 mEq.)

Cranberry juice or cocktail
Lemonade and limeade, frozen diluted
Cranberry sauce
Grape juice drink
Ripe olives
Pear nectar

GROUP II (>1.3–2.6 mEq.)

Green olives
Blueberries, canned
Applesauce, canned
Blueberries, frozen
Peach nectar
Blueberries, fresh
Pears, canned or frozen
Pineapple, canned or frozen
Raspberries, frozen
Watermelon

GROUP III (>2.6–3.8 mEq.)

Apple juice
Lime juice, fresh or canned
Apple, fresh
Strawberries, frozen
Blackberries, canned
Red or black raspberries, canned
Grape juice, bottled or canned
Peaches, frozen
Tangerines, fresh
Bing or Royal Anne cherries, canned
Pears, fresh
Peaches, canned
Grapefruit, fresh or canned
Lemon juice, fresh
Plums, canned
Pineapple, fresh
Figs, canned

GROUP IV (>3.8–5.1 mEq.)

Apricot nectar
Gooseberries, fresh
Grapes, fresh
Fruit cocktail, canned
Grapefruit juice, canned or frozen
Strawberries, fresh
Red or black raspberries, fresh
Plums, fresh
Loganberries and blackberries, fresh
Tangerine juice, canned
Japanese persimmons, fresh
Orange juice, frozen
Unsweetened cherries, frozen
Cherries, fresh
Figs, fresh
Oranges, fresh

GROUP V (>5.1–7.7 mEq.)

Peaches, fresh
Rhubarb, frozen
Papayas, fresh
Apricots, canned
Prune juice
Cantaloupe
Honeydew melon
Apricots, fresh
Nectarine

GROUP VI (>7.7–25.6 mEq.)

Bananas
Avocado
Dates
Prunes, dried
Raisins, dried
Peaches, dried
Apricots, dried

Table 4.
Potassium Content of Vegetables

Amounts listed are for ¹/₂ cup servings. Foods are listed in order of increasing potassium content.

GROUP I (1.3–3.8 mEq.)

Green snap or wax beans, canned
Green peas, canned
Corn, canned
Onions, fresh cooked
Carrots, canned
Sweet potatoes, canned
Sauerkraut, canned
Summer squash, fresh cooked
Turnip greens, frozen cooked
Eggplant, fresh cooked
Green snap beans, frozen cooked

GROUP II (>3.8–5.1 mEq.)

Green snap or wax beans, fresh cooked
Green snap beans, frozen cooked
Mung bean sprouts, fresh cooked
Onions, raw
Cucumbers, raw
Cabbage, fresh cooked
Wax beans, frozen cooked
Okra, frozen cooked
Corn cut off cob, fresh cooked
Asparagus spears, canned
Beets, canned
Rutabaga, fresh cooked
Summer squash, frozen
Okra, fresh cooked
Lettuce, crisphead varieties, raw
Asparagus, fresh cooked
Corn, frozen
Diced turnip roots, fresh cooked
Sweet potatoes, candied
Mixed vegetables, frozen cooked
Corn on the cob, fresh cooked
Green peas, fresh cooked
Mushrooms, canned
Coleslaw with mayonnaise

GROUP III (>5.1–7.7 mEq.)

Cauliflower, fresh or frozen cooked
Winter squash, frozen cooked
Beets, fresh cooked
Lima beans, canned with pork
Green sweet peppers, raw
Tomatoes, canned
Mustard greens, fresh cooked
Broccoli, frozen cooked
Kale, fresh cooked
Carrots, fresh cooked
Lima beans (immature), canned
Cabbage, raw
Tomato juice, canned
Black-eyed peas, dry cooked
Collard greens, fresh cooked
Asparagus spears, frozen
Celery, fresh cooked
Pumpkin, canned
Sweet potato, boiled in skin
Tomatoes, raw
Succotash, frozen
Spinach, canned
Chinese or celery cabbage, fresh
Winter squash, cooked and mashed
White potato mashed with milk
Red pinto beans, canned
Broccoli, fresh cooked
White potato, peeled and boiled
Tomatoes, fresh cooked
Brussel sprouts, frozen
Dry split peas, cooked

(continued)

Table 4 (Cont.)
Potassium Content of Vegetables

GROUP IV (>7.7–10.3 mEq.)

Sweet potato, baked
Swiss chard, fresh cooked
Radishes, raw
Spinach, fresh cooked
Beet greens, fresh cooked
Red pinto beans, dry cooked
Celery, raw
Carrots, raw
Spinach, chopped, frozen cooked
Black-eyed peas, frozen cooked
Black-eyed peas, canned
Spinach, leaf, frozen cooked
Black-eyed peas, fresh cooked
Parsnips, fresh cooked
Baby lima beans, frozen cooked

GROUP V (>10.3–38.5 mEq.)

Lima beans, immature, fresh cooked
Fordhook lima beans, frozen cooked
Winter squash, baked
Potato, baked
Parsnips, raw
Lima beans, mature, dry cooked
French fried potatoes, frozen cooked
French fried potatoes, fresh cooked
Potato chips

From: Clara M. Lewis, Sodium and Potassium. *Philadelphia, F. A. Davis, 1976, pp. S-153–S-155.*

APPENDIX C: DESIRABLE WEIGHTS FOR PERSONS AGE 25 AND OVER

Table 1
Men

HEIGHT (WITH SHOES ON) 1-INCH HEELS		SMALL* FRAME	MEDIUM* FRAME	LARGE* FRAME
Feet	**Inches**			
5	2	112–120	118–129	126–141
5	3	115–123	121–133	129–144
5	4	118–126	124–136	132–148
5	5	121–129	127–139	135–152
5	6	124–133	130–143	138–156
5	7	128–137	134–147	142–161
5	8	132–141	138–152	147–166
5	9	136–145	142–156	151–170
5	10	140–150	146–160	155–174
5	11	144–154	150–165	159–179
6	0	148–158	154–170	164–184
6	1	152–162	158–175	168–189
6	2	156–167	162–180	173–194
6	3	160–171	167–185	178–199
6	4	164–175	172–190	182–204

*Weight in pounds according to frame (in indoor clothing).
From: Metropolitan Life Insurance, New York (with permission).

Table 2
Women*

HEIGHT (WITH SHOES ON) 2-INCH HEELS		SMALL† FRAME	MEDIUM† FRAME	LARGE† FRAME
Feet	Inches			
4	10	92−98	96−107	104−119
4	11	94−101	98−110	106−122
5	0	96−104	101−113	109−125
5	1	99−107	104−116	112−128
5	2	102−110	107−119	115−131
5	3	105−113	110−122	118−134
5	4	108−116	113−126	121−138
5	5	111−119	116−130	125−142
5	6	114−123	120−135	129−146
5	7	118−127	124−139	133−150
5	8	122−131	128−143	137−154
5	9	126−135	132−147	141−158
5	10	130−140	136−151	145−163
5	11	134−144	140−155	149−168
6	0	138−148	144−159	153−173

*For girls between 18 and 25, subtract 1 pound for each year under 25.
†weight in pounds according to frame (in indoor clothing).
From: Metropolitan Life Insurance, New York (with permission).

APPENDIX E:
STUART PERCENTILE
CURVES FOR INFANTS
AND CHILDREN

INFANT GIRLS AND BOYS

The accompanying graphs provide for infant girls and infant boys standards of reference for body weight and recumbent length by month from birth to 28 months and for head circumference by week from birth to 28 weeks. It is based on repeated measurements at selected ages of a group of more than 100 white infant girls and 100 white infant boys of North European ancestry living under normal conditions of health and home life in Boston, Mass. The distribution of the measurements obtained from the infants at each age is expressed in percentiles, each percentile giving a value which represents a particular position in the normal range of occurrences. The number of the percentile refers to the position which a measurement of the given value would hold in any typical series of 100 infants. Thus the 10th percentile gives the value for the tenth in any hundred; that is, 9 infants of the same sex and age would be expected to be smaller in the measurement under consideration while 90 would be expected to be larger than the figure given. Similarly the 90th percentile would indicate that 89 infants might be expected to be smaller than the figure given while 10 would be larger. The 50th percentile represents the median or midposition in the customary range. Here, the 10th and 90th percentiles are presented in heavy lines to show the limits within which most infants remain. The lighter lines in the graphs divide the distributions into segments for ready recognition and description of individual differences as well as of the "regularity" of progress. The 3rd and 97th percentiles represent unusual though not necessarily abnormal findings.

In line with common usage in the United States, the charts are ruled on a scale in pounds to represent weight. They are ruled, however, in centimeters to represent length and head circumference, because this scale facilitates accuracy in measuring and recording and centimeter rules and tapes are readily available. For the convenience of those preferring them, scales for kilograms and inches are placed outside of the principal scales and paralleling them. Therefore, if weights are taken in kilograms and lengths and head circumferences in inches, they may be plotted directly without conversion by placing a ruler at the appropriate points on the outer scales of the charts.

To determine the percentile position of any measurement at a given age, the vertical age line is located and a dot is placed where this intersects the horizontal line representing the value obtained from the measurement. Vertical lines give age by 1-month intervals for weight and length and 1-week intervals for head circumference; horizontal lines give 1/2-pound, 1-cm, and 0.5-cm intervals, respectively. This permits by interpolation accurate placement for age to weeks, for weights to 2 ounces and for centimeters to 0.5 cm. Recognition of the position within or outside of the range held by an infant in respect to each measurement recorded calls attention to the relative size and build of the individual at the time. More importantly, comparisons of percentile positions held by these measurements at repeated periodic examinations, indicate adherence to or possibly significant deviation from previous percentile positions. Under normal circumstances, one expects an infant to maintain a similar position from age to age—that is, on or near one percentile line or between the same two lines. Occasional sharp deviations or gradual, but continuing shifts from one percentile position to another call for further investigation as to their causes. In all cases, readings of measurements should be checked and

From: The Children's Medical Center, Boston, Massachusetts, with permission.

STUART PERCENTILE CURVES

INFANT GIRLS

NAME   BIRTH DATE   NO.

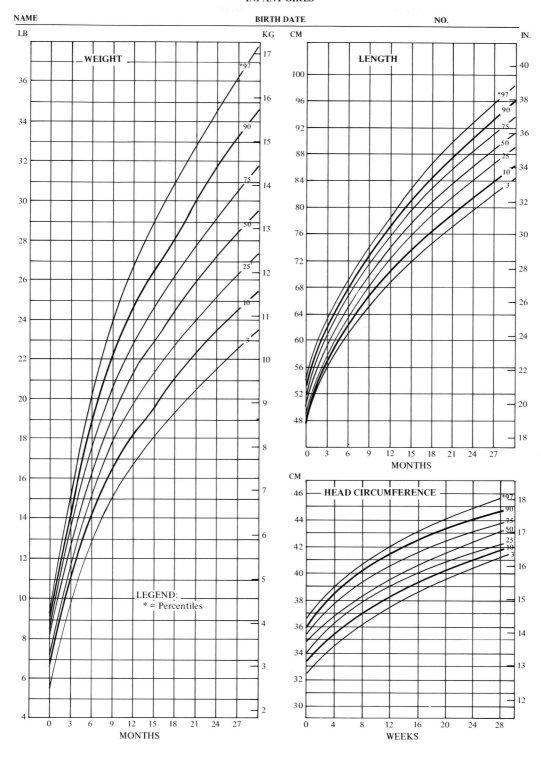

care should be taken to secure the same position of the infant at all examinations. The following procedures were used in obtaining these norms and therefore are recommended:

- *Body Weight*—The infant is weighed without clothing, preferably on special infant scales.
- *Recumbent Length*—The infant lies relaxed on a firm surface parallel to a centimeter rule or on a special infant measuring board which permits the following procedure. The soles of the feet are held firmly against a fixed upright at the zero mark on the rule, and a movable square is brought firmly against the vertex. Care must be taken to secure extension at the knees, and the head should be held so that the eyes face the ceiling.
- *Head Circumference*—This measurement is more satisfactory if taken with the infant lying on his back. The tape is passed around the head from above and placed anteriorly over the lower forehead just above the supraorbital ridges. With the position of the tape thus fixed anteriorly, the largest circumference is obtained by passing it posteriorly over the most prominent part of the occiput.

GIRLS AND BOYS

The accompanying graphs provide for girls and boys standards of reference for body weight and recumbent length at ages between 2 and 6 years and for weight and standing height from 6 to 13 years. It is based on repeated measurements at selected ages of a group of more than 100 white girls and 100 white boys of North European ancestry living under normal conditions of health and home life in Boston, Mass. The distribution of the measurements obtained from these children at each age is expressed in percentiles, each percentile giving a value which represents a particular position in the normal range of occurrences. The number of the percentile refers to the position which a measurement of the given value would hold in any typical series of 100 children. Thus the 10th percentile gives the value for the tenth in any hundred; that is, 9 children of the same sex and age would be expected to be smaller in the measurement under consideration while 90 would be expected to

be larger than the figure given. Similarly the 90th percentile would indicate that 89 children might be expected to be smaller than the figure given while 10 would be larger. The 50th percentile represents the median or midposition in the customary range. Here, the 10th and 90th percentiles are represented in heavy lines to show the limits within which most children remain. The lighter lines in the graphs divide the distribution into segments for ready recognition and description of individual differences as well as of the "regularity" of progress. The 3rd and 97th percentiles represent unusual though not necessarily abnormal findings.

In line with common usage in the United States, the charts are ruled on a scale in pounds to represent weight. They are ruled, however, in centimeters to represent length under 6 years and height thereafter, because this scale facilitates accuracy in measuring and recording and centimeter rules and tapes are readily available. For the convenience of those preferring them, scales for kilograms and inches are placed outside of the principal scales and paralleling them. Therefore, if weights are taken in kilograms and lengths and heights in inches, they may be plotted directly without conversion by placing a ruler at the appropriate points on the outer scales of the chart.

To determine the percentile position of any measurement at a given age, the vertical age line is located and a dot is placed where this intersects the horizontal line representing the value obtained from the measurement. Vertical lines give age by 2-month intervals and horizontal lines by 2-pound and 2-cm intervals. This permits by interpolation accurate placement for age to $1/2$ month and for measurements to $1/2$ pound or 0.5 cm. Recognition of the position held by a child within or outside of the range in respect to each measurement recorded calls attention to the relative size and build of the individual at the time. More importantly, comparisons of percentile positions held by these measurements at repeated periodic examinations indicate adherence to or possibly significant deviation from previous percentile positions. Under normal circumstances, one expects a child to maintain a similar position from age to age—that is, on or near one percentile line or between the same two lines. Occasionally encountered sharp deviations or more gradual but continuing shifts from one percentile position to another call for further investigation as to their causes. In all cases, readings of measurements should be checked and care should be taken to secure the same position of the child accurately at all examinations. The following procedures were used in

INFANT BOYS

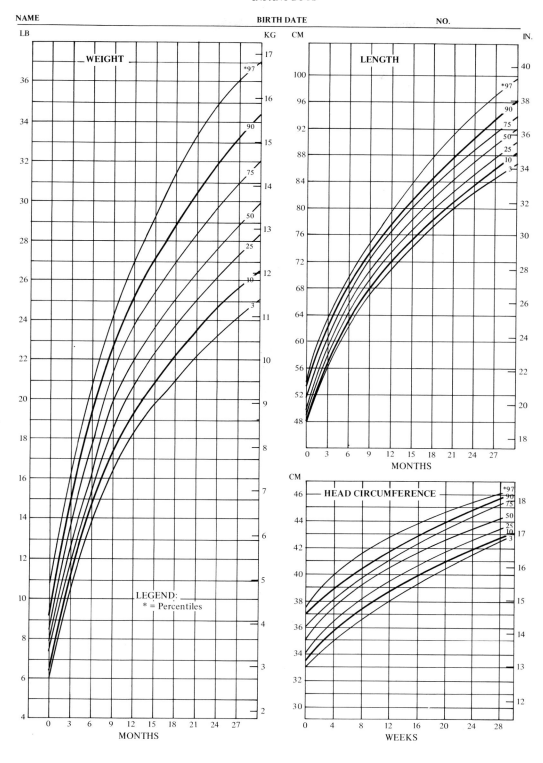

obtaining these norms and therefore are recommended:

- *Body Weight*—The child is weighed without clothing except light undergarments.
- *Recumbent Length*—The child lies relaxed on a firm surface parallel to a centimeter rule. The soles of the feet are held firmly against a fixed upright at the zero mark on the rule, and a movable square is brought firmly against the vertex. The head is held so that the eyes face the ceiling.

- *Height*—The child's heels should be near together, and heels, buttocks, and occiput should be against a firm vertical upright mounting the measuring stick. The eyes should be horizontal and approximately in the same plane as the external auditory canals. A right-angle triangle or other movable device should be placed firmly on the head at right angles to the measuring stick and the measurement read after a satisfactory position has been adopted.

GIRLS

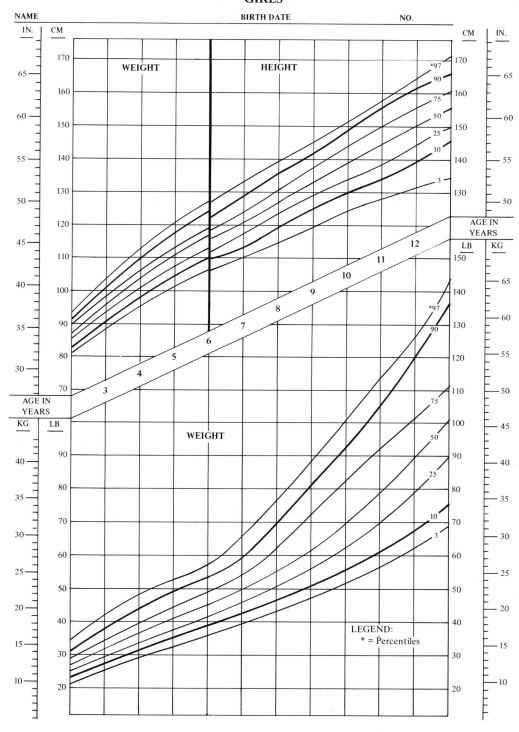

BOYS

NAME   BIRTH DATE   NO.

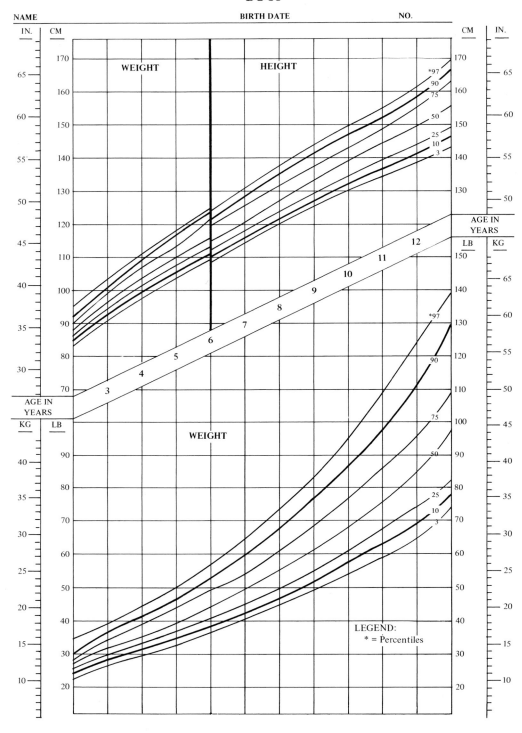

LEGEND:
* = Percentiles

APPENDIX F: NURSING ORGANIZATIONS

American Association of Colleges of Nursing
(AACN)—1969*
Washington, D.C. 20009

American Association of Critical Care Nurses
(AACN)
P. O. Box 5445
Orange, California 92667
Official Publication: *Heart and Lung: The Journal of Critical Care*

American Association of Industrial Nurses
(AAIN)—1942
79 Madison Avenue
New York, New York 10016
Official Publication: *Occupational Health Nursing*

American Association of Nurse Anesthetists
(AANA)—1931
111 East Wacker Drive
Chicago, Illinois 60601
Official Publication: *The Journal of the American Association of Nurse Anesthetists*

American Nurses' Association (ANA)—1897
2420 Pershing Road
Kansas City, Missouri 64108
Official Publication: *American Journal of Nursing*

Association of Operating Room Nurses
(AORN)—1957
10170 East Mississippi Avenue
Denver, Colorado 80231
Official Publication: *AORN Journal*

International Council of Nurses (ICN)
37 Rue de Vermont
1202 Geneva, Switzerland
Official Publication: *International Nursing Review*

National Black Nurses' Association (NBNA)—1971
P. O. Box 8295
Canton, Ohio 44711

National League for Nursing (NLN)—1952
10 Columbus Circle
New York, New York 10019

National Student Nurses Association (NSNA)—
1953
10 Columbus Circle
New York, New York, 10019
Official Publication: *Imprint*

Nurses Coalition for Political Action (N-Cap)—
1974 (Address same as ANA)

Sigma Theta Tau—1922
1232 West Michigan, Room 347
Indianapolis, Indiana 46202
Official Publication: *Image*

The American Association for Nephrology Nurses
and Technicians (AAANNT)—1969
Middle City Station, P. O. Box 2368
Philadelphia, Pennsylvania 19103

The American Association of Neurosurgical Nurses
(AANN)—1968
428 East Preston Street
Baltimore, Maryland 21203
Official Publication: *The Journal of Neurosurgical Nursing*

The American College of Nurse Midwives (ACNM)
50 East 92nd Street
New York, New York 10028
Official Publication: *The Journal of Nurse Midwifery*

The Nurses' Association of the American College of
Obstetricians and Gynecologists (NAACOG)—
1969
1 East Wacker Drive, Suite 2700
Chicago, Illinois 60601
Official Publication: *Journal of Obstetric, Gynecologic and Neonatal Nursing*

---

*Dates following organization name indicate when founded.

APPENDIX G:
RELATED PROFESSIONAL
ORGANIZATIONS

American College of Hospital Administration (ACHA)—1933*
840 North Lake Shore Drive
Chicago, Illinois 60611
Official Publication: *Hospital Administration*

American Hospital Association (AHA)—1898
840 North Lake Shore Drive
Chicago, Illinois 60611
Official Publication: *Hospitals, Journal of the American Hospital Association*

American Medical Association (AMA)—1847
840 North Lake Shore Drive
Chicago, Illinois 60611
Official Publication: *Journal of the American Medical Association* (also publishes *Todays Health* for the lay person)

---

*Dates following organization name indicate when founded.

American Nursing Home Association (ANHA)—1949
1200 15th Street N.W.
Washington, D.C. 20005
Official Publication: *Nursing Homes*

National Association for Practical Nurse Education and Service (NAPNES)—1941
122 East 42nd Street
New York, New York 10017
Official Publication: *Journal of Practical Nursing*

The American Public Health Association (APHA)—1872
1015 18th Street N.W.
Washington, D.C. 20036
Official Publication: *American Journal of Public Health*

World Health Organization (WHO)—1948
1211 Geneva, 27
Switzerland

770

APPENDIX H: RESOURCES ON HEALTH CARE NEEDS FOR THE NURSE AND THE INDIVIDUAL

Abbott Laboratories
North Chicago, Illinois 60064

Action
Washington, D.C. 20525

Administration on Aging
U.S. Department of Health, Education and Welfare
Washington, D.C. 20201

Al-Anon
Family Group Headquarters
P. O. Box 182
Madison Square Station
New York, New York 10010

American Academy of Facial, Plastic and Reconstructive Surgery, Inc.
1110 West Main Street
Durham, North Carolina 27701

American Association of Retired Persons
1909 K Street N.W.
Washington, D.C. 20049

American Cancer Society
219 East 42nd Street
New York, New York 10017

American Dental Association
211 East Chicago Avenue
Chicago, Illinois 60611

American Diabetes Association, Inc.
18 East 48th Street
New York, New York 10017

American Dietetic Association
620 North Michigan Avenue
Chicago, Illinois 60611

American Foundation for the Blind
15 West 16th Street
New York, New York 10011

American Heart Association
44 East 23rd Street
New York, New York 10010

American Lung Association
1740 Broadway
New York, New York 10019

American National Red Cross
17th and D Street, N.W.
Washington, D.C. 20006

American Orthotics and Prosthetics Association
1440 N Street N.W.
Washington, D.C. 20005

American Parkinson Disease Foundation
147 East 50th Street
New York, New York 10022

American Pyschological Association
1200 17th Street N.W.
Washington, D.C. 20036

American Speech and Hearing Association
9030 Old Georgetown Road
Washington, D.C. 20014

Bird Space Technology
Respirator Lane
Palm Springs, California 92262

Carnation Company
5045 Wilshire Boulevard
Los Angeles, California 90036

Center for Disease Control
Atlanta, Georgia 30333

Committee to Combat Huntington's Disease
Suite 2016
200 West 57th Street
New York, New York 10019

Concern for Dying
250 West 57th Street
New York, New York 10019

Cutter Laboratories
Berkeley, California 94710

Division for the Blind and Physically Handicapped
Library of Congress
Washington, D.C. 20542

Division of Enforcement and Emergency Services
Department of Transportation
National Highway Traffic Safety Administration
Department of Transportation
Washington, D.C. 20590

Eaton Laboratories
Norwich, New York 13815

Epilepsy Foundation of America
Suite 406
1828 L Street N.W.
Washington, D.C. 20036

Ethicon Inc.
Somerville, New Jersey 08876

Everest and Jennings, Inc.
1803 Pontius Avenue
Los Angeles, California 90025

C. B. Fleet Company, Inc.
Lynchburg, Virginia 24505

Gomco Surgical Manufacturing Corporation
828 East Ferry Street
Buffalo, New York 14211

Guide Dogs for the Blind, Inc.
San Rafael, California 94902

Hollister Incorporated
211 East Chicago Avenue
Chicago, Illinois 60611

Institute of Rehabilitation Medicine
400 East 34th Street
New York, New York 10016

International Association of Laryngectomees
219 East 42nd Street
New York, New York 10017

International Association for Suicide Prevention
2521 West Pico Boulevard
Los Angeles, California 90006

Leukemia Society of America, Inc.
211 East 43rd Street
New York, New York 10017

Lumex, Inc.
100 Spence Street
Bay Shore, New York 11706

Mead Johnson Laboratories, Inc.
Evansville, Indiana 44721

Metropolitan Life Insurance Company
Health and Welfare Division
1 Madison Avenue
New York, New York 10010

Muscular Dystrophy Association of America, Inc.
1790 Broadway
New York, New York 10019

Myasthenia Gravis Foundation, Inc.
New York Academy of Medicine Building
2 East 103rd Steet
New York, New York 10029

National Association of the Deaf
814 Thayer Avenue
Silver Springs, Maryland 20910

National Committee for Prevention of Child Abuse
111 East Wacker Drive
Suite 510
Chicago, Illinois 60607

National Council on Aging
1828 L Street N.W.
Washington, D.C. 20036

National Foundation—March of Dimes
1275 Mamaroneck Avenue
White Plains, New York 10605

National Heart and Lung Institute
National Institutes of Health
Bethesda, Maryland 20014

National Hemophilia Foundation
25 West 39th Street
New York, New York 10018

National Humanistic Education Center
110 Spring Street
Saratoga Springs, New York 12866

National Institute of Arthritis, Metabolism and Digestive Disease
National Institutes of Health
Bethesda, Maryland 20014

National Institute of Neurological Disease and Stroke
National Institutes of Health
Bethesda, Maryland 20014

National Kidney Foundation
116 East 27th Street
New York, New York 10016

National Multiple Sclerosis Society
257 Park Avenue South
New York, New York 10010

National Paraplegia Foundation
33 North Michigan Avenue
Chicago, Illinois 60601

National Psoriasis Foundation
Suite 250
6415 S.W. Canyon Court
Portland, Oregon 97221

National Safety Council
425 North Michigan Avenue
Chicago, Illinois 60611

National SIDS Foundation
Suite 1904
310 South Michigan Avenue
Chicago, Illinois 60604

Office of Vocational Rehabilitation
United States Department of Health, Education and Welfare
Washington, D.C. 20402

Planned Parenthood—World Population
515 Madison Avenue
New York, New York 10022

Presidents Committee on Mental Retardation
R.O.B. Building
Washington, D.C. 20201

Public Health Service
Department of Health, Education and Welfare
North Building
Washington, D.C. 20201
(P.H.S. has 6 agencies: National Institutes of Health; Health Services Administration; Center for Disease Control; Food and Drug Administration; Alcohol, Drug Abuse and Mental Health Administration; and the Health Resources Administration—one of the Health Resources subdivisions is the Division of Nursing.)

Rape Crisis Center
Box 21005
Washington, D.C. 20009

Reach to Recovery Foundation
19 West 56th Street
New York, New York 10019

Recording for the Blind, Inc.
121 East 58th Street
New York, New York 10022

Rehabilitation Services Administration
Department of Health, Education and Welfare
330 C Street S.W.
Washington, D.C. 20201

Sex Information and Education Council of the United States
1855 Broadway
New York, New York 10019

Stryker Company
843 Ocean Front
Long Beach, New York 11561

The Arthritis Foundation
1212 Avenue of the Americas
New York, New York 10036

The Foundation for Research and Education in Sickle-Cell Disease
421-431 West 120th Street
New York, New York 10027

The Society of Compassionate Friends
P. O. Box 181 LV
Lathrup Village, Michigan 48076

Travenol Laboratories, Inc.
Morton Grove, Illinois 60053

United Cerebral Palsy Association, Inc.
66 East 34th Street
New York, New York 10016

United Ostomy Association
1111 Wilshire Boulevard
Los Angeles, California 90017

Veterans Administration Prosthetic Center
Veterans Administration
252 7th Avenue
New York, New York 10001

Wyeth Laboratories
Philadelphia, Pennsylvania 19101

Zimmer, USA
727 North Detroit Street
Warsaw, Indiana 46580

APPENDIX I:
REFERENCE SOURCES
FOR NURSES

PUBLICATIONS

(Other than those listed as official publications for nursing organizations)

Canadian Nurse
50, The Driveway
Ottawa 4, Ontario, Canada

Cardiovascular Nursing
The American Heart Association
44 East 23rd Street
New York, New York 10010

Journal of Continuing Education in Nursing
6900 Grove Road
Thorofare, New Jersey 08086

Journal of Gerontological Nursing
Charles B. Slack, Inc.
6900 Grove Road
Thorofare, New Jersey 08086

Journal of Nursing Education
Charles B. Slack, Inc.
6900 Grove Road
Thorofare, New Jersey 08086

Journal of Nursing Administration
12 Lakeside Park
607 North Avenue
Wakefield, Massachusetts 01880

Journal of School Health
American School Health Association
200 East Main Street
Kent, Ohio 44240

Nursing 80 (year changes)
Intermed Communications, Inc.
132 Welsh Road
Horsham, Pennsylvania 19044

Nurse Educator
Contemporary Publishing, Inc.
12 Lakeside Park
Wakefield, Massachusetts 01880

Nursing Leadership
Charles B. Slack, Inc.
6900 Grove Road
Thorofare, New Jersey 08086

Nursing Clinics of North America
W. B. Saunders Company
West Washington Square
Philadelphia, Pennsylvania 19105

Nursing Dimensions
Nursing Resources, Inc.
12 Lakeside Park
607 North Avenue
Wakefield, Massachusetts 01880

Nursing Education Monographs
Bureau of Publications
Teachers College
Columbia University
New York, New York 10027

Nursing Forum
Nursing Publications
P. O. Box 218
Hillsdale, New Jersey 07642

Nursing Outlook
10 Columbus Circle
New York, New York 10019

Nursing Research
10 Columbus Circle
New York, New York 10019

Nursing Research Report
American Foundation of Nurses
2420 Pershing Road
Kansas City, Missouri 64108

R.N.
Oradell, New Jersey 07649

Supervisory Nurse
S-N Publications, Inc.
18 South Michigan Avenue
Chicago, Illinois 60603

Abstracts of Hospital Management Studies,
University of Michigan, Ann Arbor, Michigan 48109

American Journal of Nursing Index

International Nursing Index
American Journal of Nursing Company

Nursing Studies Index, Va. Henderson, Phila. J. B.
Lippincott

Nursing Research Index

Nursing Outlook Index

INDEXES

Cumulative Index to Nursing and Allied Health Literature
Glendale Medical Center, Glendale, California 91209

COMPUTER SERVICES

Medline

Avline

GLOSSARY OF TERMS

Absorption   The transfer of substances from the gastrointestinal tract into the tissues.

Acapnea   Low $PaCO_2$ levels while PaO_2 levels remain fairly constant.

Accountability   Professional responsibility for maintaining safe, competent skills; protecting individuals within the care situation; promoting their well-being; understanding implications of care; improving professional standards of practice; and advocating societal well-being.

Accreditation   The professional process through which a recognized group or agency determines, evaluates, and recognizes the ability of an institution, educational body, or agency to provide professional services and practice.

Acknowledgment   Fourth phase of behavior of coping with loss, characterized by recognition of implications.

Action of a drug   The particular cellular activity produced by a drug to bring about an intended response.

Active immunity   Immunity acquired by specific exposure to an antigen with a resultant formation of antibodies.

Acts of commission   Activities of care the nurse performs which result in damage to the individual or the individual's property.

Acts of omission   Activities the nurse fails to perform which result in damage to the individual or the individual's property.

Actual power   The visible influence one realistically has over others.

Adaptation   The process of compensation to stress.

Addiction   The process which occurs when prolonged use of a substance creates a physiologic dependence in body tissues.

Adhesion   The connection of two tissue surfaces which are usually not connected.

Adventitious sounds   Unexpected breath sounds produced by trapped air or secretions.

Advocate   One who works with, or on behalf of, a person or system to bring about a positive difference in the individual's or system's state or condition of health.

Aerosol   Solid or liquid particles suspended in a gas.

Affect   The emotional content of behavior.

Agent   Any biologic, chemical, physical, mechanical, or psychosocial mechanism which has the potential for creating illness.

Agnosia   The inability to use familiar objects in a purposeful and appropriate manner.

Alarm phase   First step in the General Adaptation Syndrome; sympathetic stimulation prepares the person for rapid response to stress (fight or flight phase).

Algor mortis   The loss of body heat after death.

Anabolism   The buildup of body tissue and substances.

Analgesic   Medication which relieves pain.

Anaphylactic shock   A life-threatening emergency caused by a hypersensitivity to an agent, resulting in complete circulatory and respiratory collapse.

Anemia   Reduced hemoglobin levels in the blood.

Anions   Particles which carry a negative charge.

Anorexia   A loss of appetite.

Antibody   A globulin produced by the lymphoid tissue in response to an antigen.

Antigen   Material foreign to the body and capable of inducing antibody formation.

Antisepsis   The retardation of the growth of organisms.

Anxiety   A diffuse feeling of dread and apprehension.

Apathy   Lack of interest.

Aphasia   The inability to understand and/or use written or spoken communication.

Appetite   Subjective desire for a food or food group.

Apraxia   The inability to recognize previously known, common stimuli by use of the senses.

Arrhythmia   Irregularity of the heartbeat.

Arteriosclerosis   Loss of elasticity of the blood vessel wall.

Ascribed groups   Groups whose members have voluntarily chosen to be members.

Aseptic practice   Activity which prevents infection.

Aspiration   The inhalation of fluids, food, or foreign objects into the lungs.

Assessment   The collection, organization, and analysis of information relevant to the person's health status at a given time.

Assigned groups   Groups into which members are born or involuntarily drafted.

Atelectasis   Localized alveolar collapse.

Atherosclerosis   Build-up of fatty plaques on the walls of the blood vessels.

Atrophy   The decrease in size and tone of body tissue.

Auscultation   The process of listening for sounds made by the body.

Avascularity   A lack of blood vessels.

Bacteriocidal   An agent which destroys microorganisms.

Bacteriostasis   The inhibition of the growth of microorganisms.

Basal metabolic rate (BMR)   The energy expenditure of the individual at rest; rate at which nutrients are metabolized when the individual is at rest.

Basic four food groups   Categorization of foods which provide the basic nutrients; these include the dairy; meat, fish, and poultry; fruit and vegetable; and bread and cereal groups.

Basic health care needs   Those needs which relate to the individual's state of health.

Basic human needs   The essential requirements to maintain life; promote physical and physiologic growth and psychosocial development; and achieve and maintain wellness.

Barriers to change   Any factors that impede the attainment of desired change.

Barriers to communication   Those factors which hinder the communication process.

Base of support   Foundation for stability of an object.

Bilateral   Occurring on both sides of the body.

Biologic rhythms   The unique internal rhythms of the individual which guide the pattern of life processes.

Biologic safety   The protection of the individual against invasion from potentially harmful agents and the possible sequelae of this invasion.

Biologic sex   The physical sex characteristics and chromosonal and hormonal makeup of the individual.

Body aesthetics   The personal process of maintaining one's structure and form so that self-image is maximized.

Body alignment   The anatomical relationship of one body segment to another.

Body image   The holistic picture of self as seen by an individual.

Body kinetics   The study of the movement of the human body.

Bradypnea   Decreased respiratory rate.

Breath sounds   Sounds heard from the usual movement of air through the respiratory tree.

Bruit   The rushing sound which is heard over an artery which reflects a murmur.

Buccal mucosa   Mucous membrane lining of the oral cavity.

Bureaucracy   A formalized organization of people which has as its aim maximum productivity.

Calculi   The abnormal precipitation of minerals in the body.

Carbon dioxide (CO_2) narcosis   Unconscious state due to high $PaCO_2$ levels.

Cardiac arrest   Sudden cessation of the heartbeat resulting in circulatory collapse.

Catabolism   The breakdown of food, body tissues, and substances to release energy.

Cathartic   *See* Laxative.

Catheterization   Insertion of a tube into a body orifice; usually a sterile procedure.

Cation   Particle which carries a positive charge.

Center of gravity   The point at which the mass of an object is concentrated.

Central cyanosis   The dusky or hazy-blue skin color occurring all over the body which results from inadequate oxygen uptake and increased levels of reduced hemoglobin.

Central venous pressure   Pressure of the blood in the right atrium of the heart.

Certification   The professional process of determining and evaluating that predetermined standards are met for specialized practice.

Change   The planned and goal-oriented process of assisting the individual or group in repatterning and modifying internal and external environments.

Change process   The recognition and analysis of a situation where change can take place; includes phases of unfreezing, movement, and refreezing.

Chart   The individual's written health care record.

Chemical name   Identifies chemical structure and composition of a drug.

Chronic obstructive lung disease (C.O.L.D.)   Fibrosis and loss of elasticity of lung tissue resulting from long-term obstruction of the respiratory tree.

Circadian rhythms   Rhythms which run in 24-hour cycles.

Circulatory collapse   Cardiac activity is decreased to the point where tissue perfusion is not sufficient for vital functioning.

Civil law   The branch of law which deals with the protection of individual rights and property.

Claudication   The hyperflexion of a body joint.

Clean   Surface with a minimal number of microorganisms.

Clinical specialist   A nurse who is an expert in a particular area of nursing practice.

Close-ended questions   Questions requiring a word or short phrase in response.

Clubbing   The increase in or flattening of the angle between the base of the nail and the nail.

Coagulation time   The time, in minutes, required for blood to clot.

Cognitive abilities   Those higher associative and interpretive capabilities which allow the individual to learn new behaviors and modify old ones, to reason, to conceptualize, and to utilize and generate new knowledge.

Cognitive dissonance   A state of tension which develops in an individual as a result of a communication interaction.

Colostomy   A surgical opening in the abdomen to which a portion of resected bowel has been attached.

Colostomy stoma   The portion of the bowel which protrudes externally after a colostomy.

Comfort   A relative and subjective state of well-being which cannot be directly assessed by anyone except the individual.

Communicable disease   An illness caused by a specific agent which has been transmitted to a host.

Communication   The dynamic multisensory interchange between two or more persons.

Confinement deprivation   State resulting when an individual is separated from significant others and familiar objects.

Constipation   A decrease in the frequency of bowel movements resulting in drier feces.

Consumerism   The process which individuals use to increase the control they have over decisions in their lives and their choice of products and services.

Content   A component of communication combining vocabulary and syntax.

Context   The approach of a particular communication.

Contract   A collaborative agreement between the nurse and the individual concerning the provision of nursing care.

Contracture   Musculoskeletal deformity which results when, in any group of antagonizing muscles, the stronger muscles dominate over the opposing ones.

Controlled substances   Substances which have a potential for addiction.

Cough   Forceful expiration of air following an intake of air.

Creativity   The generation of new patterns of thought and actions utilizing the ideas drawn from thinking critically in original ways.

Credentialing   The professional process for determining and maintaining competency in the practice of professional nursing.

Crepitation   The grating of two bone surfaces rubbing against each other.

Criminal law   The branch of law which applies to the welfare of society as a whole.

Crisis   A life situation in which a person's usual methods of coping with stressors are not adequate; may be situational or maturational; occurs in five phases: shock, general realization, defensive retreat, acknowledgment, and resolution.

Crisis intervention   An interactional process of mutual problem-solving.

Critical thinking   A logical pattern of thought based on knowledge, experience, problem-solving ability, and reasoning.

Crutch palsy   Damage to and paresis of the radial nerve resulting from prolonged pressure on the axilla.

Culture   The traditions, experiences, practices, beliefs, and values developed by a group of persons and passed on from generation to generation.

Cytology   The study of cell structure and function.

Decubitus ulcer   Skin lesion resulting from a decrease in oxygen and nutrient supply to an area.

Deductive reasoning   The drawing of specific conclusions from general theories or principles.

Deep pain   Pain occurring in deep viscera or tissues.

Defensive retreat   Third phase of pattern of coping with loss. Characterized by avoidance techniques to protect self from reality.

Dermatomes   Zones of innervation.

Designated power   The power given to a person by a recognized authority source.

Diarrhea   Increased frequency of bowel evacuation resulting in watery, nonformed feces.

Diastolic pressure   The resistance of blood on the arterial wall during diastole.

Diffuse pain   Generalized pain occurring throughout the whole body or a large body area.

Digestion   The breakdown and absorption of food.

Dimpling   Puckering of the skin.

Direct contact   Contact of a host with a contaminated reservoir.

Discomfort   A feeling of unease, tension, irritation, low energy, and dissatisfaction experienced when needs are not met.

Disinfection   The process of killing microorganisms but not their spores.

Distortion in body image   Any change in the self-concept which is at variance with the individual's previous, more positive one and which interferes with the individual's level of functioning.

Diverticula   Outpouching of the mucous membrane lining of a body passage (e.g., intestines); results from deviation in surrounding muscles.

Dullness   The sound produced by percussing tissues that are relatively dense, e.g., kidney, spleen, liver.

Dyspnea   The individual's subjective awareness of difficulty in breathing.

Edema   Increased fluid in the interstitial tissues resulting in pallor and swelling. A surface manifestation of obstructed venous return

Edentulousness   Absence of teeth.

Elective surgery   Surgery which is required to prevent the possible sequelae of a condition but does not require immediate treatment.

Embolus   A blood clot (thrombus) in the bloodstream.

Emergency surgery   Surgery usually performed in life-threatening situations.

Emesis   *See* Vomiting.

Empathy   The ability to share another person's feelings to the extent that one can actually put oneself in the other's place.

Empiricism   The use of facts and experiences as the basis for the interpretation and analysis of data.

Endurance   The ability to withstand movement and do work in terms of duration and absence of fatigue.

Environment   The internal or external milieu of the host which can either facilitate or hinder the individual's level of wellness.

Epispadias   Opening of the urinary meatus on the top surface of the penis.

Erythema   The increased redness of the skin resulting from increased blood flow.

Euphoria   An inappropriate feeling of well-being.

Evaluation   The ongoing measurement of the process of change and its outcomes.

Expectorate   To expel sputum from the respiratory tree.

Extension   Straightening of a body part.

Exudates   Drainages.

Facilitators of change   Any factors that increase the probability that change will occur and will be long term.

Facilitators to communication   Those factors which enhance the effectiveness of the communication process.

Fecal impaction   Collection of dry, hard stool in the lower intestine which cannot be moved through the usual elimination process.

Feedback   The cyclic process in which a stimulus results in a response or series of responses which modify the recipient's reaction to the initial stimulus.

Fibrosis   Increased density and loss of elasticity of connective tissue.

Flatness   Sound produced when solid tissue is percussed.

Flatulence   Gaseous distention of the lower intestine.

Flexion   The act of bending a body part.

Food   Any substance, solid or liquid, which is required by an organism for its growth and survival.

Formal groups   Groups which have stated rules and regulations which result in imposed norms.

Foreseeable nursing diagnosis   A statement of behavior having a high probability of future occurrence.

Fowler's position   A sitting position with the trunk at a 90-degree angle to the legs and the legs in extension.

Friction rubs   Rubbing sounds heard when inflamed pleural surfaces come in contact with each other.

Gait   The way in which an individual walks.

Gangrene   Death of tissue related to an inadequate blood supply; results from bacterial invasion of this tissue.

Gastric decompression Removal of food, fluid, secretions, and gas by means of negative pressure.

Gastric gavage The instillation of food through a nasogastric tube.

Gastric lavage The removal of stomach contents through a nasogastric tube.

Gender identity The individual's feelings of masculinity of femininity.

Generic name The identification of a drug once it has been developed.

General anesthesia The depression of the central nervous system to produce total body anesthesia.

Goal An aim or objective for action.

Grieving The holistic process experienced by an individual in response to or anticipation of an actual or perceived loss.

Group A set of people having shared needs or goals.

Group dynamics The constantly changing interaction patterns, movements, and processes present within the group.

Habituation The process resulting from prolonged use of a substance in which continued use becomes an involuntary pattern.

Hallucinations Subjective activation of the senses without objective external stimuli.

Health A dynamic process which continually changes as the interaction between the individual and the environment changes.

Health behavior The overt, conscious, learned activities which the individual carries out *and* the automatic, involuntary, internal mechanisms of the individual, in relation to maintenance of physical or emotional well-being.

Health beliefs Convictions the individual holds related to health which may not necessarily be based on fact or reality.

Health practice An activity the individual carries out as a result of health belief or definitions.

Heart rate The speed at which the heart beats, measured in beats per minute.

Heaves An abnormal rising of the chest wall during systole.

Host The individual who is susceptible to the forces of an agent.

Human needs Essential requirements to maintain life, promote physical and psychologic growth and psychosocial development, and achieve and maintain wellness.

Hunger The body's response to stimuli in the feeding center of the hypothalamus resulting in the seeking of food.

Hyperalimentation Administration of greater than optimal amount of nutrients.

Hypercalcemia Calcium ion excesses.

Hypercapnea High $Paco_2$ levels while Pao_2 levels decrease.

Hyperchloremia Chloride ion excess.

Hyperkalemia Potassium ion excess.

Hypernatremia Sodium ion excess.

Hyperplasia Increased production of cells beyond expected levels.

Hyperpnea Increased depth.

Hyperresonance Sound produced by percussion of an area where either the amount of air has increased or the amount of tissue has decreased proportionally.

Hypertension High arterial blood pressure.

Hyperventilation Increased respiratory rate and depth.

Hypertrophy The increase in size or deformity in shape of body tissue.

Hypocalcemia Calcium ion deficit.

Hypochloremia Chloride ion deficit.

Hypokalemia Potassium ion deficit.

Hyponatremia Sodium ion deficit.

Hypospadias The opening of the urinary meatus on the undersurface of the penis.

Hypotension Low arterial blood pressure.

Hypoventilation A decrease in the amount of oxygen-enriched air inspired, resulting in less oxygen being taken in and more carbon dioxide being retained.

Hypoxemia Low oxygen saturation levels in the blood.

Hypoxia Decreased oxygenation of body tissues.

Hypoxic drive Secondary stimulus to respiration resulting from lowered PaO_2 levels.

Iatrogenic malnutrition Disorder in nutrition resulting from treatment regimen or health care setting.

Illness The inability of the individual to meet needs in a way which allows functioning.

Immediate nursing diagnoses Those diagnoses based directly on behaviors the individual is presently exhibiting and for which there is verifiable data.

Immediate-range goals Present-oriented objectives which must be accomplished before successive intermediate and long-range goals can be accomplished.

Immobility deprivation A predominantly physiologic phenomenon which results from a decrease in physical movement and activity.

Independent practitioner A nurse who functions in settings other than traditional, organized health care systems and who is not under the direct aegis of others.

Indirect contact Contact which occurs when the host touches an object which has been exposed to a reservoir.

Inductive reasoning The drawing of generalizable conclusions from specific data.

Infarct Localized damage or death of tissues resulting from the occlusion of the blood supply to an area.

Infection The condition resulting when microorganisms invade the body and are not effectively counteracted by the body's defense system.

Inflammatory response An attempt by the body to neutralize, destroy, and limit the effects of tissue trauma and/or agent invasion.

Informal groups Groups which have much spontaneous interpersonal behavior with few written rules and regulations.

Infradian rhythms Rhythms which run longer than a 24-hour cycle.

Ingestion The taking-in of food.

Inspection Visualization of the individual's body surface.

Intermediate-range goals Transitional steps from specific (immediate) goals to general (long-range) goals.

Intermittent pain Pain which varies in intensity over a period of time.

Intertrigous areas Areas where two skin surfaces touch each other.

Intervention Action phase of the nursing process.

Interviewing A goal-oriented and planned communication skill used to explore thoughts, feelings, and perceptions; gather and give information; and clarify goals.

Intracranial pressure A rise in pressure which occurs whenever the volume of contents of the cranium increases.

Intractable pain Pain which is not reduced by use of traditional methods.

Intradermal drug administration Administration of substances into the dermal layer of the skin.

Intramuscular drug administration Injection of substances into the muscular tissue.

Intraoperative phase The period which begins with the induction of anesthesia and ends when the surgical procedure is completed.

Intravenous drug administration Administration of a drug directly into the bloodstream.

Intuition Perception of the meaning of an event or set of stimuli without any specific knowledge or facts about it.

Inversion Retraction of the skin.

Irrigation Instillation of fluid into a body opening for purposes of cleansing.

Ischemia A decrease in the blood supply to a body tissue.

Isolation The process of protection used to prevent contamination by microorganisms.

Kilocalorie Unit of measurement which reflects

the amount of energy required to raise 1 kg of water 1 degree centigrade.

Kinesthesis The sensation of movement.

Kyphosis Increased convexity of the posterior portion of the spine.

Labile Liable to extreme and rapidly changing emotional states.

Lateral position Side-lying position.

Laxative Oral bowel cleanser, a cathartic.

Leadership The facilitation of change through creative direction, motivation, and guidance of others toward achieving mutually accepted goals.

Learner demography Characteristics of the learner which influence the teaching—learning process.

Learning A relatively permanent change in behavior not brought about by maturation or any chance circumstances.

Lethal dose The amount of a drug which will most likely result in the individual's death.

Leukocytosis An increase in the total number of white blood cells.

Level of consciousness The individual's ability to respond to external stimuli.

Level of growth and development Physical, Physiologic, and psychosocial behavior at a given point on the life process continuum.

Licensing The legal procedure for demonstrating minimal standards of practice.

Livor mortis The mottling of dependent areas of the body after death.

Local anesthesia Blocking of peripheral nerve endings within a circumscribed area to prevent transmission of stimuli during surgery.

Localized pain Pain circumscribed in an identified area.

Long-range goals Future-oriented objectives toward which all other goals are directed.

Lordosis Increased concavity of the lumbar spine.

Loss The absence, actual or perceived, of a significant person, object, body part, function, role, or emotion which was formerly present.

Malnutrition Insufficient nutrient intake to meet an individual's needs.

Management The systematic organization and administration of institutionally set goals through delegated authority.

Mastication Chewing.

Masturbation Manual manipulation of the genital organs for sexual gratification.

Maturational crisis A series of stressful life events which arise out of the growth and development process and for which the individual's usual coping methods are inadequate.

Medical asepsis The use of equipment and supplies free of pathogenic organisms in a clean environment.

Metabolic acidosis An excess in hydrogen ions with a concurrent deficit of bicarbonate ions.

Metabolic alkalosis An excess of bicarbonate ions with a concurrent deficit of hydrogen ions.

Metabolism The sum of physicochemical processes which maintain the life of an organism.

Metastasis The spread of cancer cells from original site to other parts of the body.

Mobility The capability of moving from one location to another.

Mode of transmission In communication, the method an individual uses to send a message. In infectious process, the method by which the agent is carried to the host.

Mottling Blue-gray or purplish blotches resulting from generalized peripheral vasoconstriction.

Movement The shift of behavior towards a new and more healthful pattern within the change process.

Mucous plugs Thick, sticky globules of mucus.

Nausea Subjective feeling of being "sick to one's stomach."

Necrosis Death of body tissue resulting from a lack of oxygen and nutrients.

Negative health behavior Any pattern of observable responses which indicate an inability to meet a health care need.

Nephritis Inflammation of the nephrons of the kidney.

Neutrophilia An increase in the number of circulating neutrophils.

Nursing A process of assisting individuals (singly or in groups) in modifying and repatterning internal and external environments in order to better meet health care needs and attain high-level wellness.

Nursing audit A peer evaluation system where health care records and situations are reviewed retrospectively.

Nursing diagnosis The statement of an existing or potential negative health behavior related to those factors which may influence the health response.

Nursing history The written record of the assessment of the individual's responses to changes in health status and patterns of living.

Nursing process A tool for effecting change consisting of four phases: assessment, including nursing diagnosis; planning, including goal setting; intervention; and evaluation.

Obesity Excessive deposits of adipose tissue resulting from excessive intake of calories.

Objective data Data which are directly observable and measurable by people other than the individual.

Observation The use of the senses to identify and categorize stimuli in the environment.

Official agency *See* Public agency.

Official name The identification of a drug recognized and accepted by the U.S. Food and Drug Administration and listed in *U.S. Pharmacopia* or *National Formulary*. Frequently the same as the generic name.

Oncology The study of cancer and its treatment.

Open-ended questions Interviewing technique that encourages an individual to pursue his reactions in detail.

Open system Any grouping of living organisms which are in constant interaction with each other to form a unified whole.

Options The alternatives or choices that the individual has within a given situation.

Orthopnea Difficulty in breathing unless in the upright position.

Orthostatic hypotension Drop in arterial blood pressure upon standing.

Packed cells Blood cells without plasma.

Pain An extreme form of discomfort most often associated with physiologic dysfunction.

Pain threshold The point at which an individual first has the sensation of pain.

Pain tolerance The manner in which the individual deals with pain.

Pallor The loss of the underlying reddish hue of the skin due to superficial vasoconstriction or a deficiency of hemoglobin.

Palpebral conjunctiva Mucous membranes of the eyelids.

Paradoxical breathing Movement of one part of the lung in a direction opposite to the movement of the rest of the lung.

Paralysis Loss of muscle function.

Paresis Muscle weakness.

Partial thromboplastin time (PTT) The measurement of the relationship of intrinsic factors to the clotting time of the blood.

Passive immunity The immunity acquired when a person receives antibodies from an external source for protection against specific antigens.

Perception The use of touch to determine characteristics of body surfaces and underlying tissue.

Perceptual deprivation State resulting from an inability to recognize and interpret stimuli from the external environment.

Percussion Sound vibration produced when one surface taps or strikes another.

Perfusion Nourishment of cells by oxygen and other nutrients through circulatory integrity.

Peripheral cyanosis Dusky or hazy blue-gray skin color of the extremities occurring as a consequence of decreased cardiac output or peripheral vascular changes.

Peritonitis Inflammation of the lining of the peritoneal cavity.

Pernicious anemia   Anemia resulting from lack of the intrinsic factor for the absorption of vitamin B_{12}.

Phase of exhaustion   Third step of the General Adaptation Syndrome in which the previous adaptive responses are no longer adequate, resulting in illness or death.

Physical assessment   Gathering of objective data on the individual's physical state through inspection, palpation, percussion, and auscultation.

Physical state   The structure and form of body tissues.

Physiologic state   The functioning of body tissues and the biochemical interactions within the body.

Pitting   The depression of tissue left when moderate pressure is applied.

Planning   The creation of an organized course of action based on established goals, designed to change a negative health behavior to a more positive one by altering those factors which influence the health response.

Plasma shift   The movement of plasma from the blood into the interstitial spaces.

Pneumothorax   Collapse of lung tissue as a result of a rise in intrapleural pressure.

Polycythemia   Increased production of red blood cells.

Possible nursing diagnosis   Statement of behavior that has been known to occur in similar circumstances but for which there is not an adequate data base at present.

Postoperative phase   The period of recovery from a surgical procedure; includes the immediate, intermediate, and later periods.

Power   The influence one has over others within a reward system to bring about a change.

Precordial thump   A forceful, sharp blow to the midsternum with the lateral aspect of a closed fist; used to spontaneously stimulate the heartbeat.

Preoperative phase   The period which starts when the individual is told of the need for surgery and ends when anesthesia is induced.

Primary care nurse   Nurse who coordinates and is responsible for the care of an individual from the time of admission to a health care facility until discharge.

Primary group   A group whose members communicate with each other over a period of time in face-to-face interactions and have a high degree of influence over each other's behavior.

Primary intention healing   Healing resulting in a minimal amount of granulation and scar formation; occurs when wound edges are in close approximation and surrounding tissue is in good condition.

Primary prevention   General wellness promotion and specific protection against disease.

Private agency   *See* Proprietary agency.

Problem solving   A step-by-step process of enquiry for determining choices of action; similar to the process used in research.

Process recording   A written record of all the verbal and nonverbal interchanges between an interviewer and interviewee, with analysis of the interaction.

Profession   A discipline which requires an extensive educational practice period; has a unique body of knowledge; is autonomous in its decision-making and practice; provides a service; has its own code of ethics; and whose membership carries a degree of status.

Prone   Front-lying position.

Pruritic   Itchy condition of skin, causing individual to scratch.

Proprietary agency   An organization which is owned by individuals and run for profit; synonymous with private agency.

Proprietary name   The identification of a drug by the developing company, designated by the symbol ®.

Prothrombin time (PT)   Measurement of the rate at which blood coagulates in the presence of additives.

Proxemics   The distancing patterns of individuals.

Pruritic   Itchy.

Psychogenic pain   A sensation of pain with little or no recognized physiologic stimulation.

Psychomotor skills Those learned processes requiring manual dexterity and practice.

Psychosocial state The interactions between the individual and the environment, the individual's mood, emotional makeup, personality, and cognitive and interaction styles.

Public agency An organization which is supported and controlled by public funds; synonymous with official agency.

Pulmonary edema Buildup of fluid in the lungs which blocks the diffusion of gasses.

Pulse The wave phenomenon caused by the flow of blood through a superficial artery with each heart contraction.

Pulse deficit Any difference between apical pulse and peripheral pulse.

Pulse pressure The arithmetic difference between the systolic and diastolic arterial blood pressures.

Purulent drainage Puslike debris from dead tissues and cells indicating infection.

Pyrexia A fever or febrile condition.

Pyrogens Agents which cause a rise in body temperature.

Quadriplegia Paralysis of all four extremities.

Rales The intermittent crackling sounds produced by air moving through excessive secretions in the bronchioles and alveoli.

Range of motion (ROM) The movement capabilities of a joint measured in degrees along an axis.

Raw data Descriptions of objective and subjective information without analysis and interpretation.

Realization Second phase of behavior of coping with loss, characterized by realization of the facts but with continuing inability to cope.

Reasoning The use of inductive and/or deductive thinking to draw conclusions from a given set of stimuli or information.

Reception deprivation Impairment of receptor organs with either partial or complete loss of sensations.

Recumbent Reclining position.

Reduction Movement of unaligned bones into proper alignment.

Referred pain Pain which originates in one organ or area of the body but is perceived in another organ or area.

Refreezing Long-term solidification of a new pattern of behavior in the change process.

Regional anesthesia The blocking of afferent nerve impulses by anesthetizing large nerve bundles or transmission sites in or around the spinal cord.

Registration A voluntary process for demonstrating basic competencies in areas of professional practice.

Required surgery Surgery which is necessary but can be delayed because of the nature of the condition.

Research The systematic process of testing theories, validating assumptions, generating new information, and discovering new relationships.

Reservoir An environment conducive to the growth and multiplication of microorganisms.

Resolution Fourth and final stage of behavior of coping with loss, characterized by new attitudes, behaviors, and coping mechanisms, which allow individual to deal effectively with the situation.

Resonance The sound produced by percussing air-filled cavities.

Resistance phase Second phase of the General Adaptation Syndrome, during which the body is compensating for and counteracting the changes produced by stress.

Respiratory acidosis An excess of carbonic acid with a concurrent increase in plasma CO_2 levels.

Respiratory alkalosis A deficit of carbonic acid.

Respiratory depth The volume of air that is inhaled and exhaled with each respiration.

Respiratory effort Degree of energy required to move air in and out of the lung.

Respiratory movement The predominating pattern of muscles used in respiration.

Respiratory rate The number of respirations an individual takes per minute.

Respiratory rhythm   The pattern of recurrence of respirations.

Rest   State which occurs when an individual is relaxed but not sleeping.

Rhonchi   The continuous, low-pitched, bubbling sounds heard as air passes through narrowed bronchioles.

Rigor mortis   The stiffening of muscles after death.

Sanguineous drainage   Bloody exudate.

Satiety   The feeling of fullness and satisfaction after eating.

Scientific principle   Accepted rule or law which explains phenomena.

Scoliosis   Side or lateral deviation of the spine.

Secondary groups   Relatively loose affiliations of people which may be short-term, task-oriented, or impersonal.

Secondary intention healing   Healing occurring when wound edges are in poor approximation, surrounding tissue is in poor condition, and/or infection is present, producing extensive granulation and scar tissue.

Secondary prevention   Early diagnosis and prompt treatment of illness and disability limitation through prevention of illness sequelae.

Semi-Fowler's position   Sitting position with hips and knees flexed.

Sensitivity   Testing of organisms for vulnerability to potentially toxic agents such as antibiotics.

Sensory deprivation   Alterations in meaningful stimuli or absolute reduction or absence of stimuli in the external environment.

Sensory overload   Multisensory bombardment by stimuli in the environment.

Sensory process   The reception and integration of stimuli from the environment in order to successfully respond to the complexity of ever-changing input.

Serosanguineous drainage   Exudate which is a mixture of blood and serum; may be pink or flecked with blood depending on the proportions of blood and serum.

Serous drainage   Clear and straw-colored exudate which consists of serum without fibrinogen.

Sexual identity   The individual's identification with the male or female sex.

Sexual role behavior   The individual's manifestations of biologic sex and sexual and gender identity.

Shearing force   The movement of skin surfaces away from underlying tissues with concomitant compression of blood vessels as a result of position changes.

Shock phase   First phase of pattern of coping with loss, characterized by high level anxiety, loss of control, failure to realize implications, and general inadequacy.

Sick role   Utilization of patterns of behavior which the individual sees as consistent with "being sick."

Sickled blood cells   Abnormal, crescent-shaped red blood cells.

Sign   The objective data which is observable and measurable by people other than the individual.

Significant others   Any person or object or belief which provides the individual with feelings of safety, security, belonging, love, and esteem over a period of time.

Situational crisis   Those unexpected, stressful events for which the individual's usual coping methods are inadequate.

Sordes   Accumulation of saliva, mucus, food, organisms, and epithelial cells in the mouth.

Specific dynamic action of food   Production of energy during the metabolism of food.

Sphygmomanometer   Instrument used to externally measure arterial blood pressure.

Sputum   Secretions of the respiratory tree, including mucus, saliva, bacteria, and cellular wastes.

Sterile   Free from living microorganisms.

Sterile technique   Use of equipment and supplies that are free from all microorganisms and their spores in a clean environment.

Sterilization   Removal of all microorganisms including their spores.

Stertorous sounds Noisy or snoring respirations.

Stoma Portion of tissue protruding externally in an ostomy.

Stool Feces.

Stress The tension which results when changes occur in any component of the individual to which he or she responds holistically.

Stressor Any stress-producing force, agent, or threat to the individual's ability to meet needs satisfactorily.

Striae Lines caused by stretching of the skin.

Stricture Narrowing of a lumen or opening in the body.

Stridor Harsh, sharp sound heard on inspiration.

Subcutaneous drug administration Injection of substances into the subcutaneous tissues.

Subcutaneous emphysema Trapping of air in subcutaneous tissues of the lung and surrounding tissue.

Subjective data Data which are not directly observable or measurable by objective criteria; that which the individual tells another as perceived by the individual.

Sublingual drug administration Administration of substances under the tongue.

Suction The application of a negative pressure to create a vacuum so that secretions move from an area of higher pressure to one of lower pressure.

Superficial pain Pain occurring in cutaneous tissues or supporting structures.

Supine Back-lying position; also known as dorsal-recumbent position.

Surgery The deliberate invasion of body tissue to create a change in the structure and/or function of the body.

Surgical asepsis Use of strict sterile technique.

Sympathy A feeling for the individual without a real sense of what the person is experiencing.

Symptom The subjective data which is not directly observable or measurable by objective criteria and is perceived by the individual.

Syntax The way vocabulary is structured into coherent messages.

Systolic pressure Resistance of blood on arterial wall during systole.

Tachypnea Increased respiratory rate.

Tactile fremitus The palpable vibrations of air passing through the vocal cords.

Teacher demography The characteristics of the teacher which influence the teaching–learning process.

Teaching The facilitation of the learning process.

Teaching – learning process A planned interaction which produces a relatively permanent change in behavior not brought about by maturation or any chance circumstances.

Tenacious Adhesive, sticky, and viscous secretions.

Tertiary intention healing The incomplete healing which occurs when a wound is extensive, resulting in limited granulation.

Tertiary prevention Rehabilitation.

Therapeutic communication A conscious goal-oriented and planned process of interaction.

Therapeutic dose The minimum amount of a drug which will produce the desired action.

Therapeutic relationship A dynamic collaborative process which is established to assist an individual in meeting health care needs.

Thrills Vibratory sensations felt over the heart caused by abnormal blood flow.

Tolerance The state in which increasing amounts of a drug are needed to produce previous drug responses.

Tonus Usual state of muscle contraction.

Total parenteral nutrition Administration of all necessary nutrients by the intravenous route.

Toxic dose The amount of a drug which causes physical, physiologic, or psychosocial damage to a person.

Tumor Formation of hyperplastic cells; swelling of tissue.

Turgor   The degree of elasticity and tone of the skin.

Tympany   Sound produced when closed air-filled cavities are percussed.

Ultradian rhythms   Rhythms which run less than a 24-hour cycle.

Undescended testicle   A testicle which fails to descend from the abdominal or inguinal canal.

Unfreezing   Dissolution of previously held patterns of behavior within the change process.

Unilateral   Occurring on one side of the body.

Urgent surgery   Surgery required within a day or two after diagnosis.

Utilization   The process by which substances are used by the body.

Vaginitis   Inflammation of the mucosal lining of the vagina.

Valsalva maneuver   The increase in intraabdominal and intrathoracic pressure when the glottis is fixed.

Varicosity   Outpouching and twisting of vein walls.

Vascularity   The observable distribution of capillaries on body surfaces.

Vector   An insect or other living thing which transmits an agent from a reservoir to a host.

Vehicle   An inanimate object which carries an agent from a reservoir to a host.

Venous engorgement   Dilation of veins with resulting blood pooling.

Venous pump   Pumping action of the muscles surrounding the veins.

Voiding   Process of urination.

Voluntary agency   A nonprofit organization that is community funded and controlled.

Vomiting   Reflex action which empties the stomach upward through the esophagus rather than downward through the intestines; synonymous with emesis.

Wellness   The maximum level of functioning of a person at a given time and place.

INDEX

INDEX

Yoga, 197
  for pain relief, 642

X-rays
  chest, 410
  skull, 230
  vertebral, 230

Z-tract method, 379